# Clinical Intensive Care and Acute Medicine

This new edition provides an accessible account of the essentials of intensive care medicine. The core of the book focuses on areas common to all critically ill patients including fluid therapy, sedation, shock, infection and other central topics. This key understanding of basic pathophysiological principles provides an excellent launch pad for the section on individual diesease entities encompassing haematology, gastroenterology, nephrology, endocrinology, the respiratory system, cardiovascular pathology, poisoning and neurology. Economic and ethical issues are also covered, and the text is supported by numerous problem-oriented guidelines to help the care provider tackle real-life practical problems as encountered in the ICU. In the same spirit, wherever possible, the authors provide precise and meaningful advice, rather than bland generalisations. This new edition reflects the excitement, challenges and uniqueness of intensive care medicine, for the benefit of all residents, trainees, nursing staff and paramedics attached to the ICU.

'While the book is specifically directed at junior medical officers, it will also be useful as an aid to the part-time intensivist and postgraduate medical and nursing education. Even for those intensive care units that already have well defined protocols, this book will fulfil an invaluable educational role. This book is an essential addition to all intensive care libraries.' *Anaesthesia and Intensive Care*

'For those of us who run intensive care units (ICU), faced with trainees of varying experience whose first question on the unit is "What book should I buy?". I can now tell them – this one. I recommend this text strongly for trainees in ICU. It will also prove useful for those preparing to take a fellowship examination. It is extremely good value.' *British Journal of Surgery*

'The clinical content of the book is sound and comprehensive and the authors are clearly masters of their topic. The volume under review is certainly a worthy addition to a burgeoning literature.' *Journal of the Royal College of Physicians of London*

'I appreciated its pragmatic approach to complex problem solving. It's size, comprehensive coverage and cost should make it an attractive competitor for other well established texts in the same area.' *Anaesthetist*

'The book conveys the information with a combination of clear descriptive paragraphs and bulleted points allowing easy reference. At the end of many chapters there are 'trouble-shooting' sections that highlight specific common problems such as oliguria – problem-oriented lists that can be quickly read by the junior doctor in time of need. I like this book for its clarity and conclusion. Very definitely a useful on-call-room companion.' *Journal of the Royal Society*

# Clinical Intensive Care and Acute Medicine

## Second Edition

Ken Hillman and

Gillian Bishop

The Liverpool Health Service
Sydney

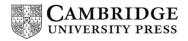

CAMBRIDGE
UNIVERSITY PRESS

PUBLISHED BY THE PRESS SYNDICATE OF THE UNIVERSITY OF CAMBRIDGE
The Pitt Building, Trumpington Street, Cambridge, United Kingdom

CAMBRIDGE UNIVERSITY PRESS
The Edinburgh Building, Cambridge CB2 2RU, UK
40 West 20th Street, New York, NY 10011–4211, USA
477 Williamstown Road, Port Melbourne, VIC 3207, Australia
Ruiz de Alarcón 13, 28014 Madrid, Spain
Dock House, The Waterfront, Cape Town 8001, South Africa

http://www.cambridge.org

First published 1996
Second edition published 2004

Printed in the United Kingdom at the University Press, Cambridge

*Typefaces* Minion 10/12pt. and Dax    *System* LATEX 2ε   [TB]

*A catalogue record for this book is available from the British Library*

*Library of Congress Cataloguing in Publication data*

ISBN 0 521 78980 X paperback
Hillman, Ken.
Clinical intensive care and acute medicine/Ken Hillman, Gillian Bishop – 2nd ed.
      p.   cm.
Includes bibliographical references and index.
ISBN 0 521 78980 X (Pbk.)
1. Critical care medicine – Handbooks, manuals, etc.   I. Bishop, Gillian.   II. Title.
[DNLM:   1. Intensive Care – methods – Handbooks.   2. Acute Disease – therapy – Handbooks.
3. Intensive Care Units – Handbooks. WX 39 H654c   2004]
RC86.8.H543   2004
616.02′8 – dc22   2003059634

Every effort has been made in preparing this book to provide accurate and up-to-date information which is in accord with accepted standards and practice at the time of publication. Nevertheless, the authors, editors and publisher can make no warranties that the information contained herein is totally free from error, not least because clinical standards are constantly changing through research and regulation. The authors, editors and publisher therefore disclaim all liability for direct or consequential damages resulting from the use of material contained in this book. Readers are strongly advised to pay careful attention to information provided by the manufacturer of any drugs or equipment that they plan to use.

# Contents

# Troubleshooting tips

# Preface to the first edition

The book is aimed at junior medical staff who rotate through intensive care units (ICUs) and other physicians who are involved in managing patients in an ICU, but not necessarily as their primary specialty. It may also prove useful to any member of the paramedical or nursing profession who is involved in acute medicine. The book initially arose from the need to give resident medical staff rotating through our own ICU a crash course in intensive care medicine. At present this subject is not universally taught to undergraduates and too often, exposure as a postgraduate turns out to be learning by experience.

Intensive care medicine is an exciting and rapidly developing specialty. There are two major problems with writing a book about it at this point of time. Firstly, it may be out of date before it is published and secondly, it may not capture the flavour of intensive care medicine. Just as a committee of specialists representing each organ may not necessarily be the best way to approach the multiorgan problems of the critically ill, then a book which only summarises the conventional wisdom of other specialties may not be the best book on intensive care medicine. It is a new specialty, drawing on the knowledge of other specialties, but also having expertise unique to itself. The specialty has its own journals and meetings as well as nursing and medical specialists. We have tried to make this book reflect the uniqueness of intensive care medicine. We have also incorporated as much recent knowledge as possible in order to prevent premature ageing.

The core of the book concentrates on areas common to all critically ill patients rather than on specific diseases. These chapters are to be found mainly in the first part of the book. It is essential to understand the basic pathophysiological principles common to all seriously ill patients before concentrating on individual disease entities. Thus, chapters such as Routine Care of the Seriously Ill, Fluids, Nutrition, Cardiovascular Failure, Respiratory Failure, Infection, Resuscitation, Sedation, Ventilation, Monitoring and Intracranial Disasters could be relevant to all seriously ill patients, no matter what the aetiology of the disease process. These chapters represent the core knowledge of intensive care medicine. We have devoted the remaining chapters to specific problems and diseases. These include Haematology, Gastroenterology, Nephrology, Endocrinology, the Respiratory System, Cardiovascular Pathology, Poisoning and Neurology. Discussion in these chapters is limited to the subject's relevance in the setting of the seriously ill. The reader is continually referred from these specific chapters to the core chapters. Finally, no matter how small the book about intensive care is, it cannot afford to dismiss economic and ethical issues. These are covered in the last chapter. Readers are encouraged to familiarise themselves with the core chapters and to refer to individual diseases as necessary. At the end of each chapter, we have included some articles and web sites for further reading. These are mainly of a review nature.

Many chapters also have problem-orientated guidelines to aid the reader. Many problems encountered by junior medical staff are common in different diseases but are not often specifically addressed. Examples include 'Fighting the Ventilator', 'Interpreting Non-Specific Opacities on the Chest Radiograph', 'The Confused Patient' and 'Sudden Hypoxia'. We have tried to identify specific areas which may assist the resident when confronted with these practical problems in the ICU. These guidelines are scattered throughout the book in relevant chapters and for easy access, a list is provided at the beginning of the book.

Because of the rapidly developing nature of intensive care medicine, we have drawn on recent publications and integrated these findings into 'accepted practice'. 'Accepted practice' is, of course, a variable and mobile concept. One of the dilemmas is always distinguishing between initial enthusiasm and a growing weight of opinion. For example, we feel there is a move away from invasive to non-invasive monitoring and have put what we consider an appropriate emphasis on that line. Similarly, we sense a tendency to use pressure-support ventilatory modes rather than simply employing controlled mandatory ventilation. Time and more research will demonstrate whether this is correct. In combining the latest information with accepted practice we have tempered the final guidelines with what we have found to work in the clinical situation. We make no apology for the clinical flavour of the book.

As much as one tries to avoid controversy in a textbook it could only be achieved by reverting to bland and vague suggestions such as 'support the patient', 'give fluids' and 'give oxygen'. We have tried wherever possible to give precise and meaningful 'bottom line messages'. In doing so, one runs the risk of giving messages which are not accepted by everyone. We have taken that risk rather than resort to vague and safe alternatives, in the knowledge that the individual specialists supervising junior medical staff are encouraged to modify management within their own unit's protocols.

Finally, we would like to gratefully acknowledge the inspiration and pleasure we have had from working with all our patients, junior medical colleagues and nursing staff in intensive care over the years.

# Preface to the second edition

The second edition of Clinical Intensive Care maintains many of its original features. It is primarily aimed at those practising Intensive Care Medicine at the bedside with practical troubleshooting tables and chapters which distil theory into relevant guidelines for management. While the whole book has been updated to include what we believe are the most important advances in acute medicine, the size of the book has been deliberately kept the same.

Intensive Care Medicine is now a mature specialty practised in every major hospital and the principles of this specialty are now being applied in the management of patients in every part of the hospital. The walls of intensive care units are becoming more virtual as their staff are being asked to consult on the seriously ill both before and after their admission to the intensive care unit. Increasingly the principles of acute medicine are part of the knowledge base of intensive care medicine and are being captured in its journals and textbooks. It seemed appropriate therefore that the title of the book changed to 'Clinical Intensive Care and Acute Medicine'. The principles of the book can be used by intensive care staff consulting on general wards as well as by other specialists caring for potentially seriously ill patients on general wards.

# Acknowledgements

Books such as this only come about as a result of inspiration and input from many sources. The list of people who fall into this category are many. First and foremost is Sue Williams, the secretary to our department who has not only typed the many drafts, but corrected them and contributed valuable advice. Other assistance in preparing the manuscript came from Jacquelene Barnes. We are indebted to Richard Barling from Cambridge University Press for his patience, inspiration and support.

Our colleagues provided a great deal of their time to review many of the chapters. Special thanks to Michael Parr, Arthas Flabouris and Antony Stewart, whose wisdom and knowledge was greatly appreciated. Thanks also to Ian Gosbell from Liverpool Hospital's microbiological department for adding a much needed dimension to the section on Infection. Stephen Deane shed clarity and perception onto our approach to the acute limb. Others to whom we owe a debt include Stephen Streat from Auckland Hospital in New Zealand for his contribution to the chapters on Trauma and Nutrition and Marcus Cremonese for his excellent illustrations.

The inspiration for this book has come from the many patients, nursing and junior medical colleagues we have been privileged to have worked with over the years. They have provided the life and meaning to the messages contained in the book and have kept us honest.

# A systematic approach to caring for the seriously ill

> - A hospital-wide system is essential for early recognition and rapid resuscitation of the seriously ill in order to limit tissue damage and optimise outcomes.
> - High dependency units (HDUs) allow a more flexible approach to managing a hospital's seriously ill population.

Intensive care medicine is no longer practised wholly within the four walls of the intensive care unit (ICU). The traditional ICU patient with multiorgan failure (MOF) being supported with artificial ventilation, dialytic therapy, multiple inotropes and complex monitoring is still strongly associated with the image of an ICU. However, the skills of intensive care physicians are increasingly being utilised in a systematic way across the entire hospital. Optimal management of patients before they are admitted to ICU has a large influence, firstly on whether the admission may have been avoided with earlier intervention and secondly on the level of support required if they were admitted; and thirdly on their eventual outcome. Patients who are allowed to develop severe shock and extensive organ dysfunction require greater resources for a longer time in the ICU than if they had been treated at an earlier stage.

Intensive care medicine is increasingly being defined by care of the seriously ill across the acute hospital, rather than within the ICU. This can be illustrated by imagining a 600-bed hospital with four intensive care beds as opposed to 40. The four beds would be occupied by severely ill patients with maximum support. Because of the severity of illness and terminal state of many of the patients, the mortality of this ICU would be high and many others throughout the hospital would suffer severe complications as a result of delayed resuscitation and the effects of prolonged ischaemia and hypoxia. Some of these patients would eventually qualify for one of the few ICU beds. Staff who work in these units may even be disdainful of the role of the 40-bed unit, where many patients may not even be intubated and ventilated, i.e. not 'real' ICUs. Forty beds may, in fact, be too many. But the real point is that if there are insufficient ICU beds, patients will eventually be admitted to the ICU when the disease state may be irreversible.

Seriously ill patients situated anywhere in a hospital need to be triaged as one does in an emergency department (ED). In fact many sick in-hospital patients may receive better treatment if they were wheeled out of the hospital and in through the ED where they would be triaged into categories according to how seriously ill they were and then receive rapid and appropriate resuscitation.

Intensive care medicine is being increasingly defined as a specialty of resuscitation and acute medicine as practised across the whole hospital. The barriers of bed limitation within the ICU should not result in inadequate resuscitation and management of the seriously ill, no matter where they are.

The problem of at-risk patients in acute hospitals is potentiated by the increasing specialisation of medicine, resulting in single organ doctors ('SODS') practising mainly ambulant medicine and not having the training, skills or experience in managing the acutely ill when organ dysfunction is rarely limited to one or even two organs. Even if medical specialists were exposed to formal training in acute hospital medicine during their training, it is difficult for 'SODS' to maintain their skills base and knowledge levels if they are mainly practising single organ medicine. Thus the acute hospital system for dealing with the seriously ill is often limited by hierarchies, ownership issues and inadequate expertise being immediately available to at-risk and seriously ill patients.

## High dependency units

The skills and infrastructure required to manage a seriously ill patient with severe and established MOF are the same as those required to manage a patient at an earlier stage, who has less severe organ dysfunction. The major difference is in the number of nursing staff required for each patient. For example, a patient on artificial ventilation, dialysis and multiple inotropes may require one or even two full-time nurses at all times, whereas a monitored patient on a continuous positive airway pressure (CPAP) mask with a thoracic epidural may be able to be managed on a nurse : patient ratio of 1 : 2 or even 1 : 3. Thus, the concept of the HDU has developed. The beds may be flexible within the same unit or separate units may exist, sometimes sharing the same staff and equipment. Entirely separate units, especially for specialty based care, also exist.

High dependency units allow a flexible approach to the management of the seriously ill within a hospital. Patients too unstable to be managed in a general ward, but not sick enough to require 1 : 1 nursing care in an ICU, can be accommodated, perhaps preventing deterioration before admission to ICU. Similarly, patients may not be quite unstable enough to justify continuing management in an ICU but may be too unstable to be managed on a general ward. Management in a HDU environment may improve patient outcome, decrease complications and hospital length of stay as well as decrease the risk of readmission to the ICU from a general ward.

**Table 1.1.** MET criteria

| Acute changes in physiology | |
| --- | --- |
| Airway | Threatened |
| Breathing | All respiratory arrests |
| | Respiratory rate < 5 |
| | Respiratory rate > 36 |
| Circulation | All cardiac arrests |
| | Pulse rate < 40 |
| | Pulse rate > 140 |
| | Systolic blood pressure < 90 |
| Neurology | Sudden fall in level of consciousness |
| | (fall in Glasgow coma scale (GCS) of > 2 points) |
| | Repeated or prolonged seizures |
| Other | Any patient who you are seriously worried about |
| | that does not fit the above criteria |

## A hospital-wide approach to the seriously ill

Apart from ICUs we expect optimum care of patients, in terms of appropriate staff and monitoring, in certain areas of the hospital. These include the ED, operating rooms and coronary care units.

However, many patients are managed in undifferentiated general wards with lower staff ratios and less monitoring. A hospital-wide system may be required to detect at-risk patients early in these environments and to provide rapid resuscitation where necessary.

## Early recognition of seriously ill patients

Even moderate degrees of ischaemia and hypoxia can cause cellular damage. More severe forms predispose to organ failure, long stays in intensive care and potentially avoidable death. The earlier ischaemia and hypoxia are detected and treated, the better the patient outcome. Such a system for early detection must be effective at all times. It could be as simple as the bedside nurse or clinician contacting someone with acute resuscitation skills as soon as they were concerned about a patient. However, this would depend on the attending staff having a high degree of awareness and knowledge about the early signs of a deteriorating patient and having the confidence and system support to immediately summon help.

An alternative is to formalise criteria which are associated with an at-risk patient. Such a system is based on the medical emergency team (MET) criteria (Table 1.1). These are mainly based on vital signs which define someone at risk. Added to the list is 'worried' so that staff are encouraged to seek assistance whenever they suspect a patient is at risk of deteriorating. The MET has replaced the cardiac arrest team in many hospitals.

**Table 1.2.** Outcome indicators for acute hospital care

| Deaths | Minus all 'not for resuscitation' patients | = | Potentially unexpected deaths |
|---|---|---|---|
| Cardiorespiratory arrests | Minus all 'not for resuscitation' patients | = | Potentially unexpected cardiorespiratory arrests |
| Intensive care admissions | Minus all elective or expected admissions from operating rooms, recovery area, emergency department. | = | Unanticipated admissions to ICU |

All events preceded by MET criteria for up to 24 h and have not been acted on are considered potentially preventable

**Table 1.3.** Distribution of outcome indicators for acute care hospitals

Individual patient details
  Senior physician ultimately responsible for patient care
  Junior medical staff caring for patients
  Ward nursing staff caring for patients
Aggregated, de-identified data
  Departmental audit activities
  Hospital audit activities
  Regional audit activities
  Inter-hospital comparison audit
  Possible involvement of health consumers

## Rapid response to the seriously ill

Ischaemia and hypoxia are potentially dangerous for patients and once detected should be rapidly reversed. The only systematic response to the seriously ill in hospitals is usually the cardiac arrest team, by which time damage may have already occurred and the resulting outcome is often poor. The MET system involves early intervention so that ischaemia and hypoxia are rapidly reversed. The MET must have at least one person who is familiar with all aspects of advanced resuscitation and can cope with all hospital emergencies in terms of knowledge and skills. A MET system assists in changing the culture of a hospital to one of a high degree of awareness of patients who may deteriorate and become seriously ill. The MET system also emphasises the fact that care of the seriously ill is a specialised area of medicine, requiring an immediate response with appropriately trained staff.

## Outcome indicators for hospital-wide care of the seriously ill

We are becoming increasingly accountable in health and that requires measuring outcomes. The performance of ICUs can be estimated using various severity of illness scoring systems. However, when assessing the care of the seriously ill across the whole hospital, different outcome indicators are required. Suggested indicators include deaths, cardiorespiratory arrests and unanticipated admissions to ICU (Table 1.2). Potential preventability can be arbitrarily defined as the presence of a MET criteria within 24 hours of one of these three adverse patient outcomes.

These indicators and measures of preventability (Tables 1.2 and 1.3) associated with them can be provided to relevant health care deliverers, providing a basis for quality assurance and improved patient care delivery. Improved management of patients before and after admission to the ICU is essential if we are to improve overall patient outcome from hospitals and to prevent patients from requiring ICU admission.

## FURTHER READING

Bristow, P. J., Hillman, K. M., Chey, T., Daffurn, K., Jacques, T. C., Norman, S. L., Bishop, G. F. and Simmons, E. G. Rates of in-hospital arrests, deaths and intensive care admissions: the effect of a medical emergency team. *Medical Journal of Australia* 173 (2000): 236–40.

Buist, M. D., Moore, G. E., Stephen, B., Waxman, B. P., Anderson, J. N. and Nguyen, T. V. Effects of a medical emergency team on reduction of incidence of and mortality from unexpected cardiac arrests in hospital: preliminary study. *British Medical Journal* 324 (2002): 387–90.

Goldhill, D. R., Worthington, L., Mulcahy, A., Tarling, M. and Sumner, A. The patient-at-risk team: identifying and managing seriously ill ward patients. *Anaesthesia* 54 (1999): 853–60.

Hillman, K., Bishop, G. and Bristow, P. Expanding the role of intensive care medicine. In *Yearbook of Intensive Care and Emergency Medicine*, ed. J.-L. Vincent, pp. 833–41. Berlin: Springer-Verlag, 1996.

Hillman, K., Bishop, G. and Bristow, P. Assessment and prevention of critical illness. In *Fundamentals of Anaesthesia and Acute Medicine: Intensive Care Medicine*, ed. J. Bion, pp. 65–78. London: BMJ Publishing Group, 1999.

Hillman, K., Alexandrou, E., Flabouris, M. *et al.* Clinical outcome indicators in acute hospital medicine. *Clinical Intensive Care* 11 (2000): 89–94.

Lee, A., Bishop, G., Hillman, K. M. and Daffurn, K. The medical emergency team. *Anaesthesia and Intensive Care* 23 (1995): 183–6.

McQuillan, P., Pilkington, S., Alan, A. *et al.* Confidential inquiry into quality of care before admission to intensive care. *British Medical Journal* 316 (1998): 1853–8.

# 2

# Organisation of an intensive care unit

## The specialty of intensive care medicine

It is generally agreed that the specialty of intensive care medicine began in Copenhagen in the early 1950s. During the poliomyelitis epidemic at that time, patients were treated by tracheostomy and prolonged manual ventilation. As a result of those measures, the mortality rate was reduced from 87% to an impressive 40%.

Although there are now many types of intensive care units (ICUs), such as medical, paediatric, respiratory, surgical, neurosurgical, cardiothoracic surgery and trauma, they all perform the same basic function: caring for the seriously ill. Caring for a group of these patients in a single space makes economic and medical sense. Our expertise in intensive care has increased enormously since the early 1950s and there are now specialised medical and nursing staff devoted solely to intensive care medicine.

Specialists working with the seriously ill may be familiar with complicated technology, physiology and pharmacology, as well as conventional medicine. However, it is even more important to become familiar with the unique requirements of critically ill patients – to develop expertise in their individual patterns of illness. These patients often do not conform to the conventional artificial divisions of medicine: 'surgical' patients develop 'medical' diseases. 'Medical' patients may develop 'surgical' diseases. The body may be looked at as a whole rather than as a series of independent organs. This requires that we break away from the tendency toward increasing medical specialisation based on individual organs. Rather than a 'superspecialty', intensive care medicine is a very broad general specialty, based on the body as an integral system, rather than an organ-based super specialty.

Advice from each of the single organ specialists must often be sought. The intensive care specialist must balance all such expert opinions and fit them into an overall strategy. What is good for one organ may be detrimental to others, as well as to the patient's overall condition. One cannot take a committee approach to the seriously ill. One doctor must take ultimate responsibility and make the final decision, and that doctor must have appropriate training in intensive care medicine and not be an absentee landlord. It matters little from what background intensivists come – anaesthetics, medicine or surgery – as long as they have highly developed clinical skills. Such skills can be gained only by spending time with seriously ill patients. The problem of territorial control by the various specialties (which specialty controls which patients) was an early feature of this specialty, but that attitude is gradually being replaced by a practice based on what is best for the patient.

Intensive care medicine arose from the need for physicians with skills in acute medicine. It is too much to expect a nurse from a general ward or a doctor who works only in another specialty to be able to cope with all of the problems unique to the critically ill. Both doctors and nurses in ICUs require specialised training, specialised books and journals for reference and specialised meetings to share their knowledge and experience. Above all, they need to be working regularly with the seriously ill. This does not mean that they should not seek advice from colleagues in other specialties, when needed, just as is done in all branches of medicine. However, a permanent clinical and administrative medical and nursing presence is essential for the best clinical practice.

## Intensive care personnel

The permanent senior medical and nursing staff must provide the continuity of care and ensure that standards are maintained within an ICU. They are responsible for the orientation, education and training of new staff. Junior medical staff usually rotate through the ICU for varying periods and this can lead to inconsistency in the care of patients unless standardisation is ensured through protocols, supervision and educational programmes.

Maintaining a constant high standard of intensive care is the greatest challenge for an ICU. The nursing staff are the mainstay in achieving that goal. They are responsible for most of the minute-to-minute monitoring and treatment. In addition to conventional nursing responsibilities, much of the clinical decision making can be decentralised to a skilled nursing staff. This requires investment in teaching, inservice programmes and audits directed at the bedside nurse. Examples of the expanded nursing role include the following.

### Weaning

The weaning process (e.g. adjusting ventilatory rates and pressures) can be carried out by the nursing staff using laboratory data and bedside monitoring.

## Drugs

Inotropes, vasodilators, sedatives, analgesics, insulin and many other drugs can be given by continuous intravenous (IV) infusion. Adjustments of infusion rates can be decided by nursing staff, based on clinical and laboratory data.

## Fluids

Transient oliguria and hypotension are common in intensive care patients. Most patients will respond to a fluid challenge. This can be done by nursing staff, with recourse to medical staff if the fluid challenge fails.

## Other aspects of ward function

The nursing staff should be integrated into all aspects of administration of the ICU, in addition to taking care of the patients and dealing with their friends and relatives. Other members of the intensive care staff may include physiotherapists, ward clerks, social workers and ward attendants. They are all essential for an efficiently run team. Although it is difficult to measure the effect on patient outcome of a well-organised team with high morale and sense of job satisfaction, most experienced intensivists value this aspect of their unit highly and invest time and energy in achieving it.

# Ward rounds and continuity

There should be at least one comprehensive ward round each day. The half-life for major decisions regarding seriously ill patients is approximately 24 hours, whereas for patients in general wards it is approximately 3–4 days. The medical staff, nursing staff and others involved in a patient's management should formulate a strategy for the next 24 hours. This is a framework around which fine-tuning can occur, depending on changes in the patient's condition and the findings on laboratory tests. Like other strategies, it must be flexible enough to allow changes according to the patient's condition. Rather than using a system that features a provisional diagnosis and final diagnosis, one must take a problem-orientated approach to seriously ill patients.

Despite the drama involved in the ups and downs of the critically ill, there are many predictable patterns. There is the initial resuscitation phase, usually begun outside the ICU. This is followed by a phase, usually within the ICU, where re-suscitation is continued and fine-tuned together with a more detailed diagnostic work-up and history taking. There follows a maintenance phase where we deal with not only the presenting problems of the patient but also complications of highly invasive management in the ICU such as nosocomial infection and intravenous line infections. If the patient survives there is a final gradual improvement phase where the challenge is to dismantle the patient from as much support as quickly as possible in order to facilitate discharge to a general ward. There are blurred boundaries, of course, between each phase and patients can move between phases during their ICU stay. The ICU team must recognise the different challenges associated with each phase and drive the patient's progress as rapidly as possible. Detailed handovers with a short- and long-term plan are essential for continuity and optimal management of the patient, especially by senior medical staff.

Apart from the on-site personnel, a senior member of the medical staff should be on call or on duty 24 hours a day for clinical or administrative consultation.

## Relatives and friends

The condition of a patient should be explained in an honest and forthright manner to relatives and friends. There is no place for false hope and avoidance of difficult explanations – even if it means admitting that many aspects of the patient's disease process are, as yet, unknown. Much of the practice of intensive care medicine is titrational (e.g. trying an inotrope or antibiotic and looking for a response, without necessarily understanding all aspects of the interactions involved), and this should be explained honestly.

It helps to have a special information pamphlet for the patient's friends and relatives that will explain certain matters:

- Relevant aspects of the hospital's function.
- Visiting policy for the ICU.
- The invasive lines and machines that may be encountered, with an explanation of their function in lay terms. Labelled photographs of the various pieces of equipment and lines, with a short description of each, can be displayed in the waiting room.

An explanation of the possible time course of the patient's illness must be given. Many relatives wish to maintain an all-night vigil during the early part of a critical illness, when the patient conceivably could remain stable for days or weeks. It is important to inform relatives of such possibilities so that they can arrange their schedules regarding sleep, work and other responsibilities. Relatives and friends should be told to prepare themselves for a marathon, rather than a 100-metre dash. It is important to provide ongoing support and counselling for relatives and friends, either by the medical and nursing staff or more specialised personnel.

## Quality assurance

Quality assurance (QA), auditing and peer review are all concepts that generally have to do with monitoring and attempting to improve current practice. The idea behind most efforts in this area is that practitioners can demonstrate to themselves and to others the quality and quantity of work they are doing.

The principles of QA and total quality management (TQM) readily lend themselves to managing an ICU. QA is not simply a matter of conducting an audit; it encompasses the principles of how an organisation should run – in our case an ICU. The Japanese have run their industries on a similar basis for decades. They call the concept 'Kaizen' or 'the continuous search for improvement' in oneself and in the system. In order to accomplish this effectively, we need to shed much of our previous conditioning and training. Decision making and autonomy must be decentralised to the bedside. The ability to make decisions comes through education. Making changes is difficult, and many who have been trained in a different way will feel uncomfortable. We need, ultimately, to reach the point at which we begin to feel comfortable with many of the unpredictable aspects of our practice, until eventually we can thrive on the non-routine. Managers must learn to authorise others to solve their problems and managers themselves must learn to find ways of saying yes, rather than finding fault and being obstructionist. The staff need to be encouraged to be autonomous and to speak out when the system is not working. We need to eliminate senseless rules and we need to carefully examine everything we do and always ask why. Rules should be replaced by guidelines and priorities. A collective rhythm must be created whereby quality can be coaxed out of the available resources, which often are inadequate. The key to an organisation's success is to master the art of orchestrating collective thinking. The common good should always be put above one's own. This system will not be the place for large egos that are easily bruised.

The principles of this new style of management include the following:

- The quality of patient care can be improved by removing the causes of problems in the system.
- Problems can be solved only after they have been identified.
- The person who is doing the job, is probably the one most knowledgeable about that job.
- People want to be involved in running the unit and doing their jobs well.
- People should be authorised and encouraged to bypass managers and solve problems themselves.
- Fear and defensive attitudes are easily instilled; it is much more difficult to get people to commit to an adventurous new vision. Supervisors and managers must be specialists who will support their people when problems arise. Authority must come from within.

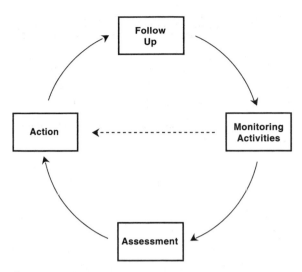

**Figure 2.1.** The quality assurance cycle.

- A structured problem-solving process, with all the relevant players being involved, will produce better solutions than an unstructured process.
- There will be a lot of resistance to implementation of this new style, both within the unit and, more importantly, outside the unit, during the period of transition. This must be resolved along the way, and, if necessary, a little pocket of excellence must be developed.

The philosophy of QA must be deployed to permeate all aspects of the running of the ICU and must be extended to all areas with which the ICU interacts. For example, the outcome for a patient who has suffered major trauma will depend as much on the system in place for initial management as on the treatment given in the ICU. All parts of the larger system must communicate in terms of QA if treatment is to be improved (Figure 2.1).

Examples of QA programmes in intensive care are as follows:

- Mortality review (exclude if death is expected).
- Review of patients' and relatives' complaints.
- Review of readmission rate to the ICU.
- Review of prolonged length of stay (e.g. > 30 days).
- Review of fire and safety practices.
- Problem identification workshops using flow charts.
- Review of nursing practices in order to eliminate outmoded practices (e.g. the way in which observations are recorded and action is taken).
- Publication of newsletters.
- Critical incident monitoring of unexpected events.

## TROUBLESHOOTING

### Assessing a seriously ill patient over the telephone

The ICU often receives calls from other areas within the hospital or from other hospitals seeking advice or requesting a transfer to the ICU. The following are some guidelines on how to handle these requests:
always be helpful, and never patronising. The ICU and its staff have equipment, skills and expertise that should be shared in a positive fashion.

#### Patient
Assess the severity of the problem.
Identify the major problem and take a quick history of the illness.
Determine the level of consciousness.
Determine the state of the airway (e.g. intubated or not).
Assess the breathing (e.g. respiratory rate, oxygenation).
Assess the circulation (e.g. blood pressure, heart rate and rhythm and urine output).
Record the relevant past history.
Determine the current treatment and the lines and monitors being used.

#### Manpower and equipment
Your advice on treatment will depend on the seniority and experience of the person to whom you are speaking. It is important not to assume that the conferring person or institution will have skills the same as your own (e.g. for intubation, central line insertion), nor should you overestimate the availability of equipment in the referring hospital (e.g. sophisticated ventilators).

#### Support
The person whom you are advising usually will have less equipment and expertise than are available in your ICU. Your advice should be aimed at stabilising the patient in the simplest and most responsible fashion, followed by support for the conferee's decision either to continue the management or to transfer the patient to ICU.

It is often helpful to monitor progress and provide encouragement by repeat telephone calls.

If the patient is transferred to your ICU, it is important to provide feedback to the referring institution regarding the patient's progress.

Honest peer review of QA cannot be imposed. If the programme is to work properly, it must have co-operation and commitment of all staff. This should lead to a system in which power is shared to produce the outcomes agreed on, rather than focusing only on the process.

## FURTHER READING

Frutiger, A., Moreno, R., Thijs, L. and Carlet, J. on behalf of the Working Group on Quality Improvement of the European Society of Intensive Care Medicine. A clinician's guide to the use of quality terminology. *Intensive Care Medicine* 24 (1998): 860–3.
Smith, G. and Nielsen, M. ABC of intensive care: criteria for admission. *British Medical Journal* 318 (1999): 1544–7.

# 3

# Routine care of the seriously ill

- The practice of good intensive care medicine is about the methodical application of basic routines.
- ABC – Always maintain a good airway, ensure adequate oxygenation and rapidly correct hypovolaemia.
- In a critically ill patient, one will miss more by not performing a thorough clinical examination than by under monitoring and under investigating.

## How to approach a patient in intensive care

When the specialty of intensive care was being defined, many of the problems were new to us. As the problems had not been documented in conventional textbooks, they had to be learnt at the bedside. Our specialty owes a lot to those first generation intensivists. It was soon learnt that complex single and multiple organ failure (MOF) often occurred in certain patterns. There are also certain features that seriously ill patients have in common. These patterns have been taken into account as part of routine care of the seriously ill patients, making the more unpredictable aspects of complex illness easier to recognise and manage. It is these common and routine aspects that are described in this chapter.

Seriously ill patients often present with complex sets of problems that make a conventional approach difficult. For example, the conventional approach of differential diagnosis, provisional diagnosis, investigations and final diagnosis is often irrelevant in seriously ill patients with multiple problems. Moreover, this approach inhibits the practice of good intensive care medicine. Not only is it rare that there will be only a single diagnosis, but in attempting to make the patient fit into our current bank of knowledge, there is the danger that the patient's unique problems will be ignored. The patient's problems are what the staff should address. Nursing and medical staff work more closely together in intensive care than in ordinary wards. As they both have to deal with the same problems, they should be documented together. For example, pressure areas and hypotension are common problems, perhaps even related, and should not be considered as separate medical and nursing problems – they are the patient's problems.

### The ward round

In order not to get lost in the morass of information available about each individual patient, there has to be some structure in your approach to them. The following is one way of doing this. Team management is crucial in intensive care and this problem-orientated approach ensures that all team members will focus on a patient's problems.

1 History: Critically ill patients are often treated before a definitive diagnosis is made and a history taken. Ambulance officers, patient's relatives and the local doctor can all give valuable information after the patient has been stabilised.
2 Handover: The problems encountered by the previous shift will help to establish a picture of the patient's current status.
3 Physical examination: Physical examination is discussed later.
4 Review of investigations, monitoring and medications. Biochemistry, haematology, arterial blood gases, monitoring, chest x-ray, CT scan, and so forth.
5 List of problems and strategy: Bring together all the information about history, examination and previous problems, and then list the current problems. The problems may be related (e.g. hypotension, oliguria, fever) and have a common cause (e.g. septicaemia). The problems need not be elaborated on, and the plan, if obvious, need not be stated in all cases unless there is some specific investigation or treatment (e.g. hypotension need not be followed in the plan by 'Find cause' or 'Correct' if it is related to an obvious cause such as septicaemia and is treated with a unit protocol). The problem sheet is meant to focus the team's thoughts on overall management strategy. It is more useful than writing reams of continuation notes and could even replace them if filed appropriately in the patient's notes. Fine-tuning is needed within this overall management plan and further problems may emerge before the next major ward round. These will need to be addressed during the course of the day. Table 3.1 outlines a quick way of reviewing patients.
6 Relatives and friends: Information given to relatives needs to be consistent. All team members should agree on the 'party line'.

## Physical assessment

It is important to thoroughly examine a 'stable' critically ill patient at least once a day. Conventional examination techniques may have to be modified as these

**Table 3.1.** A mnemonic to assist in the tasks of junior medical staff

A.  Airway
B.  Breathing
C.  Circulation
D.  Disability – GCS and focal neurology
E.  Electrolytes – results
F.  Fluids – are they appropriate?
G.  Gut – examine and nutritional assessment
H.  Haematology – results
I.  Infection – latest microbiology and white cell count
L.  Lines – are the sites clean? How long have they been in?
M.  Medications – review and interactions
R.  Relatives – what is the common message?

patients are often unconscious, usually with a plethora of monitoring equipment, invasive lines and drains attached. A sound picture can be built up only after a thorough examination of the patient, in combination with knowledge of the patient's history, monitoring trends and concurrent therapy. There is a definite art to examining the seriously ill. As with all other forms of physical assessment in medicine, a set routine guarantees that little is missed. Table 3.2 provides an outline.

## General

Address the patient by name, even if the patient is unconscious, and explain what you are going to do.

The initial routine inspection includes rapid assessment of the airway, breathing and circulation. Once you are happy that the patient is ABC stable you can proceed to the more detailed physical examination. More is missed by not looking than by not knowing and there is a lot to be seen in the seriously ill.

Stand at the end of the bed and look at the patient. Are they resting comfortably, are they distressed? Take a look at the monitor, all the lines, infusions and support equipment, e.g. dialysis and inotropes, as this will give you a good initial 'picture' of the patient. Often the diagnosis or main problem and complications can be obvious from the end of the bed.

Lift the sheet off the patient and expose as much of the body as possible. Start the general examination from the top and work down. Turn the patient into the lateral position and inspect the back of the trunk and legs. Inspect the skin for features such as jaundice, rashes and bruising. Observe early pressure areas, especially around the heels, and feel for dependent oedema.

Inspect the eyes, looking carefully for corneal ulceration as a result of drying. Inspect the mouth, nose and teeth. Inspect all invasive equipment sites such as

**Table 3.2.** Daily routine examination of patients in intensive care

1  Address the patient by name and explain what you intend to do
2  Rapidly assess the airway, breathing and circulation. If the patient is stable proceed with the
     formal examination
3  Expose the patient's whole body, placing the patient supine if possible
4  Airway and head
     Check natural airway, artificial airway (cuff, type of tube and securing method, cuff pressure,
       diameter)
     Inspect scalp, sinuses, mouth, ears, NG tube, cervical nodes, eyes (especially pupils and corneal
       abrasions)
     Check for neck stiffness
5  Neurological system
     Check GCS trends and current level of consciousness and inquire of nursing staff about GCS
       and limb movement
     Assess sedation in the light of need, as well as liver and renal functions
     Exclude seizures
     If necessary, check brainstem reflexes
     Obtain gross information using focal neurological signs and then, if necessary, make a more
       detailed examination
6  Respiratory system
     Inspect chest movement, respiratory rate and effort
     Check interaction of patient with ventilator and observe $FiO_2$, PIP, PEEP levels, ventilator
       mode, tidal and minute volumes and respiratory swings with spontaneous respiration
     Assess gas exchange (colour, oximetry, arterial blood gases)
     Auscultate the chest, especially posterior and lateral bases
     Check ICC for bubbling and fluid
     Correlate findings with chest x-ray
     Ask nursing staff about the patient's ability to cough and the type of secretions
7  Circulatory system
     Inspect precordium
     Observe neck veins
     Assess peripheral pulses and rhythm
     Exclude peripheral oedema
     Assess peripheral perfusion
     Auscultate the precordium
     Check the trends in BP, pulse rate, urine output and other more complex measurements, such
       as cardiac output, $VO_2$, and $DO_2$
8  Gastrointestinal tract
     Observe the abdomen for distension, wounds and drains
     Study the underlying surgery and recent imaging (e.g. CT scan or ultrasound)
     Palpate for tenderness, tenseness and masses
     Listen for bowel sounds
     Inquire about NG aspirate, efficacy of enteral feeding and bowel actions
9  Limbs
     Inspect for rashes, oedema and wounds
     Remove dressings, where possible and inspect wounds
     Study the underlying fractures, traction, surgery and relevant radiological appearances

**Table 3.3.** Signs peculiar to the critically ill

Bounding in the neck and precordium often indicates sepsis

An indentation ring in the skin, left after listening for bowel sounds with a stethoscope, indicates extensive peripheral oedema

Blue knees (i.e. peripheral cyanosis) is a sign of a severely compromised circulation

The silhouette of the head seen over the mediastinum on an upright chest x-ray is a poor prognostic sign and is usually followed by intubation within the next 24 hours

Attempts to breathe against the ventilator, despite what appears to be an adequate minute volume, is often due to severe metabolic acidosis

Rapid deterioration in cardiorespiratory signs can indicate a pneumothorax

surgical drains, intercostal catheters (ICCs), intravenous (IV) and intra-arterial lines and endotracheal tubes (ETTs). Remove all dressings and inspect wounds. Look for abnormal bleeding into wounds or bleeding from puncture sites. It is important to know exactly where surgical drains have been placed and for what purpose and to inspect the drainage fluid for amount and appearance. Ensure that the lines and drains are secure and working efficiently. Ask yourself if they are really needed and consider removal if there is any doubt. During the examination, ensure that the patient is not lying on equipment such as IV lines and catheters as they can cause pressure areas.

Some signs peculiar to the critically ill are listed in Table 3.3.

## Neurological assessment

The most important features of a neurological examination in the ICU are the level of consciousness, brainstem function and lateralising signs in the limbs. The patient's level of consciousness is usually monitored by the Glasgow Coma Scale (GCS). Look at the GCS trends. Further information can be gained from the nursing staff. Assess the level of consciousness in light of the amount of sedation. Sedation may take days to wear off, especially in the presence of hepatic and renal insufficiency. A consistent painful stimulus is recommended to test the level of response. Vigorous stimulation of the outer aspects of the eyebrow can cause nerve palsies and rubbing of the sternum with one's knuckles can cause unsightly bruising. The nail bed is a more suitable area to elicit a reaction to a painful stimulus. The presence of seizures should be noted. Neck stiffness, fever and photophobia suggest meningeal irritation due to the presence of blood or infection.

Reflexes, such as pupil size and reaction to light, corneal reflex, gag reflex and respiration pattern, will give an indication of brainstem function.

Information on focal neurological deficits can be grossly elicited by inquiring about movement of the limbs from the nursing staff, spontaneously and in response to pain. Limb reflexes and tone can also be elicited. A nerve stimulator may be useful in determining residual paralysis, especially after prolonged use of muscle relaxants.

## Respiratory system

Always assess the adequacy of the airway, even if the patient has an ETT or tracheostomy in place. It may be kinked or blocked. Note the diameter of the ETT, as narrow tubes can be the greatest contributors to the work of breathing. Ask the nursing staff about the nature and amount of tracheal secretions. Check the way the airway has been secured, check cuff pressures and inquire about the appropriateness of the cuff for long-term use. Monitoring of ventilator variables and gas exchange will also provide valuable information about respiratory function (see Chapter 19). Assess oxygenation, in terms of pulse oximetry and fraction of inspired oxygen ($FiO_2$). Note the breathing rate, the tidal volume, the respiratory effort and, if ventilated, the positive end-expiratory pressure (PEEP), the peak inspiratory pressure (PIP) and the breathing mode. Look for asymmetry of chest movement and position of the mediastinum, as judged by the trachea and apex beat. Observe how the patient is interacting with the ventilator.

Auscultation remains important in the ICU. The lung bases posteriorly represent areas often blind to the chest X-ray. It is essential to take trouble to auscultate these areas, especially for decreased air entry and bronchial breathing. Intrapulmonary shadows on a chest x-ray can be difficult to interpret, but bronchial breath sounds will indicate that pneumonia is more likely than acute lung injury (ALI) or pulmonary oedema. Decreased air entry, indicating collapse and rhonchi, indicating the degree of bronchospasm, are important aspects in examining the respiratory system in the critically ill. Check for chest drains and flail segments. Look for bubbling from the ICC, as well as the amount and type of drainage. The best single means of assessing respiratory status is an upright chest x-ray. Other considerations in interpreting chest x-rays in the seriously ill are discussed later (see Chapter 17). Examine the trend of arterial blood gases. Interpret the sputum microbiology.

## Cardiovascular system

There is often 'information overload' concerning cardiorespiratory variables in the ICU. Amongst all this hard data, it is important not to overlook simple vital signs such as arterial blood pressure (BP), pulse rate and rhythm, urine output and peripheral perfusion. Current values should be seen in light of previous trends. Information may also be available for cardiac output, peripheral resistance, oxygen delivery ($DO_2$) and consumption ($VO_2$) and other estimates of cardiac function derived from echocardiography. Despite the cardiovascular measurements available, careful physical examination of the patient is important. Assess peripheral pulses and auscultate the precordium for added sounds, murmurs and bruits. Examine the patient for peripheral oedema.

There are signs peculiar to the seriously ill. For example, a bounding precordium in the neck is usually seen with systemic sepsis and is due to the hyperdynamic cardiovascular status accompanying that state. This is obvious from the end of the bed. Patients with sepsis will often have tachycardia and low BP, even with normal filling pressures. Peripheral temperature is a good empirical guide to adequate circulating volume, but it is difficult to interpret in the presence of sepsis and a fever.

## Gastrointestinal tract

It is important to carefully examine the gastrointestinal tract (GIT) at least once each day. Carefully inspect the face for signs of sinusitis and the nose and mouth, especially in the presence of artificial airways and tubes, as they can make thorough inspection difficult.

The abdomen should be observed for distension, wounds and drains. Palpate for tenderness, tenseness and abnormal masses. Listen for bowel sounds and inquire about bowel actions and absorption of oral feeds. The presence of bowel sounds means that air and fluid are present, but their absence does not mean a non-functioning GIT. It is important to be familiar with all abdominal drains – where they originate and what they are draining. A clear diagram of any abdominal surgery displayed in the notes at the patient's bedside can clarify the complexities of the abdominal surgery. Carefully observe the perineum for signs of swelling, inflammation and discharge. Do not neglect to do a rectal examination if required, e.g. for a patient with diarrhoea.

## Renal and fluids

Note the adequacy of the intravascular volume as reflected by pulse rate, BP, peripheral perfusion, urine output, pulmonary artery wedge pressure (PAWP), central venous pressure (CVP) and so forth. Note the state of hydration (e.g. skin turgor, dry tongue).

Assess the fluid balance chart, noting any major losses and the sources of those losses (e.g. nasogastric [NG] losses, drains). Review the urinalysis.

Check electrolytes (sodium, potassium, calcium, phosphate and magnesium) at least once each day.

Check urea, creatinine and urine output as markers of renal function. A 4-hour creatinine clearance may be useful, especially if compared with a previous one.

The urinary catheter must be inserted using strictly aseptic technique, with urine drainage collected in a closed sterile system. There is a good argument for using Silastic catheters in seriously ill patients, as they are associated with fewer long-term complications. It is also advisable in long-term male patients to pull the penis up and tape the catheter onto the lower part of the abdomen to optimise the angle that the catheter makes in its course, thus reducing pressure around the prostate gland. The catheter should be taped to the patient's skin to prevent trauma caused by traction.

## Limbs

Attention to a patient's limbs is sometimes overlooked in the ICU. They should be carefully inspected for rashes, oedema and adequacy of perfusion. Hands, feet and nails should also be inspected. Dressings should be taken down and inspected where applicable. The details of underlying fractures should be known and close communication with orthopaedic surgeons is essential. Fractures are often associated with wounds. It is important that plaster be regularly removed or have windows cut so that the wounds can be inspected. Orthopaedic surgeons should be encouraged to pin or plate fractures, as traction makes nursing and patient care very difficult.

## Blood glucose

There is evidence that tight control of blood glucose to within normal levels improves mortality in the ICU.

## Haematology

Check for obvious oozing or bleeding. Note the results of coagulation tests and platelet counts. Check the haemoglobin and white blood cell count. Assess anti-coagulation therapy, if appropriate.

## Thromboembolism

There are many risk factors associated with the formation of venous thromboemboli in the critically ill – immobility, decreased blood flow secondary to positive-pressure ventilation (PPV), surgery or trauma and low flow states. Clinical manifestations of pulmonary emboli may not be obvious in the critically ill so a high index of suspicion should be maintained.
    Prophylaxis

- frequent turning
- mobilisation
- graded compression stockings
- subcutaneous heparin, unfractionated or low molecular weight heparin
- pneumatic full length leg compression.

## Patient positioning

Unless sitting up is contraindicated, patients in intensive care should always be sat up to an angle of at least 30°. Pressure measurements can be taken in this position

**Table 3.4.** Demonstrated to be potentially successful interventions aimed at restoring or maintaining a 'normal' state

- Rapidly restoring the airway, breathing and circulation
- Manage patient in an upright position (> 30°) whenever possible.
- Maintaining a normal blood sugar
- Encouraging spontaneous respiration
- The establishment of early enteral feeding
- Use stress ulcer prophylaxis ($H_2$ receptor blocker) only in at-risk patients (e.g. those with a history of upper GIT bleeding, long-term ventilation, coagulopathy)
- Maintaining normal airway humidification
- Maintaining normal sleep patterns for patients
- Physiotherapy and nursing interventions
- Encouraging a 'human' orientated ICU environment, e.g. flexible visiting policies, communication with patients
- Maintaining a normal temperature in intracerebral crises
- Surgery, e.g.
  - Reducing pressure in compartment syndromes – craniectomy, fasciotomy, 'open' abdomen, pleural and pericardial space drainage
  - Aggressively removing infected and necrotic tissue
  - Orthopaedic and plastic surgery
  - Restoring blood flow in vessels

as long as the transducers are correctly placed. Upright patients usually have better oxygenation, decreased work of breathing and less chance of aspirating. There is a lower incidence of nosocomial pneumonia and lower intracranial pressure (ICP) usually can be achieved in patients who are sitting upright.

As for the head down position, apart from specific purposes such as the insertion of central venous lines, a patient should not be placed with the head down, not even as a temporary measure for hypotension. Posture-related hypotension should be corrected by intravascular fluids.

In a patient with lung pathology, hypoxia can be exacerbated when the patient's position is changed. For the same reason, when assessing serial blood gases and pulse oximetry, the position of the patient at the time should be noted.

Stable, critically ill patients should be turned from side to side regularly, usually every 2 hours, always maintaining them in the upright position where possible. This helps with oxygenation and may prevent pressure sores.

## Interventions

There have been many interventions and manipulations of normal physiology used over the years in the treatment of the seriously ill, primarily aimed at restoring normality. Table 3.4 lists the interventions that have stood the test of time or have been demonstrated to be effective. There are also conditions where interventions

**Table 3.5.** Examples of interventions shown to be potentially beneficial but with possible complications

- Low tidal volumes; high $FiO_2$ and high $PaCO_2$ during artificial ventilation
- Supporting inspiration with pressure and maintaining alveolar opening with PEEP
- Monitoring – especially invasive
- Drugs, e.g. inotropes, antibiotics, bronchodilators
- Lower than normal haemoglobin

**Table 3.6.** Non-'normal' interventions/states which have doubtful beneficial effects

- Supranormal $DO_2$
- Hyperbaric oxygenation
- High serum osmolality
- Intravenous nutrition
- Hypervolaemia
- 'Magic bullets' e.g.
  - anticytokines
  - anti-inflammatories
  - immunoglobulins
  - antioxidants
  - nitric oxide
  - high-dose steroids
- High-flow continuous veno-venous haemofiltration
- Deliberate coma in intracerebral pathology

and variations on normal physiology (e.g. low tidal volumes in ALI) may help to maintain life while the disease process comes under control (Table 3.5). There are other interventions that are more doubtful or, as yet, not widely accepted as a result of insufficient evidence (Table 3.6). These lists will, of course, change over time and various interventions may move between the lists as more evidence becomes available.

## Routine monitoring, observations and investigations

Patients should have their vital signs, such as pulse rate, arterial BP, respiratory rate and urine output, measured regularly. Continuous ECG monitoring and pulse oximetry are usually necessary in all seriously ill patients. Other measurements, such as CVP, PAWP and cardiac output, may also be sometimes employed. Oxygenation and ventilation should be monitored by regularly measuring the $FiO_2$, respiratory rate and blood gases. If a patient is artificially ventilated, tidal volumes, inspiratory pressures and respiratory frequency may also require monitoring. For more details on cardiorespiratory monitoring, see Chapter 20.

The patient's level of consciousness should be charted according to a consistent scale, such as the GCS.

Central temperature, rather than oral or skin temperature, should be measured either rectally or by probe in the oesophagus or bladder.

As part of quality assurance, the staff in the ICU should continuously be asking questions: Why is this parameter being measured? does it need recording? It may be more productive to invest time and resources in educating the primary health giver (i.e. the nurse at the bedside) to act on information, rather than simply recording it. A beautiful chart, with every possible variable meticulously recorded, may not necessarily reflect a high standard of patient care. Early action, rather than simply recording abnormal observations, is preferable.

Theoretically, computers should offer more sophisticated documentation and information on trends for all intensive care measurements; charts may not be necessary in the future. However, the clinical information systems that are currently available are expensive, often duplicate what is recorded in charts and are not yet as flexible as is required.

## Routine investigations

There are certain routine tests that should be performed in all seriously ill patients. Many hospitals now have auto-analysers, which makes selective tests impractical. The following are guidelines to the minimum routine tests for the seriously ill:

### Four-hourly determinations
Blood sugar levels should be measured in all seriously ill and unconscious patients at least 4-hourly and sometimes hourly.

### Twice-daily determinations
- Arterial blood gases.
- Potassium.

### Daily determinations
- Urea and creatinine.
- Sodium and chloride.
- Haemoglobin.
- White cell count.
- Platelets.
- Magnesium.
- Calcium and phosphate.
- Chest x-ray.
- 12-lead ECG.

## Twice-weekly determinations
- So-called liver function tests (i.e. serum bilirubin, alkaline phosphatase and aminotransferase activities and serum albumin).
- Prothrombin time (PT).
- Partial thromboplastin (PTTK).

## Radiology
The stethoscope is useful for detecting chest abnormalities, but daily chest x-rays are essential. Patients should always have upright chest x-rays with every attempt made to standardise exposures, making comparisons easier. Large viewing boxes with room for representative and consecutive films should be available. Ideally, a radiologist with experience in interpreting these films, together with the intensive care team, should look at all the day's films. The interpretation of chest x-rays is discussed in more detail later (see Chapter 17).

## Microbiology
Microbiology is an important area for investigation in the seriously ill. Unlike the situation in biochemistry, the findings are never clear cut; they must be interpreted and daily consultation with a microbiologist with clinical experience is an advantage. Specific tests and routine surveillance must be carefully tracked. Antibiotic treatment should be reviewed daily and not continued nor commenced unnecessarily. Antibiotic blood levels should be monitored closely as the patient's condition changes.

# Intravascular lines

This book does not cover the anatomic and procedural aspects of cannulation. There are, however, several important points relating to intravascular lines.

## Peripheral lines
- Use large bore (>18 gauge) in ICU patients.
- Remove all resuscitation lines (e.g. those inserted in the emergency department within the first 24 hours), as they may have been placed in less than strictly aseptic conditions.
- Peripheral lines should all be changed after 48 hours, as the infection rate increases exponentially.
- Drugs with powerful α-agonist action should not be transfused through peripheral lines except in an emergency.

## Central lines
- Beware of covered patients during central line insertion – the head down position is dangerous in the seriously ill. Staff can focus their attention on pressure waveforms and technical difficulties during intravascular cannulation,

rather than the condition of the patient. Someone must be assigned to watch and monitor the patient. Pulse oximetry, continuous ECG and BP measurements should be made because of the potential for hypoxia and hypotension in the head down position. The wire used in a Seldinger technique may cause arrhythmias.

- Pulmonary artery catheters ideally should be removed between 48 and 72 hours.
- Multilumen central venous lines should be placed early if the patient has MOF, requiring multidrug support. They allow CVP measurements to be performed without interruption of essential drugs.
- Catheters should be inspected at least daily and removed if there are any signs of inflammation. There is no evidence to suggest that routine changing of central venous catheters reduces the incidence of infection. Antibiotic impregnated lines decrease the incidence of catheter-related sepsis but are expensive. They should probably be used in patients at risk of catheter-related sepsis, e.g. the immunosupressed patient.
- Femoral lines have not been demonstrated to have a higher infection rate than lines inserted in the neck and are technically easier to insert.

## Arterial lines
Keep the arterial line site in view at all times. Disconnection can lead to catastrophic haemorrhage.

- Arterial lines have a low incidence of complications and their insertion can be justified for multiple sampling of blood gases alone.
- Beware of retrogradely flushing air into the radial artery line as it can cause cerebral air embolism.

## General points
1  Some points to remember when dressing intravascular lines:
   - strict aseptic technique
   - no topical antibiotics
   - secure with a suture.
2  Beware of taking blood cultures from existing lines. The connections soon become colonised and may give misleading results.

## Intubation and tracheal care

Intubation is necessary in many seriously ill patients to:

- secure an adequate airway
- facilitate removal of secretions
- facilitate ventilation and oxygenation.

General complications of ETT and tracheostomies include:

- malposition
- dislodgement
- disconnection
- obstruction
- infection
- local trauma to larynx and trachea that can result in long-term damage
- interference with normal humidification and warming of inspired gases.

## Intubation

Be properly prepared with the necessary equipment.
Pre-oxygenate for 5 minutes with 100% oxygen.

Seriously ill patients need someone who can intubate expertly and rapidly. It is not the time for teaching. In fact, it is preferable to have a second experienced doctor on hand at the time of intubation to monitor and, if necessary, to help resuscitate the patient.

There is often a dilemma concerning which artificial airway should be used – nasotracheal tube (NTT), orotracheal tube (OTT) or tracheostomy. Each ICU will develop its own policy based on some of the following considerations.

## Orotracheal tubes

Advantages compared with NTT.

- A larger lumen tube can be passed through the mouth than through the nose, facilitating spontaneous breathing by decreasing the work of breathing.
- Insertion of an OTT is a quicker and easier technical procedure than inserting a NTT. This may be particularly important when rapid intubation is necessary.
- An OTT makes it easier to pass a suction catheter.
- An OTT does not cause local trauma and predispose to sinusitis

### Disadvantages.
- An OTT is more difficult to secure than an NTT.
- The bandage around the neck can impede venous drainage (important if there is an elevated ICP) and cut into the corners of the mouth.
- Because of difficulty in securing it, there is more movement of the OTT within the trachea.
- It is difficult to conduct mouth care in the presence of an OTT.
- There can be chronic laryngeal dysfunction and tracheal stenosis at the cuff site.
- Patients can cause occlusion by biting on the tube.

## Tracheostomy

An OTT can be left in place for 7–21 days before tracheostomy is considered. Even then, some units delay tracheostomy. A tracheostomy tube simply bypasses a part of the OTT or NTT. The tracheal tube and cuff remain in the trachea and that is the source of most morbidity and mortality. However, laryngeal dysfunction and even vocal cord paralysis can occur with an OTT. The decision to perform a tracheostomy after 7–10 days is largely dictated by unit policy and whether or not prolonged airway access will be required. If a prolonged period of intubation is anticipated, some units now perform tracheostomy within the first few days.

Tracheostomy should be performed by an experienced surgeon or intensivist when the patient is stable. The best procedure is to use the smallest incision, with the greatest preservation of cartilage, between the first and second tracheal rings. Percutaneous tracheostomy is a simple procedure that can be performed in the ICU by members of the intensive care staff. Percutaneous tracheostomies have shown, in comparative trials, to have less complications then conventional surgical tracheostomies.

### Advantages

- There is better patient tolerance than for an OTT or NTT.
- The tube is easier to secure and enhances patient mobility.
- There is no trauma to mouth, nose or larynx. Oral toilet is easier. Some patients can eat with a tracheostomy tube in place.
- It is easier to introduce suction catheters.
- A larger diameter tube is possible, decreasing dead space, resistance and the work of breathing during spontaneous breathing.

### Disadvantages

- An operation is involved, with small, but documented, rates of mortality and morbidity.
- The wound almost always becomes superficially infected.
- There can be difficulty in reinserting the tracheostomy tube if it becomes dislodged, especially in the first few days after insertion.
- There can be tracheal stenosis at the cuff site and erosion into adjacent structures.

## Nasotracheal tube

Nasotracheal tubes are used less frequently than OTT or tracheostomy. They predispose to local trauma and sinusitis and probably should be confined for use only for specific and temporary indicators.

## Minitracheostomy

Minitracheostomy tubes are available in pre-packaged kit form. They can be inserted using local anaesthetic through the cricothyroid membrane in the ICU. Minitracheostomy tubes can also be inserted through a tracheostomy stoma after the tracheostomy tube has been removed, in order to facilitate suction.

### Indications

The main indication is to facilitate suction of secretions, typically in patients with chronic lung disease and patients with copious secretions who cannot, or will not, cough.

## Care of tubes

Cut the tube off flush with the mouth or nose once the position is checked on a chest x-ray. This helps to prevent kinking, to decrease resistance and to prevent excessive movement within the trachea.

Take a chest x-ray after insertion and at least daily to verify position (see Chapter 17). When not visualised radiographically, the carina can be expected to lie on a line corresponding to approximately halfway down the aortic knob. Neck flexion and extension can cause the tip of the ETT to move up to 2 cm.

Change a tube immediately if obstruction is suspected and cannot be excluded (e.g. increased ventilatory pressures or difficulty in breathing). Simply passing a suction catheter successfully through the lumen of a tube does not guarantee that it is not obstructed. Viscous secretions can cause a ball-valve effect as the catheter passes through it. Patients with haemoptysis are particularly prone to blocking their ETT.

## Tracheal suction

- Regular suctioning of any tube is necessary, but unfortunately the procedure is always accompanied by hypoxia.
  1 Pre-oxygenate with 100% oxygen before suction.
  2 Use an ETT connector through which a suction catheter can be passed without having to disconnect the patient.
  3 Suction rapidly – do not leave the catheter down for more than 5 seconds at any one time.
  4 Avoid mechanical damage – be gentle and use soft tips with lateral holes.
- Never suction active pulmonary oedema and reduce suctioning of hypoxic patients otherwise.
- Never actively suction the trachea while the patient is being extubated – that would cause hypoxia at a critical time. Suction around the pharynx and extubate

at the height of inspiration so that the patient can clear secretions by exhaling or coughing.

## Routine care of ventilated patients

Take at least hourly measurements of tidal volume, respiratory rate and peak airway pressure. Ventilator alarms usually provide continuous monitoring of excessive pressure and notice of disconnection.

Assess lung abnormalities at least once daily with an upright chest x-ray (see Chapter 17).

The aim of ventilation is to maintain adequate gas exchange. Regular determinations of arterial blood gases, continuous pulse oximetry and clinical assessment are essential.

## Fluids

Fluid treatment can be perplexing in seriously ill patients. This topic is discussed in some detail later (see Chapter 4). Briefly, some of the difficulties faced are as follows.

- Conventional guides to fluid treatment (fluid balance chart, CVP, urine output, arterial BP, PAWP, pulse rate) are often misleading in a seriously ill patient.
- In patients who are not seriously ill, the normal compensation mechanisms, such as thirst and renal function, allow more room for error in fluid treatment. However, these mechanisms are often compromised in the critically ill. Such a patient cannot, therefore, compensate for poor fluid treatment.

The sequelae of poor fluid treatment, such as pulmonary oedema, hypotension and renal failure, will compound the existing MOF.

The following are guidelines for routine fluid treatment for seriously ill patients.

### Colloid and blood products

Colloid and blood products are confined mainly to the intravascular space. Measurements in this space (e.g. BP, pulse rate, urine output, CVP, PAWP) are much more easily accomplished than are measurements in the interstitial and intracellular spaces (e.g. tissue turgor, dry mucosa). The best method of assessing the intravascular volume is with a fluid challenge: measure intravascular parameters before and after a challenge of 200–500 ml of colloid, as a guide to fluid requirement.

**It is vital to maintain intravascular volume in seriously ill patients at all times and it is essential to avoid overexpansion of the interstitial space.**

### Crystalloid solutions

Crystalloid solutions will rehydrate the intravascular space temporarily. The majority of the infused fluid enters the intracellular and interstitial spaces. Clinical assessment of these spaces is notoriously inaccurate and the 'stress response' in the critically ill encourages salt and water retention, thus promoting peripheral and pulmonary oedema. Excessive administration of crystalloid solutions should therefore be avoided.

### Clinical guidelines

Intravenous fluids fall into three categories: fluid to resuscitate and maintain the intravascular volume, maintenance fluids and fluids to replace abnormal losses.

- Give packed cells or whole blood to keep haemoglobin above 8 g/dl. Higher values may be needed in some patients.
- Titrate the colloid solution against intravascular measurements (e.g. CVP, BP, pulse rate, urine output).
- Give 500–2500 ml of appropriate maintenance fluid over 24 hours for a normal sized adult, titrated empirically against the daily serum sodium concentration.
- If patient is normovolaemic and has a stable cardiovascular system, only maintenance fluids are necessary (e.g. 4% dextrose and 0.2-N saline at 1000–3000 ml over 24 hours).
- Abnormal losses should be replaced with a separate solution to the maintenance fluid, e.g. large NG losses should be replaced with 0.9% sodium chloride.

## Gastrointestinal tract haemorrhage

Stress ulceration is related primarily to ischaemia and can be a complication of acute illness. A low gastric pH in seriously ill patients is associated with a higher incidence of gastric bleeding than is a gastric pH of 4 or more. That has, in the past, prompted many ICUs to institute prophylactic measures to prevent stress ulceration. However, the successful institution of enteral nutrition and adequate splanchnic perfusion usually means other prophylactic measures to prevent stress ulceration are not necessary. Stress ulcer prophylaxis probably should only be considered in those critically ill patients who are at high risk such as those with a history of upper GIT bleeding or those who are ventilated for more than 48 hours or who have a coagulopathy.

### Drugs

Meta-analysis has demonstrated that $H_2$-receptor antagonists are probably superior to other drugs such as sucralfate or antacids. The incidence of nosocomial pneumonia is also less for $H_2$ antagonists.

The role of proton pump inhibitors, e.g. omeprazole is not clear.

# Nutrition

Many aspects of feeding critically ill patients remain unclear, even after more than two decades of research. These issues are discussed in more detail in Chapter 5. Some of the bottom line messages are included here.

- Enteral feeding is preferable to intravenous nutrition (IVN) and should be used whenever possible. Enteral feeding is cheaper and more efficient, encourages GIT mucosal growth and involves fewer complications.
- Many of the contraindications to enteral feeding, such as abdominal distension, high gastric aspirates and recent surgery, are only relative. Increasingly, feeding tubes are bypassing the stomach in order to facilitate feeding.
- Obligatory catabolism often occurs in the seriously ill, especially during the early, unstable period. Nutrition is therefore of doubtful benefit while a patient is being resuscitated. Moreover, IVN probably is not necessary until approximately 7–10 days after initial resuscitation.

## Daily nutrition

1. Use enteral nutrition if the gut is working.
2. Use parenteral nutrition only after demonstrated failure of enteral feeding. Do not try to achieve perfect nitrogen balance. Aggressive feeding of calories is also not necessary. Approximately 2000 kcal/day is a realistic level for adults. Other components also need to be considered:
   - Trace elements, especially zinc, should be given empirically.
   - Multivitamin preparations.
   - Folic acid.
   - Vitamin K.
   - Potassium, phosphate, magnesium and calcium must be measured frequently (at least once each day) and supplemented if necessary.

## Obesity in intensive care

Obesity is an increasing problem in the developed world. A simple definition of obesity is that the amount of fat tissue has increased to such an extent that mental and physical health are affected and life expectancy is decreased. Obesity poses the following problems in intensive care:

- 5% have obstructive sleep apnoea.
- Increased $VO_2$ and carbon dioxide production.
- Closing volume may be reached in normal tidal breathing leading to hypoxia. High incidence of basal lung collapse and pneumonia.
- Left ventricular hypertrophy and impaired systolic function.
- Increased risk of deep vein thrombosis.

- Altered drug handling.
- Direct arterial BP monitoring is necessary as BP cuffs are too inaccurate.

## Age and the seriously ill

Elderly patients are becoming increasingly common in most ICUs. Age alone should not preclude admission to intensive care. A patient's level of functioning before hospitalisation and the number of co-morbidities probably are better predictors of outcome than is age. The term 'frailty' attempts to define this lack of reserve and probably describes the final stages of ageing marked by a significant decrease in reserve. This is important in ICU because these patients require only a small acute insult to expose their lack of reserve and inability to recover. As yet, 'frailty' can only be described in general terms as weight loss, loss of strength, increased falls and inability to perform their usual tasks.

- In general, the elderly have limited physiological reserves.
- There are increasing incidences of co-existing illnesses, such as diabetes, carcinoma, heart failure and ischaemic heart disease.
- There tend to be increasing effects from tobacco and alcohol-related diseases.
- There tends to be increased use of medications that can interact with the acute illness or with the medications used to treat the acute illness or impair the ability of the body to metabolise drugs.
- Central nervous system:
  ↑predisposition to confusional states
  impaired thermoregulation
  ↑cerebral atrophy.
- Respiratory system:
  ↓functional residual capacity
  ↑closing volume
  ↑airway closure
  ↓alveoli and lung mass from age 16 years
  ↑emphysematous changes
  ↓lung compliance
  ↑alveolar-arterial gradient: $PaO_2 = 105 - 0.3$ (age in years) (mmHg)
  ↓vital capacity
  ↓inspiratory reserve
  ↓ventilatory drive to hypoxia and hypercarbia
  ↓respiratory reflexes.
- Cardiovascular system:
  ↓ability to increase heart rate
  ↑BP (systolic pressure is approximately age + 100 mmHg), less compliant ventricles, and decreased ejection fraction and cardiac index
  ↑incidence of valvular dysfunction

↑incidence of arrhythmias
↑atheroma
↑blunting of sympathetic response.
- Musculoskeletal system and skin
↓muscle mass
↓mobility
↓elasticity of skin, and more prone to pressure necrosis
↑osteoporosis.
- Renal system
↓total body water
↓glomerular filtration rate (approximately half that of a 30-year-old by age 60 years)
↑benign prostatic enlargement
↓number of nephrons.
- Gastrointestinal tract and nutrition
↓motility
↓fat stores
↓basal metabolic rate
↓hepatocyte numbers
↑glucose intolerance.
- Social and ethical considerations
Involve friends and family in decisions and discussion of the prognosis. Elderly patients have often discussed what they would like to happen in the event of a life-threatening illness.
Evaluate the patient's circumstances of living and support and the degree of independence before illness.

## Patient reaction to intensive care

### Patient

The reactions of patients in intensive care often involve anxiety, exhaustion, disorientation and lack of communication. They are to be expected and are quite normal. Reassure the patient that these reactions are expected, always acknowledge anxiety and fear and attempt to have him/her externalise their fears.

- Explanation: Medical and nursing staff should try to explain each procedure and why it is being done, in addition to orientating the patient in time and place.
- Measures for sedation and pain relief should be taken only if necessary.
- Relatives and friends should be allowed unrestricted access, in limited numbers, to the patient. They should be encouraged to touch and talk to the patient.
- Speech aids and writing devices should be fully utilised if the patient is awake and unable to speak.

# TROUBLESHOOTING

## Routine assessment of the seriously ill in the ICU

Inquire about the patient's condition from the nursing staff. Obtain a general impression of the patient's condition, level of support and monitoring from the end of the bed. The following is a checklist of some major points to be considered during routine assessment of the seriously ill in the ICU. Further details are available elsewhere.

### Central nervous system
Assess the patient's level of consciousness in the light of

- intracranial abnormalities
- sedatives and other drugs.

Look for lateralising neurological signs.

### Respiratory system
Check airway, secretions and chest drains.
Oxygenation: Assess $FiO_2$, $PaO_2$ or $SaO_2$, physical examination and chest radiograph.
Ventilation: Assess ventilatory mode, $PaCO_2$ and inspiratory pressures.

### Cardiovascular system
Determine BP, pulse rate and rhythm and peripheral perfusion.
Check for the presence of inotropes, vasopressors, vasodilators and other cardiovascular drugs.

### Fluid and renal
Urine output and other abnormal losses
Creatinine, urea and electrolytes.
Fluid input: volume and composition.

### Gastrointestinal Tract
Type of feeding and vitamins (is it being tolerated?).
Examination of abdomen.
Liver function tests.

### Haematology
Haemoglobin.
Platelets.
Clinical bleeding and coagulation profile.

### Microbiology
Temperature.
White cell count.
Results of microbiological tests and culture.
Type of antibiotics, dose, duration and appropriateness.

### Drugs
Are they all still required?
Check drug levels.

### Catheters, lines and monitoring
Appropriateness and duration.

### Devise a plan of action based on this assessment

## TROUBLESHOOTING

## Routine postoperative management following elective vascular surgery

These patients often have severe impairments of their underlying physiological reserves (e.g. previous myocardial infarction, ischaemic heart disease, chronic airflow limitation (CAL), diabetes).

As such, they are at risk for acute perioperative events, such as myocardial ischaemia and stroke.

The key to perioperative management is to maintain excellent cardiorespiratory stability.

### Ventilation

Elective postoperative ventilation is sometimes used, especially after laparotomies. Adequate pain relief, supplemental oxygen and continuous positive airway pressure (CPAP) may be as effective as elective ventilation.

### Oxygenation

Normal oxygenation should be carefully maintained in order to prevent myocardial ischaemia and to facilitate wound healing. Oxygen supplementation is almost invariably required and is not usually a problem, even in the presence of severe CAL.

### Cardiovascular system

These patients often are hypertensive and need to have their BP maintained within their own 'normal' preoperative limits. Hypotension usually responds to fluid replacement. If not, look very carefully for the cause of the hypotension, e.g. surgical bleeding, acute myocardial infarct. Check ECG and troponin levels.

A transthoracic echo will be useful. Paradoxical hypertension may occur in these patients when they are hypovolaemic.

### Fluid replacement

Patients, especially those who have had vascular surgery, including a laparotomy, often require large amounts of fluid replacement for the first 12 hours postoperatively (e.g. 2–4 L).

### Urine output

It is crucial to maintain urine output at or above $0.5 \text{ ml} \cdot \text{kg}^{-1} \cdot \text{h}^{-1}$. Fluids are usually sufficient to achieve this. If the patient has had a laparotomy check the intra-abdominal pressure.

### Pain relief

Recovery from surgery involving a lower limb or the carotid artery is not especially painful. However, it is important to provide adequate pain relief for patients following laparotomy, in order to ensure adequate ventilation and oxygenation. Horizontal abdominal incisions are less painful than the more traditional vertical ones. Techniques for pain relief include:

- epidural analgesia
- continuous narcotic infusion or patient-controlled analgesia.

### Routine postoperative monitoring

Routine postoperative monitoring should include the following:

- determinations of BP, pulse rate, respiratory rate, pulse oximetry and temperature
- neurological assessment, especially after carotid surgery
- determinations of peripheral pulses and perfusion to test adequacy of grafts
- monitoring for bleeding around graft sites.

## TROUBLESHOOTING

### Postoperative care following carotid endarterectomy

Maintain arterial BP within the patient's normal preoperative range.

Monitor the patient for postoperative myocardial ischaemia with routine 12-lead ECG, considering cardiac enzymes or troponin, symptoms and ST/T-wave changes on continuous ECG recording. Treat myocardial ischaemia aggressively.

Early signs of cerebral ischaemia (e.g. focal neurological signs) should be reported to the surgeon immediately. A surgical cause is common and surgical intervention necessary.

Test for hypoglossal neuropraxia. It is temporary and has little clinical significance but keeps the surgeons on their toes.

Early signs of bleeding around the operative site should be taken seriously. Severe obstruction of the upper airways can occur rapidly, even without obvious signs such as stridor. Intubation is extremely difficult in these circumstances and expert assistance is necessary.

Despite the occurrence of what often resembles torture in an ICU – sleep deprivation, distressing and painful procedures, disorientation – most patients have complete amnesia about their time in an ICU. This may be related to the underlying illness or the use of sedation and pain-relieving drugs. However, there can be long-term social and psychological sequelae (e.g. depression, nightmares and mood swings) after a severe illness and a stay in an ICU. This can last for many months or even years and will require dedicated support and honest explanation from health professionals, relatives and friends.

### Relatives

Relatives and friends often experience anxiety, stress and sleep deprivation to similar degrees as the patient. This is one of the most traumatic times for any family. The patient may be critically ill for days or weeks. Relatives initially have a tendency to want to maintain a 24-hour vigil. That should be discouraged. Friends and relatives should be given an instruction pamphlet explaining that patients can remain seriously ill for days or even weeks and months. The relatives should be prepared for a marathon, not a 100-metre dash. Although visiting at any time is to be encouraged, some sort of regular eating and sleeping pattern for the relatives should also be encouraged. The pamphlet should also contain a lay description of all the machines and tubes that may be supporting the patient and what the staff hope to achieve with these devices. Relatives should be encouraged to talk to medical or nursing staff about any problems or questions they may have.

Relatives often have an insatiable need for reassurance and information. Such information must be consistent and straightforward. Discussing what the family 'line' will be during the ward round with medical, nursing and social work staff, will help ensure this. A family conference is also a good way to communicate consistent information. If interpreters are required, use a formal, reliable service, not a family member; otherwise, information could become distorted or be censored during translation.

## FURTHER READING

Hillman, K., Bishop, G. and Flabouris, A. Patient examination in the intensive care unit. In *Yearbook of Intensive Care and Emergency Medicine*, ed J.-L. Vincent, pp. 942–50. Berlin: Springer Verlag, 2002.

Saint, S. and Matthay, M. A. Risk reduction in the intensive care unit. *American Journal of Medicine* 105 (1998): 515–23.

Watson, J., McBurnie, M. A., Newman, A. *et al.* Frailty and activation of the inflammation and coagulation systems with and without clinical co-morbidities: results from the cardiovascular Health Study. *Archives of Internal Medicine* 162 (2002): 2333–41.

# Fluid therapy and electrolytes

- Rapid and continual replacement of the circulating volume is one of the commonest and most important manoeuvres in intensive care.
- The intravascular space (IVS) should be continually resuscitated against 'hard' and easily measurable end-points, while the interstitial and intracellular fluid spaces are maintained using 'softer' end-points.
- Serum potassium, magnesium, and phosphate values should be measured at least daily and corrected.

## Assessment of body fluid spaces

Body fluid is distributed to three compartments – the intravascular space (IVS), the interstitial space (ISS) and the intracellular space (ICS) (Figure 4.1). The IVS and ISS together contain the extracellular fluid (ECF). The fluid in each space has a unique composition and function. The function of the IVS fluid is to carry gases, nutrients and metabolites to and from cells. The ISS bridges the gap between the cells and the capillaries. It also carries the lymph system, which transports protein, other solutes and fluid back into the circulation. Dehydration results in depletion of the ISS fluid, whereas oedema occurs when there is excessive fluid. Oedema is common in the seriously ill and can cause serious complications. The ISS fluid consists largely of sodium and water and the ICS fluid consists mainly of potassium and water.

Assessment of the ISS is more difficult than assessment of the IVS. There are many reasonably accurate measurements, such as blood pressure (BP), pulse rate, urine output and cardiac filling pressures that can reflect the volume of the IVS, whereas measurements reflecting the ISS and ICS, such as tissue turgor and the extent of dry mucosa, are relatively 'soft' in comparison.

Before any decision about fluid replacement is made, one must determine which fluid space is depleted; then the most appropriate fluid for replenishing that particular space should be given.

**Table 4.1.** Causes of hypovolaemia

1  Blood loss
2  Water and electrolyte loss, e.g.
        GIT loss
        Excessive diuresis
        Excessive sweating
3  Plasma loss, e.g.
        Burns
4  Vasodilation causing relative hypovolaemia, e.g.
        Sepsis
        Drugs

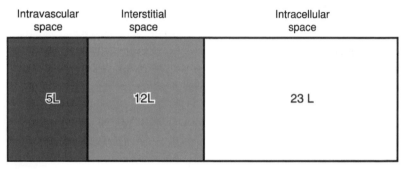

**Figure 4.1.** Volumes of the body's fluid compartments.

- IVS: approximately 70 ml/kg in adults.
- ISS: approximately 200 ml/kg in adults.
- ICS: approximately 330 ml/kg in adults.

Table 4.1 lists the causes of hypovolaemia.

## Assessment of the intravascular space

### Pulse rate

Tachycardia is a good indicator of hypovolaemia in the young when there are no other complicating factors. However, interpretation can be difficult, as tachyarrhythmias due to underlying disease, such as sepsis, pain and anxiety, or drug administration, can commonly affect heart rate in the seriously ill. Underlying cardiac disease, especially in the elderly, can also complicate the interpretation of tachycardia as an indicator of hypovolaemia. As a general rule the young respond more vigorously to hypovolaemia with a tachycardia than do the elderly.

## Arterial blood pressure

Hypotension often means hypovolaemia, whereas hypertension is rarely caused by hypervolaemia. In fact, hypovolaemia can paradoxically cause hypertension, especially in the patients who previously have been hypertensive, in children, or in the presence of autonomic dysfunction (e.g. tetanus, poliomyelitis, Guillain–Barré syndrome). However, there is a reasonably steady relationship between arterial BP and intravascular volume in seriously ill patients in intensive care. The pressure must be interpreted in the light of any artificial support by inotropes and vasopressors. Intravascular volume 'tracks' BP more accurately in the elderly than in fit young patients, where it tends to be compensated for by an active response to sympathoadrenal activity, until dangerous levels of hypovolaemia have been reached.

## Central venous pressure

Central venous pressure (CVP) is a reflection of only right-sided cardiac filling pressures; it is not an accurate indicator of left-sided cardiac pressures.

Lung abnormalities, artificial ventilation and positive end-expiratory pressure (PEEP) can cause increases in pulmonary artery pressure and right-sided heart pressures even in the presence of normal or low blood volumes (Figure 4.2). Excessive sympathetic tone accompanying hypovolaemia also can artificially increase the CVP. Thus, CVP in the presence of hypovolaemia also can be low, normal or high. Similarly, after fluid correction, it may increase, decrease or remain the same.

The CVP is, at best, useful to indicate a trend and then only when it is consistent with other measurements of intravascular volume.

## Pulmonary artery wedge pressure

The pulmonary artery wedge pressure (PAWP), measured with a pulmonary artery catheter, is a reflection of left-sided filling pressure in the heart and thus is a more accurate indicator of the systemic circulation than is CVP. As with CVP measurement, technical errors can be common.

There is little relationship between left ventricular end-diastolic volume and PAWP in seriously ill patients. This is largely because of the unpredictable relationship between left ventricular pressure and volume, or compliance, in the presence of critical illness such as multitrauma and septicaemia.

The PAWP may be difficult to interpret in artificially ventilated patients, because it increases in the presence of increased intrathoracic pressure, such as PEEP, continuous positive airway pressure (CPAP) or intermittent positive-pressure ventilation (IPPV).

Thus, PAWP is useful to indicate a trend, rather than as an absolute reading and is useful in association with, rather than in isolation from, other indications of intravascular volume. The value of pulmonary artery catheters in the ICU is currently questioned and their use is decreasing.

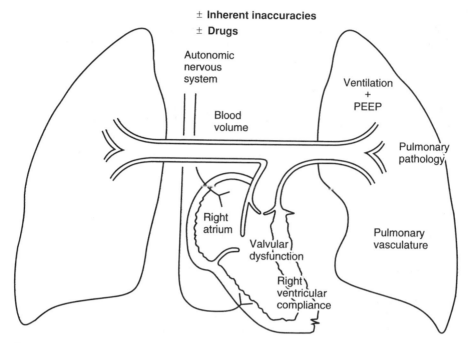

**Figure 4.2.** Determinants of central venous pressure other than blood volume (keep in mind that there may be inherent inaccuracies in the measuring of CVP, as well as the possible effects of drugs). PEEP, positive end-expiratory pressure.

### Peripheral perfusion

The ratio between core temperature and peripheral temperature reflects peripheral perfusion. The temperature in the extremities provides a rapid means for estimating peripheral perfusion. The estimation cannot, of course, allow one to differentiate between hypovolaemia and poor cardiac function.

### Urine output

Hourly urine output offers an accurate and easy means for assessing peripheral perfusion and circulating volume. However, it can be affected by drugs, including diuretics, as well as by the underlying renal function.

### Tonometry

The problem with many of our current measurements of circulating volume is that they do not reflect the adequacy of blood flow to the tissues. Tonometry indirectly measures blood flow in the mucosa of the gastrointestinal tract (GIT). The technique is described in more detail later. Tonometry was one of the first measurements to give us information about tissue perfusion in a non-invasive way. Like most measurements of the IVS its accuracy and reliability has not been established. It does reflect the new direction in monitoring – non-invasive and measuring tissue perfusion not global perfusion.

## Fluid challenge
The intravascular compartment is most accurately assessed by using the fluid challenge technique: measure all available indicators of the IVS before and after rapidly infusing a fluid bolus (200–500 ml). If they all rapidly improve, consideration should be given to a further bolus. If minimal improvement occurs, the circulating volume is close to being optimally filled.

## Assessment of the interstitial and intracellular spaces

The ISS and ICS usually are assessed together, because it is difficult to distinguish between them on clinical grounds. Although they contain the majority of the body's water, the ISS and ICS are far less accessible to estimation than is the IVS.

## Fluid balance charts
A fluid balance chart, at best, provides only a guideline to fluid needs. Limited ins and outs are recorded on a fluid balance chart (e.g. gastric aspirate, urine output, oral and intravenous intakes). The recorded fluid balance can represent less than half of the fluids actually lost or gained, as many of the fluids are inaccessible to measurement (e.g. insensible loss, water of oxidation, GIT losses from an ileus and wound oedema).

Unless the electrolyte and protein concentrations of lost body fluids are known, we cannot know from which body space a fluid was lost, nor, therefore, the most appropriate fluid with which to replace that loss.

## History
A history of fluid losses (e.g. diarrhoea, gastric contents, diuresis, excessive sweating, wound and fistula losses, hyperventilation) will provide information on the magnitude and composition of the lost fluid. For example, pancreatic fluid and bile will have electrolyte concentrations similar to those of the ISS fluid, whereas gastric losses and fluid from an osmotic diuresis will have comparatively lower sodium concentrations and higher potassium concentrations, indicating fluid losses from the ICS as well as the ISS.

## Serum sodium
The serum sodium concentration is the single most important indicator of total body water (TBW), as it usually is a reflection of body water changes rather than the absolute amount of body sodium. Thus, hyponatraemia usually represents

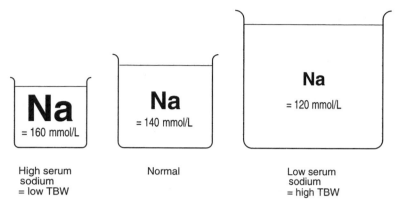

**Figure 4.3.** Interpreting serum sodium concentrations. TBW, total body water.

excessive body water and hypernatraemia usually represents depleted body water (Figure 4.3).

### Chest x-ray
A chest x-ray will provide an accurate indication of lung water, which is equivalent to the ISS of lung tissue. Regular chest x-rays constitute an efficient and accurate predictor of lung water. However, the lung water usually is the result of an underlying abnormality, such as cardiogenic pulmonary oedema or acute lung injury (ALI), rather than simple fluid overload. There is a direct relationship between intravascular pressures and the amount of lung water in a patient with either ALI or cardiogenic pulmonary oedema.

### Dry mucosa
The extent of dry mucosa is difficult to interpret in intensive care, as such patients usually are unconscious or have a high rate of gas flow from an oxygen mask.

### Tissue turgor
The tissue turgor is an estimate of both the ISS and ICS volumes. It varies enormously with age. It provides an empirical guide, at best, allowing one to estimate the extremes of 'very dry' (dehydration) or 'very wet' (oedema).

## Fluid replacement

Fluid replacement in the critically ill must be precise, as these patients often will have lost the normal mechanisms for fluid control, such as thirst and normal renal function and thus they cannot compensate for excessive or inadequate fluid volumes.

## Priorities in fluid replacement

1 The first priority, and one of the most important and common manoeuvres in intensive care, is to continually assess and correct the intravascular volume. Replacement of lost IVS fluid is essential in order to maintain normal tissue perfusion.
2 Maintain adequate haemoglobin concentration to ensure adequate oxygenation.
3 Replace electrolytes in order to maintain the distribution and volume of body water, as well as to maintain cellular function (e.g. sodium, potassium, calcium, magnesium, phosphate).
4 Replace water to maintain the ISS and the ICS.

## Intravascular space

Once measurements have verified hypovolaemia, a fluid that will be retained within the circulating volume is the most efficient form of replacement (e.g. colloid or blood). Crystalloid solutions (e.g. isotonic saline, Ringer's lactate) are distributed throughout the whole ECF and therefore are not as efficient for correcting intravascular deficits, as are colloid solutions. Where possible, colloid or blood should be titrated against the indicators of intravascular volume – BP, pulse rate, CVP, PAWP, urine output, peripheral perfusion.

In practice, all of these measurements of the intravascular volume have shortcomings and they are more useful when taken in conjunction with a fluid challenge. Appropriate readings should be taken before and after a challenge of 200–500 ml of rapidly infused fluid for adults, or aliquots of 20 ml/kg for children.

There is some evidence that early surgery is more effective than just replacing blood loss in penetrating injury to the torso. Unfortunately there is a potentially dangerous assumption that not replacing blood loss or correcting shock is acceptable. In the continual effort to make one's mark in the world, the term permissive hypotension has been devised. This is presumably based on the practice of permissive hypercarbia in order to prevent lung damage during ventilation. However permissive hypercarbia is not permissive hypoxia. Blood flow containing oxygenation is a basic premise in the practice of intensive care. Until we have unequivocal evidence that uncorrected shock and ischaemia is not only safe but beneficial we should avoid permissive hypotension and reverse shock at all times.

## Interstitial space

Most of the crystalloid solution will be distributed to the ISS, not the IVS. Thus, crystalloids are the most useful fluids for dehydrating the ISS. However, it is rare to have a depleted ISS in a seriously ill patient. In fact, oedema or expansion of the ISS usually is a much greater problem. Crystalloid solutions should therefore be used cautiously when correcting hypovolaemia.

### Pulmonary and peripheral oedema

Because crystalloids are distributed mainly to the ISS rather than the IVS, they can cause pulmonary and peripheral oedema in subclinical and overt forms. Pulmonary oedema causes decreases in oxygenation and lung compliance and peripheral oedema decreases cellular perfusion and oxygen consumption.

Salt-containing solutions (e.g. isotonic saline or Ringer's lactate solution) should be used judiciously for the correction of hypovolaemia, especially when large volumes are contemplated. Often the ISS is already overexpanded in the seriously ill, as a result of the salt and water retention that accompanies the stress response.

## Intracellular space

Assessment of the ICS is clinically difficult. Most of the body's water is contained within the ICS, but serum sodium concentration is the most important clinical indication of TBW status. Hyponatraemia usually indicates excessive TBW and hypernatraemia usually indicates inadequate TBW. Thus, water (usually in the form of 5% dextrose) can be titrated in an empirical fashion against serum sodium.

Although water losses in the seriously ill can be substantial, water gains due to secretion of antidiuretic hormone (ADH) and due to catabolism are not insignificant. As a guideline, between 500–2000 ml of 5% dextrose/24 h (20–100 ml/h) usually will be sufficient water replacement in the seriously ill.

## Approach to fluid replacement in the critically ill

**One should not use rigid and inflexible regimens and formulae for fluid replacement. Each patient should be carefully assessed and the right type of fluid in the right amount should be prescribed for that particular time in the course of that patient's illness.**

No matter what the origin of the fluid problem (e.g. shock, dehydration, excessive GIT losses, diabetic ketoacidosis, polyuria), the general principles for fluid and electrolyte replacements are the same.

1  Correct the circulating volume with colloid or blood. Restore organ perfusion and oxygen-carrying capacity of the blood as soon as possible. Often a continuous infusion of colloid (50–200 ml/h) is required in the seriously ill in order to maintain a normal circulating volume. In disorders such as septicaemia or pancreatitis, higher infusion rates are sometimes required.
2  Rehydrate the interstitial and intracellular compartments as appropriate in view of the patient's clinical status and biochemistry (e.g. serum electrolyte composition). This is usually achieved by titrating 5% dextrose empirically

against the serum sodium concentration. An empirical hourly rate (20–100 ml/h is usually sufficient) can be charted once each day according to the daily serum concentration. More may be necessary in the presence of large fluid losses and hypernatraemia.

3 If a patient is relatively stable, a solution containing sodium and water can be used as maintenance fluid. Such solutions usually contain dextrose and saline in varying amounts to achieve isotonicity (Table 4.2). The sodium concentration is usually between 30 and 70 mmol/L. Such a maintenance solution should be given at a rate between 50–150 ml/h (1200–3000 ml/day). Compositions of commonly used IV fluids are given in Table 4.3.

4 If there are excessive losses from one particular part of the body, then extra infusion of fluid of the appropriate composition will be required. For example, fluid losses from diarrhoea, from a small bowel fistula and from an osmotic diuresis will all have different electrolyte concentrations (Table 4.3). Moreover, the amount recorded as draining from a particular site may represent only a small percentage of the real losses. For example, whereas a bowel leak may drain a substantial amount, fluid can also be lost into the intra-abdominal cavity and thus not recorded. As a general rule, we assume that losses are actually greater than those recorded.

## Perioperative fluids

The principles of fluid replacement are the same in the perioperative period as for critically ill patients, no matter what the cause of the fluid loss or from which space it occurs.

1 Rapidly and aggressively correct hypovolaemia with blood or colloid.

2 Maintain TBW by infusing 5% dextrose at a rate to maintain the serum sodium concentration within normal limits.

3 When the patient becomes stabilised, a maintenance fluid can be used: 4% dextrose at $20–40 \ ml \cdot kg^{-1} \cdot day^{-1}$ plus 0.18% NaCl, or a similar combination of dextrose and saline.

4 Replacement fluid: Most body secretions (e.g. urine, gastric fluid, large intestinal fluid) contain relatively low concentrations of sodium. A dextrose/saline combination (Na 30–70 mmol/L) can be used to replace excessive losses of most body fluids. Some body fluids (e.g. bile and pancreatic juice) contain higher amounts of sodium and may need crystalloids (e.g. isotonic saline or Ringer's lactate) in order to replace losses.

### Manipulation of fluid spaces

The distribution of infused fluid can be predicted on the basis of its colloid oncotic pressure (COP) and sodium content. For example, fluid with a COP the same as that of plasma will largely remain in the IVS. Isotonic saline will largely

**Table 4.2.** Compositions of commonly used intravenous solutions

| | Na (mmol/L) | K (mmol/L) | Ca (mmol/L) | Mg (mmol/L) | Cl (mmol/L) | Lactate (mmol/L) | Dextrose (g/100 ml) | pH | Osmolality |
|---|---|---|---|---|---|---|---|---|---|
| 0.9% NaCl | 154 | – | – | – | 154 | – | – | 5.0 | 308 |
| 0.45% saline (N/2) | 77 | – | – | – | 77 | – | – | 5.2 | 154 |
| Hartmann's Solution (Ringers lactate) | 131 | 5 | 1 | 1 | 112 | 29 | – | 5.2 | 280 |
| 4.0% dextrose in 0.18% NaCl | 31 | – | – | – | 31 | – | 4.0 | 4.0 | 282 |
| 5.0% dextrose | – | – | – | – | – | – | 5.0 | 4.0 | 278 |
| 2.5% dextrose in 0.45 saline (N/2) | 75 | – | – | – | 75 | – | 2.5 | 4.0 | 280 |
| 3.75% dextrose in 0.225% NaCl (N/4) | 37.5 | – | – | – | 37.5 | – | 3.75 | 4.0 | 280 |

Reprinted by permission of Butterworth Heinmann Ltd. Hillman, K. M. Fluids and electrolytes. In Scurr C, Feldman S, Soni N. *Scientific Foundations of Anaesthesia, The Basis of Intensive Care*, 4th edn., ed. C. Scurr, S. Feldman and N. Soni, p. 460. London: Butterworth Heinmann, 1990.

**Table 4.3.** Volumes and electrolyte concentrations of various body fluids

|  | Volume (L/day) | Sodium (mmoL) | Potassium (mmol/L) | Chloride (mmol/L) | Bicarbonate (mmol/L) |
|---|---|---|---|---|---|
| Saliva | 1–2 | 30 | 20 | 35 | 15 |
| Gastric juice | 2 | 50 | 10 | 150 | – |
| Bile | 1.5 | 140 | 5 | 100 | 30 |
| Pancreatic fluid | 1.0 | 140 | 5 | 30 | 120 |
| Small intestine fluid | 3.5–4.0 | 100 | 5 | 100 | 25 |
| Large intestine fluid | 0.5 | 80 | 15 | 50 | – |
| Diarrhoeal fluid |  | 80 | 30 | 60 | 25 |
| Sweat | 0–3 | 50 | 10 | 50 | – |

remain within the ISS. A 5% dextrose solution will be distributed equally over all three body fluid compartments. Dextrose/saline-containing solutions will be distributed over all three compartments; the amount going to the ISS is dependent on the sodium concentration in that fluid. Artificial elimination of fluid from the body spaces, such as via haemofiltration, follows the same principles. The IVS is more amenable to manipulation than are the ISS and ICS. For example, the circulating volume can be artificially vasodilated or vasoconstricted with drug combinations.

## Intravascular space
• Replace fluid losses with blood or colloid.
• The size of the intravascular compartment can also be manipulated by drugs that act either directly on smooth muscle or indirectly via the autonomic nervous system and adrenergic receptors – vasodilators and vasopressors.

## Interstitial and intracellular space
• Assessment of these spaces is more difficult than the IVS.
• Use isotonic saline to replace ISS losses; use water in an isotonic form to replace losses from the ICS.
• Excess fluid from the ISS and ICS can be removed by dialytic techniques, such as haemodialysis and ultrafiltration, or with drugs, such as diuretics or aldosterone and angiotensin antagonists.

## Fluid manipulation across body spaces
Fluids can be encouraged to move from one compartment to another by a combination of strategies. For example, a patient with peripheral oedema in the presence of hypovolaemia and hypotension can be given a solution containing colloid osmotic particles, which will exert an oncotic pressure, causing the interstitial fluid to move into the IVS. Simultaneously, a diuretic or ultrafiltration can be used to decrease the ISS. Similarly, glucose, insulin and potassium can be given to

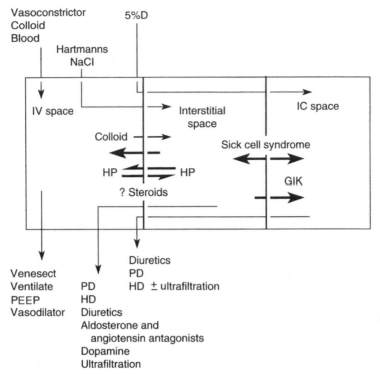

**Figure 4.4.** Manipulation of fluid compartments. Representation of the different fluid compartments and how they may be manipulated. Following access through vascular cannulation, the various fluids are distributed mainly to one compartment or another. Similarly, by the use of various drugs or techniques, fluid can be removed from the fluid compartments. Fluid can also be encouraged to move from one compartment to another. The following key is used: PD, peritoneal dialysis; HD, haemodialysis; GIK, glucose, insulin, and potassium; HP, hydrostatic pressure; PEEP, positive end-expiratory pressure; IV, intravascular.

Reprinted by permission of Hillman, K. Fluids and electrolytes. In: *Scientific Foundations of Anaesthesia, The Basis of Intensive Care, 4th edn*, ed. C. Scurr, S. Feldman and N. Soni, pp. 448–62. Oxford: Heinemann Medical Books, 1990.

move water into the ICS (Figure 4.4). By considering each fluid compartment separately, one can devise the right fluid for each space, or, alternatively, the right strategy when there is excessive fluid in any individual space.

## Hypertonic saline solutions

The place of hypertonic saline solutions is not clear, apart from in the management of hyponatraemia. However, they are used empirically in many situations, e.g. prehospital trauma, head injury and ALI. There is little firm evidence supporting their widespread use and problems include hypernatraemia, hyperosmolality and peripheral oedema.

## Colloid or crystalloid?

This is largely an irrelevant question. The controversy as to whether crystalloid or colloid solutions should be used arose because of the false assumptions that both fluids performed the same function, that they were distributed to the same body fluid spaces, and that the same measurements could be used as guidelines to their use. None of those assumptions were true. Using blood or colloid is the most efficient way of replacing intravascular volume, because the majority of it will be distributed to that space. Crystalloid, on the other hand, will mainly be distributed to the ISS.

When measurements of the IVS are used for fluid replacement (e.g. BP, pulse rate, CVP, PAWP) then a fluid that will be largely distributed to that space should ideally be used (e.g. blood or colloid solutions). As crystalloid solutions are distributed mainly to the ISS, they should be titrated against the assessment of that space (e.g. tissue turgor).

When choosing a colloid solution, there are studies which suggest that colloid solutions, in particular albumin-based fluids, may be associated with worse outcomes. The controversy surrounding this issue may soon be resolved by a large randomised controlled trial comparing albumin and crystalloid.

Crystalloid solutions (solutions containing isotonic amounts of sodium) are mainly distributed to the ISS, not to the IVS, and therefore are inefficient for intravascular volume replacement. In excessive amounts, crystalloids can cause pulmonary, peripheral and perhaps even cerebral oedema (Figure 4.5). Critically ill patients are stressed and, because of associated neuroendocrine responses, they retain sodium and water. This protects the ISS more than the ICS or IVS, exacerbating peripheral and pulmonary oedema.

The ISS should be kept 'dry' for optimum gas exchange in the lungs and for exchange of gases, substrates, and metabolites at a capillary level. Moreover, optimum lymphatic function depends on a 'dry' ISS. This is difficult to achieve when crystalloid solutions are used in the seriously ill. **Colloid or blood should be used to replenish the IVS on the basis of intravascular measurements. Crystalloid and hypotonic solutions should be used to maintain the other fluid spaces on the basis of biochemical and clinical assessment.**

## Special problems

### Syndrome of inappropriate secretion of antidiuretic hormone

Hyponatraemia is common in ICUs and there are many causes. The syndrome of inappropriate secretion of antidiuretic hormone (SIADH) is usually a diagnosis of exclusion. Increased serum osmolality, stress and hypovolaemia cause release of ADH, which, in turn, causes water retention. All of these conditions are common in the seriously ill. Hypovolaemia will cause ADH release

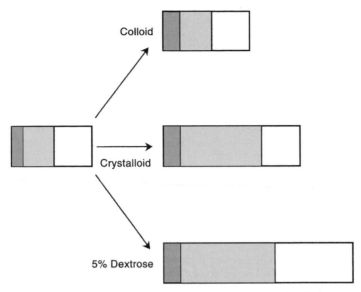

**Figure 4.5.** Correction of hypovolaemia with various fluids. The box on the left represents a hypothetical hypovolaemic patient. It can be seen that with the use of 5% dextrose to resuscitate the patient, massive expansions of the ICS and ISS will also occur. Similarly, with the use of a crystalloid, there will be significant expansion of the ISS. It is more efficient to use a colloid as the fluid, as less is required, and there are fewer complications because of less oedema.

even if the patient is hypo-osmolar. Most ADH release in the critically ill is appropriate.

Inappropriate ADH release implies that ADH is released in the face of a normal initial intravascular volume and osmolality.

Inappropriate ADH release is rare and is associated with acute infections, acute psychiatric conditions, carcinoma, neurological disorders, endocrine disorders and some drugs.

## Approach
- Correct any reversible aspect of the primary disease.
- Correct any abnormalities of the circulating volume and serum osmolality; then reduce water intake according to the clinical state, serum osmolality and serum sodium concentrations.
- Administer demeclocycline (600–1200 mg/24 h); lithium and frusemide have been used in resistant cases.

### Diabetes insipidus

When the patient is conscious this syndrome is characterised by polyuria, thirst and polydipsia secondary to plasma hyperosmolality and occurs when there is

**Table 4.4.** Comparison of SIADH and diabetes insipidus

|  | SIADH | Diabetes insipidus |
|---|---|---|
| Pathophysiology | ADH release inappropriate to the volume/osmolar state | Too little ADH, or insensitive to ADH |
| Alerting sign | Hyponatraemia | Polyuria |
| Serum osmolality | < 275 mOsmol/L | > 310 mOsmol/L |
| Urine osmolality | > 100 mOsmol/L | < 200 mOsmol/L |
| Urinary sodium | > 20 mmol/L | > 20 mmol/L |

an absolute or relative deficiency of ADH (Table 4.4). However, most cases in the ICU are neurogenic and the patients present with polyuria in the presence of serious cerebral injury.

## Nephrogenic
The nephrogenic form is rare – the renal concentrating mechanism is not responsive to ADH.

## Neurogenic
The neurogenic form is common – often follows neurosurgery, head injury or other cerebral insults. It results in polyuria which often is severe.

## Diagnosis
Take a history and conduct a physical examination. Determine

- urine volume and osmolality
- plasma osmolality
- glucose, electrolyte and calcium concentrations.

In diabetes insipidus, the plasma osmolality is usually greater than 310 mOsm/kg (often > 350), whereas the urine osmolality is usually less than 200 mOsm/kg (often < 100).

In the acute setting, a therapeutic trial of desmopressin acetate (DDAVP) may be indicated: in patients with neurogenic diabetes insipidus, urine output, as well as urine and plasma osmolarities, will be corrected. In patients with nephrogenic diabetes, the polyuria will not respond to DDAVP. Water deprivation tests are more suitable for ambulant patients with chronic diabetes insipidus, rather than those in an intensive care unit (ICU).

## Management
Exclude other causes of polyuria (e.g. associated with hyperglycaemia, mannitol or other diuretics). Correct hypovolaemia with colloid and replenish other body spaces as appropriate.

**It is particularly important to treat polyuria in an unconscious patient because the thirst mechanism is impaired and dehydration might otherwise occur.**

Use DDAVP parenterally rather than nasally in the acute situation. Give 1–5 units intramuscularly (IM) every 4–6 hours, according to control of polyuria. DDAVP is a potent drug, and care must be taken to avoid overdose and water intoxication. Alternatively, use a continuous IV infusion of vasopressin (1–2 units/h initially and then titrate against urine output). When using vasopressin, beware of myocardial ischaemia, which can be reversed by nitrates. Other complications include diarrhoea, nausea and abdominal cramps.

Measure the urinary electrolytes and replace the urinary losses with the most appropriate solution – usually a dextrose/saline solution. Maintain the plasma osmolarity and serum sodium concentration within normal ranges.

## Electrolytes

### Sodium

Sodium is the principal extracellular ion. Its turnover is approximately 150 mmol/24 h. The normal kidney will slowly (over 3–5 days) adjust to widely varying sodium intakes.

Stressed and seriously ill patients have a neuroendocrine adaptation to retain water and sodium. Excessive sodium as a result of replacement and retention is common and will cause ISS expansion with pulmonary and peripheral oedema.

#### Hyponatraemia

Hyponatraemia does not necessarily imply either hypo-osmolality, nor sodium depletion. Hyponatraemia can occur with decreased, normal, or even increased total body sodium. In the seriously ill, hyponatraemia is commonly due to excess body water, but rarely due to too little sodium. Clinical evaluation of the patient's fluid status will assist in the diagnosis. Hyponatraemia can occur with any acute illness, in association with liver disease and alcoholism, or as a result of water intoxication.

Rarely, hyponatraemia can be spurious, as a result of hyperlipidaemia or hyperproteinaemia. It can also occur in association with hyperglycaemia as a result of intracellular water moving into the ISS.

Hyponatraemia is rarely a problem in chronic states, as long as the serum sodium concentration is above 120 mmol/L.

Symptoms are related to the rate of change as well as to the absolute level – mild (weakness, dysarthria and confusion) or severe (seizures, coma, central pontine myelinolysis and cerebral oedema). Rapid correction of the hyponatraemia may also precipitate these symptoms.

Treatment: The goals of treatment in acute hyponatraemia are to reduce excessive water and increase the plasma sodium concentration.

- Correction of hyponatraemia must be slow, unless the patient is in a coma or is having convulsions. Permanent cerebral damage can occur secondary to rapid correction.
- Treat any underlying cause (e.g. cardiac failure).
- Aim to increase the serum sodium by no more than 10 mmol/24 h, even when a level of 120 mmol/L has been reached.
- Correction to more than 130 mmol/L is rarely necessary.
- In symptomatic cases (e.g. seizures or coma), consider using hypertonic saline (514 mmol/L) in conjunction with a diuretic such as mannitol or frusemide. Initially correct the serum sodium concentration to no more than 120 mmol/L.
- Water restriction will reverse most cases of mild hyponatraemia ($>$125 mmol/L) in patients who are asymptomatic.

## Hypernatraemia

Hypernatraemia is almost always due to a deficit in body water (e.g. from GIT losses, skin losses or osmotic diuresis). It is rarely due to excess total body sodium. Hypernatraemia can cause central nervous system symptoms.
Treatment:

- Correct the underlying cause.
- A slow rehydration with 5% dextrose (100–200 ml/h) will correct most cases.
- Rarely, dialysis may be necessary.

## Potassium

Potassium is the principal intracellular ion. It is an important determinant of the resting membrane potential. Its turnover is approximately 50–100 mmol/24 h.

Unlike the case for sodium, the body's mechanisms for retaining potassium are underdeveloped. Small shifts in serum concentrations can be dangerous.

## Hypokalaemia

Hypokalaemia is common in the ICU.
**Hypokalaemia is a potent cause of both supraventricular and ventricular arrhythmias.**
Hypokalaemia can also cause coma and neuromyopathy.

Acute hypokalaemia is more arrhythmogenic than the chronic form. The ECG changes include flat or inverted T-waves, ST segment depression and U waves (Figure 4.6).

Many patients on long-term diuretics or oral theophylline preparations will be hypokalaemic on admission.

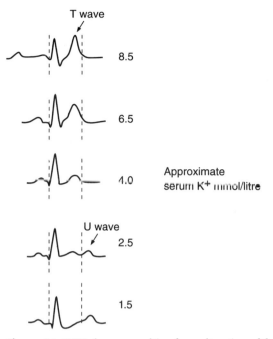

**Figure 4.6.** ECG changes resulting from alteration of the serum potassium concentration. Reprinted by permission of Blackwell Scientific Publications Inc. Hutton, P. and Cooper, G. *Guidelines in Clinical Anaesthesia* (1985): 254.

Hypokalaemia also accompanies drugs with $\beta_2$-agonist activity (e.g. adrenaline, salbutamol).

Causes of hypokalaemia

Losses:

- The kidney is the main source of clinically significant hypokalaemia in the seriously ill.
- Diuretics (e.g. frusemide or mannitol), diabetic ketoacidosis and diabetes insipidus.
- GIT loss (e.g. diarrhoea) and excessive nasogastric losses.

Intracellular shift:

- Correction of metabolic acidosis.
- Insulin-treated hyperglycaemia.
- Aminophylline.
- Catecholamines with $\beta_2$ activity.

Treatment:

- Cardiac arrhythmias, including supraventricular and ventricular, are more common with hypokalaemia, even at the lower limits of 'normal'.

- Keep the serum potassium more than 4 mmol/L.
- Intravenous potassium (5–40 mmol/h) should be given via a central line and the rate readjusted regularly with frequent monitoring of serum levels until the hypokalaemia is corrected.

## Hyperkalaemia

The ECG changes include T-wave elevation, prolongation of the PR interval, widening of the QRS complex and deepening of the S-wave (Figure 4.6). Patients are prone to cardiac tachyarrhythmias, peripheral paraesthesia, profound muscle weakness and eventually asystole.

Causes:

- Failure of excretion, renal insufficiency.
- Cellular damage and potassium release: crush injury, burns, rhabdomyolysis, haemolysis, succinylcholine administration.
- Potassium shift from cells as a result of severe acidosis.

Treatment:

1 Protect the heart from life-threatening arrhythmias.
   - Calcium: 10 ml of 10% solution (calcium chloride).
   - Sodium bicarbonate: 100 mmol (100 ml of 8.4% solution) – also drives potassium intracellularly.
2 Shift potassium intracellularly.
   - Glucose: 100 ml of 50% glucose, with 20 units of soluble insulin. By driving potassium intracellularly, this acts as a temporary measure.
3 Remove potassium.
   - Ion-exchange resin: calcium resonium, 30–60 g, 2–6 hourly, either orally or rectally, will decrease the serum potassium.
   - Dialysis may be urgently required in severe or resistant hyperkalaemia.

## Chloride

Chloride is the principal anion in the body. Its concentration varies in different body fluid spaces. The chloride concentration is largely dependent on the concentration of other organic anions:

- Plasma: 104 mmol/L.
- Interstitial fluid: 117 mmol/L.
- Cells vary from 2 mmol/L in skeletal muscle to 90 mmol/L in erythrocytes.

The turnover of chloride is approximately 135 mmol/day. The plasma concentration of chloride tends to vary in the same direction as that of sodium and in the opposite direction to that of bicarbonate (i.e. increased sodium is associated with increased chloride and increased bicarbonate is associated with decreased chloride).

### Hypochloraemia (serum concentration < 95 mmol/L)
Hypochloraemia accompanies losses from the GIT and kidneys; it can be caused by dilution and accompanies certain disease states.

Causes:

- Large gastric aspirate
- Metabolic alkalosis
- Respiratory acidosis (chronic)
- Over-hydration with hypotonic solutions.
- Diuretic therapy
- Inappropriate ADH release
- Burns

Treatment: The treatment is the same as for hyponatraemia. Remember to correct the serum potassium concentration.

### Hyperchloraemia (serum concentration > 110 mmol/L)
Hyperchloraemia in intensive care often accompanies respiratory alkalosis, hypovolaemia or a metabolic acidosis. Artefactual readings may be due to sampling blood close to an IV line or may be secondary to replenishment with hyperosmolar solutions containing chloride.

Causes:

- Hyperchloraemic metabolic acidosis
- Respiratory alkalosis
- Dehydration and hypovolaemia
- Renal disease
- Diabetes insipidus
- Hypertonic saline infusion or large volumes of 0.9% NaCl
- Bromide intoxication

Treatment:
Chloride disturbances often are markers of other abnormalities in the seriously ill and usually no specific treatment is indicated. However, it is important to determine the cause of the abnormal chloride concentration and treat the underlying disease.

## Calcium

Calcium is an essential component of a 'universal messenger system'. Calcium is essential for the integrity of cell membranes (muscles, nerves), as well as for a range of other functions: complement activity; clotting; secretion of exocrine, endocrine and neurocrine products; transport and secretion of fluids and electrolytes; growth of cells.

About 99% of the body's calcium is found in bones and teeth. Only a small amount is present in body fluids and cells. Circulating calcium can be in either the protein-bound form (about 45%), where it is mainly bound to albumin, in the form of non-ionised salts with phosphate, sulphate and citrate (5–10%); or in the active form, as ionised calcium (about 50%). Acidosis decreases its protein binding (increasing ionised calcium) and alkalosis increases its protein binding (decreasing ionised calcium). A low serum concentration of albumin will also affect the total calcium concentration. Measurement of ionised calcium is therefore necessary to evaluate the physiologically active fraction.

Circulating calcium is closely regulated by parathyroid hormone (PTH) and vitamin D through their effects on bone, kidney and the GIT. The influence of severe illness on calcium homeostasis is not clear. Normally, calcium is controlled within narrow limits by a complex and efficient feedback system. Its daily turnover is approximately 5–15 mmol.

## Hypocalcaemia

Hypocalcaemia is very common in the ICU – predisposing factors being sepsis, alkalaemia, chelation (e.g. citrate in blood products) and renal failure. It can also result from acute deposition of calcium into soft tissue (e.g. following rhabdomyolysis), as well as from PTH deficiency, hypomagnesaemia, vitamin D deficiency, acute pancreatitis or anticonvulsant treatment (phenytoin, phenobarbital).

Always measure the ionised calcium concentration, not the total serum calcium, because correlation between the two is poor.

Hypocalcaemia can cause increased neuronal membrane irritability and tetany, central nervous system symptoms such as seizures and even heart failure and arrhythmias.

The ECG changes include a prolonged QT interval as a result of a prolonged ST segment.

Treatment:

- Correct the serum magnesium and phosphate concentrations.
- Give 10 ml of 10% calcium chloride solution (IV) over 10 minutes. Beware of treating hypocalcaemia in patients with rhabdomyolysis, as it can predispose to precipitation of calcium in muscle and soft tissues.
- A vitamin D supplement may also be required.

## Hypercalcaemia

Hypercalcaemia is commonly associated with hyperparathyroidism (usually mild, < 3.5 mmol/L) or malignancies (can be severe > 4.0 mmol/L) (Table 4.5). Distinguishing between the two causes usually is not difficult and the diagnosis is readily confirmed by measurement of serum PTH.

**Table 4.5.** Causes of hypercalcaemia

Primary hyperparathyroidism – confirmed by measurement of serum PTH
Underlying malignancy – assays of PTH related protein are available
Non-parathyroid endocrine disorders (e.g. thyrotoxicosis, phaeochromocytoma, adrenal insufficiency)
Granulomatous diseases (e.g. sarcoidosis, tuberculosis)
Drugs (e.g. thiazide diuretics, lithium)
Miscellaneous (e.g. immobilisation, milk-alkali syndrome, vitamin A and D intoxication, IVN acute and chronic renal insufficiency)

Hypercalcaemia can result in muscle weakness, polydipsia and polyuria, as well as GIT symptoms (anorexia, nausea, vomiting, constipation) and central nervous system disturbances (lethargy, depression).

Treatment guidelines:

1 Resuscitate (airway, breathing, circulation).
2 Identify and treat the underlying disorder. The following measures are only temporary and the underlying disorder must be addressed (Table 4.5).
3 Correct other obvious fluid (e.g. dehydration) and electrolyte problems.
4 Enhance renal excretion: calciuresis with 2.5–4 L of isotonic saline daily, plus a loop diuretic (e.g. frusemide at 10–50 mg IV 2-hourly.

Avoid thiazide diuretics as they can enhance calcium reabsorption from the distal tubule.

Hydration and calciuresis with normal saline and diuretic are adequate for most cases of moderate hypercalcaemia.

Severe or refractory hypercalcaemia: Give calcitonin at 4 units/kg IV, then 4 units/kg IM at 12–24 hour intervals. Calcitonin acts rapidly and is relatively safe. It is the drug of first choice in severe hypercalcaemia (> 4.0 mmol/L) or if the patient is symptomatic. Calcitonin acts as an osteoclast inhibitor and also increases renal excretion of calcium.

Give mithramycin 25 μg/kg IV over 4–6 hours, repeated every 24–48 hours if there is no hepatic or renal dysfunction, thrombocytopaenia or coagulopathy. Mithramycin is a useful drug for severe hypercalcaemia, as it is rapid acting.

Disphosphonates inhibit osteoclasts and accelerate bone resorption. These can be considered when mithramycin is contraindicated or when the need to reduce calcium levels is less urgent (e.g. etidronate at 7.5 mg/kg IV over 8 hours for 3–7 days). Disphosphonates together with hydration will reduce calcium concentrations in 90% of patients with malignancies.

The place of gallium nitrate is not clear. It appears to be as potent as the disphosphonates and mithramycin but less toxic than the latter.

Other measures:

- Corticosteroids (e.g. prednisolone 60 mg/24 h) should be considered in the presence of severe hypercalcaemia, especially if an underlying malignancy is suspected.
- Give phosphate, 50 mmol over 12 hours, only as an emergency measure. This treatment can cause precipitation of calcium salts. Phosphate should be limited to patients with life-threatening hypercalcaemia in whom other measures have failed.
- Haemodialysis, using a low calcium dialysate, should also be considered in severe unresponsive cases. This treatment can be dangerous as it can cause precipitation of calcium salts. It should be limited to patients with life-threatening hypercalcaemia when other measures have failed.

## Magnesium

Magnesium is the second most common intracellular cation and is essential for many enzyme systems. The average daily requirements are approximately 3 mmol/day. Often, more is required in the critically ill (e.g. 10–20 mmol/24 h).

### Hypomagnesaemia

Always think of hypomagnesaemia when there is hypokalaemia, especially in the presence of polyuria (e.g. diuretics, diabetes). Hypomagnesaemia is often seen in association with chronic diuretic treatment, alcoholism, malnutrition or intravenous nutrition (IVN) without magnesium supplements. Significant losses of magnesium can also occur with diarrhoea, ileus, gastric suction, as well as from other GIT losses.

Hypomagnesaemia is common in the seriously ill and is often unrecognised. The most important sequelae are ventricular and supraventricular arrhythmias, neuromuscular excitability, GIT and central nervous system abnormalities and heart failure. It is difficult to separate the clinical syndrome of hypomagnesaemia from hypokalaemia and hypocalcaemia, as they often occur together. Moreover, there is no direct relationship between intracellular and extracellular magnesium concentrations.

Treatment:

- Give magnesium: 20 mmol diluted in 100 ml of 5% dextrose IV over 30 minutes, repeat as necessary until the condition is corrected.
- Use a maintenance dosage with daily monitoring.

### Hypermagnesaemia

Hypermagnesaemia is rare in intensive care. Sometimes it is seen in association with renal insufficiency or occurs as a result of magnesium-containing antacids. It is associated with impaired neuromuscular activity and depression of the central nervous system and cardiovascular system. It can be associated with magnesium treatment (e.g. pre-eclampsia)

## TROUBLESHOOTING

### Hyponatraemia

Is it a true result?

- Check the sample is not proximal to an IV line.
- Hyperlipidaemia
- Hyperproteinaemia ⎫ all decrease the serum sodium
- Hyperglycaemia ⎭

Check the urinary sodium.
Check the patient's extracellular volume (ECV) status.

| | | |
|---|---|---|
| Urinary sodium > 20 mmol/L | – ECV low | Diuretics |
| | | Cerebral salt wasting |
| | | Tubular disease |
| | – ECV normal | SIADH |
| | | Drugs |
| | | Chronic renal failure |
| Urinary sodium < 20 mmol/L | – ECV low | Extrarenal sodium loss e.g. diarrhoea |
| | – ECV normal | Water intoxication |
| | | Psychogenic polydipsia |
| | – ECV high (oedematous) | Cirrhosis |
| | | Heart failure |
| | | Nephrotic syndrome |

Treatment:

- Give calcium 5 mmol IV, or isotonic saline plus 5 mmol calcium/L, 6 hourly
  +
  frusemide, 20 mg IV, 4 hourly.
- Use haemodialysis if the condition is resistant and is associated with symptoms.

### Phosphate

Phosphate is a major intracellular anion – an important buffer and an integral part of adenosine triphosphate (ATP) and phospholipids. The daily requirements are at least 20 mmol/24 h.

### Hypophosphataemia

Hypophosphataemia is common in the ICU. Hypophosphataemia can cause severe respiratory and muscle weakness, as well as central nervous system depression. It can mimic polyneuritis and lead to profound coma. It can also cause erythrocyte and leucocyte dysfunction, predisposing to infection, as well as myocardial dysfunction and rhabdomyolysis. Hypophosphataemia is commonly associated with chronic alcoholism, acute severe asthma, malnutrition and diabetic ketoacidosis.

Treatment:

- Give 20–60 mmol of phosphate over 6 hours as an IV infusion, repeated as necessary.
- Up to 10 mmol/h can be given safely, followed by up to 20–60 mmol/24 h to maintain a normal concentration according to daily measurements.

## Hyperphosphataemia

Hyperphosphataemia is usually seen in the presence of renal failure or in association with hypercatabolic states, chemotherapy or cell destruction (e.g. rhabdomyolysis).

Treatment:

- The only reliable way to decrease the serum phosphate concentration is to restore renal function or use dialysis. Commence oral aluminium hydroxide (30 ml every 8 hours) or calcium carbonate (600 mg every 8 hours).

## FURTHER READING

Adrogue, H. J. and Madias, N. E. Hypernatremia. *New England Journal of Medicine* 342 (2000): 1493–9.

Boldt, J. Volume therapy in the intensive care patient – we are still confused, but . . . *Intensive Care Medicine* 26 (2000): 1181–92.

Cochrane Injuries Group Albumin Reviewers. Human albumin administration in critically ill patients: systematic review of randomised controlled trials. *British Medical Journal* 317 (1998): 235–40.

Hillman, K., Bishop, G. and Bristow, P. Fluid resuscitation. Focus on: physiology and pathophysiology of fluids and electrolytes. *Current Anaesthesia and Critical Care* 7 (1996): 187–91.

Schierhout, G. and Roberts, I. Fluid resuscitation with colloid or crystalloid solutions in critically ill patients: a systemic review of randomised trials. *British Medical Journal* 316 (1998): 961–4.

Worthley, L. I. G. Osmolar disorders. *Critical Care and Resuscitation* 1 (1999): 45–54.

# 5

# Nutrition and metabolism

> • Giving substrates to a severely catabolic patient does not guarantee their utilisation.
> • Enteral feeding is safer, cheaper and more beneficial than parenteral feeding.
> • The usual contraindications to enteral feeding, such as recent surgery and an ileus are relative, not absolute.

## Metabolic responses to illness and substrate utilisation

Nutritional support for the critically ill is aimed at preventing malnutrition and its consequences. These include increased morbidity, prolonged length of stay, increased infectious complications and decreased wound healing. Malnutrition is also associated with a suppression of immune function, particularly cell-mediated immunity, complement activity and the bactericidal function of neutrophils.

The metabolic consequences of illness and injury differ markedly from that of starvation. In starvation the body tries to decrease its metabolic rate, in critical illness the metabolic rate increases 2–3 times.

This leads to the picture often seen in intensive care patients, severe muscle wasting and preservation of body fat, hyperglycaemia as well as sodium and water retention. Lean body mass is lost at a rate 2–3 times higher than in starvation. There is relative glucose intolerance, insulin levels rise and lipolysis is reduced. A neuroendocrine response characterised by increased sympathetic activity and enhanced secretion of cortisol, glucagon and growth hormone, also counteracts the effects of insulin.

Disuse atrophy also accounts for much muscle wasting in seriously ill patients who usually move very little. The wasting of a limb encased in a full length plaster cast is indicative of how disuse atrophy occurs, even in a mobile, well-nourished patient. This wasting is not altered by supplying substrates.

Critically ill patients do not respond well to nutritional manipulation and the more severe the stress response, the more difficult it is to guarantee substrate utilisation.

## Nutritional assessment

As in many areas of nutrition in the ICU, there is little information available on simple and effective ways to assess current nutritional status and needs. Commonly used parameters include:

- premorbid history (e.g. length of starvation period)
- patient's weight
- anthropometric determinations (e.g. triceps skin fold)
- biochemical markers (e.g. serum albumin, transferrin and pre-albumin).

The Harris Benedict equation can be used to estimate caloric requirements. In critically ill patients it overestimates by approximately 20–30%. Achieving a positive nitrogen balance is difficult. Metabolic measurement 'carts' are used to estimate oxygen consumption ($VO_2$), thus indirectly giving some information on caloric requirements (kcal/day $= VO_2 \times 7$). However, such carts are expensive and difficult to use and the information is not easily interpreted. There is no evidence that measurements improve outcome compared with an educated guess.

Simple observation using the 'Hansel-and-Gretel' squeeze test (the short-sighted witch squeezed Hansel's finger to assess his weight gain) is probably as effective as more complex tests.

## Enteral nutrition

If the patient has an intact or partially intact gastrointestinal tract (GIT), enteral feeding should be used. The only absolute contraindications to enteral feeding are:

- complete bowel obstruction
- mesenteric ischaemia.

Other conditions may allow some enteral feeding, perhaps supplemented by intravenous nutrition (IVN):

- partial bowel obstruction
- severe diarrhoea
- severe pancreatitis
- high output fistulas.

**Table 5.1.** Enteral vs parenteral nutrition

Advantages of enteral nutrition
  Preserves immune function
  Less costly
  Blunts hypermetabolic response
  Central venous access not required
  Decreases the risk of GIT bleeding and stress ulceration
  Preserves GIT function, including motility and integrity of GIT mucosa
  Few serious complications
Advantages of IVN
  Provision of food when GIT not working
Disadvantages of enteral nutrition
  Difficult to establish feeding because of gastric atony
  Depends on intact working gut
Disadvantages of IVN
  Central access
  Gut mucosal atrophy
  Increased infections

After an acute insult (e.g. trauma or surgery), gastric and colonic atony occurs, but motility in the remainder of the small bowel is restored quickly (within 12 hours) and early feeding may be possible with duodenal or jejunal tube placement in order to bypass the stomach. Bowel sounds are not good indicators of when to start enteral nutrition; gas, which is necessary to generate bowel sounds, is present mainly in the stomach and colon, not in the small bowel. The presence or absence of bowel sounds is not indicative of small bowel activity.

Enteral nutrition has many real advantages (Table 5.1). Intravenous nutrition will not maintain the integrity of the gut mucosal barrier as enteral nutrition does – an advantage for enteral nutrition as important as its nutritive values.

Despite all the advantages, enteral feeding has a high number of gastrointestinal complications and is frustratingly difficult to achieve in some patients. Problems include high aspirates, whether or not nutrients are being absorbed and transported along the bowel, bloating and diarrhoea. It also takes longer to establish full feeding via the enteral route than intravenously. There is a risk of passive regurgitation and aspiration in the presence of gastroparesis. If in doubt, put food colouring in the feeds in order to test for aspiration. Sitting patients upright helps prevent aspiration.

Most feeds have the following characteristics:

- isomolar composition
- 1 kcal/ml
- protein content < 20% of total calories
- long chain triglycerides ± medium chain triglycerides

- some vitamin and trace elements
- additional substances including fibre

### Immunonutrition

Arginine, glutamine, omega-3 fatty acids and nucleotides have been shown to marginally improve immune function in some models.

Glutamine is the preferred substrate for enterocytes and adding glutamine to enteral nutrition may reduce bacterial translocation. Short chain fatty acids may confer a similar advantage on the colonocytes.

Enteral foods, including some or all of these substances have been studied in the critically ill. When compared with standard enteral food, there is no effect on mortality but a marginal decrease in infection rates, ventilator days and hospital length of stay. This is most obvious in surgical patients. As with most new therapies immunonutrition is expensive and probably not justified.

## Clinical guidelines

### Failure of gastric emptying and ileus

The stomach appears to guard the GIT from enteral feeding in the seriously ill. Our grandmothers expressed this reflex in the advice to – 'feed a cold, starve a fever'. In other words, when we are very ill, we do not have an appetite and often suffer nausea and vomiting. Teleologically, the body may just demonstrate its immediate priority is not feeding when it is seriously threatened.

Other factors may contribute to the specific failure of gastric emptying and general paresis of the GIT during serious illness. These include mechanical ventilation, decreased splanchnic blood flow, recent surgery, intracranial disorders and drugs such as opiates and anticholinergics.

### Promotility agents

Gastroparesis in critically ill patients may be improved by the use of prokinetic agents such as metoclopramide, cisapride and erythromycin.

Metoclopramide (dose 10 mg IV/6-hourly) acts by antagonising the gut inhibitory neurotransmitter, dopamine and sensitising the gut to acetylcholine. It has been shown to improve gastric emptying in the critically ill in some studies.

Cisapride (dose start 10 mg/6-hourly, nasogastrically) enhances cholinergic motor activity throughout the whole gut. However, it is associated with potential complications such as serious cardiac arrhythmias and is contraindicated in patients with prolonged QT interval. It can also potentially interact with many other drugs used in the ICU as it shares the microsomal P-450 enzyme system. It has been shown to improve gastric emptying in the critically ill in some studies but probably should be avoided in the critically ill.

Erythromycin (dose 500 mg IV/6-hourly) is a macrolide antibiotic that increases gastric motility by acting on motilin receptors in the GIT. Erythromycin can also cause torsades de point in combination with drugs causing a prolonged QT interval such as amiodarone and cisapride. It has been shown to improve gastric emptying in the critically ill in some studies.

Conclusion: Because of its side effects, cisapride may not be as safe as the other two drugs. The merit of using an antibiotic to enhance feeding with the possibility of bacterial resistance, can be debated. None of these drugs is particularly effective and increasingly procedures to bypass the stomach with a jejunal feeding tube are used.

## Placement of a jejunal feeding tube

A jejunal tube overcomes many of the problems associated with gastroparesis. Jejunal motility and absorption is usually spared in even the most seriously ill patients.

There are many suggested ways of non-invasively placing an oro- and naso-jejunal tube. If the patient needs a laparotomy for an indication which may be associated with problems in nasogastric (NG) feeding, one can be inserted either as a jejunostomy tube or via nasojejunal placement at operation. Otherwise they can be inserted at the bedside using fluoscopy or endoscopy. Both techniques require skill and experience. Some tubes can be designed to migrate. A small injection of radio-opaque dye can confirm the position.

## Feeding guidelines

When to start enteral feeding is contentious. The following are some common sense guidelines:

- There is no benefit in starting enteral feeding before the patient is haemodynamically stable.
- If the patient is likely to have an oral diet within 3–4 days there is little benefit.
- If the patient was malnourished before this illness and/or is not likely to have a normal diet for 4 days or more, then enteral feeding should be commenced.

Early enteral nutrition has theoretical merit and may decrease infectious complications in some critically ill patients.

A common problem is excess aspirate, especially if a NG tube is used. Remember the stomach normally excretes approximately 40 ml/h and this must be taken into account when estimating if there is total or partial gastroparesis. It is also normal to have some residual aspirate. If the aspirates are more than 200–300 ml, then reduce rate by 50% for 6 hours and resume, progressively increasing the rate over 24 hours. Monitor gastric residues twice a day.

## Diarrhoea

Diarrhoea is common and can be a problem; usually it is partially osmotic and partially due to malabsorption. Check feeds are not becoming infected. Do not stop feeding, as the problem will recur when you start again. Bulking agents may help. Bloody diarrhoea points to mesenteric ischaemia. Diarrhoea continuing for more than three days, particularly associated with broad spectrum antibiotics, should be tested for *Clostridium difficile* toxin A and B.

## Intravenous nutrition

Parenteral nutrition should be considered only for patients who cannot tolerate food enterally. It is effective in patients with isolated GIT abnormalities, but its broader place in the seriously ill is far from clear. It is probably no coincidence that there has been an enormous amount of information published on the subject of IVN and that it is an expensive product which is aggressively marketed.

During the acute phase of critical illness (as contrasted with isolated GIT disorders), we still know little about what substrates in IVN are actually used for metabolism. Nor do we know to what extent the catabolic process is obligatory and whether or not it is affected by IVN. While IVN can improve some biochemical indices, we do not know if IVN actually influences outcomes in patients with serious illness. There is good evidence now that IVN should only be considered when every attempt at enteral feeding has either failed or is not possible. If some enteral feeding is possible use IVN as a supplement only.

### Clinical guidelines

Some guidelines for IVN are discussed next, but the bottom line messages are far from clear.

#### Indications
Intravenous nutrition supplementation may be considered in the following conditions:

- when enteral feeding is not possible
- abnormalities of the GIT that would limit enteral feeding (e.g. high output fistulae, malabsorption syndrome, inflammatory bowel disease, prolonged obstruction).

#### Protein metabolism
The main goal of nitrogen supply is to limit muscle catabolism and supply the liver with amino acids to synthesise proteins – especially those involved in the immune system:

Normal protein requirement: $0.4 \text{ g} \cdot \text{kg}^{-1} \cdot \text{day}^{-1}$.
Recommended in the ICU:    $0.7–2.0 \text{ g} \cdot \text{kg}^{-1} \cdot \text{day}^{-1}$.
(1 g of nitrogen approximately equals 6.25 g of protein or 7.5 g amino acids).

Use synthetic L-amino acid mixtures:

    Essential: non-essential ratio approximately 2:5.

    Branched-chain: total amino acid ratio approximately 1:4.

Branched-chain amino acids (leucine, isoleucine, valine) are metabolised mainly by skeletal muscles. There is no good evidence for their use at high levels in hypermetabolic states.

Give albumin separately, if needed.

## Energy metabolism

Stressed patients (apart from those with burns) are not as hypermetabolic as was once thought. Energy expenditure in patients with septicaemia is 1.5–1.75 times the normal level. They therefore do not require large amounts of calories. This is due to the fact that while the basal energy requirements are increased, the energy actively expended is reduced. Whereas exogenous substrates do not prevent gluconeogenesis, they may reduce it. The clearing of blood glucose does not necessarily mean that the glucose has been oxidised or utilised in metabolic pathways. Using insulin to decrease the blood sugar concentration by moving it intracellularly does not necessarily guarantee utilisation.

The caloric requirements increase as the metabolic rate of the patient increases (e.g. patients with burns may require up to 70 kcal $. kg^{-1} . day^{-1}$), twice the basal energy rate.

The ideal ratio of calories from fat and carbohydrate is unknown. While IVN regimes without lipids have decreased the risk of infectious complications, some fat is required for essential fatty acids. Current recommendations are 5% of the total calories as lipids. Lipid solutions are approximately five times more expensive than dextrose solutions.

Hyperglycaemia can be due to stress, administration of steroids or catecholamines, diabetes or sepsis. Glucose is not well tolerated in the seriously ill. Hyperglycaemia and hepatic steatosis may occur if excessive glucose is administered. A non-diabetic patient should not require an insulin infusion to maintain a normal blood sugar – reduce the glucose infusion rate if necessary.

## Electrolytes (see Chapter 4)

Acute illness often leads to deficits in magnesium, phosphate and potassium. Their concentrations should be measured daily and supplements should be given as necessary.

## Vitamins

The exact vitamin requirements of the seriously ill have not been well documented. Recommendations are given in the form of theoretical estimates for each day or, more practically, there is regular administration of a commercial preparation.

A preparation of water-soluble vitamins should be given daily. Vitamins A, D and K should be added intramuscularly if not included otherwise. Adequate vitamin E will come from 500 ml of Intralipid per week.

Intramuscular injection of 5 mg folic acid/day is necessary for the seriously ill. This is much higher than the recommended doses for normal patients, because of rapid cell turnover. Fat-soluble vitamins (except for vitamin K) probably are not necessary in the short term (less than 2 weeks).

## Trace elements

Humans need trace amounts of iron, aluminium, zinc, copper, chromium, selenium, iodine and cobalt. Vanadium, fluoride, iodide, manganese, silicon and molybdenum probably should also be replaced over the long term (more than 3 months).

Zinc is important in many enzyme systems and is the only trace element that must be included in IVN in the short term (less than 2 weeks).

High concentrations of aluminium can occur in association with antacid treatment and excessive administration of plasma protein solutions.

Information on trace elements is sparse. Most sources emphasise the importance of trace elements but stop short of recommending practical guidelines as to how much of each should be given and when they should be commenced. One of the difficulties is monitoring and interpreting the concentrations. Some trace elements occur as contaminations in intravenous (IV) fluid and in blood products. Over the long term (more than 2 weeks), consideration should be given to adding trace elements to IVN regimes, especially in the face of abnormal GIT losses and malnutrition.

### Monitoring

Formal assessment of nutritional status (e.g. muscle power, nitrogen balance, anthropometric parameters) usually is not required in seriously ill patients, nor are serum albumin and immune status tests (e.g. anergy) accurate guides to nutritional status. Because indirect calorimetry is expensive and difficult to interpret, it is not practical for many ICUs.

Basic monitoring of IVN:

Daily:

- fluid balance
- serum electrolytes
- serum urea/creatinine
- arterial blood gases
- blood glucose.

Twice weekly:

- liver function tests
- calcium, phosphate, magnesium
- complete blood count
- prothrombin time.

Special:

- serum/urine osmolalities
- serum lipids
- serum urate
- serum zinc and copper
- serum $B_{12}$ and folate
- iron studies
- microbiological cultures as necessary.

## Recommendations

- There is no evidence that IVN improves mortality or decreases major complications.
- Keep it simple and cheap.
- Energy requirements are basal rate $\times$ 1.25 (surgery) up to 1.75 (sepsis and trauma).
- This energy requirement should be composed of 1.5–2.0 g protein $kg^{-1}$ $day^{-1}$, minimal fat (500 ml of 20% Intralipid 1–2 times $week^{-1}$) and the remaining calories from glucose.
- There are many commercial preparations available, as components, premixed in one bag and also solutions that do not require a central line. Each unit should use the mix that is the safest and most cost-effective in their hands.

Nutrition should support metabolic pathways without forcing them in abnormal and possibly detrimental directions.

Intravenous nutrition should not be commenced until the patient is fully resuscitated. It works best when patients are metabolically normal. However, that is rarely the case in the seriously ill and thus the guidelines are empirical

Aminoacid and dextrose solutions are hypertonic and should be delivered through a central line. Most lipid solutions are isotonic.

The most important practical limitation to IVN concerns fluid. Seriously ill patients often have neuroendocrine systems adapted to retain salt and water, or they may have renal insufficiency, which may limit water excretion. Both can predispose to water retention.

Pulmonary and peripheral oedema will accompany water retention, especially in combination with excessive fluid administration. Seriously ill patients with normal renal function often cannot tolerate more than 1000 ml of water/day (see

**Table 5.2.** Potential complications of IVN

---

Complications associated with central line insertion (e.g. thrombosis, infection, pneumothorax, haemorrhage)

Hyperlipidaemia and hypertriglyceridaemia

Electrolyte disturbances

Hyperosmolality

Hyperglycaemia

Acid base disturbances

Vitamin and trace element deficiencies

Hypercarbia

Fatty liver

---

Chapter 4). Haemofiltration, with or without dialysis, can make more 'space' for fluid. It may be useful in conjunction with IVN.

Individual ICUs should establish their own protocols for IVN delivery as well as for insertion of central venous lines, catheter dressing and care and routine monitoring of the biochemistry. Until we know more, the guidelines for IVN use will remain largely empirical. Potential complications of IVN are listed in Table 5.2.

## Nutrition for specific organ failure

### Acute renal failure

Acute renal failure is associated with hypermetabolism – a measured energy expenditure of 20–50% above normal. Provisions for adequate nutrition are hampered by volume restrictions, electrolyte problems and rising concentrations of blood urea. Special IVN solutions and manipulations of feeding regimes (e.g. increasing the calorie-to-nitrogen ratio) can limit the increase in blood urea.

Early dialysis or filtration will solve the electrolyte, urea and volume overload problems. Aminoacids, glucose and vitamins are all removed by dialysis.

### Hepatic failure

There is a lot of confusion in this area, mainly concerning support for patients with acute and chronic liver failure. As a bottom line, whereas administration of branched-chain amino acids will increase the number of people who will awaken from hepatic encephalopathy, they can confer no morbidity/mortality advantage over balanced, standard amino acid solutions. Fat solutions probably should be restricted to 125–250 ml of 20% emulsion/day. Hypertonic glucose should supply the bulk of the calories.

### Preoperative nutrition

The advantages of increasing the preoperative nutrition outweigh the disadvantages (e.g. catheter-related sepsis) only for a very small population of severely

**TROUBLESHOOTING**

## Failure of enteral feeding

### Aspirated secretions

The stomach produces gastric secretions at a rate of 40 ml/h.

Feeding has failed when the aspirate is greater than 100 ml/h or is greater than double the amount of feed put into the stomach.

If the amounts of aspirated secretions are high, do not cease feeding, simply reduce to 10–20 ml/h. Enteral feed acts as gastric protection.

Metoclopramide, cisapride or erythromycin may help overcome gastroparesis.

High doses of narcotics may slow GIT activity. As an alternative, consider epidural analgesia for pain relief.

Detection of bowel sounds is not necessary before feeding starts or for effective feeding.

Bypass the stomach: nasojejunal tubes can be used for early feeding. If the patient requires a laparotomy, consider a feeding jejunostomy at the same time.

### Vomiting

Stop feeding and check for the reason (e.g. bowel obstruction, gastric dilation, drug effects).

### Diarrhoea

Halve the rate, do not stop. If feeding is stopped, diarrhoea will only recur when feeding is started again.

Check for *Clostridium difficile* toxin.

Fibre, bulking agents, codeine or Lomotil may help.

malnourished patients, who are having operations that routinely have a high complication rate.

## FURTHER READING

Bengmark, S. Gut microbial ecology in critical illness: is there a role for prebiotics, and synbiotics. *Current Opinion in Critical Care* 8 (2000): 145–51.

Davies, A. R., Froomes, P. R. A., French, C. J., Bellomo, R., Gutteridge, G., Nyulasi, I., Walker, R. and Sewell, R. B. Randomized comparison of nasojejunal and nasogastric feeding in critically ill patients. *Critical Care Medicine* 30 (2002): 586–90.

Frost, P., Edwards, N. and Bihari, D. Gastric emptying in the critically ill – the way forward? *Intensive Care Medicine* 23 (1997): 243–5.

Heyland, D. K., MacDonald, S., Keefe, L. and Drover, J. W. Total parenteral nutrition in the critically ill patient: a meta-analysis. *Journal of the American Medical Association* 280 (1998): 2013–9.

Klein, S., Kinney, J. and Jeejeebhoy, K. Nutritional support in clinical practice. *Journal of Parenteral and Enteral Nutrition* 21 (1997): 133–56.

Jolliet, P. and Prichard, C. Immunonutrition in the critically ill. *Intensive Care Medicine* 25 (1999): 631–3.

Jolliet, P., Pichard C., Biolog, G., Chiolero, R., Grimble, G., Leverve, X., Nitenberg, G., Novak, I., Planas, M., Preiser, J.-C., Roth, E., Schols, A.-M. and Wernerman, J. (Working Group on Nutrition and Metabolism, ESICM). Enteral nutrition in intensive care patients: a practical approach. *Intensive Care Medicine* 24 (1998): 848–59.

Souba, W. W. Nutritional support. *New England Journal of Medicine* 336 (1997): 41–8.

Thorborg, P. Enteral nutrition: how do we get more of the good and less of the bad and ugly? *Critical Care Medicine* 29 (2001): 1633–4.

Weissman, C. Artificial nutrition in the critically ill. *Intensive Care Medicine* 24 (1998): 984–5.

Zaloga, G. P. and Marik, P. Promotility agents in the intensive care unit. *Critical Care Medicine* 28 (2000): 2657–8.

# 6

# Acid–base balance

> • Arterial blood gases reflect oxygenation ($PaO_2$) ventilation ($PaCO_2$) and acid–base status (pH).
> • In general, the pH value reflects the primary disorder, not the compensation.
> • Specific therapy is rarely required – correct the underlying disorder.

The body attempts to keep its hydrogen ion concentration tightly controlled as acid–base disturbances affect the basic molecules of metabolism – enzymes. Severe alkalosis is as harmful as severe acidosis. Acid–base homeostasis depends on chemical reactions involving buffers, in combination with intact renal and respiratory function. There is no neural or endocrine control. In order to diagnose any acid–base disorder, the hydrogen ion concentration or pH value, $PaCO_2$ and bicarbonate concentration must be determined. The relationship between pH and hydrogen ion concentration is logarithmic not linear (Table 6.1). It is also important to remember, when interpreting acid–base disorders that an immediate reaction with body buffers is followed by a rapid compensatory respiratory response and/or slow renal adaption.

Although in the following guidelines we consider metabolic and respiratory disorders separately, severely ill patients often have combined disturbances, whose interpretations can be complicated by the presence of artificial ventilation and drugs. It is vital to consider the underlying cause of the disorder before actively treating the acidosis or alkalosis.

Table 6.2 provides guidelines to blood gas analysis.

## Body pH regulation

### Buffers

Although many reactions in the body can influence hydrogen ion concentration, the pH value remains remarkably stable. This is achieved initially by the body's

**Table 6.1.** Variation of [H$^+$] with pH

| pH units | Hydrogen ion concentration (nmol/L) |
|----------|-------------------------------------|
| 3.0 | 1 000 000 |
| 6.0 | 1000 |
| 7.0 | 100 |
| 7.1 | 80 |
| 7.4 | 40 |
| 7.7 | 20 |
| 8.0 | 10 |
| 9.0 | 1 |

**Table 6.2.** Interpretation of arterial blood gas findings

1 Look at PaO$_2$. Rapidly correct it if it is abnormal.
2 Look at the pH value:
   Acidosis     H$^+$ > 44 nmol/L, pH < 7.35
   Alkalosis     H$^+$ < 35 nmol/L, pH > 7.45
3 Is the acidosis respiratory or metabolic?
   Respiratory: PaCO$_2$ > 45 mmHg (> 6 kPa)
   Metabolic: HCO$_3$ < 22 mmol/L
4 Is the alkalosis respiratory or metabolic?
   Respiratory: PaCO$_2$ < 35 mm Hg (< 4.7 kPa)
   Metabolic: HCO$_3$ > 26 mmol/L
5 Is there any compensation? The compensation is the
   opposite of the original disorder (e.g. the compensation for
   metabolic acidosis is respiratory alkalosis).

natural buffers and then by renal and respiratory adjustments of bicarbonate and PaCO$_2$ (Figure 6.1). Buffers are present in both extracellular fluid and intracellular fluid. Buffers minimise the change in hydrogen ion concentration when a strong base or acid is added. Their effectiveness will depend on the buffer concentration, pKa (the pH of a system when the acid and its anion are in equal concentrations), and whether or not the buffers can be influenced by renal and respiratory function (Figure 6.1).

## Bicarbonate – carbonic acid (HCO$_3$/H$_2$CO$_3$)

The carbonic acid bicarbonate (H$_2$CO$_3$/HCO$_3$) buffer system plays a central role in acid–base balance because of its prevalence and its relation to physiological regulatory mechanisms. Although the pKa value of 6.1 of this buffering system is well outside the body's normal pH value, it is a very effective buffer as it is 'open ended', the equation can go in both directions, with the kidney influencing one

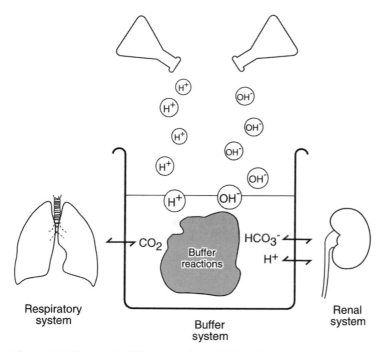

**Figure 6.1.** The body's ability to regulate acid–base balance depends on the lungs, kidneys, and chemical buffers.

end and the lungs the other.

$$[H^+] + [HCO_3^-] \leftrightarrow [H_2CO_3] \leftrightarrow [H_2O] + [CO_2]$$

Renal mechanisms regulate the bicarbonate concentration and respiratory mechanisms adjust the PaCO$_2$. It thus becomes the most important of the body's buffering systems – all other systems adjust according to this pair.

### Other buffers

Haemoglobin: Haemoglobin handles carbonic acid by utilising the imidazole group of histidine. By virtue of the large numbers of imidazole groups, haemoglobin provides a large buffering capacity.

Protein: Both extracellular and intracellular proteins are efficient buffering systems.

Phosphate: Phosphate has an effective pKa of 6.8 and is an important source of intracellular buffering.

## Renal response

Compared with the respiratory contribution to acid–base balance, the renal response to pH disturbances is slow and works through bicarbonate rather than carbonic acid. The kidney can adjust to excreting large acid loads (up to 600–700 mmol of $H^+$/day). Mechanisms include excretion of titratable acid, excretion of ammonia, secretion of hydrogen ion and excretion and reabsorption of filtered bicarbonate.

## Respiratory response

Normal carbon dioxide ($CO_2$) production is about 13 000 mmol/day. The ventilatory response to changing hydrogen ion levels is rapid and precise.

## Acidosis

### Respiratory acidosis

Respiratory acidosis is initiated by an increase in $PaCO_2$. The immediate consequence is an increase in plasma acidity. There is an initial small increase in plasma bicarbonate concentration and if the hypercapnia becomes more chronic, renal absorption of bicarbonate results in a further increase in plasma bicarbonate concentration.

### Clinical manifestations
Acute hypercapnia induces peripheral and cerebral vasodilatation, stimulates the sympathetic nervous system and increases cardiac output. Cerebral dysfunction occurs as hypercapnia becomes more severe.

### Causes
Inadequate $CO_2$ removal: (see also hypoventilation, and acute respiratory failure).

- Obstructed airway.
- Lung abnormalities (e.g. chronic airway disease).
- Central or neuromuscular abnormalities (e.g. drug-induced hypoventilation, Guillain–Barré syndrome, exhaustion as a result of acute respiratory failure).
- Mechanical failure – related to inefficient action of the muscles of respiration (e.g. kyphoscoliosis, obesity, pain, flail chest, pneumothorax).
- An increase in dead space, relative to tidal volume.

Excess $CO_2$ production: e.g. hypermetabolism secondary to fever, excessive parenteral glucose or rapid injection of sodium bicarbonate, which forms $CO_2$.

## Treatment

1 Correct any underlying cause (e.g. obstructed airway or excessive opiates).
2 Artificially ventilate (especially patients with hypoventilation and acute hypercarbia).

Exceptions: Many patients who have acute respiratory failure and who are being artificially ventilated are deliberately under-ventilated with low tidal volumes to limit peak inspiratory pressures. This technique is called elective hypoventilation or permissive hypercarbia. High inspiratory volumes and pressures can cause complications such as cardiovascular impairment and pulmonary barotrauma.

Artificially ventilated patients with chronic lung disease and hypercarbia who have acute exacerbations of their disease should be ventilated only to correct the $PaCO_2$ to their 'normal' levels. Values lower than that can alter the pH of the cerebrospinal fluid (CSF) and make it difficult to wean the patient.

## Metabolic acidosis

Metabolic acidosis is initiated by a reduction in plasma bicarbonate concentration which then causes an increase in plasma acidity. That is followed by compensatory hyperventilation and a reduction in $PaCO_2$.

### Clinical manifestations
• Respiratory system: compensatory hyperventilation or Kussmaul respiration.
• Cardiovascular system: possible myocardial depression, arterial vasodilatation and direct venoconstriction.
• Oxygen transport: rightward shift in oxyhaemoglobin dissociation curve making dissociation easier.

### Causes
Excessive hydrogen ion production or administration (e.g. lactic acidosis, ketoacidosis, salicylic acid, lysine, ammonium chloride).
Loss of bicarbonate (e.g. small bowel loss [especially pancreatic fistulae], diarrhoea, renal tubular acidosis, carbonic anhydrase inhibition).
Failure to excrete hydrogen ion (e.g. sulphate and phosphate acids associated with renal failure and renal tubular acidosis).

Metabolic acidosis is split into two categories depending on the anion gap (Table 6.3). The main positively charged ions (sodium and potassium) and the negatively charged ions (bicarbonate and chloride) usually have a gap of less than 18 mmol/L, made up mainly of protein. In a high anion gap metabolic acidosis, unmeasured anions (e.g. lactate in septic shock) increase the gap.

**Table 6.3.** Anion gap

---

1  Calculate: $(Na^+ + K^+) - (Cl^- + HCO_3^-)$
2  High anion gap metabolic acidosis ($>18$ mmol/L)
   Sepsis entails the presence of lactate
   Renal failure involves phosphate and sulphate
   Diabetic ketoacidosis involves acetoacetate and $\beta$-hydroxybutyrate
   Presence of methanol, ethanol, ethylene glycol involves formate, lactate, oxalate
3  Normal anion gap metabolic acidosis $< 18$ mmol/L
   Renal tubular acidosis entails loss of $HCO_3$ in urine
   Gastrointestinal losses cause loss of $HCO_3$ from the gut

---

Normal anion gap metabolic acidosis occurs when bicarbonate is lost from the body or used in buffering and is replaced by chloride. For example, in severe diarrhoea or after resuscitation with fluids containing a high concentration of chloride, such as normal saline (chloride concentration of 150 mmol/L).

## Treatment

The most common cause of acidosis in the ICU is lactic acidosis resulting from inadequate perfusion and oxygenation. Although acidosis causes negative inotropic effects in vitro, it is not necessary to correct the arterial pH to 'normal' in the clinical setting, as even with severe acidosis the effect on myocardial contractility may not be as depressant as once thought. A pH of 7.20 ($H^+$ 63.1 nmol/L) is well tolerated.

- Correct reversible causes such as diabetic ketoacidosis (see Chapter 29).
- Restore adequate circulation and oxygenation.
- Alkali: Usually the foregoing measures are sufficient and bicarbonate is not necessary. Treatment of the acidosis per se is not as important as treatment of the cause of the acidosis. The bicarbonate may 'buy time' while waiting for definitive treatment.
- Dialysis may be required for intractable acidosis or where renal failure is anticipated.

Complications of bicarbonate therapy: Bicarbonate is sometimes given to seriously ill patients, especially during cardiopulmonary resuscitation (CPR). It may result in a rebound alkalosis and hypernatraemia. During CPR, give bicarbonate only for severe acute acidosis (e.g. at least a pH of $< 7.0$): start with 1 mmol/kg, wait 20 minutes, repeat arterial blood gas determinations and give another 1 mmol/kg if needed. Correcting the metabolic acidosis using formulae based on base deficits and weight is inaccurate and causes overcorrection. If bicarbonate is necessary, it should be given as a slow infusion, rather than as a bolus. This allows adequate time for elimination of the $CO_2$ generated from the reaction between the hydrogen ion and bicarbonate. Overcorrection with sodium bicarbonate can result in:

- sodium and osmolar loading
- reduced availability of calcium
- reduced oxygen availability, by shifting the oxyhaemoglobin curve to the left
- a paradoxical decrease in intracellular pH.

Bicarbonate may be used in intensive care in severe hyperkalaemia and to alkalinise the urine in rhabdomyolysis.

# Alkalosis

## Respiratory alkalosis

Respiratory alkalosis is a result of a reduction in $PaCO_2$ that alkalinises the body fluids. With changes in renal absorption of bicarbonate, the degree of alkalinisation is gradually modified.

### Causes
Hypocarbia and alkalosis are commonly associated with the early stages of acute respiratory failure (see Chapter 16), liver failure and central nervous system disorders. They may be present before any other sign of organ dysfunction. However, another common cause in the ICU is inadvertent or deliberate hyperventilation.

Hypocarbia can also occur with hypometabolism and decreased $CO_2$ production, such as after barbiturate overdose, brain death or hypothermia.

## Clinical manifestations

As with respiratory acidosis, central nervous system dysfunction is the most prominent clinical feature of respiratory alkalosis. Acute hypocapnia decreases cerebral blood flow, causing light-headedness, confusion and even seizures.

### Treatment
- Correct any underlying cause.
- Decrease the minute volume of the ventilator.

## Metabolic alkalosis

Metabolic alkalosis is initiated by an increase in plasma bicarbonate or a loss of hydrogen ions. This gives rise to a compensatory decrease in alveolar ventilation. Alkalosis will disturb enzyme activities and body function to the same extent as acidosis.

### Clinical manifestations

Central nervous system manifestations include lethargy, confusion, muscle twitching and seizures. Hypokalaemia occurs as potassium shifts into cells.

### Causes

Loss of acids:

- From the gastrointestinal tract: nasogastric suctioning and vomiting, diarrhoea, villous adenoma.
- From the kidney: diuretics, hypermineralocorticoid states such as occur with corticosteroid use or hyperaldosteronism, Conn's syndrome, Cushing's syndrome.

Gain in alkali:

- Antacid treatment, milk alkali syndrome, excessive bicarbonate administration, metabolism of organic anions (lactate, citrate, acetate).
- Compensation for respiratory acidosis.

### Treatment

Metabolic alkaloses are split into those that are chloride responsive – loss of chloride from the GIT or hydrogen ions from the kidney secondary to diuretics – and those that are chloride resistant: Conn's and Cushing's syndrome.

- Correct any reversible cause.
- Correct factors which maintain the alkalosis:
    decreased extracellular fluid volume
    hypokalaemia, hypomagnesaemia, hypochloraemia
    mineralocorticoids
    stress.
- Drugs
    Only rarely do drugs need to be given.
    Give acetazolamide, 500 mg IV once or twice daily.

If still alkalotic, give diluted HCl (0.1 mol) at a rate of 0.2 mmol [$H^+$]/kg/h through a central venous line until pH returns toward normal (only in cases of severe resistant alkalosis).

Avoid ammonium chloride and arginine monohydrochloride infusions, as they both require hepatic conversion and good renal function for full activity and are more difficult to titrate against pH.

## Mixed disorders

Many acid–base disturbances in the ICU are mixed (e.g. a patient with chronic lung disease who retains $CO_2$ (a respiratory acidosis), has a myocardial infarction and develops shock and a metabolic acidosis). Useful points for interpretation are included in the troubleshooting section.

It must be remembered that there can be variations from these predictions and that predicted changes do not necessarily exclude mixed or complex disorders (e.g. acute hypocapnia superimposed on chronic respiratory acidosis could mimic the findings of uncomplicated metabolic alkalosis). Careful analysis of the history, clinical findings and response to treatment will usually allow one to sort out these dilemmas.

## TROUBLESHOOTING

### Arterial blood gas tricks

#### Arterial or venous?
There is no infallible rule for quickly telling if the sample is arterial or venous. Assume that it is arterial and check against the oximetry findings.

#### Primary disorder or compensation?
In general, the pH reflects the primary disorder, not the compensation.

#### Metabolic acidosis
Check the anion gap.
The two figures in the fractional part of the pH value should equal the $PaCO_2$ if the disorder is fully compensated (pH range 7.10–7.30): if pH is 7.25, $PaCO_2$ should be 25 mmHg).

#### Respiratory acidosis
For every 10 mmHg change in the $PaCO_2$ the pH will change by 0.08 units.
Acute: The $HCO_3$ concentration will increase 1 mmol/L for each increase in $PaCO_2$ of 10 mmHg (1.3 kPa).
Chronic: The $HCO_3$ concentration will increase 4 mmol/L for each increase in $PaCO_2$ of 10 mmHg (1.3 kPa).

#### Metabolic alkalosis
$PaCO_2$ will increase 7 mmHg (1.0 kPa) for each increase in $HCO_3$ concentration of 10 mmol/L.

#### Respiratory alkalosis
The $HCO_3$ concentration will decrease 2 mmol/L for each decrease in $PaCO_2$ of 10 mmHg (1.3 kPa).

#### Results
Results may not be accurate below a temperature of 35 °C.

## FURTHER READING

Adrogue, H. J. and Madias, N. E. Medical progress: Management of life-threatening acid–base disorders: first of two parts. *New England Journal of Medicine* 338 (1998): 26–34.

Adrogue, H. J. and Madias, N. E. Medical progress: management of life-threatening acid–base disorders: second of two parts. *New England Journal of Medicine* 338 (1998): 107–11.

Gluck, S. L. Acid–base. *Lancet* 352 (1998): 474–9.

Gutierrez, G. and Wulf, M. E. Lactic acidosis in sepsis: a commentary. *Intensive Care Medicine* 22 (1996): 6–16.

Kellum, J. A. Metabolic acidosis in the critically ill: lessons from physical chemistry. *Kidney International* 66 (1998): 581–6.

Thomson, W. S. T, Adams, J. F. and Cowan, R. A. (ed.). *Clinical Acid–Base Balance*. Oxford: University Press, 1997.

Walmsley, R. N. and White, G. H. (ed.). *A Guide to Diagnostic Clinical Chemistry*, 4th edn. Melbourne: Blackwell Scientific Publications, 1994.

Zaritsky, A. Unmeasured anions: Déjà vu all over again? *Critical Care Medicine* 27 (1999): 1672–3.

# 7

# Sedation, analgesia and muscle relaxants

- Make sure that sedation is for the good of the patient and not for the benefit of the staff.
- Optimal pain relief is every patient's right in intensive care.
- Muscle relaxation is rarely required in the critically ill.

## Assessing the need for sedation

The word 'sedation' and 'sedatives' are used here in the broadest sense (i.e. in the sense of producing a sleep-like state). Drugs such as opiates obviously have other properties such as pain relief (Table 7.1). Drugs should never be used as substitutes for sympathetic explanation and reassurance. This is particularly important when patients are emerging from coma – pathological or drug induced. It is often tempting to sedate these patients in order to make the patients look 'tidy' and to facilitate management for the staff. Explanation and reassurance will often make sedation unnecessary. Nor should sedation be used when the cause of agitation or confusion is unknown. Withdrawal from alcohol or drugs, hypoxia, electrolyte disorders and many other abnormalities can cause confusion and agitation. These must be excluded before one resorts to sedation.

Patients should be allowed to sleep whenever possible. Sleep is important for optimum physiological functioning and immune competence. Drugs do not necessarily ensure that a patient will get adequate sleep. Sleep deprivation is to be avoided, even if it means a less rigorous approach to routine tests, monitoring and therapy.

When a patient's pain is not amenable to regional or epidural analgesia, liberal pharmacological pain relief should be provided. Patients should not suffer pain in an ICU. Opiates used in the right dosages do not necessarily inhibit spontaneous

**Table 7.1.** Sedation in intensive care

---

1  Assess need

   Sedation should not be a substitute for explanation and reassurance by medical and
   nursing staff

   Adjust ventilatory strategies to encourage spontaneous breathing, instead of sedating
   and paralysing patients to make them conform with the ventilator

2  Pain relief and sedation

   Local analgesia: If possible, use an epidural or regional local anaesthetic technique for
   pain relief

   Opiate: Use either intermittent doses or continuous IV infusion (e.g. morphine
   infusion at 2–20 mg/h for pain relief as well as sedation)

   Benzodiazepines: Either add intermittent prn IV doses of benzodiazepine if anxiolysis
   is inadequate (e.g. midazolam 1–2.5 mg) or a benzodiazepine infusion (midazolam
   50 mg in 50 ml) titrated to a sedation score

3  Measure the effect

   Decide on the level of analgesia and sedation required, measure the levels frequently
   and titrate the drugs to achieve that level

---

respiration. Conscious and co-operative patients can use patient-controlled analgesia very successfully.

Sedation should not be used to facilitate positive-pressure ventilation in cases where patients could otherwise breathe spontaneously, facilitated by techniques such as continuous positive airway pressure (CPAP) or intermittent mandatory ventilation (IMV) (see Chapter 18).

The pharmacokinetics of drugs used in the ICU can be unpredictable because of factors such as depressed hepatic and renal function, as well as increased volume of drug distribution. Analgesia and sedative drugs should not be mixed in the same syringe; each patient has different needs for pain relief and sedation.

## Assessing the level of analgesia and sedation

The level of analgesia and sedation should be set for each patient and the effects of the analgesic and sedative drugs should be evaluated often using a rating scale. The goal is good analgesia and the lightest level of sedation compatible with patient safety and comfort. A linear analogue scale from 1–10 is an effective way of assessing pain and a sedation score such as the Ramsay score distinguishes between coma and a dangerous level of agitation (Table 7.2).

In patients who are receiving neuromuscular blocking drugs it can be difficult to assess their level of sedation. A monitor called the Bispectral index (BIS) records a 4-channel EEG, uses complicated statistics and previous analyses of EEG patterns from people at all levels of sedation to produce a number from

**Table 7.2.** Sedation score

---

1  Agitated or restless or both
2  Co-operative, orientated, calm
3  Obeys commands
4  Rouses quickly to a loud voice
5  Rouses slowly to a loud voice
6  No response

---

1 to 100. A fully awake patient scores 100 and 40 correlates with deep sedation. Its role in ICU is uncertain and there is doubt about what physiological phenomena it is measuring!

## Features of the main sedative groups

### Opiates

- Pain relief, euphoria and drowsiness.
- Predictable cardiovascular and respiratory depression.
- The longer the half-life, the cheaper the drug.
- Dependence, despite high dosages, is rare.
- Tolerance and increased plasma clearance can gradually occur.
- May contribute to the ileus and psuedo-obstruction commonly seen in seriously ill patients.
- Variable actions are usually affected by both renal and hepatic function.
- No clinical evidence of immune depression.
- No direct effect on intracranial pressure (ICP).

### Benzodiazepines

- Provide sedation, anxiolysis and amnesia and contribute to muscle relaxation.
- Variable responses.
- Unpredictable cardiovascular and respiratory depression, especially with bolus doses.
- Variable length of action (e.g. very prolonged action of diazepam). This may or may not be a disadvantage in the ICU.
- Well-documented incidence of withdrawal-symptoms, such as seizures after long-term use (more than 1 week) of short-acting drugs such as midazolam.
- Thrombophlebitis in small veins with diazepam.

## Ketamine

- Minimum cardiovascular and respiratory effects.
- Analgesia as well as sedation.
- Incidence of unpleasant dreams and psychological disturbances.
- Increases ICP.

## Propofol

- Short acting, rapidly metabolised intravenous (IV) anaesthetic agent which is in the form of an emulsion.
- Expensive.
- No analgesia.
- Rapid metabolism and lack of accumulation may make it suitable for use as a continuous infusion in the ICU, especially as an adjunct in the management of coma. It is sometimes used to cover the period of agitation as longer-acting agents gradually wear off.
- Causes hypotension.
- Requires special handling as the fat emulsion becomes contaminated easily.
- Despite earlier reservations about the long-term use of this drug in adult intensive care, there have been few adverse reports apart for hypotension, hyperlipidaemia and possible pancreatitis.

# Choice of drug

Assess whether the proposed sedation is for the benefit of the patient or the staff. It can be tempting to use excessive sedation in order to maintain and control artificial ventilation, instead of weaning the patient to CPAP as soon as possible.

**When sedation is necessary, opiates and benzodiazepines remain the mainstay of sedation in intensive care.**

**The ideal level of analgesia and sedation should be determined for the patient and assessed using sedation and analgesia scales.**

## Pain relief

Where possible, use epidural or regional local anaesthetic blocks, since they permit greater patient co-operation and facilitate spontaneous breathing. If this is not possible, titrate an IV narcotic infusion against pain. Patient-controlled analgesia is possible in some patients.

## Anxiolysis

If a patient needs more sedation, or if it is believed that anxiolysis or amnesia is also necessary, benzodiazepines can be used in addition to, or instead of, narcotics.

## Liver and renal dysfunctions

Drug metabolism is compromised in the presence of renal or hepatic failure. Drugs such as morphine, which have traditionally been thought to be metabolised by the liver, have significantly prolonged actions in the presence of renal failure. In a patient with acute liver failure, sedation often is not needed because of the accompanying encephalopathy. These patients often have cerebral oedema and elevated ICPs; sedative drugs that cause increases in ICP should therefore be avoided.

## Immune depression

As the risk of immune depression is possible with anaesthetic induction agents, their use should be confined to cases of severe increases in ICP that are refractory to conventional treatment, status epilepticus unresponsive to conventional treatment and short-term procedures requiring anaesthesia in the ICU.

## Tolerance

Because of enzyme induction, sedation invariably will have to be increased over time. At the end of a number of weeks the drug requirement, especially when narcotics are being used, can be extremely high.

### Choice of narcotics

All of the opiates have effective pain relieving and sedative properties. Each ICU will have its favourite opiate. If the differences among them are marginal, cost should be considered. Pethidine and morphine cost approximately the same; fentanyl and phenoperidine are at least eight times more expensive. Pethidine probably should be avoided in the ICU as its metabolite, norpethidine can accumulate and, at high dosages, can cause epileptiform activity, irritability and hallucinations.

### Choice of benzodiazepines

Although diazepam has been used extensively in ICUs for many years, it can have a very prolonged action, especially in the presence of hepatic and renal dysfunctions. The metabolites of diazepam are also pharmacologically active. Lorazepam, oxazepam and temazepam are intermediate-acting benzodiazepines, while midazolam is a short-acting benzodiazepine. These may be used for short procedures or as sedative infusions. However, seriously ill patients do not metabolise drugs in the same way as normal patients and so-called short-acting benzodiazepines also accumulate over the long-term. Whereas long-acting benzodiazepines may not be suitable for a short anaesthetic procedure, they may be satisfactory for use in long-term seriously ill patients. Moreover, the long-acting benzodiazepines usually are less expensive than the short-acting varieties.

## Mode of delivery

Sedatives should be given intravenously in the ICU – they will be more reliably absorbed. The drugs can be given either as required or via a continuous IV infusion.

### Continuous IV infusions

Infusions are an easy, effective and flexible technique for drug delivery. They should be titrated against an end-point – pain relief and anxiolysis. Infusions result in less total drug being used. Aggressive marketing has popularised the use of volumetric infusion pumps for continuous IV infusions. The simple motorised infusion syringe pump may have more advantages: it is cheaper and does not require dedicated and expensive giving sets; it is easy to operate and can use high concentrations of drugs in standard syringes; it is small and can be more easily placed in the overcrowded area around a patient's bed. The high degree of accuracy claimed by the manufacturers of volumetric infusion pumps is not necessarily an advantage when titrating against physiological end-points such as pain relief or anxiolysis.

### Patient-controlled analgesia

Patient-controlled analgesia gives effective pain relief with less drug use and increased patient satisfaction. Patients must be awake and co-operative to use this technique. Take into account their analgesia requirements, renal and hepatic function before deciding on the settings. A baseline infusion rate may not be required.

### Oral analgesia

Oral analgesics are effective adjuncts and opiate sparing. Simple analgesics such as paracetamol have few side effects.

Non-steroidal anti-inflammatory drugs are effective for pleuritic pain and fractures. Use with caution in patients with a past history of gastrointestinal bleeding and not at all in patients with current gastrointestinal bleeding, renal compromise or coagulopathy.

Tramadol is a centrally acting synthetic analgesic with opioid-like effects. Use with caution in the elderly and those with renal impairment. Dose 50–100 mg IV or orally 4–6 hourly. Side effects include nausea and dizziness.

## Complications of sedation

### Airway obstruction and loss of cough reflex

All sedatives will cause a decrease in a patient's level of consciousness, with depressed upper airway reflexes and possible airway obstruction. This is not a problem when a patient has an artificial airway. If there is any doubt about the patency of the airway, sedation should be avoided until it is secured.

### Respiratory depression

Opiates, particularly, cause respiratory depression. Because of the high numbers of trained staff in ICUs and the predictable nature of respiratory depression, this does not present the same problem that it might on a general ward with fewer nursing staff. Opiates should be titrated against pain relief and respiratory depression.

### Cardiovascular depression

Like respiratory depression, this well-documented side effect of many sedative drugs is not necessarily a contraindication to their use in the ICU. Hypotension usually is related to vasodilatation, rather than cardiac depression; it is dosage dependent and predictable and is easily reversed with a fluid infusion. Even in the presence of severe multiorgan failure and hypotension, drugs such as benzodiazepines and opiates can be used to sedate patients as long as the intravascular volume is optimal.

### Immune depression

Anaesthetic induction agents used as continuous sedation in intensive care have been associated with profound immune depression especially barbiturates and etomidate. We are awaiting a definitive answer for propofol. Other sedatives such as narcotics and benzodiazepines have not been associated with immune depression in the clinical setting.

## Allergic reactions

Even mild allergic reactions are quite rare with commonly used sedative drugs.

## Addiction and dependence

Whereas narcotics often are grudgingly dispensed in meagre doses on general wards for fear of dependence, they are often used in 'industrial' doses for long periods in the ICU. Despite this, addiction or psychological dependence is rare. Physical withdrawal symptoms are only rarely seen when narcotics and benzodiazepines are used in large amounts over long periods. Such symptoms can be modified by gradually reducing the dosage.

Similarly, physical and psychological withdrawal symptoms have not been reported often for the other commonly used sedatives. It is possible that there are degrees of withdrawal reactions for many sedative drugs that have been disguised by the concurrent illness and gradual drug withdrawal. Pre-existing psychosocial circumstances and an active decision to take the drug may be more important in the development of drug dependence.

Long-term use of short-acting benzodiazepines (e.g. midazolam for 2–3 weeks) can provoke epileptic seizures on their withdrawal. Patients thought to be at risk should be changed to long-acting benzodiazepines (e.g. diazepam for 3–4 days) prior to stopping benzodiazepines altogether.

## Changes in intracranial pressure

Simply sedating a patient (preventing movement, especially coughing and straining) will decrease the ICP. There are also some sedatives that can independently reduce the ICP. These are mainly IV anaesthetic induction agents such as thiopentone and propofol. Ketamine will increase the ICP and should be avoided in the presence of intracranial abnormalities that are likely to increase the ICP.

## Phlebitis

Many of the commonly used sedatives, apart from opiates, cause phlebitis; this is usually overcome by delivering the drug through a central venous catheter.

## Muscle relaxants

Muscle relaxants are most commonly used in an ICU to facilitate ventilation. Sometimes this is necessary as in patients with severe hypoxia or high ICP. However, most patients when given judicious analgesia with or without sedation and with appropriate ventilatory support (pressure-support ventilation) will not require muscle relaxation for ventilation.

Muscle relaxants also prevent assessment of neurological status and detection of epilepsy and they can preclude spontaneous breathing in the event of a disconnection from ventilatory support. Muscle relaxants should never be used without adequate sedation.

Muscle relaxants have also been implicated in the aetiology of polyneuropathy in the critically ill.

## Mode of delivery and monitoring

Muscle relaxants can be given as a continuous infusion or in intermittent doses. Excessive amounts should be avoided, as unpredictable rates of drug metabolism and excretion can lead to prolonged paralysis. Neuromuscular blockade can be monitored clinically using end-points such as patient movement, respiratory effort or coughing. Prolonged neuromuscular blockade should be monitored by measuring the muscle responses to peripheral nerve stimulation, e.g. train of four. This may avoid prolonged weakness after the use of neuromuscular blocking agents.

## Choice of drug

- Pancuronium is relatively inexpensive and has little effect on cardiovascular stability, but it can potentiate tachyarrhythmias. The dose is usually 0.1 mg/kg as an intubating dose and 2 mg IV as a bolus dose to maintain relaxation.
- Vecuronium (0.08–0.1 mg/kg as an intubating dose, 75–100 μg/kg per h for infusion) has a short half-life. It has no cardiovascular side effects and is eliminated by both renal excretion (10–20%) and hepatic metabolism. Accumulation of 3-desacetylvecuronium may be responsible for decreased infusion rates needed with long-term vecuronium use, especially in the elderly.
- Rocuronium: An analogue of vecuronium. Its real advantage is as a rapidly acting non-depolarising neuromuscular blocker which at a dose of 0.6 mg/kg has ideal intubating conditions in 60 seconds. It is cardiovascularly stable and has no cumulative effect on infusion. The infusion rate is 0.15 mg/kg.
- Atracurium (0.5 mg/kg IV as an intubating dose) is expensive, but it has the advantage of not being dependent on renal or hepatic function for degradation and has a relatively short action. However, atracurium may not be suitable for long-term use in the ICU, as laudanosine (a metabolite of atracurium) may accumulate, causing seizures at high concentrations.
- Cis-Atracurium: A stereoisomer of atracurium. The intubating dose is 0.15 mg/kg. Further doses to be given at 0.03 mg/kg.

## Other forms of pain relief

### Regional or epidural analgesia using local anaesthetics

Regional and epidural analgesia is eminently suitable for seriously ill patients. The local anaesthetic agents and opiates used are relatively safe and provide excellent pain relief. The techniques are specialised and, like all other procedures, are best performed by experienced operators. Both regional and epidural analgesia can be provided by continuous infusion techniques or by intermittent boluses with long-acting agents. They should be considered for pain in association with:

- flail chest
- fractured ribs
- postoperative states, especially following laparotomy and thoracotomy
- pelvic and limb injuries.

Complete thoracic and abdominal pain relief will aid deep breathing, coughing ability and physiotherapy and may improve oxygenation and obviate artificial ventilation.

### Epidural analgesia

Exclude any patient with an unstable cardiovascular system, incomplete resuscitation, spinal trauma, overlying skin infection, coagulopathies, previous laminectomy or head injury, as well as any patient who is unconscious, unwilling or unco-operative. If the patient is on heparin, low molecular weight heparin or an antiplatelet agent then these will need to be stopped prior to performing the local block and stopped again prior to the epidural being removed. Recommendations differ if the anticoagulant is for prophylaxis of venous thrombosis or therapeutic. Following removal of the epidural, neurological evaluation should be carried out for at least 24 hours. The quicker an epidural haematoma is found and treated the less likely there is to be neurological sequelae.

The epidural should provide analgesia to the painful area, but no higher than T4. The level of the block should be assessed 4 hourly and after any bolus doses or change in infusion rate. This is best done with temperature rather than pain!

The level of insertion should be at the lower limit of the site that needs blocking. Lumbar epidurals with large volumes of dilute local anaesthetic are rarely successful if a high thoracic block is needed. Ensure the patient is normovolaemic and fluid loaded before using local anaesthetic agents, as sympathetic blockade may unmask hypovolaemia.

Techniques: Many different protocols are used, and each unit should develop its own. The following are several established techniques that can be adapted; the variations have to do with such issues as continuous or intermittent, with or without narcotics, long-acting or short-acting agents.

## TROUBLESHOOTING

### The confused patient in the ICU: Approach

**Rapidly exclude reversible factors:**
- hypoxia
- hypercarbia
- hypotension
- hypertension
- rarer causes (electrolyte disturbances, hypoglycaemia, renal or liver failure, vitamin and co-factor deficiencies, generalised sepsis and intracranial abnormalities).

### History
Elicit past history of disease and drugs, particularly alcohol and sedative dependence.

### Relieve pain
### Reassure
Encourage visitors and staff to talk to the patient, explaining the underlying disease and orientating the patient as to time and place.

### Sleep
Encourage sleep, with as little disturbance as possible to the patients while they are sleeping.

### Secure lines
Secure lines and tubes to minimise patient interference.

### Restraint
Bed rails, finger tapes and even manacles may be sometimes necessary.

### Sedation
Additional sedation may be necessary when reasonable causes have been excluded and other measures have failed.

### Psychiatric consultation
Psychiatric consultation may help in some cases when patients become more co-operative.

Local anaesthetics:

- Bolus dose: bupivicaine 0.5%, plain or with 1:20 000 solution of adrenaline, 5–8 ml, depending on level of analgesia required.
- Continuous infusion: bupivicaine, 0.125–0.25%. Start immediately after the bolus dose. The infusion rate will depend on the level of analgesia required.

## TROUBLESHOOTING

### The confused patient in the ICU: Causes

**Metabolic**
Uraemia, electrolyte abnormalities, vitamin and co-factor deficiencies, hypoglycaemia and hyperglycaemia.

**Global hypoperfusion or hypoxia**
**Drugs**
Withdrawal from alcohol, sedatives, opiates, hypnotics, barbiturates.
Idiosyncratic reaction to sedation.
Direct effect (e.g. ketamine or breakdown products of pethidine).
Drug overdose (e.g. hallucinogenics, tricyclic antidepressants, phenothiazines, theophylline and anticholinergics).

**Systemic infection** (e.g. septicaemia).

**Pain** (e.g. full stomach or bladder).

**Fever**

**Underlying chronic disease**
Psychiatric (e.g. psychosis, schizophrenia).
Chronic organic brain disease (e.g. collagen disease).
Endocrine disease, thyroid and parathyroid disorders.

**Intracranial problem** (e.g. trauma, infection, epilepsy, strokes, tumour, abscess, haematoma).
**Acute postcardiac bypass confusional state**
**Fat emboli**
**Hypertensive encephalopathy**
**'ICU psychosis'**
A diagnosis of exclusion, due to a combination of disorientation, drugs, sleep deprivation, etc. The elderly and very young are prone to confusional states in ICU.

Continuous infusions will provide more satisfactory pain relief and less cardio-vascular effects. The recommended amount of bupivicaine to avoid toxicity is:

- no more than 2 mg/kg as a bolus
  or
- no more than 400 mg/day.

Tachyphylaxis can occur with the use of bupivicaine, necessitating more frequent increases in dosage.
    Ropivicaine has less cardiac toxicity than bupivicaine.

Local anaesthetic ± narcotics: Mixtures of narcotics and local anaesthetics are very successful. Bupivicaine concentrations tend to vary between 0.125 and 0.2%. Fentanyl is the commonest narcotic used and its concentrations range between 2 and 4 $\mu$g/ml. The mixture we use is

bupivicaine 0.5% – 20 ml  
fentanyl 200 $\mu$g  } given at 5–8 ml/h  
normal saline 26 ml

This mixture gives

bupivicaine concentration, 0.2%  
fentanyl, 4 $\mu$g/ml

Commercial packs are also available.

Epidural narcotics alone offer little advantage over IV narcotics.

In the ICU, epidural and systemic narcotics are often used together (e.g. for flail chest plus fractured upper limbs), as the patient can be closely watched for respiratory depression. If this occurs, a small dose of naloxone (50–100 $\mu$g IV) will reverse the respiratory depression. Decrease the epidural infusion rate or decrease the narcotic concentration in the solution.

Pruritus, nausea and vomiting can also be reversed with 50–100 $\mu$g of naloxone IV while continuing the epidural infusion.

Inadequate pain relief: Check the delivery system for leakages or mechanical faults. Check the epidural concentration; a bolus 2–4 ml of infusion solution plus a higher infusion rate may be required.

## FURTHER READING

Buggy, D. J. and Smith, G. Epidural anaesthesia and analgesia: better outcome after major surgery? *British Medical Journal* 319 (1999): 530–1.

Rosser, D. and Bion, J. (ed.). Measuring sedation in the ICU: guidelines on the scales? *British Journal of Anaesthesia* 83 (1999): 693–4.

Stevens, D. S. and Edwards, W. T. Management of pain in intensive care setting. *Surgical Clinics of North America* 79 (1999): 371–86.

Society of Critical Care Medicine Working Group. Management of the agitated intensive care patient. *Critical Care Medicine* 30 (2002): (Suppl.) S97–123.

Sydow, M. and Neumann, P. Sedation for the critically ill. *Intensive Care Medicine* 25 (1999): 634–6.

Young, C. Sedation in intensive care. *Critical Care Medicine* 28 (2000): 854–66.

# 8

# Shock and anaphylaxis

- Ischaemia and shock overlap. Even minor ischaemia can adversely affect cellular function.
- 'Normal' vital signs and monitoring may not ensure adequate oxygen delivery ($DO_2$).
- Hypovolaemia (relative or absolute) is the commonest cause of tissue ischaemia and the easiest to correct.

## General features of shock

Shock can be defined as a state of inadequate cellular sustenance associated with inadequate or inappropriate tissue perfusion resulting in abnormal cellular metabolism. This can occur as a result of inadequate $DO_2$, maldistribution of blood flow, a low perfusion pressure, or, as usually is the case, a combination of all three. Shock is associated with anaerobic metabolism, oxygen debt and tissue acidosis.

Shock predisposes to multiorgan failure (MOF) (see Chapter 9), manifested by coma, ileus, diarrhoea, liver malfunction and jaundice, renal insufficiency, coagulopathy and acute lung injury (ALI).

The common denominator and earliest manifestation of shock is reduced oxygen consumption ($VO_2$). This is caused by low flow in haemorrhagic or cardiogenic shock, a cellular or metabolic deficit in septic shock and by maldistribution of flow in all types of shock.

The term 'compensated shock' suggests that the blood pressure (BP) is maintained at the expense of peripheral shutdown and ischaemia to many tissues.

It is becoming increasingly recognised that compensated shock is difficult to detect clinically, but can have deleterious effects. Measurements of parameters such as BP and pulse rate may be normal in these circumstances because of a redistribution of blood flow to vital organs, such as the brain and heart, and away from the so-called non-vital organs, such as skin and the gastrointestinal

**Table 8.1.** Classic haemodynamic patterns in shock

| Type of shock | Cardiac output | Left ventricular volume | Systemic vascular resistance |
|---|---|---|---|
| Hypovolaemia | ↓ | ↓↓ | ↑↑ |
| Cardiogenic | ↓↓ | ↑↑ | ↑ |
| Septic | ↑↑ | ↓↓ | ↓↓↓ |
| Anaphylactic | ↓ | ↓↓ | ↓↓ |
| Neurogenic | ↓ | ↓↓ | ↓↓↓ |

tract. It may be appropriate to employ measurements of tissue perfusion, such as monitoring the pH of the gastric mucosa (tonometry), as well as global measurements of $DO_2$. The state of compensated shock is associated with relatively normal estimates of global $DO_2$ in the presence of local ischaemia in many tissues. Compensated shock is associated with inadequate resuscitation and with high rates of morbidity and mortality. For example, decreased splanchnic blood flow is associated with potentially serious sequelae, such as bacteraemia, endotoxaemia and MOF. Oxygen free radicals and other damaging substances are produced during hypoperfusion. The threshold of $DO_2$ at which this occurs has not been defined and each tissue may have a different threshold. These oxygen free radicals and mediators are released from damaged cells on reperfusion and result in activation of macrophages and membrane injury – the 'ischaemia-reperfusion' injury.

There is an increasing tendency to 'hyper-resuscitate' or over-resuscitate patients suspected of having hypoperfusion or compensated shock in order to ensure adequate $DO_2$ to all cells.

## Classification of shock

There are many classifications of shock, some based on clinical entities and some on pathophysiology. This is somewhat unreal, as there is a large overlap between some of the groups, especially in their more severe forms and one or more processes may be involved simultaneously (Table 8.1). All forms of shock can eventually result in profound cellular dysfunction and death – so-called irreversible shock. Irreversibility is difficult to define and may depend on inappropriate management as much as on the clinical state.

The following is a clinically useful initial approach to shock in association with the classical causes of shock (Table 8.1).

- The patient's history is very important in determining the cause.
- Hypotension is often the first sign of shock.
- BP = cardiac output × systemic vascular resistance (SVR).
- Firstly, determine whether the problem is mainly one of decreased SVR or decreased cardiac output.

- If cardiac output is decreased, is that associated with a high (heart failure) or a low (hypovolaemia) filling pressure?

## Hypovolaemic shock

Hypovolaemic shock is related to decreased intravascular volume, secondary to loss of:

- blood (e.g. trauma)
- plasma (e.g. burns)
- water and electrolytes (e.g. vomiting, diarrhoea).

## Cardiogenic shock

Cardiogenic shock is related to 'pump' failure from many possible causes.
   Inside the heart:

- valve dysfunction
- papillae rupture
- myocardial infarct
- arrhythmias
- tamponade.

   Outside the heart:

- pulmonary embolus.

## Septic Shock

Septic shock has both central (myocardial) and peripheral circulatory problems.

- A major feature of septic shock is vasodilatation of the circulation causing relative hypovolaemia, which responds rapidly to fluid replacement.
- Peripheral circulation (e.g. redistribution, arterial to venous shunts).
- Leaky capillaries in both the periphery and lungs.
- Depressed myocardial contractility

## Anaphylactic shock

Anaphylactic shock is secondary to vasoactive mediator release:

- vasodilatation and hypotension
- leaky capillaries, leading to loss of intravascular volume
- severe bronchospasm.

## Neurogenic shock

Neurogenic shock involves loss of sympathetic tone, leading to vasodilatation.

## Adverse effects of shock

### Central nervous system
Confusion, restlessness and depressed level of consciousness with permanent damage in the presence of severe and prolonged ischaemia.

### Lung
Acute lung injury (ALI).

### Myocardium
Depressed myocardial contractility.

### Kidney
Oliguria and renal failure.

### Gastrointestinal tract
Stress ulceration, ileus, diarrhoea and ischaemia. Ischaemia of the GIT encourages bacterial translocation, endotoxaemia and MOF.

### Liver
Elevation of hepatic transaminases and bilirubin.

### Coagulation
Disseminated intravascular coagulation.

### Other tissue damage
Other systems (e.g. skin, muscle, immune system) are almost certainly involved as well, but the end-points of damage are difficult to measure.

## Management

As in all acute situations in the ICU, diagnosis and treatment go hand in hand. Airway, breathing and circulation must be secured first.

### Airway
If in any doubt, intubate.

### Breathing
Always maintain a high fraction of inspired oxygen ($FiO_2$) in shocked patients, even if respiratory function appears normal. This is to enhance $DO_2$ and to compensate for V/Q inequalities and the tissue hypoxia that accompanies low flow states.

Use artificial respiratory support – continuous positive airway pressure (CPAP), bilevel positive airways pressure (BiPAP) or intermittent positive-pressure ventilation (IPPV) – where necessary (see Chapter 18). Apply other principles of treatment for acute respiratory failure as necessary (see Chapter 16).

## Circulation

Hypovolaemia is the commonest cause of shock and the most easily reversed.

Fluid: Simple measurements should be used initially to monitor resuscitation (e.g. BP, pulse rate, skin perfusion and urine output) (see Chapter 20). As the intravascular volume is corrected, it can be fine-tuned using more complex, time-consuming measurements of parameters such as central venous pressure (CVP), pulmonary artery wedge pressure (PAWP), cardiac output and arterial blood gases (ABG). A fluid challenge, using 200–500 ml aliquots titrated against the relative changes in all relevant intravascular volume measurements, rather than a single absolute measurement, is the most accurate way of replacing intravascular fluid (see Chapter 4).

Inotropes: If hypotension persists despite optimising intravascular volume, inotrope support and/or a vasopressor may be needed. A particular drug or combination of drugs at a certain concentration will suit a particular patient at a particular time in that illness. The principles of choosing an inotrope are outlined elsewhere.

A useful first choice for hypotension, that is not responsive to fluid, is adrenaline or noradrenaline (4 mg in 100 ml of 5% dextrose), titrated against BP.

Adequate haemoglobin concentration: Red blood cells must be rapidly replaced in actively bleeding patients. If necessary, group-specific blood, which normally can be obtained more quickly than cross-matched blood, should be used in severe bleeding to ensure adequate oxygenation of the tissues.

## Reversible elements

Rapid correction of reversible and treatable factors is the most important step in the management of shock

Correct any reversible factors (e.g. bleeding, intra-abdominal sepsis, pulmonary embolism, pericardial tamponade, rupture of heart valve).

## Fine-tuning of shock

Ischaemia merges with shock and compensated shock represents inadequate resuscitation. After the patient has initially been resuscitated, evidence of residual ischaemia must be monitored and corrected.

Evidence of ischaemia can be detected clinically (e.g. cold peripheries and oliguria) and by more sophisticated measurements, such as those of $DO_2$ and $VO_2$, serum lactate, ABGs and GIT mucosal pH, as measured by a gastric tonometer.

## Specific forms of shock

Hypovolaemic shock, cardiogenic shock, septic shock and neurogenic shock are discussed in more detail elsewhere. Only anaphylactic shock will be discussed here.

# Anaphylaxis

Both anaphylactic and anaphylactoid reactions are characterised by sudden and dramatic changes in vascular tone, permeability and bronchial hyper-reactivity. This is due to the release of vasoactive mediators such as histamine, kinins and prostaglandins. The clinical manifestations of anaphylactoid reactions and anaphylactic reactions are identical. Anaphylactic reactions are usually attributed to participation of IgE antibodies (i.e. previous exposure to the antigen) whereas in anaphylactoid reactions vasoactive mediator release is via a non-immunoglobin mediated pathway, e.g. complement activation or direct mediator release.

## Clinical manifestations

- Skin: erythema, urticaria, pruritus, angioedema.
- Respiratory: bronchospasm, laryngeal oedema.
- Gastrointestinal: vomiting, abdominal cramps, diarrhoea.
- Cardiovascular: hypotension, tachycardia, arrhythmias, vasodilatation, decreased myocardial contractility.
- General: apprehension, metallic taste, coughing, paraesthesias, arthralgia, clouding of consciousness and clotting abnormalities.

These changes are variable; less than 20% of patients have a rash, 33% have bronchospasm and 86% have cardiovascular collapse. The reaction can be immediate or delayed.

## Management

### Oxygen
Oxygen in high concentrations, via a face mask, should always be given.

### Adrenaline
Adrenaline is the drug of choice for anaphylaxis:

- Initially give 0.5 ml of 1:1000 adrenaline intramuscularly (IM).
- Commence an IV adrenaline infusion (4 mg in 100 ml of 5% dextrose) titrated against the systemic blood pressure.

- If the patient has an unrecordable BP and is about to have a cardiac arrest then give 10 ml of 1 : 10 000 adrenaline intravenously (IV) over 5 minutes. Repeat as required or increase the IV adrenaline infusion rate.

### Plasma expansion
Because of vasodilatation and leakage of plasma protein, colloid should be used to correct the volume of the intravascular compartment. It must be given rapidly, initially 10–20 ml/kg. Larger volumes may be required.

### Bronchospasm
Apart from adrenaline, other measures that are used for asthma may be necessary (e.g. salbutamol). Intubation and ventilation may be required for severe bronchospasm. The same ventilatory techniques as for severe asthma should be used.

### Other drugs
Steroids are of uncertain benefit. Hydrocortisone 100–200 mg slowly IV may be given in severe or recurrent reactions. It may also be useful in asthmatics.

The role of antihistamines in the acute setting is uncertain, but probably of little benefit. Chlorpheniramine 10–20 mg IM may be given.

### Monitoring
- Patients should be monitored closely in the ICU until stable. Fine-tuning of the cardiorespiratory system can be accomplished after resuscitation. Measurement of cardiac filling pressures, e.g. CVP and PAWP and continuous inotrope infusions may be useful.
- Monitor BP, saturation, ECG and blood gases.

### Further management
Take blood for determination of complement, antibody concentrations and mast cell tryptase in order to identify possible precipitating agents (e.g. anaesthetic agents). Skin testing at a later date may further clarify the causative agent.

Counsel the patient and relatives about future reactions to the same stimulus. Inform relevant medical practitioners of the event and consider a hyposensitisation programme.

## FURTHER READING

Aranow, J. S. and Fink, M. P. Determinants of intestinal barrier failure in critical illness. *British Journal of Anaesthesia* 77 (1996): 71–81.
Ewan, P. W. Anaphylaxis. *British Medical Journal* 316 (1998): 1442–6.

Hasdai, D., Topol, E. J., Califf, R. M., Berger, P. B. and Holmes, D. R. Jr. Cardiogenic shock complicating acute coronary syndromes. *Lancet* 356 (2000): 749–56.

Landry, D. W. and Oliver, J. A. Mechanisms of disease: the pathogenesis of vasodilatory shock. *New England Journal of Medicine* 345 (2001): 588–95.

Porter, J. M. and Ivatury, R. R. In search of the optimal end points of resuscitation in trauma patients: a review. *Journal of Trauma-Injury Infection and Critical Care* 44 (1998): 908–14.

Project Team, Resuscitation Council (UK). Emergency medical treatment of anaphylactic reactions. *Journal of Accident and Emergency Medicine* 16 (1998): 243–7.

Williams, S. G., Wright, D. J. and Tan, L. B. Management of cardiogenic shock complicating acute myocardial infarction: towards evidence based medical practice. *Heart* 83 (2000): 621–6.

# 9

# Multiorgan failure

- Early aggressive resuscitation may prevent multiorgan failure (MOF).
- The clinical presentation of MOF is determined by the host's response as much as the triggering factor.
- Aggressive investigation and treatment of the cause are the most important steps.

Multiorgan failure (MOF) is considered to be a discrete entity or syndrome in the critically ill. It is a process, rather than an event, and it develops over time in response not only to an initial stimulus, such as sepsis, multitrauma, inflammation, severe burns, major surgery or shock, but also to the host's response to that particular stimulus. In fact, the host's response may be a more important determinant of the development of MOF than is the initial stimulus. Another name, the systemic inflammatory response syndrome (SIRS) is often used to describe this inflammatory response and to emphasise the importance of the host reaction rather than the exact nature of the insult. Multiorgan failure does not necessarily mean the total failure of every individual organ, but rather relative dysfunction. Failure or dysfunction of certain organs can be difficult to quantitate and so the extent of system disintegration may be underestimated. For example, renal function is estimated on the basis of relatively firm end-points, such as a rising serum creatinine concentration or oliguria, whereas there is no equivalent biochemical test for gastrointestinal tract function and thus softer clinical end-points must be used. Patterns of organ dysfunction are variable from one patient to another.

## Manifestations of multiorgan failure

### Respiratory system

Acute lung injury (ALI) is usually defined as hypoxia in the appropriate clinical setting, with bilateral pulmonary infiltrates and a normal left atrial pressure.

### Cardiovascular system

Peripheral dilatation, high cardiac output, supraventricular arrhythmias, impaired contractility or low output failure.

Cardiovascular parameters seen in MOF can depend on the patient's underlying heart function as much as the acute insult.

### Central nervous system

Encephalopathy and coma.

### Renal system

Acute renal failure, with impaired glomerular filtration and tubular function.

### Gastrointestinal tract

Stress ulceration, decreased gastric emptying, ileus and diarrhoea.

### Hepatobiliary system

Increase in bilirubin and increases in liver enzymes.

### Pancreas

Mild to moderate pancreatitis.

### Haematological

Anaemia, coagulopathy, thrombocytopaenia, as well as impairment of bone marrow function.

### Metabolic

Oxygen consumption may rise or fall; increased energy expenditure; increased gluconeogenesis from protein and consequent hyperglycaemia; increased fat oxidation; and failure to prevent catabolism by nutritional support.

### Other factors

Other organs and tissues are probably also involved (e.g. skin, muscle, bone) but these dysfunctions are even more difficult to measure and define.

## Quantification of organ dysfunction

There have been attempts to quantify the extent of MOF in order to help predict outcome as well as to classify and compare a similar population of patients. The scoring systems include cardiovascular (using blood pressure, heart rate and response to fluid and/or pressures); respiratory system (using $PaO_2/FiO_2$); renal system (using creatinine, urea and/or urine output); and the central nervous system (using the Glasgow Coma Scale). One of the more widely used is the Sequential Organ Failure Assessment (SOFA) system.

## Pathophysiology

Multiorgan failure is generally considered to be a syndrome with many causes but a similar final common pathway. Animal studies have demonstrated that the physiological alterations associated with MOF are produced by a complex cascade of more than 100 separate molecular mediators, including cytokines, eicosanoids, complement components, platelet activating factor (PAF) and intermediates of nitrogen and oxygen metabolism. These mediators have overlapping biological effects and are released from host cells, mainly macrophages, in response to a variety of stimuli. Experimental administration of some of these mediators, including tumour necrosis factor (TNF), interleukin-1 (IL-1), IL-2 and IL-6, produces a picture that in many ways simulates MOF. The levels of mediators in the circulation do not correlate with the clinical responses. The response to insults by mediators have important biological advantages by neutralising the insult, while at the same time often causing serious damage to the host.

The pathogenesis of MOF may be more closely related to an uncontrolled host response to an initiating stimulus, such as sepsis, than to uncontrolled infection and unchecked bacterial multiplication. Thus, MOF probably results from a systemic inflammatory response, rather than a pure infection. Although MOF was initially thought to be triggered by bacteria, it is now apparent that many stimuli, including tissue ischaemia, can initiate the inflammatory response. The clinical findings and mediator responses do not currently allow one to differentiate between infectious and non-infectious causes of MOF. In addition to ischaemic injury, reperfusion of ischaemic areas will result in an additional injury, mediated by inflammatory cells. Ischaemia of the GIT mucosa may also play an important role in MOF. The intestinal mucosal barrier is particularly vulnerable during ischaemia because of an increased demand for oxygen in the face of decreased oxygen supply. The compromised mucosa is unable to prevent translocation of bacteria, which leads to further stimulation of inflammatory mediators throughout the body. It has been suggested that the compromised GIT mucosa is the 'motor' of MOF.

The antecedents of the syndrome – trauma, burns, inflammation, major surgery, ischaemia, shock and infection – are associated with a complex spectrum of immunological abnormalities. The result is a dynamic process due to the interplay of the initial stimulus and the host reaction. Management must therefore be directed to restoration of normal physiological status as rapidly as possible, rather than relying on simplistic solutions such as broad-spectrum antibiotics. In the future, there is the possibility of specific treatments directed against the many mediators of MOF. These include TNF, IL-1, IL-10, interferon-$\gamma$, transforming growth factor $\beta$ (TGF-$\beta$), prostaglandins, PAF and nitric oxide (NO). However, there is increasing disillusionment with a 'magic bullet' for MOF and management is now aimed at prevention, in terms of correcting hypoxia and ischaemia at the earliest possible stage.

## Management

Treatment of sepsis is often considered the model for management of MOF. The principles of management for sepsis are the same for MOF and are discussed in detail elsewhere. The following are guidelines for the management of MOF.

### Prevention

- Rapid resuscitation: Restore the circulating blood volume, arterial BP and blood flow; maintain oxygen delivery ($DO_2$) to the cells.
- Prevention of sepsis.
- Rapid diagnosis and treatment of sepsis.

### Support

- Maintain $DO_2$ to the cells (see Chapter 16):
    adequate arterial oxygenation
    adequate haemoglobin concentration
    adequate cardiac output.
- There may be an abnormal relationship between $DO_2$ and oxygen consumption ($VO_2$) in patients with MOF. Even at high rates of $DO_2$, there may be a dependence of $VO_2$ on $DO_2$. The more oxygen supplied, the more that is utilised. However, there is little convincing evidence to aim for higher rather than 'normal' $DO_2$ in patients with MOF.
- Maintain adequate perfusion pressure.
- Minimise peripheral oedema to encourage capillary blood flow and $VO_2$.
- Avoid high intrathoracic pressures associated with artificial ventilatory support to prevent lung damage and encourage extrathoracic organ blood flow.

- Commence early enteral nutrition and in appropriate patients commence stress ulcer prophylaxis.
- Replace coagulation factors and platelets.

## Definitive treatment

**Aggressively investigate and remove or treat the source of sepsis or other causes of the MOF. Definitive treatment is the most important step.**

### Drugs

Drugs such as steroids, non-steroidal anti-inflammatory agents, heparin, branched-chain amino acids, desferroxamine, allopurinol, prostaglandins and monoclonal antibodies have all been tried or are currently being investigated for use with MOF. As yet, none can be unequivocally recommended.

## Outcome

There have been few large and epidemiologically sound studies on MOF and thus far it has been difficult to define the syndrome and determine what constitutes organ failure. More extensive trials will be required before we shall have precise information on how the high mortality associated with this syndrome can be reduced. However, we know that it is not only the number of failing organ systems that determines the outcome but also the degree of dysfunction within each system.

The removal of inflammatory mediators by techniques such as continuous renal replacement therapy and plasma filtration can be achieved. So far this has not resulted in improved outcomes.

## FURTHER READING

Bernard, G. R. Quantification of organ dysfunction: seeking standardization. *Critical Care Medicine* 26 (1998): 1767–8.

De Vriese, A. S., Vanholder, R. C., Pascual, M., Lameire, N. H. and Colardyn, F. A. Can inflammatory cytokines be removed efficiently by continuous renal replacement therapies? *Intensive Care Medicine* 25 (1999): 903–10.

Holmes, C. L. Plasmafiltration in sepsis: removing the evil humors. *Critical Care Medicine* 27 (1999): 2287–9.

Leverve, X. M. From tissue perfusion to metabolic marker: assessing organ competition and co-operation in critically ill patients? *Intensive Care Medicine* 25 (1999): 890–2.

Marik, P. E. Intestinal mucosal permeability: mechanisms and implications for treatment. *Critical Care Medicine* 27 (1999): 1650–1.

# 10

# Cardiopulmonary resuscitation

- Immediate cardioversion is the best treatment for ventricular fibrillation and pulseless ventricular tachycardia.
- Pupil size and reactions are unreliable indicators of cerebral function during cardiopulmonary resuscitation (CPR).
- Up to half of all patients who experience in-hospital cardiac arrests had major physiological abnormalities beforehand. These should be identified and treated early.

## Initial management in the hospital setting

Firstly, determine that the patient is unconscious: shake the patient and attempt to communicate. Call for help and lie the patient flat.

Identify the rhythm immediately:

- If ventricular fibrillation (VF) (Figure 10.1) or ventricular tachycardia (VT) (Figure 10.2) is the first rhythm encountered, up to three DC shocks should be delivered as soon as possible, at energy settings of 200 J, 200 J and then 360 J (Figure 10.3).
- If the rhythm is other than VF, immediately proceed to the non-VF/VT protocol (Figure 10.3).

If the rhythm cannot be identified immediately:

- Gain control of the airway, commence basic CPR and establish intravenous (IV) access while waiting for rhythm monitoring equipment to arrive.

### Airway

The three basic airway manoeuvres are head tilt, chin lift and jaw thrust. The airway must be cleared of any foreign matter or obstruction with finger sweeps

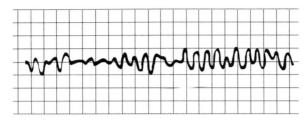

**Figure 10.1.** Ventricular fibrillation.

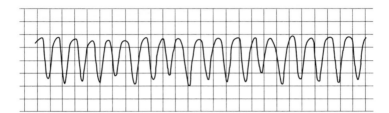

**Figure 10.2.** Ventricular tachycardia.

(community) or suction (hospital) and positioning. Initially use mouth-to-mask or bag-and-mask ventilation. Intubation with a tracheal tube will give better control of the airway. If intubation is difficult, do not persevere – ensure adequate ventilation and oxygenation with a simpler technique such as a laryngeal mask.

## Ventilation

For most relatively untrained nursing and medical staff, the use of self-inflating bags probably is not as efficient as mouth-to-mask techniques with supplemental oxygen. When using mouth-to-mask ventilation, pause to allow chest compression. The period of lung inflation should be 1.5–2 seconds/breath. This will increase the likelihood of lung inflation, rather than gastric distension.

## Circulation

Check for a carotid or femoral pulse. If there is no pulse or only a weak pulse and the blood pressure is too low to be measured, start external chest compression (Figure 10.4).

Measure two finger breadths up from the xiphi sternum. Place the heel of your hand on the lower sternum. Place your other hand on top of the first, keeping the heel of the hand on the chest and the fingers off.

With your shoulders directly over the patient, use your body weight (not your arm muscles) to depress the sternum.

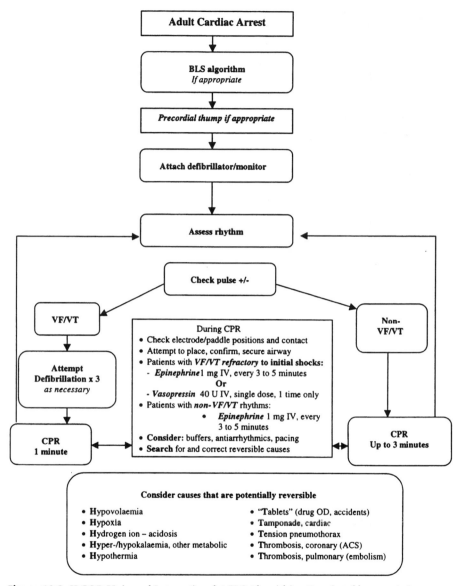

**Figure 10.3.** ILCOR Universal International ACLS Algorithim. Reprinted by permission of *Resuscitation* 46(1–3) (2000): 1–488.

- Compress at a rate of approximately 100 times/minute.
- Depress the sternum 4–5 cm each time.
- Use equal compression and relaxation times.
- The ratio of 15 compressions to 2 ventilations is used until the airway is secured with an endotracheal tube (ETT).

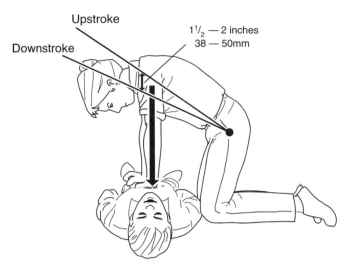

**Figure 10.4.** External cardiac compression.

## Reversible causes

Check for and correct reversible causes:

5 H's:
Hypoxaemia
Hypovolaemia
Hypothermia
Hydrogen ion – acidosis
Hyper/hypokalaemia and metabolic disorders

5 T's:
Tamponade
Tension pneumothorax
Toxins/poisons/drugs
Thrombosis – coronary
Thrombosis – pulmonary embolism

Effective CPR, at best, will give a cardiac output that will be 25–30% of normal, a systolic blood pressure (BP) of 60–80 mmHg and a diastolic pressure of approximately 40 mmHg. Cardiac output will decline with time. After 15 minutes, it will be only 15% of normal.

The 'chest thump' as an initial manoeuvre to convert VF may be used in monitored VF/pulseless VT arrests as it will occasionally result in conversion. However, the 'chest thump' should not delay the administration of DC shock.

## IV access

The initial IV access should be via a large peripheral vein (e.g. antecubital fossa). Central lines are not required; their insertion would only interrupt the performance of external chest compression. Intravenous fluids usually are not required during CPR but a slow running drip will facilitate drug infusion.

If IV access cannot be gained, some drugs including adrenaline and lignocaine can be administered via the ETT or intraosseously in children. Dosages 2–2.5 times normal should be used. Sodium bicarbonate and calcium should not be administered via the ETT. A central line is preferable for administration of inotropes. The external jugular is a rapid option. If peripheral access is used, flush with a large volume of fluid (e.g. 20 ml) after the inotrope bolus. Intracardiac drugs should not be used.

## Defibrillation

Defibrillation depolarises the myocardium and allows the most rapid natural pacemaker, the sinoatrial node, to drive the heart's rhythm. Immediate defibrillation is the treatment of choice for VF or VT (Figure 10.3). If VF or VT without an output is the first rhythm encountered, up to three sequential countershocks of 200 J, 200 J and then 360 J should be delivered, with no CPR in between. If the DC shock can be delivered within 3 minutes, up to 80% of patients will revert. After 5 minutes, defibrillation rarely results in spontaneous reversion. This emphasises the importance of early DC shock. The use of sequential shocks without a pause for CPR takes advantage of the accumulated decrease in transthoracic impedance. More current is therefore applied to the heart. However, excessive current can damage the heart. Energy levels of more than 360 J are seldom required. Repeated shocks may be necessary, but ensure that correctable factors are corrected (e.g. adequate oxygenation, as well as potassium and magnesium concentrations).

The defibrillator operator is responsible for determining that staff members are clear of the bed at the time of defibrillation.

Staff members must familiarise themselves with their hospital's defibrillators and have some basic knowledge about troubleshooting. The commonest reasons for defibrillator malfunction include batteries without sufficient charge, poor contact with the patient and inadvertent use of the synchronisation mode. This mode should be used only for cardioversion of arrhythmias with adequate circulation.

Most current defibrillators have a monophasic waveform, i.e. deliver current in one direction. Defibrillators with a biphasic waveform require lower energy to defibrillate and also do not require an increasing current with each shock. Some automatic external defibrillators (AEDs) deliver a biphasic waveform. The place of biphasic defibrillators is uncertain at present.

## Drugs

### Adrenaline

Adrenaline is widely used in ALS algorithms. Its $\alpha$ vasoconstrictor action diverts the blood flow, increasing the flow to vital organs and increasing coronary and cerebral perfusion pressures. Adverse effects include increased myocardial oxygen consumption ($VO_2$), subendocardial ischaemia and arrhythmia. Adrenaline is still the first line drug for use in patients who have VF/VT unresponsive to defibrillation, asystole and pulseless electrical activity (PEA). There is little evidence to show it improves outcome and the optimal dose is uncertain.

It must be emphasised that adequate chest compression is critical if one is to gain the full beneficial effects of vasoconstrictors.

Guidelines:

1 mg IV every 3 minutes.
A higher dose (5 mg) may be given after failure of the standard algorithm.

### Vasopressin

The naturally occurring antidiuretic hormone vasopressin is a vasoconstrictor at high doses via the $V_1$ receptor. High endogenous levels of vasopressin in survivors versus non-survivors of cardiac arrest lead to its initial use. However, there is no good evidence it improves outcome.

Guidelines:

It is recommended by some to be used in VF/VT refractory to shock and adrenaline. One dose only at 40 units. The half-life of vasopressin is 10–70 minutes.

### Sodium bicarbonate

The indications for the use of sodium bicarbonate in CPR are few; they include pre-existing metabolic acidosis, hyperkalaemia and overdosage with tricyclic drugs. It may also be useful in prolonged CPR (e.g. more than 20 minutes). Bicarbonate treatment is often associated with complications such as hypernatraemia, hyperosmolality, hypocalcaemia, paradoxical intracellular acidosis, impaired release of oxygen from haemoglobin and rebound alkalosis.

Guidelines:

Give sodium bicarbonate (50 mmol) IV as a bolus dose and then use regular arterial blood gas determinations to guide further treatment. However, during prolonged CPR, arterial blood gases do not necessarily reflect the degree of intracellular acidosis.

### Calcium chloride

Calcium is indicated for hyperkalaemia and hypocalcaemia and in cases in which it is suspected that there is toxicity due to calcium channel blocking drugs.

Guidelines:

Give calcium chloride (10%) 2–4 mg/kg. Repeat after 10 minutes if necessary.

## Lignocaine

Lignocaine is no longer the first choice antiarrhythmic for VT. With normal cardiac function procainamide or sotalol are preferred. With abnormal cardiac function amiodarone is the preferred drug.

Guidelines:

Give 1–1.5 mg/kg bolus in a cardiac arrest.
Not more than 3 mg/kg in total.

## Amiodarone

Amiodarone is useful in both supraventricular and ventricular arrhythmia, particularly in patients with impaired left ventricular function.

Guidelines:

150 mg IV over 10 minutes then an infusion of 1 mg/min for 6 hours.

## Other inotropes

Combinations of other drugs, such as dobutamine, dopamine, noradrenaline and isoprenaline, may have a place in 'fine-tuning' cardiovascular function after spontaneous circulation has been re-established.

## Further management

**Continue CPR: when conducting tests, procedures or reviewing an ECG, do not interrupt the CPR for more than a few seconds.**

A spontaneous palpable pulse is the best evidence that cardiac output has returned. Immediately resume CPR if the pulse is not detected.

## Brain resuscitation

The most effective way to maintain cerebral function is to provide efficient CPR. There is no evidence to support the use of barbiturates, calcium channel blockers or steroids in this setting. Inducing hypothermia following successful resuscitation is currently being studied. Initial studies show improved neurologic outcome.

## When to stop

The decision when to stop is largely governed by 'when to start'. The physical conditions of many patients are not suitable for commencement of CPR and, whenever possible, that should be clarified for each patient before

**Table 10.1.** Poor Prognostic indicators after CPR

No CPR given until 4 minutes or more had elapsed
No defibrillation during the first 8 minutes or more
Age of patient greater than 75 years and arrest lasting 5 minutes or longer
Severe underlying disease (e.g. malignancy)
Initial rhythm asystole or pulseless electrical activity.
Unwitnessed arrest of unknown duration

cardiorespiratory arrest occurs. The purpose of CPR is to prevent sudden, unexpected death, not to prolong meaningless life.

Brainstem signs such as pupil size and reaction to light are unreliable indicators of neurological status during CPR.

If there is a delay of greater than 4 minutes before basic CPR is initiated and a delay of more than 8 minutes before defibrillation, the outcome is generally very poor (Table 10.1).

Prolonging CPR beyond 15 minutes has resulted in a survival rate of less than 5% and except in exceptional circumstances, such as primary hypothermia or drug overdose, CPR beyond 30 minutes is rarely successful.

## Post-cardiopulmonary resuscitation

After resuscitation, a significant amount of organ damage due to ischaemia and/or reperfusion may occur.

It is important to correct as many 'correctables' as possible, in order to optimise tissue perfusion (e.g. serum potassium and magnesium, blood glucose [hyperglycaemia may exacerbate focal ischaemia] and temperature).

Maintain oxygenation and ventilation. The aim of ventilation should be to achieve normal levels of $PaCO_2$.

Obtain a post-resuscitation chest x-ray to exclude pulmonary barotrauma, aspiration pneumonia, gastric dilatation and check the position of the ETT and invasive monitoring devices in the thorax (e.g. temporary pacemakers, central venous catheters).

Regarding neurological damage, most studies have shown that if there is to be full neurological recovery, it will occur within the first 48 hours after cardiac arrest. Otherwise there will be varying degrees of permanent damage resulting from the global ischaemia at the time of arrest.

## Prevention of cardiopulmonary arrests

Up to half of all patients who experience in-hospital cardiac arrest can be shown to have had severe and identifiable abnormalities before arrest. These include tachypnoea, hypotension, oliguria and decreased level of consciousness. Because of the increased monitoring and awareness in ICUs, it probably is no coincidence that patients in intensive care rarely experience unexpected cardiorespiratory arrest. It is therefore important that the entire staff of a hospital become better educated in how to recognise patients who are rapidly deteriorating. Despite considerable advances in our knowledge of cardiac arrest, outcomes have not improved markedly over the past two decades. There is some evidence that the cardiac arrest team would be more successful being rapidly deployed to patients who were at high risk of having an arrest, rather than to those who had actually arrested.

## FURTHER READING

Special Issue International Guidelines 2000 for CPR and ECC – a consensus on science. *Resuscitation* 46(1–3) (2000): 1–448.

The American Heart Association in Collaboration with the International Liaison Committee on Resuscitation (ILCOR). Guidelines for cardiopulmonary resuscitation and emergency cardiovascular care. International consensus on science. *Circulation* 102 (2000) (Suppl). 1–384. Also at http://www.circulationaha.org

Other sites:  http://www.resus.org.uk/siteindex.htm
http://www.erc.edu/

So, H. Y., Buckley, T. A. and Oh, T. E. 1994. Factors affecting outcome following cardiopulmonary resuscitation. *Anaesthesia and Intensive Care* 22 (1994): 647–58.

**Table 11.1.** Physiological responses to temperature changes

Hypothermia
    Skin vessel vasoconstriction
    Muscle vessel vasodilatation
    Tachypnoea
    Hypertension
    Shivering
    Increased metabolic rate
Hyperthermia
    Skin vasodilatation
    Sweating
    Increased minute volume

rather than peripheral temperature, is essential in patients with hyperthermia and hypothermia. Patients who have cardiorespiratory instability, resulting in unpredictable skin blood flow, should also have their core temperatures, rather than peripheral temperatures, recorded.

Simple glass thermometers are suitable for routine measurements of oral or axillary temperature in otherwise stable patients. They usually read 0.4–0.7 °C below simultaneously recorded core temperatures. There is little difference in accuracy or ease of use between mercury thermometers and electronic systems for measuring non-core temperatures. However, electronic thermistor type devices are needed for measuring core temperature. It is important to routinely maintain and test these devices for accurate calibration.

## Hypothermia

Hypothermia is said to occur when the body's core temperature is 35 °C or less. It is a medical emergency (Table 11.2). Among patients with core temperatures lower than 32 °C there is high mortality.

Hypothermia can result from

1 Exposure – when cold stress exceeds the body's maximum heat production.
2 Exhaustion – which results from depletion of the body's available energy sources.
3 Failure of central temperature regulation – which is seen mainly in elderly patients and the newborn.

It is important for every ICU to have a thermometer capable of measuring core temperatures below 35 °C.

**Table 11.2.** Clinical effects of core hypothermia

---

36 °C: Increased metabolic rate, in an attempt to balance heat loss; shivering, vasoconstriction.

32 °C: Decreased metabolic activity, consciousness clouded, pupils dilated, shivering ceases, temperature control lost, bradycardia, J waves on ECG.

31 °C: Blood pressure difficult to measure; increasing metabolic acidosis.

30 °C: Increasing muscular rigidity, slow pulse and respiration, metabolic rate 50% of normal.

28 °C: Ventricular fibrillation may develop if the heart is irritated.

26 °C: Unconscious

    Pupils unreactive    Resuscitation may still be effective at this stage.

    No deep tendon reflexes

    Respiratory arrest

24 °C: Spontaneous VF, pulmonary oedema, severe coagulopathy.

20 °C: Asystole.

---

The authors are grateful to Dr R. Lee for his permission to reprint the above table.

## Causes of hypothermia

- Loss of consciousness (e.g. cerebrovascular events, head trauma).
- Metabolic and endocrine (e.g. acute diabetic emergencies, myxoedema, pituitary and adrenal failure).
- Accidental hypothermia – in association with low ambient temperature (e.g. mountaineering and immersion accidents).
- Surgery – intraoperative hypothermia is common, especially during prolonged procedures involving open body cavities.
- Drugs – especially alcohol and drugs associated with self-poisoning.

Hypothermia is potentiated in

- the elderly
- the newborn
- the acutely ill (e.g. patients with pneumonia and renal failure)
- patients with cardiovascular instability (e.g. congestive heart failure, myocardial infarction, septicaemia).

## Clinical features

Adaptive mechanisms such as tachypnoea, tachycardia and muscle rigidity gradually give way to slowing of respiration, bradycardia, hypotension and coma (Table 11.2). ECG changes include QT prolongation, T-wave inversion, J waves and an increase in the PR interval (Figure 11.1). Ventricular fibrillation (VF)

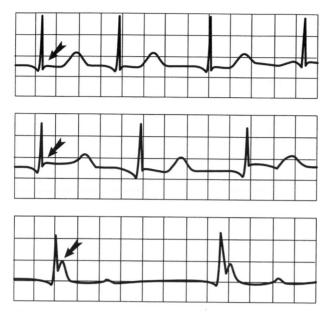

**Figure 11.1.** ECG changes associated with hypothermia. As the temperature decreases (from top to bottom), the heart rate slows and the QT and PR intervals become more prolonged. J waves (arrows) appear at a temperature of about 35 °C (top) and become more prominent at 25 °C (bottom).
Reprinted by permission of Little Brown and Company. Curley, F. J. and Irwin, R. S. Disorders of temperature control. Part I hypothermia. In *Intensive Care Medicine*, 2nd edn, ed. J. M. Rippe, R. S. Irwin, J. J. Alpert and M. P. Fink, pp. 658–73. New York: Little Brown and Company, 1991.

usually occurs when the core temperature drops below 25 °C. The VF is often resistant to treatment until the core temperature is increased.

## Management

### Immediate
Hypothermia is a medical emergency and should be managed in an appropriately monitored area.

Airway: Intubate if the patient is unconscious or has decreased airway reflexes.

Breathing: All patients require high flow oxygen, especially if they are shivering. Bradypnoea is usually associated with a core temperature of less than 30 °C. Early intubation and artificial ventilation will assist with oxygenation and rewarming.

Circulation: If there is no palpable pulse, perform cardiopulmonary resuscitation (CPR). As a general rule, for every 10 °C decrease in body temperature, the time during which there can be hope of recovery from circulatory arrest without CPR can be doubled. This refers only to primary hypothermia (i.e. people who are instantly cooled to a low temperature). It does not apply to people who have become hypothermic secondary to cardiac arrest (secondary hypothermia). Hypotension requires warmed intravenous fluid. Catecholamines are often required. Antiarrhythmics and cardioversion may be ineffective at low temperatures. Treatment of arrhythmias must therefore include aggressive rewarming.

Monitoring: Use continuous ECG monitoring, pulse oximetry, vital signs and other cardiorespiratory monitoring where appropriate.

Investigations: Immediate investigations must include arterial blood gases, blood sugar, electrolytes, microbiology, chest x-ray and 12-lead ECG. Measurement of core temperature with a low reading thermometer is mandatory.

Coagulopathy: Hypothermia causes marked disturbances of the enzymes involved in the coagulation cascade, thus predisposing the patient to bleeding. The abnormalities will not be detected if coagulation profiles are constructed at 37 °C. The tests must be performed at the patient's core temperature.

## Rewarming

Core temperature > 30 °C. External warming: External rewarming is achieved by covering the patient using hot air blankets and giving warm IV fluids and warmed humidified oxygen. More active techniques such as immersing a patient in hot water are unsound and not necessary. A temperature rise of 0.5 °C/h should be the target.

Core temperature < 30 °C. Active core rewarming: Surface rewarming is contraindicated when the core temperature is less than 30 °C as it would cause shunting of blood to the dilating skin circulation. The vasodilatation would exacerbate hypotension and cause a further decrease in core temperature, both of which could precipitate VF. Active core rewarming can be achieved in various ways.

- Delivering warmed humidified gases.
- Delivering warmed parenteral fluids.
- Peritoneal dialysis (4–8 L/h at a temperature of 37–42 °C).
- Circulating water, heated to 42 °C, through a closed irrigation system inserted into the oesophagus or stomach at a rate of about 3 L/h.
- The technique of choice for severe hypothermia probably is haemoperfusion. This procedure employs extracorporeal circulation by a continuous arteriovenous or venovenous technique. The blood is warmed as it flows past a dialysis solution warmed to 40 °C.

Active measures can be ceased when the temperature reaches 35 °C.

## Outcome

The mortality amongst hospitalised patients with core temperatures lower than 30 °C can vary from 20% to 85%, depending on the age of the patient, the

**Table 11.3.** Non-infectious causes of fever in the ICU

Aspiration
Acute lung injury
Pulmonary emboli and fat emboli
Deep vein thrombosis
Myocardial infarct
Cerebral infarction /haemorrhage
Subarachnoid haemorrhage
Other forms of brain injury
Acalculous cholecystitis
Alcohol/drug withdrawal
Blood or platelet transfusions
Gout
Neoplasms
Drug reactions are an uncommon cause of fever

associated underlying condition and the severity of hypothermia. Meticulous supportive care and the use of sound resuscitative techniques are just as important as the rewarming technique.

## Hyperthermia

### Fever

Fever is a common problem in seriously ill patients. The increased temperature is in response to cytokines released from mononuclear cells which act on the hypothalamus and reset central temperature control. This is the body's attempt to rid itself of invading pathogens. The diagnostic dilemma is to determine if the fever has an infectious or non-infectious cause. The 'big five' causes of infection in the ICU are the lungs, bloodstream, abdomen, urine catheters and wounds. Other sites such as sinusitis, endocarditis and osteomyelitis are not as common. Non-infectious causes are listed in Table 11.3.

### Effects of fever

- Increased metabolic rate (approximately 10% for each 1 °C rise in temperature).
- Increases in oxygen consumption ($VO_2$), pulse rate and cardiac output.
- Increased protein breakdown.
- Improved bacteriocidal action – enhanced antibody and cytokine production.
- Improved wound healing.

## Management

Determine the cause of the fever – infectious or non-infectious. A general guideline, made to be broken, is that non-infectious causes of a fever rarely reach a temperature of greater than 38.9 °C. Atelectasis does not cause a fever unless it is infected.

Fever is beneficial for host defences; patients with a fever have an improved outcome. As a guideline, the temperature should not be reduced by either physical or drug means unless the patient has an acute brain injury, limited cardiovascular reserve or the temperature is over 40 °C.

### Surface cooling

Ice packs, cooling blankets and fans have been used to cool patients. However, as a result of peripheral vasoconstriction, secondary to surface cooling by those methods, a paradoxical increase in core temperature can occur. Evaporative techniques (e.g. fans and tepid sponging) are more efficient than convective techniques (e.g. ice packs and cooling blankets). Care must be taken that a fan not be directed at the patient's face, as corneal drying and ulceration can occur if the eyes of a semiconscious patient are partially opened.

### Antipyretic drugs

Paracetamol, non-steroidal anti-inflammatory drugs and aspirin can all lower body temperature. The drug may have to be given rectally if oral absorption is not possible (e.g. indomethacin, 100 mg/rectum).

## Heatstroke

Heatstroke can occur as a result of increased heat production by the body or decreased heat loss or a combination of the two. It occurs particularly in certain groups and certain situations.

- The elderly.
- Athletes participating in endurance sports, particularly in warm temperatures.
- People with underlying cardiovascular disease.
- Hot ambient temperature (e.g. young children confined in cars).
- Infants with febrile illnesses who are wrapped too warmly.
- As a result of drugs such as anticholinergics and alcohol.

## Clinical features

A spectrum of damage will occur as the temperature increases. Heat exhaustion represents failure of the body to maintain a normal core temperature. Heatstroke can then rapidly supervene and it includes the following features, especially when the core temperature exceeds 42 °C.

- tachycardia
- muscle cramps
- hypotension
- hypovolaemia
- weakness
- widespread cellular damage causing rhabdomyolysis, renal failure, hepatic failure, coagulopathy and thrombocytopaenia.
- disorientation
- delirium
- severe vomiting and diarrhoea
- convulsions
- coma

**The severity of tissue damage will be determined by the duration and degree of hyperthermia. Rapid cooling is essential.**

### Management

Heatstroke is a medical emergency. Treatment must be prompt.

Airway and breathing: If the patient is unconscious or is having a seizure, or if there is doubt about the airway, intubation and ventilation should be performed.

Oxygen: Initially 100% oxygen should be delivered and then the inspired oxygen should be adjusted according to the patient's oxygenation.

Circulation: Hypovolaemia and hypotension are common. Rapid resuscitation with fluid is required. Cardiac damage may have occurred, necessitating catecholamine infusion in order to support the circulation.

Monitor core temperature: Use a high reading thermometer.

Investigations: Conduct baseline measurements: arterial blood gases, electrolytes, renal and liver function tests, blood glucose, haemoglobin, platelet count, coagulation profile and creatinine kinase.

### Cooling

As the severity of tissue damage will be determined by the degree and duration of hyperthermia, rapid cooling is paramount. At the site of injury, this involves removing clothing, moving to a shaded area, wetting the skin and actively fanning. The temperature must be rapidly dropped to less than 40 °C. Higher core temperatures may exacerbate the cellular damage.

Convection: Although measures such as immersion in cold water or packing the body in ice have been successfully employed, they can precipitate vasoconstriction and shivering, both of which will increase core temperature.

Evaporation: Evaporation is a more efficient method for cooling. This involves repeated or continuous wetting of the whole body while simultaneously fanning with air. An atomised spray or water spray will make the process even more efficient. Alpha-adrenergic blocking drugs such as chlorpromazine can enhance peripheral dilatation and cooling. However, these drugs should not be given until the cardiovascular system is stable.

Conduction: Gastric or bladder lavage with cold fluid will reduce the core temperature.

Extracorporeal techniques: Techniques such as continuous haemofiltration may be suitable for rapid cooling. The lines and filter can be surrounded by cool fluid. The patient may also be dialysed against cooled dialysate.

## Other measures
- Monitor urine output.
- Give blood products, as necessary, to correct any coagulopathy.
- Urgent dialysis may be necessary to correct acid base, potassium or phosphate disturbances. Intravenous calcium and phosphate replacement can cause widespread precipitation in many tissues, especially muscle, and should be avoided acutely.
- Mannitol at 0.3 g/kg may prevent precipitation of myoglobin in renal tubules.
- Treat convulsions, shivering and excessive muscle activity in order to limit further temperature increases.
- Dantrolene has been shown to be ineffective for treatment of heatstroke.

# Malignant hyperthermia

Malignant hyperthermia (MH) is a condition that occurs in association with the use of anaesthesia in genetically susceptible patients. It is an inherited disorder of calcium transport and calcium binding by cell membranes, associated with hyperpyrexia and hypermetabolism.

## Clinical features

Malignant hyperthermia typically occurs after induction of anaesthesia, especially with succinylcholine and volatile anaesthetic agents. These patients develop rigidity and hypermetabolism. Poor relaxation and exaggerated fasciculation can occur after succinylcholine. Other features include a steady rise in the end-tidal $CO_2$, tachycardia, fluctuations in blood pressure (BP), arrhythmias, sweating, tachypnoea, cyanosis and skin mottling.

Cardiac arrest, secondary to ventricular arrhythmia, can occur and later complications can include coagulopathy, acute renal failure, rhabdomyolysis, pulmonary oedema and cerebral oedema.

Non-anaesthetic related reactions are much less common but can be triggered by vigorous exercise, hot weather, muscle trauma, infection, shivering and, perhaps, emotional stress.

## Laboratory abnormalities
- Marked metabolic acidosis.
- Respiratory acidosis.
- Hyperkalaemia.
- Hypermagnesaemia.
- Acute renal failure.
- Massive rise in creatinine phosphokinase (CPK).
- Myoglobin in urine and serum.
- Coagulopathy and thrombocytopaenia.

## Diagnosis
The clinical diagnosis must be made immediately because of the life-threatening nature of this condition.

A definitive diagnosis requires eliciting a family history and muscle biopsy studies.

## Management

1  An effective treatment protocol and appropriate drugs must be readily available at all sites where anaesthetics are used.
2  Cease the use of suspected anaesthetic agents. Commence narcotics if anaesthesia is still needed. Induction agents and local anaesthetics may also be used. Terminate surgery as soon as possible.
3  Give 100% oxygen and hyperventilate.
4  Change to a vapour-free anaesthetic machine or non-rebreathing circuit.
5  Dantrolene: Initially give 2 mg/kg measuring end-points such as central temperature, heart rate and muscle rigidity. Subsequent doses may be required every 5 minutes up to 10 mg/kg. Further doses every 10–15 hours (half-life 10 h) should be continued until all evidence of MH has disappeared. It is important that dantrolene is given early while there is still muscle perfusion.
6  Institute cooling, as described previously. In summary, this may include:
    - cooled IV fluids
    - spraying with water and fanning
    - intragastric or intraperitoneal cooling
    - an extracorporeal circuit for cooling (e.g. haemoperfusion circuit with cooled filter or cardiopulmonary bypass).

7 Monitoring
  - ECG
  - BP
  - urinary output
  - central temperature

Frequent monitoring of the following:
  - arterial blood gases
  - electrolytes
  - blood sugar
  - renal function tests
  - coagulation tests
  - haematocrit.

8 Sodium bicarbonate (1 mmol/kg) may be necessary.
9 Arrhythmias: Procainamide, propranolol and verapamil have all been used successfully.
10 Avoid cardiac glycosides, calcium, quinidine and catecholamines, as they may perpetuate MH.

Further management: These patients must be tested and have the condition carefully explained to them so that they can avoid the use of precipitating agents during any future anaesthesia. The families must also be screened and counselled.

## Neuroleptic malignant syndrome

Neuroleptic malignant syndrome (NMS) is a rare idiosyncratic reaction to certain drugs such as the phenothiazines and butyrophenones. It has many features in common with MH – fever, rigidity and a high CPK. Dantrolene is useful in both and each has abnormal muscle contractility tests. There are two theories of the aetiology, a central hypothalamic disorder plus or minus a peripheral muscular mechanism.

There are major and minor diagnostic criteria:

Major criteria are hyperthermia, rigidity and a high CPK.
Minor criteria are hypertension, tachycardia, tachypnoea and change in level of consciousness.

### Clinical features

- Slow onset (24–72 h) of increased muscle rigidity and akinesia, involuntary movements and fluctuating tremor. Extrapyramidal symptoms are features of NMS, especially lead pipe rigidity.
- Hyperpyrexia, usually more than 39 °C.
- Variable levels of consciousness (normal to coma).

- Autonomic dysfunction (e.g. tachycardia, tachypnoea, labile BP, diaphoresis and incontinence).
- Differential diagnosis includes any febrile illness superimposed on a neuroleptic-induced dystonic reaction, neuroleptic-related heatstroke, MH and severe dystonic reactions.

## Laboratory abnormalities

- Rhabdomyolysis is almost always present with an increased CPK concentration.
- Myoglobin is present in blood and urine.
- Acute renal failure occurs in about half of all cases.
- Leucocytosis is common.
- Abnormal liver function tests.

## Drugs implicated in NMS

- Phenothiazines.
- Thioxanthenes.
- Amantadine.
- Novel antipsychotic drugs, clozapine and risperidone.
- Butyrophenones.

Neuroleptic malignant syndrome can occur after first use of the causative drug or at any time during its administration, even years after it has been commenced. Neuroleptic malignant syndrome is likely to recur if the drugs are given again. These patients probably should not have drugs that predispose to MH.

## Management

- Cease giving any likely offending drug and transfer the patient to an ICU.
- Control the airway, breathing and circulation as for heatstroke.
- Cooling should be instituted as for heatstroke, if necessary.
- Dantrolene sodium has been reported as being successful in NMS, probably because of the similarity between this syndrome and MH. It has been used in dosages of 1–10 mg/kg, either orally or IV, as a single dose or for several days.
- Bromocriptine (oral dosage 7.5–30 mg/day for several days) has also been used successfully. There are theoretical synergistic effects when dantrolene and bromocriptine are used together and no serious side effects have been reported.

Outcome: The mortality has been found to be up to 20–30%.

## FURTHER READING

Campbell, I. T. (ed.) Thermoregulation in critical illness. *British Journal of Anaesthesia* 78 (1997): 121–5.

Circiumaru, B., Baldock, G. and Cohen, J. A prospective study of fever in the intensive care unit. *Intensive Care Medicine* 25 (1999): 668–73.

Cunha, B. A. (ed.) Fever in the intensive care unit. *Intensive Care Medicine* 25 (1999): 648–51.

Erickson, R. S. The continuing question of how best to measure body temperature. *Critical Care Medicine* 27 (1999): 2307–10.

Faenza, S. Hypothermia: an adverse effect or a missing partner? *Intensive Care Medicine* 23 (1997): 1015–7.

Marik, P. E. Fever in the ICU. *Chest* 117 (2000): 855–69.

O'Grady, N. P., Barie, P. S. Bartlett, J. *et al.* Practice parameters for evaluating new fever in critically ill adult patients. Task Force of the American College of Critical Care Medicine of the Society of Critical Care Medicine in collaboration with the Infectious Disease Society of America. *Critical Care Medicine* 26 (1998): 392–408.

# 12

# Transport of the seriously ill

- Experienced personnel must transport patients.
- Equipment should be simple and robust.
- The level of monitoring during transport must be at least as comprehensive as in the ICU.

It is crucial to maintain the same high standards of intensive care for seriously ill patients during transport as during their stay in the ICU. This necessitates the following:

1  A high standard of medical and nursing care must be maintained during the transport. The staff not only must be skilled in caring for seriously ill patients but also must have had specific experience in transporting these patients.
2  Equipment and monitoring must be appropriate. The level of monitoring must be at least as comprehensive during transport as when the patient is in the ICU. In determining the equipment and drug supply, one not only must take into account the immediate support for the patient but also must be prepared for the unexpected, such as blocked endotracheal tubes (ETTs), ventilator failure, increased need for sedation and cardiorespiratory deterioration.

**It is in the interest of every intensivist to ensure the most efficient and rapid transfer of patients to and from other sites or institutions. Suboptimal treatment and deterioration during transfer can adversely affect the patient's ultimate outcome.**

Equally, it is crucial to maintain high standards during transport within the hospital. It is no longer good enough to send the least experienced and most junior members of staff on these journeys. Transport of the seriously ill requires experienced staff.

# Retrieval

## Primary retrieval

Primary retrieval involves transportation from the site of an incident to a site of definitive medical treatment. It often includes rescue or extraction from difficult terrain or from damaged vehicles. Primary retrieval usually is performed by ambulance personnel or a paramedical service. Depending on the level of sophistication of that service, medical personnel may also be involved.

## Secondary retrieval

Secondary retrieval involves transport of a patient from a primary centre to a secondary or referral centre. With increasing rationalisation and centralisation of expensive resources in the ICU, secondary retrieval is becoming more common.

# Retrieval system

A retrieval network must be well organised and must have adequate facilities for data collection and peer review in order to monitor the efficiency of the system.

## Communication

A comprehensive and integrated communication network is essential. The referring and receiving hospitals need to communicate with each other and with the retrieval team and transport facility. Often there is a co-ordination centre to facilitate communication.

## Retrieval teams

It is essential that the retrieval team includes medical staff who not only can deliver intensive care medicine equal to the standard of the receiving centre, but also are familiar with the problems associated with various modes of retrieval (e.g. aviation medicine). The team should also include a nurse or assistant with experience in intensive care medicine and retrieval.

## Education, data collection and peer review

There is no point in devoting all effort and resources solely to the medical retrieval system and the receiving centre. The basic principles of initial resuscitation must be implemented at the site of first contact with the patient. This involves a comprehensive education system, data collection facilities and peer review in order to locate and correct weak points in the system.

## Stabilisation

A patient must be resuscitated before transport is undertaken. If, for example, in a patient with multitrauma, the abdomen is expanding and it is difficult to maintain the arterial blood pressure with intravenous fluid, an immediate laparotomy is needed *before* transport. If the patient is unconscious and there is doubt about the airway, intubation should be carried out *before* transport. Pneumothoraces must be drained and other life-threatening conditions corrected. Procedures such as these are best attended to before transport. Detection and treatment of such conditions are difficult in the back of an ambulance or during air transport. Once such problems are under control, the attending team can then devote attention to monitoring and maintaining cardiorespiratory stability during transport.

Before transport, the medical team must attend to the following matters.

Airway: Intubate if there is any doubt.

Ventilation: Institute artificial ventilatory support with an appropriate fraction of inspired oxygen ($FiO_2$), especially in the presence of head or chest injuries.

Circulation: Ensure adequate fluid resuscitation with blood if necessary. Take adequate reserves of further blood or fluid for use during transport. Arrhythmias should be diagnosed and treated and the circulation supported with inotropes if necessary.

History: The history of the event is important, as it may point to potential injuries or other associated injuries (e.g. high speed motor vehicle crash and widened mediastinum).

Examination: The patient must be thoroughly examined from head to foot, noting vital signs (e.g. arterial BP, respiratory rate, pulse rate, temperature, urine output, peripheral perfusion), assessing stability and looking for other injuries.

Venous access: Short, wide-base cannulae are more appropriate than central lines for use during transport. Measurement of central venous pressure (CVP) is not necessary during initial resuscitation and transport. If inotropes or other drugs such as concentrated potassium are needed, then a long line from the cubital fossa, rather than a central line placed from the upper chest or neck, should be inserted in order to avoid the possible complication of pneumothorax, especially during flight.

Mechanics of fluid infusion: Under normal circumstances, a hydrostatic head of more than 75 cm$H_2O$ is sufficient for adequate fluid flow into a peripheral vein. A motorised syringe pump with optional battery pack is the most appropriate method for delivering concentrated drugs such as inotropes, vasodilators and drugs for sedation and pain relief.

Pleural drains: A chest x-ray to confirm placement of drain lines must be performed before transport. A flutter valve, such as the Heimlich design, is usually used, rather than an underwater drainage system. Although the Heimlich valve is more convenient and overcomes the problem of having to place the underwater drain below the patient during transport, the lips of the flutter valve can become blocked if it is contaminated by blood or other fluid.

## Cardiorespiratory monitoring

Monitoring can be difficult during transport. Outside noise, vibration and movement can make even simple clinical observations very difficult (e.g. chest rising with respiration and palpable pulse). Monitoring equipment can be similarly affected. However, there are now robust, portable, battery-operated monitors that work reliably under these conditions. The minimum equipment list should include capabilities for the following:

- Continuous ECG monitoring.
- Invasive/non-invasive determination of the BP, adult and paediatric cuffs.
- Pulse oximetry, with finger and multisite sensors.
- End tidal $CO_2$ determination, especially for ventilated head injury patients.
- Disconnect alarm.
- Airway pressure monitoring.
- Oxygen failure alarm.

## Other equipment

Intubating equipment (laryngoscopes, adult and paediatric, Guedel airways, Magill forceps).
ETTs (neonate to adult sizes).
Emergency percutaneous airway set.
Chest drains (Heimlich valves, paediatric to adult sizes).
Portable suction equipment and catheters.
Manual ventilating system.
Oxygen masks.
Portable oxygen.
Disposable humidifiers.
Defibrillator and spare batteries.
Syringe pumps, battery powered.
IV fluids, cannulae, giving sets.
Syringes, needles, non-return valves.
Nasogastric (NG) tubes and bags.
Urinary catheters and bags.

**Table 12.1.** List of drugs needed for transport of the seriously ill

| | | | | |
|---|---|---|---|---|
| adrenaline | 1: 10 000 | 10 ml × 5 | thiopentone | 500 mg | |
| adrenaline | 1: 1000 | 1 ml × 5 | water | 20 ml | |
| amiodarone | 300 mg | | salbutamol | 500 μg | |
| atropine | 1.2 mg | | dextrose | 50% | 50 ml |
| calcium | 1 g | | NaHCO$_3$ | 8.4% | 50 ml |
| frusemide | 40 mg | | neostigmine | 2.5 mg | |
| lignocaine | 150 mg | | morphine | 10 mg | |
| dopamine | 200 mg | | naloxone | 4 mg | |
| isoprenaline | 1.0 mg | | midazolam | 5 mg | |
| magnesium sulphate | 20 mmol | | diazepam | 10 mg | |
| verapamil | 20 mg | | vecuronium | 10 mg powder | |
| metoprolol | 5 mg | | ketamine | 200 mg | |
| NaCl (flushing) | 10 ml | | suxamethonium | 200 mg | |
| potassium chloride | 10 mmol | 10 ml | (replace weekly in | | |
| digoxin | 500 μg | | summer and | | |
| | | | biweekly in cooler | | |
| | | | weather) | | |

## Drugs

Table 12.1 contains the minimum ranges of drugs needed for transport of the seriously ill. The numbers of the various ampoules of the drugs carried will depend on the length of the journey and the type of patient.

## Mode of transport

The decision to use road transport, fixed wing aircraft, helicopters or even water transport depends on many factors. The patient's condition and the urgency for definitive treatment or investigation are the most important factors. However, other factors include distance between the two points, local geography, weather and visibility, adequacy of roads, facilities for air transport and comparative costs.

## Intrahospital transport

The principles of transport, whether travelling thousands of kilometres between hospitals or taking a patient from the ICU to the computerised tomography (CT) unit, are the same. The patient must be stabilised before transport and the clinician accompanying the patient must be experienced in the principles of intensive care medicine as well as transport. The list of drugs and equipment to be carried during intrahospital transport is almost the same as for retrieval. Some items, such as

**TROUBLESHOOTING**

## Transporting the ICU patient around the hospital

### Checklist
Do we really need to subject the patient to transport?
Why is the patient having this investigation?
How will it change their case if it is positive/negative?
A  Airway – stable/secured.
B  Breathing – will the patient be able to be ventilated on a transport ventilator?
   Oxygen/air cylinders full?
   Check arterial blood gases and latest chest x-ray.
   Check chest drains are well secured.
C  Circulation – is the rhythm stable?
   What cardiovascular system parameters are being aimed for?
   If the BP drops – fluid or inotropes?
   Extra syringes of all inotropes and extra pump.
D  Central nervous system – does the patient need extra analgesia/sedation?
   How will you monitor the intracranial pressure during transport?
E  Check the latest laboratory results.
F  Secure the patient well.
G  Check drugs – what they are, when they need to be given?

### Monitoring
Minimum:
Disconnect alarm.
   $SaO_2$ $ETCO_2$.
   Reliable BP.
   ECG.
   Intracranial pressure (if being monitored).
Before you move the patient, check you know where everything is, the patient is
stable and you have enough help – extra nurses, wardsmen, consultant if required!

NG tubes and urinary catheters, are, of course, unnecessary for intrahospital
transport, but appropriate equipment and drugs must accompany the patient in
case of an emergency or equipment failure. A standard form of monitoring and a
dedicated mobile bed will make intrahospital transport a simple and safe routine,
rather than a hazardous venture.

### FURTHER READING

Joint Faculty of Intensive Care Medicine, Australian and New Zealand College of Anaesthetists. Policy Documents. Minimum standards for transport of the critically ill. (1996)
www.fic.anzca.edu.au/policy/index.htm.

Ferdinande, P., on behalf of the Working Group on Neurosurgical Intensive Care of the European Society of Intensive Care Medicine. Recommendations for intra-hospital transport of the severely head injured patient. *Intensive Care Medicine* 25 (1999): 1441–3.

The Intensive Care Society. *Guidelines for Transport of the Critically Ill.* London: The Intensive Care Society, 1997.

# 13

# Infection

- Endogenous sources of nosocomial infections are far more common than an exogenous source.
- The use of antibiotics is only one part of the management of sepsis. The source of the sepsis must be relentlessly sought and treated.
- Avoid broad-spectrum antibiotics and prolonged antimicrobial treatment where possible.

## Source of infection

### Primary infection

Infections acquired outside the hospital are considered to be primary or community-acquired infections. Such infections include pneumonia, tetanus, acute epiglottitis, urinary tract infection (UTI) and meningoencephalitis. These are usually well-defined entities with accepted norms for their diagnoses and treatment.

### Nosocomial infection

Nosocomial infections are hospital-acquired infections and represent a major problem, especially in the ICU. Our current knowledge about the diagnosis and treatment of these disorders is not as extensive as our knowledge of primary infections.

#### Exogenous infection

Exogenous infections originate from the hospital environment. Patients can acquire such infections either by an airborne route or by direct contact. The ICU is an environment where significant cross infection can occur. This is usually discovered when several patients develop infection with a particular species of organism, such as methicillin resistant *Staphylococcus aureus* (MRSA) or resistant gram-negative rods.

**Essential precautions: The single most important intervention to reduce cross infection is hand washing before and after contact with each patient.** The compliance with hand washing is poor with all health-care workers but doctors are amongst the worst offenders. Strict aseptic conditions for all invasive procedures are also essential.

Equivocal precautions:

- Plastic aprons.
- Isolation rooms.
- Laminar flow ventilation.
- Individual stethoscope for each patient.

Very doubtful precautions:

- Shoe covers, sticky or disinfectant mats.
- Surface disinfectant on floors.
- Changing clothes before entering the ICU.
- Routine examinations of environmental cultures.
- Routine changing of infusion systems every 24 hours.
- Inline bacterial filters.
- Nose and throat cultures from staff, except during epidemics.
- Routine sterilisation of internal ventilatory machinery between patients.
- Banning of flowers in the ward.
- Disinfection of sinks and drains.

## Endogenous infection

These are the most important kinds of nosocomial infections in the ICU, and they account for most episodes of septicaemia. They pose one of the most common and most serious problems amongst the critically ill.

The normal microbial flora of the human body includes organisms found in the alimentary tract, upper respiratory tract, female genital tract and skin. The three stages of endogenous infection in the ICU are colonisation of normally sterile areas, followed by colonisation of major organ systems such as the respiratory tract and bladder and, finally, overt infection.

Colonisation: presence of microorganisms without tissue invasion and injury.

Infection: invasion of tissues by microorganisms with tissue injury.

A patient's own organisms usually cause nosocomial infections. For example, coliforms colonise the gastrointestinal tract, exacerbated by alkalinisation of the stomach (Table 13.1). Antibiotics, especially broad-spectrum antibiotics, change the microbial environment by selectively killing some organisms. Thus the original flora is replaced by a new range of otherwise harmless organisms, such as

**Table 13.1.** Common organisms causing nosocomial infections

Staphylococci
   *Staphylococcus aureus*
   MRSA
Coagulase negative *Staphylococcus* spp.
*Streptococcus pyogenes*
*Enterococcus* spp.
Coliforms
   *Escherichia coli*
   *Klebsiella* spp.
   *Proteus* spp.
   *Enterobacter* spp.
   *Serratia* spp.
   *Acinetobacter* spp.
*Pseudomonas* spp.
Fungi

**Table 13.2.** Nosocomial infection sites

| Site | Approximate incidence (%) |
| --- | --- |
| Urinary tract | 30 |
| Generalised septicaemia | 20 |
| Pneumonia | 20 |
| Skin and subcutaneous tissue | 10 |
| Upper respiratory tract (including sinusitis) | 10 |
| Wound infection | 10 |

fungi and *Pseudomonas* species, that often are resistant to antimicrobials. These microorganisms are equally as dangerous to a seriously ill patient as the organisms for which the antibiotics were originally prescribed, and often they are markers of unwise use of antibiotics. The host may have been immunocompromised as a result of invasive procedures, malnutrition and immunosuppressive drugs (Table 13.2), rendering such a patient more susceptible to infection from other benign organisms. The microbiological ecology of the patient should be carefully considered and empirical antibiotic treatment with broad-spectrum antibiotics should be avoided wherever possible. Although most clinicians and microbiologists will agree with these principles, in practice they are often ignored.

## Guidelines for controlling nosocomial infection
• Determine the incidence and type of nosocomial infections in your ICU.
• Rigorously encourage hand washing before and after treatment of each patient.

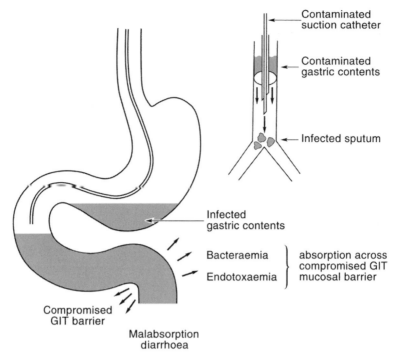

**Figure 13.1.** Potential complications of bacterial overgrowth in the stomach. GIT, gastrointestinal tract.

- Limit the number of invasive procedures and the insertion times for intravascular devices.
- Resuscitate early and aggressively. Examine cultures of sputum, urine and blood routinely, as well as those for wounds, cerebrospinal fluid (CSF), peritoneal fluid and other sites when necessary.
- Always manage the patient sitting up to avoid nosocomial pneumonia (Figure 13.1).
- Make every effort to culture organisms before antibiotics are given.
- Use narrow spectrum antibiotics where possible.
- If antibiotics are having no effect within 3–5 days, stop and reculture. Differentiate between normal flora, harmless colonisation (particularly *Pseudomonas* species and fungi) and clinically significant infections.
- The use of antibiotics will change the microbial ecology and encourage the development of resistance. Use them sparingly, for short, sharp bursts.
- Review the findings from cultures and rationalise antibiotic treatment daily.
- Everyone pays lip service to good microbiological practice and wise use of antibiotics. It is crucial to incorporate all these principles into your own clinical practice.

**Table 13.3.** Some suggested definitions related to sepsis

Although there are no universally agreed definitions for clinical syndromes related to sepsis, here are some guidelines.

Bacteraemia: positive blood culture.

Sepsis: the systemic response to infection (e.g. tachypnoea [respiratory rate > 20 breaths/ min], tachycardia [HR > 90/min], hyperthermia [> 39 °C] or hypothermia [< 35.5 °C]).

Sepsis syndrome: sepsis with evidence of organ dysfunction (e.g. altered level of consciousness, hypoxia, renal failure, jaundice).

Septic shock: sepsis syndrome with hypotension, despite adequate fluid resuscitation, along with evidence of reduced perfusion (e.g. oliguria, lactic acidosis).

Septicaemia: used interchangeably with 'sepsis', 'sepsis syndrome' and 'septic shock'.

Refractory septic shock: septic shock unresponsive to fluids and inotropes.

Systemic inflammatory response syndrome (SIRS): two or more of the following:

Temperature > 38.0 °C, or temperature < 36 °C
Heart rate > 90 beats/min
Respiratory rate > 20/min or $PaCO_2$ < 32 mmHg (4.5 kPa)
White cell count > 12 × $10^9$/L, or more than 10% immature forms

- Limit perioperative prophylactic antibiotic regimens to less than 24 hours. Single-dose prophylaxis is appropriate in most cases.
- Avoid routine use of systemic antibiotics for prevention of postoperative pneumonia.
- Improve immune status of patient if possible (e.g. nutrition, prevention of renal failure, rapid resuscitation, avoidance of drugs that could compromise immune function, such as barbiturates, anaesthetic agents and corticosteroids).
- Work closely with your own microbiology department and encourage daily ward rounds with a specialist in infectious diseases if possible.

## Septicaemia

The term 'septic' shock strikes fear in the heart of even the bravest intensivist. The mortality from septic shock remains around 50%. The term 'septic shock', 'septic syndrome', 'sepsis' and 'septicaemia' are often used interchangeably (Table 13.3). The term usually refers to evidence of infection accompanied by signs of systemic involvement and altered organ perfusion such as an altered level of consciousness, hypoxia and oliguria. Positive findings from blood cultures are not necessarily the rule. In fact, sepsis can occur in association with bacteraemia, viraemia, fungaemia or endotoxaemia or, indeed, without evidence of any microbes at all. It remains one of the most common and most difficult

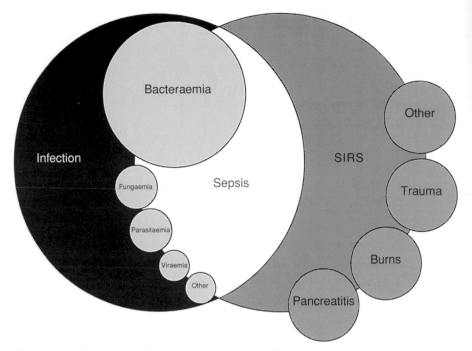

**Figure 13.2.** The inter-relationship among systemic inflammatory response syndrome (SIRS), sepsis and infection. Reprinted by permission of ACCP/SCCM Consensus Conference. Bone, R.C. Definitions for sepsis and organ failure and guidelines for the use of innovative therapies in sepsis. *Chest* 101 (1992): 1644–55.

disorders to treat in intensive care. Cases of sepsis or septicaemia represent inflammatory responses to a variety of insults including non-infectious insults such as pancreatitis, ischaemia, multitrauma, tissue injury, haemorrhagic shock and immune-mediated organ injury. It has been suggested that because the host responses are the same, regardless of whether the cause is infective or non-infective, the term should be changed to 'systemic inflammatory response syndrome (SIRS) (Figure 13.2). The terms 'sepsis' and 'septicaemia' will be used synonymously in this chapter. There are, however, efforts being made to agree on stricter terminology (Table 13.3). Sepsis is characterised by a pro-inflammatory response and simultaneously, an anti-inflammatory response, aimed at dampening the initial pro-inflammatory insult. The pro-inflammatory response results in activation of multiple biological cascades including:

- Inflammatory mediators (e.g. cytokines, chemokines, lipid mediators).
- Coagulation/fibrinolysis system.

The anti-inflammatory response may predominate in some patients resulting in 'immune paralysis' which may worsen outcome. On the other hand, if the

**Table 13.4.** Features of septicaemia

Clinical
 Decreased level of consciousness or confusion
 Fever or hypothermia
 Hypotension
 Tachycardia and bounding precordium
 Tachypnoea
 Oliguria
 Jaundice
 Ileus
 Stress ulceration
Laboratory and monitoring
 Manifestations of organ failure
 Respiratory (e.g. hypoxia)
 Kidney (e.g. increased urea and creatinine)
 Cardiac (e.g. supraventricular tachycardia)
 Liver (e.g. increased bilirubin)
 Metabolic (e.g. hyperglycaemia)
 Haematological (e.g. 'toxic' changes in white cells)

pro-inflammatory response is allowed to dominate unchecked, complications such as multiorgan failure (MOF) may result.

## Clinical features of septicaemia

The pathophysiology of septicaemia involves all systems. Consequently, sepsis usually presents as MOF. The initial sign in sepsis is peripheral vasodilatation, with a compensatory increase in cardiac output. Other cardiovascular changes occur before hypotension. These include increases in cardiac output; increases in pulmonary vascular resistance; decreases in systemic vascular resistance; and disturbances in oxygen delivery ($O_2$) and oxygen consumption ($VO_2$). These changes continue throughout the septic episode (Table 13.4). Low cardiac output in sepsis is rare, even in the latter stages.

**Consistent clinical signs of sepsis are a bounding precordium and a pulsating neck, often visible from the end of the bed.**

Patients with sepsis develop abnormalities of cardiac function, even in the early hyperdynamic phase and in the presence of a high cardiac output. Manifestations of depressed myocardial function include ventricular dilatation, diminished left and right ejection fractions and altered diastolic pressure volume relationships. The mechanism of depressed myocardial function has not, as yet, been fully elucidated, but the inflammatory mediators of sepsis may be involved. Processes other than peripheral vasodilatation which occur in the peripheral circulation, include redistribution of blood flow, intravascular pooling, increased

**Table 13.5.** Haemodynamic response to sepsis

| | |
|---|---|
| Cardiac function | ↓ Blood pressure |
| | ↑ Cardiac index, ↓ SVR, ↓ LV ejection fraction |
| | ↓ Left ventricular end-diastolic volume |
| | ↓↓ Preload |
| |     Loss of vasomotor tone, splanchnic pooling |
| |     ↑ Microvascular permeability, ↓ circulating blood volume |
| | ↓ Contractility |
| |     Myocardial depressant factor |
| |     Often masked by ↓ LV afterload |
| | ↓ Coronary blood flow |
| Regional distribution of blood flow | Loss of vasomotor tone |
| | Vasodilatation |
| | Redistribution of blood flow (balance between local tissue mechanisms and central mechanisms is disturbed and local autoregulation malfunctions) |
| Micro-circulation | Vasodilatation |
| | Microemboli |
| | Endothelial cell injury |
| | Tissue $O_2$ extraction is decreased, diffusion distance for oxygen is increased capillary recruitment |

microvascular permeability and microembolisation (Table 13.5). Despite elevations in cardiac output and $DO_2$, tissues cannot extract adequate oxygen. Cells produce lactate and other signs of tissue dysfunction begin to appear.

The exact mechanism for ineffective peripheral tissue metabolism is unknown. The proposed mechanisms have included inadequate fluid resuscitation, anatomic shunting, enzyme inhibition, a left shift of the oxygen dissociation curve and a primary inability of cells to utilise oxygen. Currently, the major dysfunction is thought to be at the microcirculatory level – vasodilatation, microembolisation and endothelial cell injury. Tissue oedema resulting from cellular injury and inappropriate fluid administration can further impair oxygen diffusion by increasing the diffusion distances and compressing capillaries. A reduced capacity for peripheral extraction of oxygen is the likely basis for the postulated abnormal dependence of $VO_2$ on the supply. The exact relationship between $DO_2$ and $VO_2$ in the presence of sepsis has not yet been determined.

Large numbers of mediators have been suggested as being activated by the presence of microorganisms. These mediators may be responsible for much of the pathophysiology of sepsis. These include cytokines, eicosanoids, complement, cyclo-oxygenase and lipo-oxygenase products and effector substances from granulocytes and platelets (Figure 13.3). This area of research is one of the most active in intensive care. However, the clinical implications are, as yet, unclear. For more details, see the publications cited at the end of this chapter.

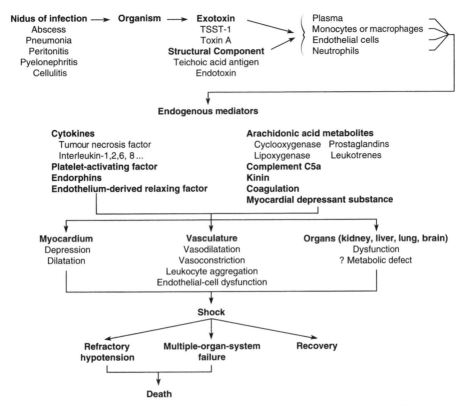

**Figure 13.3.** Pathogenic sequence of events in patients with septic shock. Reprinted by permission of Parrillo, J.E. Pathogenetic mechanisms of septic shock. *New England Journal of Medicine* 328 (1993): 1471–7.

Free radical nitric oxide (NO) is produced from arginine and mediates vascular relaxation via cyclic guanosine monophosphate (cGMP). It is suggested that cytokines can induce the enzyme NO synthase (NOS), leading to excess production of NO and hence profound hypotension unresponsive to catecholamines. Trials using NOS inhibitors to reverse the vasodilatation of sepsis have so far not resulted in improved outcomes.

## Other features

### Temperature disturbances
Fever is common, but it is not an inevitable sign of sepsis. Central temperature should be measured 4-hourly and plotted graphically, so that a swinging fever can be detected – this is a valuable guide to an occult source of sepsis. Fever can also be associated with drugs (including antibiotics), malignancy or non-infective

inflammatory process. However, hypothermia occurs in up to 10% of patients with sepsis and is associated with a worse prognosis.

### Nausea, vomiting, diarrhoea
These are very common features of sepsis in conscious patients and may be manifested as increased nasogastric (NG) aspirate in the unconscious.

### Clouding of the level of consciousness
Consciousness is almost always depressed in patients with sepsis, even before the arterial blood pressure falls. The blood–brain barrier is damaged and the cerebral metabolic rate increases. These changes are reversible.

### Hyperventilation and hypoxia
The development of acute lung injury (ALI) is often a marker of infection. It is a common accompaniment of septic shock and MOF (see Chapter 9). Tachypnoea and respiratory alkalosis are amongst the first signs of systemic sepsis.

### Supraventricular arrhythmias
Atrial fibrillation (AF) and supraventricular tachycardia (SVT) occur in at least 40% of all patients with septic episodes.

### Jaundice
Jaundice occurs frequently during septic episodes and is related to hepatocellular dysfunction. It is of uncertain aetiology and is reversible, resolving as the sepsis resolves. Biliary obstruction and alcalculous cholecystitis must be considered in the differential diagnosis if the underlying cause of sepsis is not obvious.

### Gastrointestinal bleeding
Signs of sepsis include a low gastric pH and mucosal bleeding. Restoration of the circulating volume is crucial. Prophylactic treatment should be instituted and NG feeding should be commenced whenever possible.

### Metabolic disturbances
Glucose intolerance: Glucose intolerance is very common during sepsis. Insulin usually is not necessary unless the serum glucose is more than 10 mmol/L, when neutrophil function can be compromised. Hyperglycaemia is primarily caused by gluconeogenesis, although there is also a relative insulin resistance.

Catabolism, proteolysis or 'auto-cannibalism' and wasting are universal features of sepsis and cannot be greatly modified by parenteral nutrition (see Chapter 5).

Fat: Increasing lipolysis and increasing concentrations of free fatty acids are initial features, followed by decreased triglyceride clearance.

## Coagulation disorders

Thrombocytopaenia: Thrombocytopaenia is common and is due to marrow suppression and increased peripheral consumption. Though often severe ($< 30\ 000/mm^3$), it is reversible, usually is not clinically significant and does not require transfusion.

Coagulopathy: Coagulopathy is very common, but rarely severe, except in specific types of septicaemia such as meningococcal or pneumococcal infection. Fibrin levels are often increased, partial thromboplastin time is increased and fibrin degradation products (FDPs) or $d$-dimer levels are equivocal. The associated disseminated intravascular coagulopathy is usually mild, rarely requires active management and resolves when the sepsis is controlled.

## Renal insufficiency

Renal failure is a frequent and dreaded accompaniment of sepsis. The pathophysiology is uncertain. It often presents as oliguria and uraemia, but it can also be non-oliguric (see Chapter 26).

## Diagnosis

The diagnosis of sepsis is made on the basis of a cluster of the foregoing features, especially in combination with a defect in the host's defence mechanisms such as occurs in the presence of acute renal failure and granulocytopaenia. Immune depression is also a feature of the critically ill or nutritionally depleted patients. The presentation of sepsis is quite variable, with some features being more prominent than others in different patients. The history of the event is very important even if not immediately available. Take the time to get a detailed description from relatives, emergency department staff and ward staff. Pay particular attention to operation and anaesthetic notes, past microbiology and antibiotic history. This history will make finding a source easier. Entities such as 'cold' (vasoconstricted) or 'warm' (vasodilated) shock are host mediated, not organism mediated. Often, 'cold' sepsis simply represents an inadequately resuscitated, hypovolaemic patient. The diagnosis of septicaemia is made clinically. Investigations support the diagnosis.

## Blood cultures

The sensitivity of blood cultures is maximised by taking 30–40 ml/episode of bacteraemia. This necessitates several sets percutaneously. Taking more than 50 ml only gives marginally more sensitivity and is discouraged. Sterilisation of the skin before taking blood for culture is critical. Isolation of skin organisms such as coagulase negative staphylococci (*Staphylococcus epidermidis*) creates diagnostic uncertainty. Skin organisms are the usual cause of contaminants, but may also be a significant cause of certain types of infections, especially central line infections. It is desirable to minimise contamination with good skin preparation.

Povidone iodine takes several minutes to act. Alcohol base solutions of chlorhexidine or iodine are preferred, as they act immediately and have been shown to significantly reduce contamination rates of blood cultures.

The findings from blood cultures are positive in less than 30% of patients with septicaemia, either because of concurrent antibiotic treatment or because the host response may be triggered by non-microbial factors.

### White cells

The whole white cell count (WCC) is often elevated in sepsis but can be within normal range or reduced. Leucopaenia indicates a poor prognosis. A consistent finding in the presence of sepsis is 'toxic' changes in the white cells – toxic granulation, vacuolation, Dohle bodies, disintegrated or 'moth eaten' appearance of neutrophils. Even when the WCC is normal in the presence of sepsis, these changes are almost invariable.

## Other investigations

Identification of a septic source is paramount. Further investigations are performed in order to identify the septic site.

### Relevant cultures (e.g. sputum, urine, CSF, wound, dialysate)

Specialised techniques may be necessary to isolate lung organisms.

### Chest x-ray

Pneumonia or a lung abscess can be a primary source of infection. Acute lung injury is a non-specific accompaniment of sepsis from any site.

### Invasive catheters

Take a culture from the tip or intradermal section.

### Sinusitis

Perform a lateral skull x-ray, CT scan or ultrasound to exclude sinusitis associated with a NG tube or nasotracheal (NT) tube. This is often overlooked and is a frequent cause of fever in ICU.

### C-reactive protein

C-reactive protein is a sensitive marker of sepsis, especially if a baseline value is known.

### Serology

Serology usually involves testing for a rise in antibody titre. The difference between acute phase and convalescent phase serology findings usually has to be more than four-fold. An elevated IgM antibody – (an acute phase specimen) may also be diagnostic. It is important that acute phase and convalescent phase sera be titrated together in order to minimise laboratory error. Serology may be important when pneumonia, meningoencephalitis and myocarditis are thought to be involved in the septic syndrome. Unfortunately, serology is usually useful only retrospectively.

## Imaging: ultrasound or CT scan

Imaging is mandatory if an abdominal source of infection is suspected. A CT scan of the chest may sometimes demonstrate an abscess or consolidation not seen on chest x-ray.

## Nuclear medicine

Leucocyte or gallium scan are non-specific markers of an inflammatory response.

## Diagnostic surgery

**Early and aggressive surgery is often necessary for diagnosis and treatment – especially in the presence of intra-abdominal sepsis.**

## Routine monitoring

The following are suggested guidelines for monitoring patients with septicaemia:

- Vital signs: BP, pulse rate, respiratory rate and temperature.
- Continuous ECG and pulse oximetry.
- Urine output, hourly.
- Arterial blood gases and pH, twice daily.
- Blood sugar, 4-hourly.
- Chest x-ray, daily.
- ECG, daily.
- Platelet count, prothrombin time, fibrinogen, FDPs or *d*-dimers, daily.
- Renal function tests, daily.
- Liver function tests, daily.
- Invasive monitoring – e.g. monitoring intravascular filling with central venous pressure (CVP), pulmonary artery wedge pressure (PAWP).

## Definitive management (Table 13.6)

### Underlying cause

**Identify and remove underlying cause. Drainage or removal of the source of sepsis is currently the most important aspect of treatment in septicaemia.** No stone can be left unturned in the search for the septic source, even if that means multiple laparotomies or drainage procedures. Necrotic tissue as well as infected tissue must be widely excised.

**Table 13.6.** Management of septicaemia

---

Preventive
  Rapid and efficient resuscitation
  Handwashing between patients
  Aseptic techniques
  Strict and firmly enforced antibiotic policies
  Avoid gastric alkalinisation for stress ulcer prophylaxis
  Avoid immunosuppressive drugs and support immune system
Definitive
  Drainage or removal of the source of sepsis
  Antimicrobials
Supportive
  Fluid – often needed in large amounts to maintain adequate circulating volume
  Maintain haemoglobin >10 g/dl
  Maintain PaO$_2$ to at least 60 mmHg (7.2 kPa)
    High flow mask
    CPAP
    Artificial ventilation
Provide catecholamine support once intravascular volume is corrected.
  Adrenaline/noradrenaline is a common first line choice for hypotension
  *or*
  Dobutamine for low output states
  Digoxin, amiodorone or verapamil for supraventricular tachyarrhythmias
  Prevention of stress ulceration
  Nutritional support
  Early dialysis if there is renal insufficiency

---

## Antimicrobials

Antibiotics are discussed in more detail later in this chapter. Although antibiotics have an undisputed role in certain primary or community-acquired infections, their role in nosocomial infections is less clear. Any antibiotic will have some influence on the flora found in patients in the hospital and in the community at large. They lead to the selection of resistant organisms, which in turn demand agents with an even broader spectrum. However, wide-spectrum antibiotics have traditionally been commenced in a blind fashion, after blood and other cultures have been taken. They have proved to be disappointing in the ICU, unless definite bacteria have been isolated. Even then they are valueless, unless the source of infection is attended to. If no specific bacteria are found, broad-spectrum antibiotics are worth a trial for a definite and limited period. If there is no response, they should be stopped and further attempts should be made to isolate the organism. Increasingly the concept of 'non-bacterial septicaemia' is being accepted. In these cases we must question the validity of continuing blind antibiotic therapy.

## Corticosteroids
Large doses are ineffective and harmful. There may be a role for small doses of hydrocortisone in patients with demonstrated adrenal insufficiency.

## Continuous haemofiltration/haemodialysis
These techniques have been demonstrated to improve some aspects of organ function and survival in animal trials, presumably by filtering molecules which are implicated in sepsis. Studies demonstrating efficacy in sepsis are awaited.

## Other drugs
Human recombinant activated protein C has been shown to improve mortality in patients with proven infection causing severe sepsis with at least one organ failure and a high risk of death. Care should be exercised in patients with increased risk of bleeding. The drug should not be used in patients who have a high risk of imminent death and it should only be employed after attempted full resuscitation. The absolute reduction in mortality, while significant, is not large. Use has so far been restricted because of the drug's extremely high cost.

Monoclonal antibodies directed against bacterial lipopolysaccharide or endotoxin have so far been ineffective. Similarly, anti-cytokines are ineffective. In view of the complexity of sepsis and the fact that a single key mediator has not, as yet, been identified, it is unlikely that a single 'magic bullet' will be successful.

Steroids are recommended for patients with severe sepsis, unresponsive to catecholamines and who do not respond to a short synacthen test.

## Supportive management

There is no guarantee that oxygen and substrates will be delivered through the disordered microcirculation and even if they are, utilisation by damaged cells may be impaired. Nevertheless, the mainstay of supportive treatment, as with other forms of shock, is to optimise arterial oxygen content and tissue perfusion and to match $DO_2$ delivery with $VO_2$ (see Chapters 8 and 16).

### Arterial oxygen content
**Oxygen delivery = Cardiac output × (Haemoglobin concentration × Oxygen saturation × 1.34)**

Haemoglobin: Maintain haemoglobin >10 g/dl. Patients without acute coronary syndromes may tolerate haemoglobin as low as 8 g/dl.

Oxygenation: Adequate tissue concentration of oxygen is important for the prevention and control of infection. Oxygen transport to the mitochondria from the capillaries is driven by a pressure gradient. The $PaO_2$ should be kept as close as possible to 'normal'. Although we often accept partial pressures of around 60 mmHg (8 kPa), pressures close to the normal of 100 mmHg (13.3 kPa) are necessary for optimal wound healing and resistance to bacteria.

Monitor oxygen with regular determinations of mixed venous oxygen saturation and lactate concentrations may also be useful.

High flow oxygen delivered via a conventional mask might be sufficient.

Continuous positive airway pressure (CPAP) has many advantages over artificial ventilation. Spontaneous respiration, either with a special mask or via an endotracheal tube (ETT), should be maintained if possible.

If adequate ventilation is not possible with CPAP, artificial ventilation with positive end-expiratory pressure (PEEP) may be necessary. Where possible, techniques such as 'pressure limited' ventilation or intermittent mandatory ventilation (IMV) should be used, rather than intermittent positive-pressure ventilation (IPPV) and PEEP, in order to decrease the deleterious effects of increased intrathoracic pressure.

Patients should be nursed in an upright position in most cases, in order to achieve optimum oxygenation.

Maintain euvolaemic dehydration: That is, maintain a normal intravascular volume while minimising interstitial overload in order to minimise tissue oedema and maximise $DO_2$.

### Tissue perfusion

**The key to cardiovascular support in patients with septicaemia is fluid volume replacement, as the primary abnormality is vasodilatation.**

It is crucial that one aggressively corrects cardiovascular impairment, as oxygen utilisation is dependent on adequate tissue perfusion. It is not enough to correct the intravascular volume to 'normal' levels, as the circulation is vasodilated. Large infusions of fluid are usually necessary to achieve adequate cellular perfusion.

Fluids: Colloid or blood, depending on the haemoglobin concentration, is the most efficient means of resuscitating the intravascular space. Colloid or blood will correct intravascular volume deficits more rapidly than crystalloids, will stay in the circulation longer and will not cause as much pulmonary and peripheral oedema.

Large amounts (200–800 ml/h) of fluid may be needed to support the circulation in patients with sepsis. Average requirements are about 100–200 ml/h.

The fluid challenge technique is the most effective means of estimating the intravascular volume. Both before and after a bolus (200–500 ml) of fluid, measure as many indicators of intravascular volume as possible (e.g. pulse rate, BP, CVP, PAWP, urine output and peripheral perfusion). The patient's response will give an indication of the degree of hypovolaemia.

Cardiovascular measurements: Regular or continuous measurements of pulse rate, BP, urine output and CVP are essential for manipulation of the cardiovascular system in patients with sepsis. Pulmonary artery wedge pressure does not correlate well with left ventricular filling in patients with sepsis, but like CVP, it is useful to show a trend and as a guide to filling pressures.

Hypovolaemia, vasodilatation and, more rarely, pump failure may occur simultaneously in the presence of sepsis. Determinations of cardiac output and PAWP may therefore be useful. Determinations of $VO_2$ and $DO_2$ may be of help in optimising cardiovascular support. Dual oximetry and continuous measurement of mixed venous oxygen saturation ($SvO_2$) may sometimes be useful for determining adequate $DO_2$.

Inotropes and vasopressors: Cardiac output, even in the advanced stages of sepsis, is usually high and the peripheral vascular resistance low. In the presence of reduced tissue perfusion, this represents a therapeutic dilemma. Maintaining intravascular volume with fluid in the face of vasodilatation is the most important manoeuvre.

Inotropes such as dobutamine and dopexamine cause vasodilatation and increased cardiac output, which are already features of sepsis. However, in the presence of demonstrated inadequacies of cardiac output and $DO_2$ and after correction of hypovolaemia and hypotension, these drugs may have a limited role. Simultaneous estimations of $DO_2$ and demand may provide firmer indications for the use of drugs such as dobutamine and dopexamine.

When hypotension is the main cardiovascular problem in a patient with septicaemia, a drug with combined inotropic and vasopressor activities, such as adrenaline or noradrenaline, may be indicated. In moderate dosages, they seem to increase the perfusion pressure for vital organs such as the heart, kidneys and brain, without causing decreases in peripheral perfusion or renal blood flow.

- Adrenaline, 5–20 mg in 500 ml, titrated against the patient's responses, commencing at 0.5 $\mu g \cdot kg^{-1} \cdot min^{-1}$ · Very high dosages may be necessary to maintain the BP in patients with severe sepsis.
- Noradrenaline, 4–20 mg/500 ml, titrated against patient's responses as for adrenaline.
- Dobutamine, up to 10 $\mu g \cdot kg^{-1} \cdot min^{-1}$, is usually used to improve cardiac output, in an attempt to match $DO_2$ with $VO_2$.

Dopamine in higher doses has $\beta$ and $\alpha$ spectra that are simulated by other equally effective and cheaper drugs (e.g. adrenaline). There may also be a place for vasopressin or one of its analogues (e.g. terlipressin) in patients with refractory hypotension unresponsive to noradrenaline.

After the intravascular volume has been corrected, a combination of these catecholamines may be necessary to maintain perfusion pressure and tissue blood flow.

If the intravascular volume is maintained, peripheral perfusion will usually remain adequate despite the use of drugs with intense vasoconstrictive properties. Occasionally there may still be ischaemia (e.g. gangrenous hands, with palpable radial pulses) especially in infections such as meningococcal septicaemia. Drugs that might seem to be conceptually appealing in this situation have been universally disappointing (e.g. heparin, aprotinin, vasodilators, prostaglandins). There is a resurgence of interest in corticosteroids in severe sepsis unresponsive to other treatment, especially if there is doubt about adrenal function.

## Supraventricular arrhythmias

Arrhythmias such as sinus tachycardia, SVT and AF are very common in patients with sepsis. They often cause further cardiovascular compromise. Management is discussed elsewhere.

## Other measures

Use NG feeding if tolerated; otherwise use intravenous nutrition (IVN). If gastric feeding is not tolerated, prokinetic agents can be used or small bowel feeding attempted. Enteral immunonutrition may improve outcome in sepsis. Stress ulcer prophylaxis should be commenced if gastric feeding is not tolerated. Blood sugar levels should be controlled between 6 and 10 mmol/1. Vitamins should be given and early dialysis should be considered if acute renal failure supervenes. Prophylaxis for venous thromboembolism should be used for septic patients. Low dose unfractionated or low molecular weight heparins can both be used. The addition of intermittent pneumatic compression or compression stockings may add extra benefit.

## Outcome

Despite the use of powerful antimicrobials and sophisticated life-support systems, there continues to be a high incidence of septic shock with a mortality rate that has remained around 50% for over 20 years.

# Approach to the unidentified infection

Patients in the ICU often have signs of sepsis such as fever, leucocytosis, hyperglycaemia, decreased level of consciousness, hypoxia, hyperventilation or jaundice. None of these by itself necessarily means that a patient is septic. The diagnosis of septicaemia is based on clinical criteria and the difficulties associated with that limitation can be compounded by the fact that isolation of an offending microbe often is not possible. There must be a methodical and relentless search for the cause of infection (Table 13.7).

## Blood culture

If possible, the diagnosis of sepsis should be confirmed by culture of an organism. A search for the organism or site of sepsis must be made, including blood and other routine cultures. Blood cultures should be taken from at least two sites using an aerobic and anaerobic bottle. This will aid interpretation should skin

**Table 13.7.** Approach to unidentified infection

---

1 Conduct a physical examination looking for features of septicaemia and possible sources. Examine the mouth, teeth, wounds, catheter sites, heart sounds, abdomen, pressure areas and peritoneal fluid if relevant. Examine the chest and listen for bronchial breath sounds. Examine the patient's back for perianal infections, pressure areas and epididymitis in association with prolonged catheterisation.

2 Examine cultures from wounds, blood, sputum and urine – check Gram stain as well as culture and sensitivity.

3 Chest x-ray for evidence of pneumonia.

4 If an intra-abdominal source of sepsis is suspected, an ultrasound or CT scan may be helpful.

5 Do not hesitate to re-explore wounds and perform repeated laparotomies for diagnostic and therapeutic purposes if conventional investigations are negative.

6 Change intravascular lines and send for culture. Consider other invasive sites.

7 Consider other causes for fever, leucocytosis (e.g. pulmonary embolus).

8 Exclude acalculous choleystitis.

9 A CT scan of the chest will sometimes demonstrate an abscess or consolidation not seen on chest x-ray.

10 Lateral skull x-ray, CT scan or ultrasound to exclude sinusitis associated with the NG or nasotracheal tubes.

11 Exclude endocarditis or endovascular infection, particularly on venous side of circulation with echocardiography.

12 Strategies such as endobronchial brushing, use of protected catheter culture, transbronchial biopsy or open lung biopsy may be necessary for unidentified pulmonary lesions.

13 Indium III leucocyte scanning may be useful for soft tissue infection, intra-abdominal sepsis or where there are no localising signs.

14 Viral infections – especially CMV and hepatitis B post blood product transfusion. Examine paired serum cultures and/or use microscopy if suspected.

---

organisms be isolated. There is little value in collecting more than four sets of blood cultures for one infective episode, unless infective endocarditis is suspected when at least six sets should be taken.

## Review of invasive lines

The diagnosis of catheter-related sepsis is made on the following basis:

1 Obvious clinical signs of local infection. Clinical signs usually occur late and are more common with peripheral catheters than with central venous catheters. As such, they are not necessarily good indicators of line-related sepsis.

2 Isolation of the same organism from blood cultures and from the removed catheter segment is indicative of line-associated sepsis. The infected catheter segment is often the intracutaneous segment, not the tip. Remember that the catheter itself does not become infected. Biofilms consisting of multilayered thicknesses of bacteria probably are deposited on many inorganic surfaces, such as vascular and urinary catheters. Removing the catheter does not

necessarily equate with removing the infection, especially if there is associated skin infection. The intradermal segment or intravenous (IV) thrombus will remain contaminated. Another catheter should not, therefore, be inserted in the same site, if it is obviously infected.

Change the catheter if there is any doubt and culture the organisms from it. There are, as yet, insufficient data to be dogmatic about changing catheters routinely.

Review other invasive sites (e.g. extraventricular drains, peritoneal dialysate, pacemakers).

Peripheral intravascular lines should be changed routinely after 48 hours.

## Pulmonary infections

Intrapulmonary shadowing seen on a chest x-ray is not specific. It can be related to many different conditions, such as pulmonary oedema, ALI and aspiration, and these cannot be specifically differentiated from pneumonia on the basis of a chest x-ray alone. A common dilemma in intensive care is to decide whether or not a patient with chest x-ray shadowing and other signs of infection has pneumonia. Pneumonia, in isolation, especially if it is nosocomial, rarely causes the clinical picture of severe systemic sepsis. Chest x-ray shadows that clear quickly, or shift position are less likely to be associated with pneumonia.

Positive findings on sputum cultures are common and usually reflect colonisation rather than infection. This is especially common with gram-negative rods including *Pseudomonas* spp., also with *Candida albicans* and *Staphylococcus aureus* (including MRSA).

Although sputum cultures from intubated patients are routinely examined, they correlate very poorly with the organism that causes pneumonia. This is probably because the sputum of intubated patients rapidly becomes colonised.

Transtracheal specimens, bronchial washings, specimens from transbronchial biopsy and 'guarded' bronchial specimens are more useful, but these secretions still can reflect airway colonisation, rather than the actual infected lung tissue.

Blood culture is an important way to isolate organisms that cause pneumonia. It is the only common specimen that is specific, but it has low sensitivity.

Biopsy via a bronchoscope or open lung biopsy, thus obtaining tissue from an obviously infected area, may be indicated in severe unresponsive pneumonia of unknown origin. However, other concomitant factors (e.g. coagulopathy and positive-pressure ventilation) may make this procedure hazardous.

### Common organisms
Community-acquired pneumonia:

*Streptococcus pneumoniae*
Legionnaires' disease

**Table 13.8.** Causes of immunosupression

Primary immunodeficiency
e.g. T-cell dysfunction
      Antibody production dysfunction
Diseases affecting immunity
e.g. Leukaemia, lymphoma, HIV, diabetes, liver and renal failure
Iatrogenic immunosupression
e.g. Drugs such as steroids or cytotoxics
      Invasive lines
Miscellaneous
e.g. Nutritional deficiency
      Elderly
      Injury

Viral pneumonia
*Staphylococcus aureus*
*Haemophilus influenzae*
*Mycoplasma pneumoniae*
Other atypical pneumonias (e.g. Q fever, psittacosis).

Aspiration pneumonia: Bacterial pneumonia following aspiration is not common and prophylactic antibiotics are not indicated. Where infection is present, it is usually with coliforms from oral flora.

Immunosuppressed patients: The type and severity of the immunosuppression has a major impact on the likely pathogens (Table 13.8).

HIV-positive patients: pneumocystis pneumonia, *Streptococcus pneumoniae*, *Haemophilus influenzae*, *Staphylococcus aureus*, viruses, fungi.

Neutropaenic patients: *Streptococcus pneumoniae*, *Haemophilus influenzae*, *Pseudomonas* spp., other resistant gram-negative rods, fungi such as aspergillus.

Nosocomial pneumonia: commonly coliforms or *Staphylococcus aureus*, including MRSA.

## Urinary tract infections

Colonisation of indwelling catheters invariably occurs and this predisposes to an increased incidence of urinary tract infection (UTI). The finding of bacteria and even cells in the urine does not necessarily equate with infection and treatment. Antibiotics should be commenced only if systemic infection is present and the urinary tract is thought to be the source.

Common hospital-acquired UTI organisms include *Escherichia coli*, *Klebsiella* spp., *Proteus* spp., *Serratia* spp., *Pseudomonas* spp., enterococci, *Staphylococcus aureus* and *Candida albicans*.

Frequent catheter changes will not reduce the incidence of bacteriuria and infection.

Urinary samples should be obtained by aspirating through prepared tubing, not from the collecting bag.

## Wounds

Wounds are often colonised by coliforms but usually they are not significant. In orthopaedic wounds *Staphylococcus aureus* and *Streptococcus pyogenes* can cause clinically significant infections. Abdominal wounds associated with bowel perforation can become infected with *Staphylococcus aureus*, streptococci, coliforms and anaerobes. Routine wound swabs are very difficult to interpret. Wound aspirates and tissue biopsies will give more accurate information. Findings from blood cultures are rarely positive.

## Occult infections

The search for occult infections includes a thorough physical examination. The following are some causes of occult infection in the ICU.

### Abdominal sepsis

Abdominal sepsis can occur as intra-abdominal abscess or acalculous cholecystitis.

### Fungal septicaemia

Long-term patients, especially on broad-spectrum antibiotics, can develop fungal septicaemia. The use of special blood cultures will allow more rapid diagnosis of fungaemia. However, findings from blood cultures are often negative in patients with systemic fungal infections.

### Lung abscess

Especially if associated with aspiration, lung abscess usually can be diagnosed on the basis of chest x-ray or CT scan.

### Sinusitis

Sinusitis is especially seen in association with nasotracheal intubation or NG tubes and after facial trauma. This is a common site of infection that often is overlooked. Fluid levels can be seen on routine lateral facial views, CT scan or on ultrasound. Sinusitis can cause meningitis, epidural and subdural abscesses, intracranial abscesses, lateral or cavernous sinus thrombosis and osteomyelitis. Orbital cellulitis may indicate infection of the sphenoid or ethnoid sinuses. The causative organisms usually are mixed aerobes and anaerobes, including *Staphyloccocus aureus*, from the upper respiratory tract. Although drainage and tube removal are the most important steps, chloramphenicol, penicillin and/or metronidazole are suitable antimicrobial agents.

## Tooth abscess
Tooth abscess can occur especially in long-term patients. Routinely inspect the oral cavity.

## Epididymitis
Epididymitis can occur in association with prolonged catheterisation.

## Brain abscess or meningitis
These can occur especially in association with head injuries.

## Perirectal abscess
Remember to inspect the patient's back.

## Decubitus ulcer
Remember to inspect the patient's back.

## Heart valves
Because of instrumentation of the heart, especially with pulmonary artery catheters, vegetations can grow on the heart valves. Although uncommon, these can become infected. Murmurs are rarely helpful in the diagnosis of right-sided endocarditis, which is commonly found in abusers of IV drugs, as well as in association with vascular catheterisation. If infection is suspected, transoephageal echocardiography is indicated.

# Antimicrobials

The patient's intact immune system is the most effective antimicrobial. Antibiotics are merely adjunct therapy – microbial debulking agents, buying time while the immune system becomes activated.

There is little difficulty in choosing the correct antimicrobial agent when the organism has been identified and its sensitivities are known. Unfortunately, that situation is uncommon in the seriously ill. The clinical setting in an ICU often is a microbiological nightmare (e.g. a septic patient with multiple intravascular lines, an ETT, a urinary catheter, pre-existing intrapulmonary shadowing of uncertain origin, having recently had an operation and often already on multiple 'blind' antibiotics).

Positive culture of organisms in these circumstances is almost impossible and even if an organism can be isolated, it will not be for at least 24 hours. This results in the use of 'best guess' antimicrobials, ideal for drug companies pushing the latest and most expensive antibiotics. The guidelines for how long these antibiotics should be used are either non-existent or empirical.

Antibiotics are only a small part of managing infections in intensive care. It is equally, if not more important, to identify and remove where possible the source of infection. At best antibiotics reduce the load of organisms so that the body's own immune system can overcome the infection.

## Principles of antimicrobial treatment in intensive care

Community-acquired infections should be treated according to the expected sensitivity of the organism implicated.

Nosocomial or hospital-acquired infections raise complex issues that vary from one hospital to another. Individual ICUs should study their own patterns of organisms and their sensitivities.

**Close co-operation with specialists in infectious diseases and microbiology is essential.**

Most systemic infections in intensive care are caused by the following organisms:

Nosocomial infections
> *Klebsiella* spp.
> *Proteus* spp.
> *Enterobacter* spp.
> *Citrobacter* spp.
> *Serratia* spp.
> *Pseudomonas* spp.
> *Acinetobacter* spp.
> *Candida* spp.
> *Staphylococcus aureus*

Community-acquired infections
> *Streptococcus pneumoniae*
> *Haemophilus influenzae*
> *Moraxella catarrhalis*
> *Escherichia coli*
> *Staphylococcus aureus*
> *Streptococcus pyogenes*

Consider the underlying disease (e.g. diabetics are often infected with mixed aerobes, burn patients and patients with leukaemia often have *Pseudomonas* spp.).

The nature of the antimicrobial must be known:

- tissue penetration
- optimum dose
- dosage interval
- toxic effects
- spectrum
- interactions.

Use monotherapy where possible. Cost is becoming increasingly important in all facets of medicine. We should no longer feel embarrassed about comparing the costs of antimicrobials and opting for the cheaper one whenever it is appropriate.

Antibiotics will alter the normal flora, encouraging overgrowth by organisms such as *Staphyloccocus aureus*, *Candida* spp. and *Pseudomonas* spp., especially in the respiratory tract and urinary tract. Broad-spectrum antibiotics encourage this phenomenon to a greater extent than do the more specific antibiotics.

Use empirical antibiotic treatment for 72 hours and monitor for clinical improvement in those patients from whom no organisms have been isolated. As in many other areas of intensive care, a titrational or challenge approach is most appropriate (i.e. commence best-guess antimicrobials and monitor clinical responses). If there has been no improvement, go to the next step:

1  Consider an occult source of sepsis. Surgery has a more important role than antibiotics in these cases.
2  Consider a non-microbial cause of the septic picture such as SIRS.
3  Consider other causes of fever or raised white cells.
4  Consider that inappropriate antibiotic treatment may have been selected (e.g. inadequate dose, spectrum or tissue penetration).

If there has been no improvement after 72 hours and there is no obvious occult infection, cease giving antibiotics, reculture and monitor the patient's progress. Another antimicrobial combination can be empirically commenced at a later stage, if indicated, rather than simply adding one antibiotic after the other.

There is no agreement on the duration of treatment or antibiotic 'course' in intensive care. Antibiotics vary in their time to reach maximum efficiency. For example, β-lactams and glycopeptides take 48–72 hours for maximum effectiveness, whereas aminoglycosides and quinolones will have peak bactericidal activity within 8 hours. As a guideline, if the antimicrobial has shown an effect within 3 days, cease the drug within 5–7 days. If there has been no effect at all, consider stopping after 3 days.

The original diagnosis of bacterial infection should also be examined (e.g. fever and leucocytosis do not necessarily mean infection). Consider other possibilities such as drug reactions, cytomegalovirus infection following transfusion (see p.   ), an occult source of sepsis, pancreatitis and other non-bacterial infections.

Once-daily IV doses of aminoglycosides are more bactericidal than are divided daily doses.

## Prophylactic antimicrobials with surgery

Prophylactic antibiotics should be used only with a procedure that commonly leads to infection (e.g. large bowel resection, contaminated tissue resection) or when an infection could cause devastating results (infection of prosthetic heart valve, implantation of foreign materials such as intracranial shunts and joint prostheses).

The antimicrobials selected should have a record of activity against the likely pathogens. Staphylococci should be covered for in procedures such as insertion of prostheses. Anaerobes and coliforms need to be covered for in gastrointestinal and genitourinary surgery.

Antimicrobials should be given about the time of induction of anaesthesia and for no more than 24 hours.

## Practical guidelines to prescribing antimicrobials

It is beyond the scope of this book to describe detailed antimicrobial guidelines for every infection and to discuss the pharmacology of every drug. Infection is common in intensive care and antimicrobials are widely used and very expensive. Staff working in ICUs should therefore familiarise themselves with this complex and rapidly changing area and work closely with their own microbiology department.

Clinical, laboratory and radiological findings will often give some indication of the source of infection.

Patterns of nosocomial infections within a particular ICU will offer further guidelines.

Immunocompromised hosts often require broader coverage against common gram-positive and gram-negative bacteria, including *Pseudomonas* spp.

### Pencillin allergy

Many patients labelled 'penicillin allergic' are not. For example, patients may have experienced a GIT problem when given a penicillin, which they may call 'allergy'. It is quite common for viral infections to cause rashes: if a penicillin was prescribed for a patient with a viral illness and a rash develops, they may mistakenly assume they are allergic to penicillin. It is necessary to explore exactly what happened when the patient took penicillin. Penicillins are often the most active agents against infections that require admissions to an ICU.

If patients describe a rash from penicillin, they may develop a similar rash when given a cephalosporin or carbapenem. However, it is highly unlikely they will develop anaphylaxis. However, if elements of a Type 1 reaction occurred with the administration of a penicillin such as facial swelling, difficulty breathing or full-blown anaphylaxis, there is a 5–10% chance of cephalosporins or carbapenem causing a Type 1 reaction. Consequently, a non β-lactam regimen is recommended. Note that the monobactam, aztreonam is the only β-lactam that does not cross-react with penicillin in patients with Type 1 reactions to penicillin and may safely be given to patients who develop anaphylaxis to penicillin.

If a patient has an infection such as endocarditis where the outcome is better when a penicillin is used, the patient can be desensitised to penicillin. In cases where it is unclear if the patient may have had a Type 1 reaction to penicillin and

**Table 13.9.** Commonly prescribed antibiotic doses

| | |
|---|---|
| Amphotericin | 1 mg/kg/24 hours |
| Ampicillin | 1–2 g IV 6-hourly |
| Cephalothin | 1–2 g IV 6-hourly |
| Cephazolin | 0.5–1 g IV 8-hourly |
| Cefotaxime | 1 g IV 8-hourly |
| Cefriaxone | 1–2 g IV daily |
| Ceftazidime | 2 g IV 8-hourly |
| Cephalothin | 1–2 g IV 6-hourly |
| Ciprofloxacin | 200–300 mg IV 12-hourly. |
| Clindamycin | 300–600 mg IV 6-hourly |
| Erythromycin | 0.5–1 g IV 6-hourly |
| Flucloxacillin | 1–2 g IV 6-hourly |
| Fluconazole | 100–200 mg IV once daily |
| Gentamicin | 3–5 mg/kg IV as once daily dose; monitor trough. Aim for a trough < 2 mg/L and a peak of 6–8 mg/L |
| Metronidazole | 500 mg IV 8-hourly |
| Penicillin | $2–3 \times 10^6$ units IV 6-hourly |
| Rifampicin | 600 mg orally 12-hourly |
| Timentin | 3.1 g IV 6-hourly |
| Vancomycin | 0.5–1g IV 12-hourly, monitored third daily with levels (trough < 15 mg/L; peak 20–40 mg/L) |

it is desirable to treat with a pencillin, skin testing can be carried out. If this is negative, then penicillin can be given without causing anaphylaxis. Advice from an immunologist should be sought in these settings.

## Approach to patients with infections of uncertain aetiology

The following guidelines are only for the initial 'blind' phase of antimicrobial treatment (Table 13.9). They must be adjusted according to microbiological findings, sensitivity patterns and local nosocomial pathogens.

### Septicaemia

Septicaemia of unknown origin can be treated as follows until microbiology findings are available:

Penicillin (e.g. ampicillin)
*plus*
gentamicin
±
metronidazole for abdominal or gynaecological infection
±

flucloxacillin (especially for community-acquired septicaemia). If MRSA is prevalent in a unit and the infection is nosocomial, substitute vancomycin.

### Pneumonia
Severe community acquired:

erythromycin
±
penicillin
*or*
cefotaxime
*or*
ceftriaxone.

Because of the high incidence of penicillin-resistant *Streptococci pneumoniae* and *Haemophilus influenzae* sensitivity, cefotaxime and cefriaxone are increasingly being used as first-line drugs.

Aspiration pneumonia: Aspiration pneumonia should be suspected in alcoholics, IV drug users, the debilitated and in the presence of a decreased level of consciousness. Mixed mouth organisms are common and require anaerobic cover.

benzylpenicillin
*plus*
metronidazole
*or*
timentin (ticarcillin plus clavulanate)
If allergic to penicillin, then ciprofloxacin plus metronidazole

Infection is rare after aspiration, e.g. on induction of anaesthesia. Antibiotics should not be commenced.

Hospital-acquired pneumonia:

gentamicin
±
ceftazidime
*or*
timentin
*or*
ciprofloxacin.

### Urinary tract infection
ampicillin
*plus*
gentamicin.

If allergic to penicillins, substitute cephalothin.

## Intra-abdominal infection

Ampicillin
*plus*
gentamicin
*plus*
metronidazole.

## Intravascular cannula infection

Remove the cannula and culture its adherent material. Possible organisms include *Staphylococcus aureus* and *S. epidermidis*. However, up to 30% of cannulae infections are gram-negative in origin and nearly always resistant to ampicillin and cephalosporins. Aminoglycosides should be used until culture results are available.

Flucloxacillin
*plus*
gentamicin.

If MRSA is prevalent, use vancomycin. If *Staphylococcus aureus* is grown in a blood culture and associated with an infected IV cannula, a transthoracic echocardiogram (TOE) and bone scan should be performed looking for sites of seeding. In this setting, antibiotics should be continued for 14 days if both tests are negative and for 6 weeks if one or other is positive.

## Neutropaenic patients

Liaise closely with microbiologists, as the host and invading organisms often present a challenge. These patients are susceptible to *Pseudomonas* spp., *Staphylococcus aureus*, fungi or coliforms, especially from the GIT. Because *Pseudomonas* spp. are associated with a high mortality, two agents should be used. The following regimen is for febrile neutropaenic patients in whom the source of infection is unknown. These recommendations should be modified as more precise information arrives from culture studies. Initial regimen before culture and sensitivities:

Gentamicin
*plus*
timentin.

If there is penicillin allergy, substitute ceftazidime. Do not use ceftriaxone or cefotaxime as their cover for pseudomonads is inadequate.

If the patient remains unresponsive, add:

vancomycin.

If the patient does not respond, give empirical antifungal therapy:

amphotericin B.

Some renal impairment is inevitable with amphotericin B. It can be reduced by maintaining intravascular volume and normal BP. The liposomal preparation should be used if creatinine increases significantly. Potassium and magnesium IV supplement should be used routinely. The infusion rate should be over at least 4 hours in order to prevent cardiac arrhythmias. Paracetamol or hydrocortisone may reduce associated rigors.

Continue until the neutropaenia resolves and liaise closely with the microbiology department. Do not use fluconazole or other antifungal agents in this situation.

The foregoing drugs for neutropaenic febrile patients should be used only initially, followed by a change to specific antimicrobials when an organism has been isolated. The use of antibiotics for empirical treatment should be based on analyses of the sensitivity patterns of the organisms that are causing infections in that particular haematology/oncology unit.

## Specific organisms

*Staphylococcus aureus*
flucloxacillin.

If penicillin allergy, use:
cephalothin
*or*
cephazolin.
If allergic to cephalosporin and penicillin use vancomycin.
Also use vancomycin according to local prevalence of MRSA.

*Streptococcus pyogenes*
clindamycin
*plus*
penicillin.

Alternatively:

First generation cephalosporin.
vancomycin.

### Pneumococcus
Penicillin
Pneumococci are increasingly resistant to penicillins and cephalosporins but can be partially overcome by increasing doses.
If allergic to penicillins use cephazolin.

### MRSA
Vancomycin causes marked thrombophlebitis – use a central line. Try to break the cycle of vancomycin needing a central line and a central line predisposing to

MRSA. Remove the central line as soon as possible and reinsert only if proven MRSA infection. Peripherally inserted central lines are effective in this setting.

### Pseudomonas aeruginosa

Regimens need to include two agents active against *Pseudomonas* spp., especially if septic shock is present. The mortality is > 80% if one antibiotic is given and 50% if a combination of β-lactam and aminoglycoside is used. A combination of β-lactam and quinolone is probably also effective.

Gentamicin
*plus*
timentin.

Alternatively, ceftazidine or meropenem can be substituted.

## Anaerobic infections

Anaerobes are a common part of the normal flora, especially in the GIT and help to prevent the overgrowth of coliforms. Anti-anaerobic drugs should therefore only be used when there is a strong suspicion of anaerobic infection such as in intra-abdominal infections, infection of the female genital tract, brain abscesses, some cases of aspiration pneumonia, gas gangrene or soft tissue infection.

The most active agent against anaerobes is metronidazole. A β-lactam/β-lactamase combination such as ticarcillin/clavulanate and carbapenems is also highly active against anaerobes. Clindamycin has less activity. β-lactamases are now prevalent amongst anaerobes in all sites and so penicillins alone are no longer recommended.

## Coliforms

Coliforms (Enterobacteriaceae) are part of the normal bowel flora. They cause urinary infections as single bacterial species infections. They are usually present with anaerobes and enterococci as mixed infections in intra-abdominal sepsis. These facts need to be borne in mind when selecting empiric antibiotic regimens.

Virtually all coliforms are resistant to ampicillin. Ampicillin remains useful for enterococci. If cephalosporins are used for mixed infections involving coliforms, you can expect enterococci to emerge, as they are intrinsically resistant to cephalosporins. Ampicillin is therefore used to stop enterococci selection; not to cover the coliforms. This is particularly important now that vancomycin-resistant enterococci have emerged in many ICUs.

If the patient has bacteraemia with coliforms, especially if shock is present, two agents active against the organism are recommended to enhance bacterial killing. Generally a combination of a β-lactam and aminoglycoside is given, e.g.

ceftriaxone plus gentamicin. If it is not desirable to use an aminoglycoside, use a combination of β-lactam and quinolone.

If the sepsis does not involve bacteraemia, single agent therapy works well. As most intra-abdominal infections are mixed, ampicillin and metronidazole are required to cover enterococci and anaerobes respectively.

The choice of antibiotic treatment depends on the sensitivities. Initial therapy:

gentamicin
*plus*
ampicillin
*plus*
metronidazole.

## Specific antibiotics

Suggested adult doses are given in Table 13.9. These may need to be modified in renal failure or hepatic dysfunction.

### Aminoglycosides

Aminoglycosides have narrow therapeutic ranges and need to be monitored closely, as they can cause nephrotoxicity and ototoxicity. Those can be potentiated when aminoglycosides are used with other drugs such as cephalosporins and frusemide. Their main value is their broad-spectrum activity against coliforms, pseudomonads and other gram-negative aerobic bacteria. They have excellent tissue penetration and are also the most rapidly bactericidal agents which is particularly important in bacteraemia. Aminoglycosides usually should be given as once-a-day doses, rather than in divided doses, as they are more efficacious and probably less toxic. The only exception to this is in endocarditis where they should be given 8-hourly.

Recommended serum concentrations (μg/ml) are as follows:

|  | Peak | Trough |
|---|---|---|
| gentamicin | 6–8 | <2 |
| tobramicin | 6–8 | <2 |
| amikacin | 20–25 | <10 |

Aminoglycosides such as tobramicin, amikacin and netilmicin should be reserved for serious infections that are resistant to gentamicin. However, resistance to gentamicin is very rare. Each ICU should determine its prevailing resistance patterns to various aminoglycosides.

## Beta-lactams

Penicillins, cephalosporins, carbapenems and monobactams are structurally related and share bactericidal activity primarily directed at the bacterial cell wall. β-lactams can also be combined with an inhibitor of β-lactamase.

## Penicillins

Narrow-spectrum penicillins: Examples include benzylpenicillin which is still active against streptococci, including *Streptococcus pneumoniae* and *Neisseria meningitidis*.

Antistaphylococcal penicillin: Because most strains of *Staphylococcus aureus* are resistant to penicillin G by virtue of β-lactamase production, treatment requires other agents (e.g. flucloxacillin or dicloxacillin). Increasingly, resistance to these compounds is being seen, especially in the hospital setting. In some hospitals up to 50% of staphyloccci isolated are resistant to methicillin.

Moderate-spectrum penicillins: Ampicillin and amoxycillin remain useful in intensive care mainly because of their activity against enterococci, but are destroyed by β-lactamase-producing strains. They also are usually active against *Haemophilus influenzae,* as well as some strains of *Escherichia coli* and *Proteus mirabilis.* Because about 50% of *Escherichia coli* isolates causing a UTI are resistant to ampicillin, it is inappropriate for the empirical treatment of UTI.

Broad-spectrum penicillins (antipseudomonal activity): Ticarcillin and piperacillin have wider ranges of activity than do ampicillin and amoxycillin against coliforms, in particular against the *Pseudomonas* spp. However, their clinical efficacy may be insufficient when they are used alone to treat *Pseudomonas* spp. infections and their gram-negative spectra are not as broad as those of the aminoglycosides. It is recommended, therefore, that they be used with an aminoglycoside. It is thus difficult to assess their true effectiveness in intensive care.

Penicillin/β-lactamase inhibitor combinations: The β-lactamase inhibitors clavulanate, sulbactam and tazobactam inhibit the enzyme produced by *Staphylococcus aureus* and *Bacteroides fragilis* and also the ubiquitous TEM enzyme, found in *Escherichia coli, Neisseria gonorrhoea* and *Haemophilus influenzae*. These three drugs possess little inherent antibacterial activity but when given with broader spectrum penicillins, they significantly extend their spectra of activity.

Examples include amoxycillin/clavulanate, ticarcillin/clavulanate, piperacillin/tazobactam. These are very broad-spectrum agents, covering staphylococci, streptococci, coliforms, pseudomonads and anaerobes. These combinations do not cover MRSA and enterococci.

## Cephalosporins

The deficiencies in cephalosporin coverage include MRSA, enterococci (enterococci are predictably selected out with these agents), *Listeria* monocytogenes and anaerobes. Widespread use of cephalosporins, especially third and fourth generation cephalosporins, puts substantial selection pressure on organisms both in the individual patient and in the flora throughout the ICU. For this reason, it is desirable to restrict their use. Outbreaks of resistant organisms such as MRSA, *Klebsiella* spp. and *Acinetobacter* spp. will often require curtailing the use of third-generation cephalosporins.

There are five classes of cephalosporins in clinical use:

First generation: Good gram-positive activity and some activity against coliforms. Useful substitute for pencillin or flucloxacillin in patients with penicillin allergy who have infections with streptococci and/or staphylococci, so long as the allergy is not anaphylaxis.

Second generation: Have 'niche' uses: cefaclor is widely used for respiratory tract infections, cefotetan is used in hepatobiliary surgery due to its high penetration into bile. Cefoxitin and cefotetan have some anti-anaerobic activity, but this action is inferior to agents such as metronidazole.

Third generation: Ceftriaxone and cefotaxime are usual agents having some activity against group A streptococci, excellent activity against *Streptococcus pneumoniae* and coliforms such as *Escherichia coli, Proteus mirabilis* and *Klebsiella* spp. They are not recommended for the 'ESCAPPM'(enterobacter, serratia, citrobacter, acinetobacter, *Proteus vulgaris*, Providentia, Morganella) group of nosocomial gram-negative rods.

Ceftazidime has excellent activity against *Pseudomonas aeruginosa* as well as *Escherichia coli, Proteus mirabilis* and *Klebsiella* spp. It is also not recommended for the 'ESCAPPM' group of nosocomial gram-negative rods. Note that ceftazidime has no useful gram-positive activity and must be used with other agents if gram-positive cover is required in a mixed infection.

Fourth generation: Cefepime and cefpirome. These agents have very broad-spectrum activity. Sensitive bacteria include staphylococci, streptococci, coliforms and pseudomonas. They also supposedly have activity against members of the 'ESCAPPM' group. They have no anti-anaerobic activity and are not useful for MRSA or enterocci.

It is tempting to resort to the cephalosporins because of their relative safety and their antibacterial spectra include gram-positive and gram-negative activities.

Because the activities of the first and second generation cephalosporins are unpredictable against gram-negative bacteria, they should not be employed for empirical, single-drug treatment. The third generation cephalosporins feature broad-spectrum, high antimicrobial potencies and excellent tissue penetration. However, several gaps are evident in the overall coverage afforded by all these drugs. For example, some enterococci, *Pseudomonas* spp. and anaerobes are resistant to third-generation cephalosporins (apart from ceftazidime). Their activity against *Staphylococcus aureus* precludes their use as single drugs against this organism. They cannot, therefore, be recommended for single-drug, empirical treatment. Because they are often used in combination with other antibiotics, such as the aminoglycosides, it is difficult to assess their independent usefulness in seriously ill patients. Cephalosporins are, however, useful in infections caused by sensitive organisms. Specifically, cefotaxime/ceftriaxone are the drugs of choice for most cases of bacterial meningitis because of their excellent tissue penetration.

## Monobactams

Aztreonam is a member of the family of monobactams. It is a highly active compound against the majority of gram-negative bacteria, but has no activity against gram-positive organisms and anaerobes. Its main usefulness is in the treatment of gram-negative rod infections for patients who are allergic to β-lactams, especially if the allergy is a Type I reaction, as cross-hypersensitivity does not occur.

## Carbapenems

Imipenem/cilastatin is the prototype of this class. Due to inactivation by a renal dipeptidase, it is formulated with cilastatin. These are amongst the widest spectrum antibiotics available. They have activity against gram-negative bacteria comparable with that of the aminoglycosides. They have excellent activity against anaerobes and many gram-positive cocci. However, they are not active against MRSA, *Enterococcus faecium*, *Mycoplasma*, *Stenotrophomonas*, *Chlamydia* and some species of *Pseudomonas*. Unusual and highly resistant bacteria such as *Stenotrophomonas maltophilia* are often selected out by this agent. Imipenem is renowned for inducing seizures, especially in the setting of a reduced seizure threshold and renal insufficiency. Meropenem has better CSF levels and is far less likely to cause fitting in these two situations. Meropenem is somewhat more active against gram-negative and less active against gram-positive than imipenem and because it is resistant to renal dipeptidase, it can be given alone.

## Nitroimidazoles

Metronidazole and timidazole cover includes *Bacteroides fragilis*, gram-positive anaerobes and anaerobic protozoa.

## Macrolides

These include erythromycin and roxithromycin. Their cover includes gram-positive cocci, *Haemophilus influenzae*, *Legionella*, *Mycoplasma*, gram-negative cocci and some anaerobes.

## Glycopeptides

Vancomycin and teicoplanin are active against a wide range of gram-positive organisms. Vancomycin is particularly useful in intensive care for the treatment of MRSA and infections due to *Staphylococcus epidermidis* or *Corynebacterium* spp. associated with prosthetic heart valves. Oral vancomycin is useful in patients with antibiotic-associated colitis due to *Clostridium difficile*. The use of vancomycin is associated with the emergence of vancomycin-resistant enterococci (VRE). For this reason, vancomycin should not be used for prophylaxis and only used for treatment if MRSA is proven or highly likely to be the cause of infection.

## Quinolones

Examples include norfloxacin, ciprofloxacin, enoxacin and ofloxacin. These agents have some theoretical attractions. They are bactericidal, with wide distributions throughout the body and have little effect on anaerobic gut flora. The newer agents have a wide spectra of activity, including some gram-positive cocci and many gram-negative bacteria. However, they are expensive and their place in the treatment of the seriously ill has not yet been defined. Their greatest usefulness may be in providing an alternative for infections with antibiotic-resistant coliforms and in situations where aminoglycosides are contraindicated. Fourth generation quinolones have offered promise in serious infections such as meningitis with penicillin-resistant *Streptococcus pneumoniae*. Unfortunately some have been withdrawn from the market due to serious and occasionally lethal toxicity.

## The 'latest' antibiotics

Today there is considerable pressure to use the latest and most expensive antibiotics. Many have been marketed and touted as being broad-spectrum replacements for aminoglycosides, as having stability against β-lactamases and as being relatively free of serious side effects. However, we need to temper our enthusiasm about their possible role in the ICU. Some comments about their clinical use in intensive care include:

- There is a danger that if they are overused, superinfections and resistances will become more common.
- Apart from their use as the first-line treatment for gram-negative meningitis, third generation cephalosporins should be used as reserve antibiotics for cases in which there are definite bacteriological indications.
- Often the 'latest' drugs are prescribed because they are currently fashionable and because of the pressure of product promotion, rather than logic.
- The full extent of the toxicity may not be appreciated, as was the case with some newer quinolones.
- The 'latest' drugs are invariably more expensive.

Scepticism and caution should be exercised when considering the use of the latest broad-spectrum antibiotics, such as imipenem/cilastatin, fourth generation cephalosporins, aztreonam and the quinolone derivatives. The mortality from septicaemia remains relatively unchanged, despite the introduction of broader spectrum antimicrobials. Many other aspects of management are equally as important as the use of antibiotics, if not more important, especially in the presence of 'non-bacterial' septicaemia. It appears that many of the more recent broad-spectrum antibiotics are expensive and still largely unproven adjuncts to treatment.

## Intra-abdominal sepsis

There is no strict dividing line between generalised intra-abdominal sepsis and abscess or peritonitis. 'Intra-abdominal sepsis' is a term that loosely refers to a generalised infection and/or localised collections. Intra-abdominal collections or abscesses can be found intraperitoneally, retroperitoneally or within viscera.

The most important principle in the management of intra-abdominal sepsis is removal and drainage. Antibiotics have a limited role in controlling the associated systemic infection. Otherwise, the role of intensive care is to keep the patient alive until the source of the sepsis can be found and evacuated.

The message to reluctant surgeons is this: Rather than viewing patients with intra-abdominal sepsis as being too sick for surgery, they should be viewed as too sick not to have surgery. Intra-abdominal infection remains a common and catastrophic event, entailing high mortality, often associated with MOF (see Chapter 9).

### Peritonitis

Contamination of the peritoneal cavity usually results in abdominal pain, guarding and rebound tenderness. These signs can become masked or modified in the elderly, in postoperative patients and in immunocompromised patients.

#### Diagnosis

The diagnosis of peritonitis is supported by a leucocytosis with toxic changes, fever and other signs of systemic sepsis. Radiological findings include free abdominal gas and/or fluid. Abdominal ultrasound or CT scan may demonstrate a source of the peritonitis. Blood cultures and routine investigations should be performed.

#### Management

Supportive care: The patient should be urgently prepared for surgery. Rapidly restore the intravascular volume and give blood if necessary, according to intravascular measurements such as arterial BP, pulse rate, CVP, PAWP and hourly urine output (see Chapter 19).

Other forms of support, such as inotropes, may be necessary as for generalised sepsis.

**Surgery: Immediate surgery is the most important step in the management of peritonitis.** The underlying source of contamination must be eliminated. **Radical surgical debridement,** as in any other form of infection, is required. The surgical team should send specimens for microbiological evaluation to aid the diagnosis.

Meticulous inspection and lavage of the intra-abdominal cavity are necessary. Postoperative drainage is essential.

The role of antibiotics in the lavage fluid and the advisability of continuous postoperative lavage have not been established.

Continuing resuscitation and general care of the seriously ill are required until all signs of infection have disappeared. Unfortunately, infection sometimes persists in the form of generalised intra-abdominal sepsis or localised collections and repeated laparotomies may be necessary.

Antibiotics:

Gentamicin
*plus*
metronidazole to cover anaerobic bacteria
*plus*
ampicillin to cover enterococci.

Then tailor antibiotic treatment according to the organisms and sensitivities identified. Continue for 5 days postoperatively, then reassess.

**If fever or signs of sepsis continue postoperatively, reinvestigation of the source and further aggressive surgical intervention are required – not additional antibiotics.**


## Intra-abdominal sepsis

'Intra-abdominal sepsis' is used here not only to refer to peritonitis but also as a general term encompassing abscesses and generalised infections, as well as possible peritoneal involvement.

### Diagnosis

Frequently there are no abdominal signs to be found in a patient with an intra-abdominal abscess. Systemic signs and symptoms of generalised sepsis are usually more prominent than local signs. These include the same features seen with septicaemia.

A septic patient may have a classic 'swinging' fever. Also, there may be changes in the patient's mental status, as well as glucose intolerance, a decrease in gastric mucosal pH, cardiovascular decompensation, hypoxia and ALI or other signs of MOF.

**An immediate, aggressive search must be made for the source of sepsis.**

Ultrasound: The sensitivity and specificity of abdominal ultrasound will vary according to many factors, including the experience of the operator, the quality of equipment and the presence of gas, drainage tubes and dressings, all of which can obscure the image. The use of portable real time ultrasound and the possibility of fine needle aspiration for diagnosis and even treatment may prevent unnecessary surgery in some cases. However, extensive debridement at laparotomy is often necessary.

CT scan: A CT scan may be more suitable than ultrasound for use in the seriously ill and postoperative patients, because it is not as strongly affected by gas and other artefacts. Oral and IV contrast should be given as part of the CT examination in order to enhance collections. The CT can also provide better views of certain areas, such as the retroperitoneal space. Percutaneous drainage in conjunction with CT scanning can also be performed. However, for CT, patients must be transported to an area of the hospital where routine monitoring can be difficult and facilities for continuous supportive care not ideal.

Radionuclide imaging: Although imaging with gallium citrate is unrewarding for investigating collections in the seriously ill, imaging with indium-III-labelled leucocytes is sometimes useful. However, there can be false-positive findings with indium III, because the leucocytes are attracted to areas of inflammation and vascularity, as well as definite infective foci. The labelled leucocytes may be taken up by the spleen and liver, but not normally by the kidneys or bowel. There can be false-negative findings when imaging chronic infective sites such as those involved in osteomyelitis.

Surgery: **Laparotomy in this setting is often an essential diagnostic tool**. If the patient remains septic and the abdomen is suspected as a continuing source of sepsis, laparotomy is mandatory.

## Treatment

**Drainage of the pus and debridement of necrotic tissue is essential**. This can sometimes be achieved with fine needle aspiration, but more often requires surgery, preferably by a surgeon with experience in this area.

Meticulous exploration of the wound and abdominal cavity is mandatory. Extensive debridement and adequate drainage are essential. It is usually not enough to percutaneously drain the contents of an intra-abdominal abscess as the cavity wall itself can be inflamed or necrotic and a source of continuing sepsis.

If there are any further signs of continuing sepsis,
**Re-investigation and re-exploration are mandatory.**

To aid re-exploration, some authors have proposed:

- Leaving the abdominal cavity open and packing it, or
- partially closing the abdominal cavity with material such as Marlex mesh.

These approaches are especially useful if the patient has high intra-abdominal pressure.

Antibiotics: Studies of blood cultures and other routine microbiological cultures should be performed in an attempt to isolate the organism.

If there are no positive cultures, empirical antibiotic treatment, as for peritonitis, should be commenced while the source of sepsis is being sought.

Other management principles:

- General supportive measures, as for septicaemia.

erythematous, oedematous and painful. Local drainage procedures are usually effective.

Following contaminated surgery, wound infections usually involve polymicrobial flora of the resected organ. The incubation period of gram-negative wound infections is 7–14 days. They produce more diffuse signs than do the staphylococcal manifestations, such as fever, tachycardia and bacteraemia. These infections should be treated with local drainage procedures as well as antibiotics.

Infections usually occur beginning on the fourth postoperative day. Wound infections occurring within the first 48 hours characteristically are caused by either clostridial or β-haemolytic streptococci. They can rapidly cause systemic symptoms and are associated with a high mortality. Aggressive wound care, including debridement as well as broad-spectrum high-dose antibiotic coverage, is essential.

Surgery: **Wound infections can be sources of life-threatening, generalised septicaemia. If there is any doubt, the wound must be re-explored and drained.**

### Necrotising fasciitis

Necrotising fasciitis is a relatively rare, potentially fatal necrotising infection of the subcutaneous tissue and superficial fascia with secondary necrosis of the overlying skin.

This infection can be due to virulent strains of *Streptococcus pyogenes* and/or *Staphylococcus aureus* but can also be due to a mixed infection with anaerobes and coliforms.

The skin rapidly becomes warm, oedematous, painful and discoloured.

The area of necrotic tissue can eventually be estimated on the basis of the anaesthesia of the overlying skin due to subcutaneous nerve destruction.

Magnetics resonance imaging (MRI) scanning is the investigation of choice – this is the most sensitive test to detect deep infective complications such as necrotising fasciitis, myositis and osteomyelitis. The early diagnosis of these conditions is essential to prompt early surgical intervention.

The extent of underlying necrosis cannot be fully appreciated by simply examining the overlying skin.

**The most important aspect of management is radical and repeated surgical excision, as well as aggressive debridement of the necrotic tissue.**

Suggested initial empirical antibiotic therapy:

benzylpenicillin
*plus*
gentamicin
*plus*
metronidazole.

## Legionnaires' disease

Legionnaires' disease often occurs as sporadic epidemics caused by inhalation of infected droplets from air conditioning, cooling towers or contaminated hotwater plumbing. Nosocomial Legionnaires' disease can also occur from the same sources. The disease is more common in people with underlying pulmonary disease and/or T-cell immunodeficiency. Legionnaires' disease is probably underdiagnosed. It is more easily recognised when it presents with a severe multilobar pneumonia together with systemic manifestations.

### Presentation
These patients present with pulmonary complaints such as coughing and purulent or blood-stained sputum.

Extrapulmonary manifestations can include very high fever, rigors, diarrhoea, myalgia, arthralgia, renal failure, myocarditis, headache and clouded sensorium.

### Diagnosis
Direct fluorescent antibody (DFA) tests on sputum have high numbers of false negatives and false positives and may not cover the many different serotypes. However, if the pretest probability of the disease is high, i.e. full constellation of clinical and laboratory features, it may offer rapid supportive evidence. A DFA should not be performed if the pretest probability is low.

Culture of the organism from sputum or bronchoscopy specimens has 100% specificity. Unfortunately it is insensitive and takes up to 2 weeks to be positive.

Urinary antigen test – 99% sensitive for *Legionella pneumophila* serogroup 1. However this represents only 40–50% of Legionnaires' disease in some countries.

Serology is quite sensitive, but can take up to 6 weeks to show positive findings.

### Treatment
Ciprofloxin
*or*
erythromycin
±
rifampicin, 600 mg orally, 12-hourly.

## Toxic shock syndrome

Toxic shock syndrome (TSS) is often associated with the use of tampons by women; it can follow nasal packing and can accompany influenza episodes and staphylococcal infection, as well as pharyngitis, tracheitis, pneumonitis and pulmonary abscess. It can also occur in association with streptococcal infections.

## Diagnosis

Criteria for diagnosis of TSS:

Temperature > 39 °C.
Systolic BP < 90 mmHg.
Rash with subsequent desquamation, especially of the palms and soles.

Together with three or more of the following:

- Vomiting or diarrhoea
- Myalgia or CPK > 5 times the upper limit of normal.
- Mucous membrane hyperaemia.
- Creatinine ≥ twice the upper limit of normal with pyuria in absence of a UTI.
- Bilirubin or AST or ALT ≥ twice the upper limit of normal.
- Platelets $<100 \times 10^9$/L.
- Disorientation without focal neurological signs.

All of the above should be in the presence of negative tests for rocky mountain spotted fever, leptospirosis or measles. Staphylococcal TSS toxin-1 (TSST-1) and staphylococcal enterotoxin-B are the implicated toxins. Routine cultures for staphylococci and streptococci should be performed and, if possible, assays for the staphylococcal toxin should be performed.

## Treatment

- Correction of shock.
- Antistaphylococcal antibiotics.
- Supportive measures, as for septicaemia.

# Human Immunodeficiency Virus infection

The Human Immunodeficiency Virus (HIV) is a human RNA virus with an enzyme that enables it to make a DNA copy of its RNA genome. The DNA genome then integrates with the genome of the host cell. Consequently, with every replication of the host cell, viral replication is assured. For that reason, infection with HIV is presumed to be life-long.

The HIV selectively destroys a subset of T lymphocytes – the helper T lymphocytes. The percentage and absolute number of these cells gradually diminish over months to years and the infected person becomes susceptible to opportunistic infections and neoplasms, the onset of which defines the diagnosis of Acquired Immunodeficiency Syndrome (AIDS).

Acquired Immunodeficiency Syndrome is part of the final stage of a spectrum of infection involving HIV. Acquired Immunodeficiency Syndrome is HIV infection plus either an opportunistic infection and/or malignancy.

Acquired Immunodeficiency Syndrome patients may present with Kaposi's sarcoma, pneumonia (usually caused by *Pneumocystitis carinii*), fever, lymphadenopathy, malaise, tiredness, loss of weight, diarrhoea, dysphagia and retrosternal pain. Neurological presentations include meningitis (usually caused by *Cryptococcus neoformans*), facial lesions (*Toxoplasma gondii*, lymphoma or cryptococcal abscess) and progressive dementia (HIV encephalopathy). The most common neoplasms are Kaposi's sarcoma and non-Hodgkin's lymphoma.

In the absence of antiretroviral intervention, approximately 50% of HIV-infected persons will develop AIDS over a period of 10 years. Accurate figures for any longer period are not as yet known.

## Diagnosis

Antibodies against HIV usually can be detected within 6 weeks following infection. The antibodies are tested using an enzyme linked immunosorbent assay (ELISA) or western immunoblot (WB). The ELISA test is currently used for screening because of its excellent specificity and sensitivity, and the WB test is used to confirm anti-HIV status. The HIV viral load assay is also widely available.

## Implications in intensive care

The HIV can be transmitted by contact with infected blood or blood products and through the transplantation of infected organs, bone grafts or tissue.

There have been a few cases in which HIV has been transmitted by needlestick injury. The risk of transmission rises with the size of the viral load. The type of injury also determines the risk. The highest risk injury is as a result of a deep penetrating wound with a hollow bore needle contaminated with HIV-infected blood.

The onus is on the health-care worker to reduce their risk of sustaining a needlestick injury. Resheathing of needles is the most common way to sustain a significant needlestick injury. This practice should be banned.

All procedures involving sharps should be done under direct vision and in such a way that accidental injury is unlikely. If sharps are being used, a sharps disposable container should be located next to the health-care worker and the sharps disposed of immediately after use. It is good practice to dispose of all sharps yourself so that the person cleaning up after you does not risk a needlestick injury. Put all sharps in the special containers.

Adoption of needleless systems for venepuncture, cannulation and injections reduce the risk of needlestick injury and have been shown to be cost-effective.

Currently there is no evidence to suggest that HIV can be transmitted to hospital staff by contact with the secretions from patients, but precautions are still mandatory.

Highly active antiretroviral therapy (HAART) significantly prolongs survival and has altered the clinical spectrum of disease. It is now unusual for people to present with *pneumocystis carinii* pneumonia (PCP).

The treatment of severe PCP is worthwhile because if the patient survives the acute episode of PCP, they are likely to enjoy several years of quality life, especially if they are given HAART.

## Precautions

Every health-care facility must define its policies and address the issues related to general precautions for health-care workers. No additional measures are necessary for patients with potentially transmittable diseases such as hepatitis or HIV infection.

- Universal precautions: All blood and body fluids should be treated as being potential sources of infection.
- Handling of needles and sharps: Work practices that will minimise the handling of sharp instruments and objects should be developed (e.g. the use of staples or clips instead of sutures for surgery). Used needles should not be resheathed by hand. Neither should they be removed from disposable syringes by hand, nor bent or manipulated in any way by hand. Persons handling a sharp must be responsible for its proper disposal. Sharp items should be disposed of in a puncture-resistant container.
- The staff should be educated about the factors associated with transmission of disease and actions to be taken should accidental exposure occur.
- There must be adequate facilities (e.g. for handwashing and decontamination).
- Safe systems are needed (e.g. personal protective equipment and equipment to avoid needlestick injury).
- There should be a system for the reporting of accidents (e.g. needlestick injuries) and follow up, including counselling.
- Vaccination programmes should be kept current.
- Policies on confidentiality and notification should be clearly stated.

Gloves should be worn for direct or potential contact with blood or body fluids. A combination of mask and protective eyewear or face shield should be worn when aerosolisation or splattering of blood is envisaged. Protective apparel (e.g. gowns, aprons and overshoes) should be worn during procedures in which blood is likely to be splashed (e.g. autopsies, trauma and surgical procedures)

## Management of exposure to body fluids
- Promptly wash away contaminating fluid.
- Encourage bleeding. Wash with soap and copious amounts of water.
- Report the incident.

- The source patient should be informed and consent must be gained for serologic testing for evidence of HIV antibody and hepatitis B and C.
- Baseline HIV, hepatitis B and C serology should be performed on the health-care worker with follow up at 3 and 6 months.
- Any febrile illness occurring within 12 weeks of exposure should be reported.
- Exposed individuals initially found to be seronegative, should be retested after 6 weeks and at periodic intervals thereafter.
- Counselling should be available for exposed individuals. If this is not immediately available, counselling should be organised for the next working day.

Source patient – unknown status: Whether to give antiretroviral treatment depends on the likelihood of HIV positivity. If unlikely, it is not required. If likely, e.g. gay male with probable PCP, then treatment should be given.

Hepatitis B immune globulin should be given if the health-care worker is non-immune or not known to be immune.

Prophylaxis against hepatitis C is not available.

Source patient – HIV positive: Seek counselling and the exposed person requires antiretroviral treatment as soon as possible.

As combination antiretroviral treatment can stop viral replication and has a synergistic effect on slowing the progression of HIV infection, triple antiretroviral therapy is recommended.

If the source is in the late stages of HIV infection and especially if they have had treatment with antiretrovirals, drug-resistant HIV is possible. In this case, advice from an HIV specialist needs to be sought immediately as an antiretroviral regimen will need to be tailored to deal with possible drug resistance.

Source patient – hepatitis B surface antigen (HB$_s$Ag) positive: If the health-care worker is non-immune, give hepatitis B immune globulin and institute vaccination. If the serostatus of the health-care worker is unknown, give hepatitis B immune globulin unless testing for the antibody to the surface antigen (anti-HB$_s$ can be performed within 24 hours).

Source patient – hepatitis C positive: There is a significant risk of acquisition of the hepatitis C virus (HCV) if the health-care worker is HCV negative. Perform liver function tests and HCV status at 6 weeks. If acute hepatitis C develops, treat with interferon. Ribavirin can also be added. This may abort the infection and possibly prevent chronic hepatitis C.

## Viral infections

### Importance in intensive care

Viral infections can sometimes present as primary diseases in patients, such as herpes encephalitis (see Chapter 23). Secondary infections can occur as a result of reactivations of viruses from a latent state, often in immunocompromised hosts.

Though the chances are small, there is always the potential danger that staff members can contract viral diseases after contact with patients, such as hepatitis transmission and HIV.

## Diagnosis of viral infections

Laboratory diagnosis of a viral infection usually comes too late to influence management and even with more rapid diagnostic techniques, definitive treatment is limited.

The diagnostic techniques available include rapid methods such as DFA, cell culture, serology and tissue biopsy with electron microscopy. Polymerase chain reaction (PCR) and other molecular methods are proving helpful in selected patients. Close co-operation with the microbiologist is needed in this rapidly developing area.

## Treatment

Because of the parasitic association of viruses and the host cells, drugs that interfere with the viral cycle often are also toxic to the host.

Most viral infections are not currently treatable. Treatable infections occur with the following viruses (Table 13.10):

Herpes simplex virus (HSV) 1 and 2
Cytomegalovirus (CMV)
HIV
HCV and hepatitis B Virus (HBV)
Influenza

Hence if any of the above are possible, they should be excluded. This is particularly so in immunocompromised hosts.

Acyclovir: Active against HSV-1, HSV-2 and *varicella zoster virus* (VZV). Can be given orally, but absorption inadequate to treat severe zoster. Dose for severe varicella and encephalitis is 10 mg/kg/8 hourly. Causes significant nausea and vomiting and can crystallise in nephrons to cause renal failure; ensure patient is well hydrated.

## Viral hepatitis

### Hepatitis A virus
Hepatitis A virus (HAV) is transmitted by the orofaecal route and produces the classic short incubation infectious hepatitis. Active and passive vaccination is available. Contacts *must* be given passive immunisation with normal human gammaglobulin, as this confers immediate immunity and is proven to prevent secondary cases. Active vaccination *must not* be used in this situation as it takes several weeks for immunity to develop and its efficacy in preventing hepatitis A in

**Table 13.10.** Viral infections in intensive care

| Virus | Antiviral | Comments |
| --- | --- | --- |
| HSV1 and 2 | Acyclovir<br>Famciclovir<br>Valaciclovir | Especially effective in immuno-compromised hosts |
| CMV | Ganciclovir<br>Foscarnet | Only used in immunocompromised hosts; quite toxic |
| HIV | Antinucleotide RT inhibitors<br>Protease inhibitors<br>Non-nucleotide RT inhibitors | HAART considerably prolongs survival; long list of side effects and drug interactions |
| HCV | Interferon<br>Ribavirin | Effective in chronic and acute infection<br>Ribavirin increases the efficacy of Interferon. Unfortunately Interferon is very expensive |
| HBV | Interferon | Some effect in chronic infection |
| Influenza | Amantidine<br>Relenza | Amantidine is useful in aborting outbreaks of Influenza A; unfortunately it has severe neurological side effects and its efficacy in severe pneumonia is doubtful. Relenza is quite effective in mild to moderate infections. Only available as inhalational caplets and cannot be given to intubated patients |
| Measles | Ribavirin | Will shorten duration of infectivity and illness. Probably useful in severe infections such as measles and pneumonia. |

contacts is unknown. Mortality of HAV is approximately 5%. There is no antiviral treatment. Management consists of supportive care and with liver transplantation in fulminant cases.

## Hepatitis B virus

Hepatitis B virus causes long incubation serum hepatitis and can be transmitted by chronic carriers who usually are asymptomatic. It has become a major health problem throughout the world and is now responsible for almost half of all cases of hepatitis. The presence of its viral HBsAg in serum signifies infection, whereas IgG antibody to the surface antigen (anti-HBs) indicates past infection and may indicate immunity. Protection of the staff is particularly important in the ICU as secretions from patients seropositive for HBsAg are infectious.

The patients who are particularly at risk of being HBsAg-positive are people from certain racial groups, drug addicts, those who have received multiple blood transfusions, homosexually active men and patients on long-term haemodialysis. All health-care workers in direct patient contact are advised to be actively immunised against hepatitis B infection – 90% will develop antibodies which will confer almost 100% immunity. An initial course of three intramuscular doses (0, 1 and 6 months) is recommended. All health-care workers are now being encouraged to become immunised. General precautions apply when dealing with patients who are HBsAg.

### Hepatitis C virus

Hepatitis C virus may be responsible for many of the cases of so-called non-A, non-B hepatitis transmitted by blood transfusions, in addition to being associated with chronic active hepatitis, cirrhosis and hepatocellular carcinoma. All donor blood should be screened for antibodies to HCV. Interferon therapy may be useful in preventing acute hepatitis C from becoming chronic. No vaccine is currently available.

### Non-A, non-B, non-C hepatitis

Non-A, non-B, non-C hepatitis is a diagnosis of exclusion, as no specific test is available. Now that hepatitis C has been separated from the previous non-A, non-B (NANB) hepatitis classification, it remains to be seen whether or not there will be one or more distinct viruses responsible for NANB hepatitis.

### Delta hepatitis (hepatitis D virus)

Delta hepatitis is caused by hepatitis D virus (HDV), which consists of a delta inner core encapsulated by the surface Ag of hepatitis B virus. The HDV is defective and requires active HBV infection in order to replicate. It can occur only in patients with hepatitis B, either simultaneously or as a superinfection that often makes the primary infection worse. Delta hepatitis infection can be indirectly prevented by vaccinating with hepatitis B vaccine.

### Hepatitis E virus

Hepatitis E virus (HEV) is another recently identified RNA virus responsible for enterically transmitted hepatitis. It is common in developing countries and should be considered a possibility in travellers with a clinical picture of hepatitis A who are negative for HAV IgM.

## Fungal infections

Systemic fungal infections in the ICU usually are associated with prolonged use of broad-spectrum antibiotics or long-term IV feeding or they can occur as complications in immunocompromised hosts. The diagnosis of disseminated fungal infection needs to be considered in severely immunocompromised hosts, especially patients with prolonged neutropaenia, transplants and HIV infection. The two most common are caused by *Candida* spp. and *Aspergillus* spp. However, other species of yeasts and filamentous fungi are being seen with increasing frequency.

### *Candida*

*Candida* spp. compose part of the normal human flora and can become a dominant coloniser as a result of broad-spectrum antibiotic therapy. It is usually seen as a benign infection of mucosal surfaces and invasive infections are often secondary to central line infections. Catheter-related candidiasis is usually associated with the administration of IVN. Hepatosplenic candidiasis occurs in patients with prolonged absolute neutropaenia. It is unusual for mucosal candidiasis to disseminate.

**Systemic *Candida* infection is a difficult diagnosis to make and, as a result, it is often delayed. It entails very high mortality and its treatment involves a high incidence of complications.**

### Diagnosis

Positive blood cultures are found in only 40–50% of cases. An increased yield of positive cultures can be obtained if lysis centrifugation techniques are used. Clinical evidence of generalised infections should be sought, including biopsy and culture of infected tissues. Specific funduscopic signs can be seen in approximately 30% of cases.

Risk factors include:

Colonisation >2 sites.
Complicated abdominal surgery.
Antibiotics >14 days.
IV catheters.
IVN.

Serological tests and PCR have so far proven disappointing.

The diagnosis is usually made clinically, with or without laboratory confirmation.

### Prophylaxis:

Nystatin, 500 000 units, 6-hourly, orally (NG).
Nystatin mouthwashes may decrease the incidence of fungaemia in patients at risk.

### Treatment:

Because the treatment carries its own high risks, it should not be commenced unless there is a strong index of suspicion (e.g. neutropaenic patients or seriously ill patients not responding to multiple antibiotics).

Empirical antifungal treatment is often used in the febrile neutropaenic host who has not responded to maximum antibacterial treatment.

Treatment of mucosal candidiasis: Fluconazole.
Treatment of systemic candidiasis: Ophthalmology review is mandatory.
If catheter related, remove catheter and culture tip.

**TROUBLESHOOTING**

## Unresponsive sepsis – some considerations

**Surgical drainage necessary**
e.g.   intra-abdominal sepsis
          sinusitis
          acalculus cholecystitis

**Intravascular device infection?**
**Immunosuppression?**
e.g.   leucopaenia

**Another infection source?**
e.g.   tuberculosis

**Non-microbial inflammation?**
e.g.   necrotic tissue
          non-infective SIRS
          vasculitis

**Other cause for fever?**
e.g.   pulmonary embolus, transfusion reaction

**Superinfection?**
e.g.   fungal infection

**Atheromatous or cholesterol emboli?**
**Inadequate therapy?**

If non-neutropaenic host; fluconazole is just as efficacious as amphotericin B and
   is less toxic. Dose 400 mg IV or PO, once daily.
If neutropaenic, use amphotericin B.
Amphotericin B: continue until there is clinical improvement.
Lipid formulations of amphotericin are less toxic but have limited availability and
   are extremely expensive.
Toxic effects.

## Aspergillosis

Unlike infections caused by *Candida* spp., aspergillosis is primarily an exogenous
infection and dissemination is usually from a pulmonary source. It is the second most common infection caused by a fungal genus in immunocompromised
hosts (apart from patients with AIDS in whom *Cryptococcus* is more common).

**TROUBLESHOOTING**

## Is it an autoimmune disease?

When you keep adding or changing antibiotics, think of a non-microbial inflammatory disease.

Autoimmune disease, particularly vasculitis manifests as fever accompanied by single or multiorgan dysfunction and needs to be differentiated from unresponsive septicaemia.

### Autoimmune diseases

Systemic lupus erythematosus (SLE)
Polymyositis
Dermatomyositis
Chronic active hepatitis
Rheumatoid arthritis
Glomerulonephritis
Sjögren's syndrome
Wegeners' granulomatosis
Goodpasture's syndrome

### Common presentations of autoimmune disease

Fever
Psychosis, confusion, seizures
Anaemia, pancytopaenia
Haemoptysis, dyspnoea
Myocarditis
Jaundice
Cutaneous vasculitis, palpable purpura
Arthralgia, swollen joints
Pain and polymyositis

Aspergilloma formation and allergic aspergillosis do not usually occur in seriously ill patients.

## Diagnosis

Although the growth of *Aspergillus* spp. in tracheal aspirates can be a normal finding, in an immunocompromised patient such a finding should be treated with a high index of suspicion.

Blood cultures are rarely positive for *Aspergillus* spp.

## Treatment

Treatment is with amphotericin. Itraconazole also has activity and can be used in the maintenance stage of treatment. New agents such as voriconazole show considerable promise.

The combination of amphotericin B with an azole (e.g. fluconazole or itraconazole) is antagonistic and should not be used.

## TROUBLESHOOTING

### Screening investigations for autoimmune diseases

Haemoglobin and full blood count.

### Antinuclear antigen (ANA)

A positive result is suggestive of:

SLE
polymyositis
dermatomyositis
Sjögrens syndrome
rheumatoid arthritis

However, false positives are common.

### Double stranded DNA

If positive, suggestive of SLE.

### Extractable nuclear antigen

Diagnosis depending on which type of antigen is positive.

### Rheumatoid factor

Indicator of active rheumatoid arthritis.

### Complement levels C3, C4, CH50

If low suggests a complement activating disease is present.

### Antineutrophil cytoplasmic antibody (ANCA)

If positive, indicates Wegener's or crescentic glomerulonephritis. cANCA indicative of Wegener's and pANCA indicative of microscopic polyangitis syndrome.

### Antiglomerular basement membrane antibody (anti-GBMAb)

Indicates Goodpasture's syndrome.

### Creatinine phosphokinase

If high, consistent with polymyositis.

### Antimitochondrial antibody

Indicates primary biliary cirrhosis.

### Anti-smooth muscle antibody

Indicates chronic active hepatitis.

### Cryoglobulin

Consistent with essential mixed cryoglobulaemia.

## TROUBLESHOOTING

### Microbiology: some tips on interpreting results

Microbiology findings, unlike biochemical parameters, are open to interpretation as to their relevance and what, if any, clinical action should be taken. Liaise closely with microbiologists about the relevance of positive findings and the trends in surveillance.

The following should be considered:

Does the patient have a clinical infection?
Are the microbiology results relevant to the clinical findings?
If the results are relevant, the most appropriate treatment should be chosen.

#### Blood cultures
Very useful if positive.
Approximately 50% of positive cultures are due to contamination.

#### Sputum
There is little correlation between the microorganisms that cause pneumonia and the organisms found in the sputum of seriously ill patients. The diagnosis is clinical. Positive blood cultures and other techniques are more accurate.
*Streptococcus pneumoniae* may be present in patients with acute bronchitis or can even be found in the throat of a normal carrier, in addition to being a cause of pneumonia. *Haemophilus influenzae* and *Moraxella catarrhalis* are common colonisers in chronic airflow limitation and may not be clinically significant.
*Staphylococcus aureus* is often associated with the presence of a NG tube and chronic bronchitis.
Mixed growth of non-haemolytic streptococci and *Neisseria* spp. is usual in the normal throat flora.
Coliforms, including *Escherichia coli* and *Klebsiella*, are common colonisers, especially in the seriously ill.

#### Wounds
*Staphylococcus aureus* in a pure heavy growth from an inflamed wound is suggestive of a wound infection. However, scanty or light growth could represent colonisation. *Streptococcus pyogenes*, even in small numbers, is probably significant.
Other organisms, even in high numbers, may simply be colonisers of wounds:

Coagulase negative staphylococci almost always a coloniser
Diptheroids virtually always a coloniser
Enterococci
Gram-negative aerobes including:
*Pseudomonas*
Coliforms

#### Urine
A pure growth of more than $10^8$ viable bacteria/L in a midstream specimen with elevated red and/or white cells is suggestive of a UTI. Catheter samples invariably have red and white cells and colonisation, and so a diagnosis of UTI on that basis alone is inappropriate. There must be other signs of systemic infection.

## FURTHER READING

### General

Bion, J. F. and Brun-Buisson, C. Infection and critical illness: genetic and environmental aspects of susceptibility and resistance. *Intensive Care Medicine* 26 (2000): (Suppl.) S1–144.

Brun-Buisson, C., Doyon, F., Carlet J, Dellamonica, P., Gouin, F., Lepoutre, A., Mercier, J-C., Offenstadt, G. and Regnier, B. for the French ICU Group for Severe Sepsis. Incidence, risk factors, and outcome of severe sepsis and septic shock in adults: a multicenter prospective study in Intensive Care Units. *Journal of the American Medical Association* 274 (1995): 968–74.

Glauser, M. P. Pathophysiologic basis of sepsis. Consideration for future strategies of intervention. *Critical Care Medicine* 28 (2000): S4–S8.

Marik, P. E. Fever in the ICU. *Chest* 117 (2000): 855.

### Septicaemia

Adrie, C. and Pinsky, M. R. The inflammatory balance in human sepsis. *Intensive Care Medicine* 26 (2000): 364–75.

Anderson, I. D., Fearon, K. C. H. and Grant, I. S. Laparotomy for abdominal sepsis in the critically ill. *British Journal of Surgery* 83 (1996): 535–39.

Annane, D. Corticosteroids for septic shock. *Critical Care Medicine* 29 (2001): (Suppl.) S117–20.

Bernard, G. R., Vincent, J.-L., Laterre, P.-F. *et al* for the PROWESS Study Group. Efficacy and Safety of recombinant human activated protein C for severe sepsis. *New England Journal of Medicine* 344 (2001): 699–709.

Bone, R. C., Grodzin, C. J. and Balk, R. A. Sepsis: A new hypothesis for pathogenesis of the disease process. *Chest* 112 (1997): 235–43.

Martin, C., Viviand, S., Leone, M. and Thirion, X. Effect of norepinephrine on the outcome of septic shock. *Critical Care Medicine* 28 (2000): 2758–65.

Opal, S. and Cohen, J. Clinical Gram-positive sepsis: Does it fundamentally differ from Gram-negative bacterial sepsis? *Critical Care Medicine* 27 (1999): 1608–16.

Pugin, J. Sepsis and the immune response. *Intensive Care Medicine* 25 (1999): 1027–28.

Steel, A. and Bihari, D. Choice of catecholamine: does it matter? *Current Opinion in Critical Care* 6 (2000): 347–53.

Wheeler, A. P. and Bernard, G. R. Treating patients with severe sepsis. *New England Journal of Medicine* 340 (1999): 207–14.

### Antimicrobials

Fowler, R. A., Cheung, A. M. and Marshall, J. C. Selective decontamination of the digestive tract in critically ill patients. *Intensive Care Medicine* 25 (1999): 1323–6.

Garbino, J., Romand, J.-A., Suter, P. M. and Pittet, D. Use of 'biotics in patients receiving intensive care. *Clinical Intensive Care* 9 (1998): 25–35.

Jenkins, S. G. Mechanisms of bacterial antibiotic resistance. *New Horizons* 4 (1996): 321–2.

Proctor, R. A. New drugs for the treatment of septic shock. *Critical Care Medicine* 29 (2001): 1650–1.

Teba, L. Polymerase chain reaction: a new chapter in critical care diagnosis. *Critical Care Medicine* 27 (1999): 860–1.

## Intra-abdominal sepsis

Anderson, I. D., Fearon, K. C. H. and Grant, I. S. Laparotomy for abdominal sepsis in the critically ill. *British Journal of Surgery* 83 (1996): 535–9.

Evans, H. L., Raymond, D. P., Pelletier, S. J., Crabtree, T. D., Pruett, T. L. and Sawyer, R. G. Diagnosis of intra-abdominal infection in the critically ill patient. *Current Opinion in Critical Care* 7 (2001): 117–21.

Seiler, C. A., Brugger, L., Forssmann U. *et al.* Conservative surgical treatment of diffuse peritonitis. *Surgery* 127 (2000): 178–84.

## Other infections

Geiss, H. K. Nosocomial sinusitis. *Intensive Care Medicine* 25 (1999): 1037–9.

Lane, H. C. and Fauci, A. S. Bioterrorism on the home front. A new challenge for American medicine. *Journal of the American Medical Association* 286 (2001): 2595–7.

Rosenberg, A. L., Seneff, M. G., Atiyeh, L., Wagner, R., Bojanowski L. and Zimmerman, J. The importance of bacterial sepsis in intensive care unit patients with acquired immunodeficiency syndrome: Implications for future care in the age of increasing antiretroviral resistance. *Critical Care Medicine* 29 (2001): 548–56.

Rosenstein, N. E., Perkins, B. A., Stephens, D. S., Popovic, T. and Hughes, J. M. Meningoccal disease. *New England Journal of Medicine* 344 (2001): 1378–88.

Seiler, C. A., Brugger, L., Forssmann, U., Baer, H. U. and Buchler, M. W. Conservative surgical treatment of diffuse peritonitis. *Surgery* 127 (2000): 178–84.

# 14

# Trauma

- The key to good results in trauma patients is rapid resuscitation and definitive care.
- A systematic, standardised team approach is required for optimal assessment, resuscitation and definitive treatment of patients.
- Whereas it is common to undertransfuse hypovolaemic patients, it is almost impossible to overtransfuse them.

## Multitrauma

### The golden hour

What happens during the first hour or 'golden hour' following severe trauma will largely determine the patient's eventual outcome. Rapid resuscitation is essential. Restoration of the circulation is one of the key goals in managing patients with major trauma. In the presence of significant hypovolaemia, blood is redirected to the so-called vital organs – the brain, heart and kidneys. The so-called non-vital organs suffer relative ischaemia. This has important implications for the splanchnic circulation. Hypoperfusion of the gastrointestinal tract (GIT) predisposes to bacterial translocation and endotoxin absorption across a compromised mucosal barrier. This is compounded by ischaemia of the reticuloendothelial system, particularly the liver, which otherwise would filter bacteria and toxins from the portal circulation. It has been proposed that bacterial translocation predisposes to the multiorgan failure (MOF) frequently seen after multitrauma. It is crucial, therefore, to rapidly restore the circulation. This means not only maintaining a normal blood pressure (BP) but also guaranteeing perfusion to the non-vital organs, particularly the GIT.

**Table 14.1.** Assessment guidelines for multitrauma

---

Primary survey: assessment of ABCs

1 Airway and cervical spine control:
   Use chin-lift and jaw-thrust manoeuvres; then oropharyngeal airway and intubate
      if in doubt
   Protect the cervical spine
2 Breathing:
   All patients should be given the maximum $FiO_2$ initially
   Artificially ventilate if in doubt
   Evacuate pneumothoraces and haemopneumothoraces
3 Circulation, with haemorrhage control:
   Use at least two large IV cannulae – rapid fluid replacement
   Do not hesitate to use group-specific blood
   Give inotropes, if necessary, and exclude cardiac tamponade
   Do not place patient head down
4 Disability: Conduct a brief neurological evaluation
5 Exposure: Completely undress the patient

Ensure that the ABC parameters have been stabilised before proceeding to the secondary
   survey.
Rapidly and simultaneously assess (history and examination) and resuscitate

Secondary survey

1 Head and skull (including ears)
2 Maxillofacial injuries
3 Neck
4 Chest
5 Abdomen/pelvis
6 Back, perineum and rectum – log-roll the patient
7 Extremities
8 Complete neurological examination
9 Appropriate x-rays, laboratory tests and special studies
10 'Tubes and fingers' in every orifice.

Summarise findings and plan the next stage of treatment

---

## Initial assessment and management (Table 14.1)

### Airway

Initial attempts to establish an airway include chin-lift and jaw-thrust manoeuvres. Blood and secretions should be sucked out, foreign bodies removed and an oropharyngeal airway inserted, if necessary. If there is any doubt about the airway, intubate, especially if the patient is unconscious or has facial injuries.

Special attention should be given to the possibility of a fracture of the cervical spine. The patient's head should be immobilised when establishing or maintaining

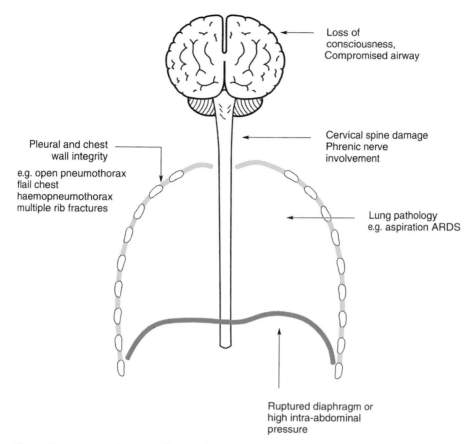

Loss of consciousness, Compromised airway

Cervical spine damage Phrenic nerve involvement

Pleural and chest wall integrity

e.g. open pneumothorax flail chest haemopneumothorax multiple rib fractures

Lung pathology e.g. aspiration ARDS

Ruptured diaphragm or high intra-abdominal pressure

**Figure 14.1.** Factors that can affect ventilation in patients with multitrauma.

an airway. Maintain the cervical spine in a neutral position. This can be facilitated by having an assistant hold the patient's head in the neutral position during intubation. Other ways of immobilising the cervical spine when damage is suspected, or has not been excluded, include the use of semirigid cervical collars, sandbags and taping the head to a spinal board.

### Breathing

Ensure adequate ventilation. The patient's breathing may be compromised by a decreased level of consciousness, airway obstruction, pneumothoraces, haemothoraces, diaphragmatic injury, multiple rib fractures, flail chest, cervical spine damage, phrenic nerve damage or increased intra-abdominal pressure (Figure 14.1).

If there is any doubt about the patient's breathing – intubate and ventilate.

**Table 14.2.** Five sites of major blood loss

---

1  External: Conduct an examination and take a history
2  Chest: Loss will be obvious on the chest x-ray or as loss from an intercostal catheter
3  Abdomen: Use lavage or clinical examination
4  Retroperitoneum: This is a diagnosis of exclusion, if 1–3 are negative. Retroperitoneal losses are often associated with a fractured pelvis
5  Major fracture: Examine femur, pelvis and pelvic x-ray

---

If ventilation remains a problem, rule out the possibility of a tension pneumothorax, which would worsen with positive-pressure ventilation.

Rapidly drain any significant collections of air or blood in the pleural cavity.

All patients who are in shock are hypoxic and need oxygenation with as high a fraction of inspired oxygen ($FiO_2$) as can be administered, as well as monitoring with pulse oximetry.

## Circulation

Restore the blood volume – hypovolaemia is the most common cause of hypotension in trauma (Table 14.2). It is difficult to overtransfuse hypovolaemic patients, but it is extremely common to undertransfuse them. Never place a shocked patient in the head down position. Leg elevation is a better temporary measure for hypotension. However, the best treatment for hypovolaemia is rapid fluid replacement. Always use two large (at least 16 gauge) peripheral cannulae. Control obvious sources of external haemorrhage and consider urgent definitive surgical control of bleeding. Rule out the possibility of cardiac tamponade.

Early definitive surgery rather than fluid replacement has been demonstrated to be advantageous for penetrating wounds of the torso. Extrapolation to other settings is potentially dangerous. Elective hypotension, as it is sometimes called, to control bleeding, is the same as elective ischaemia or shock. Intravascular restoration of the circulation should occur while urgent surgery is planned and performed. Both should occur together and not be considered as self exclusive.

Type of fluid for initial intravascular volume replacement: There may be advantages in using colloid or even hypertonic saline rather than crystalloid solution, in cases of severe hypovolaemia (see Chapter 8). However, the real challenge is to replenish the circulating volume as rapidly as possible. Because a saline cross match for ABO compatibility (type specific) can be performed in less than 10 minutes, rapidly cross-matched (group-specific) blood should be used early in cases of severe bleeding until fully cross-matched blood is available. Fully cross-matched blood (99.9% serologically safe) is only marginally safer than group-specific ABO compatible blood (99.4% serologically safe).

**Table 14.3.** Immediate investigations for patients suffering severe multitrauma

| |
|---|
| Immediate blood cross match and baseline values for biochemistry, arterial blood gases and haematology |
| Chest x-ray (if there is a widened mediastinum or other signs of ruptured thoracic aorta, an immediate aortogram is necessary) |
| Lateral x-ray of cervical spine |
| Pelvic x-ray |
| Diagnostic peritoneal lavage or abdominal ultrasound |
| Cranial CT scan – for all patients with significant neurological impairments or deteriorating neurological signs |

## Initial monitoring (Table 14.3)

As a first step, it is important to simultaneously assess and rapidly resuscitate. Do not spend time on complicated monitoring or investigations until the patient is adequately resuscitated.

### Respiration
- Adequacy of airway and chest movement.
- Airway pressure if the patient is ventilated.
- Colour.
- Respiratory rate.
- Chest x-ray.
- Pulse oximetry (non-invasive, continuous, easily obtained estimate of oxygenation that can, however, be compromised by poor peripheral perfusion.

### Circulation
- Pulse rate will more accurately 'track' hypovolaemia in the young than in the elderly.
- Blood pressure: Because of well-developed sympatheticoadrenal responses, a young, fit patient often will maintain good arterial BP until just before circulatory collapse, whereas in the elderly, BP tracks the circulation more accurately.
- Urine output: Beware of inappropriate polyuria secondary to use of alcohol, mannitol or intravenous contrast solution.
- Arterial blood gases, particularly arterial pH, can reflect the status of the circulation. Failure to correct metabolic acidosis usually reflects hypovolaemia.
- Skin perfusion, as estimated by skin temperature, will provide a simple indication of hypovolaemia in multitrauma patients. It may be difficult to estimate when a patient has central hypothermia, when there is a low ambient temperature or when the local arterial blood supply is compromised.

- ECG monitoring is easy to perform and can be useful during the early stages of resuscitation, even as a continuous readout of pulse rate.

## Later monitoring

When a patient is stable, measurement of central venous pressure (CVP) may be useful for estimating fluid replacement. However, the only value in having a central line initially is to facilitate fluid administration, not to measure intravascular pressures. Even then it is preferable to use a large diameter cannula. When the patient has been initially resuscitated, measurements such as pulmonary artery wedge pressure (PAWP), cardiac output, oxygen delivery ($DO_2$) and oxygen consumption ($VO_2$) may be useful for fine-tuning the circulation. The use of a pulmonary artery catheter has not improved the outcome in patients with trauma, nor indeed in intensive care generally. The place of tonometry (measurement of gastric mucosal pH) following major trauma has not been determined.

## Further assessment and management

### History
A history of the incident should be sought, especially from the first person on the scene, as well as from the patient, if possible and others who witnessed the incident that caused the trauma.

### Examination
A top-to-bottom examination of the patient should be performed: Determine the level of consciousness using the Glasgow Coma Scale (GCS) and document any lateralising signs. Look for external scalp lacerations (which can cause significant roadside blood loss), otorrhoea, rhinorrhoea, facial fractures (use palpation), flail segments and fractured ribs. Examine the neck for tenderness, penetrating wounds, pulses and bruits, venous distension, tracheal position and evidence of subcutaneous air. Remove all clothing and carefully examine the abdomen and pelvis. Perform rectal and vaginal examinations. Always examine the patient's back. All this should take only minutes. Finally, assess the limbs. Do not x-ray limbs at this stage; wait until the patient is adequately resuscitated. Radiography is time-consuming. Limb fractures usually are obvious and are not immediately life-threatening.

### The next steps
Continue to reassess the airway, ventilation, oxygenation and circulation during the initial examination. **Keep the patient warm.**

**Table 14.4.** Features to be noted on a lateral cervical spine view

All seven vertebral bodies must be clearly seen, including C7 to T1 junction
Evaluate alignments of the posterior cervical line, the four lordotic curves, the anterior
   longitudinal ligament line, the posterior longitudinal ligament line; the spinolaminal
   line and the tips of the spinous processes
Evaluate the predental space (< 3 mm in adults, 4–5 mm in children)
Evaluate each vertebra for fractures and increased or decreased density (e.g. compression
   fracture)
Evaluate the intervertebral and interspinous spaces (an angulation of more than 11° at a
   single space is abnormal)
Evaluate fanning of the spinous processes, suggestive of posterior ligament disruption
Evaluate prevertebral soft tissue distance (< 7 mm at C2 and < 5 mm at C2–C4)
Evaluate the atlanto-occipital region for possible dislocation

Laboratory tests: Take blood for cross matching, if necessary, and for other determinations: haemoglobin, haematocrit, white cells, platelets, urea, creatinine and electrolytes.

Cervical spine x-ray: Obtain a lateral view of the cervical spine (Table 14.4). If all seven bodies cannot be seen, maintain spinal immobilisation until the initial resuscitation is complete when further views can be contemplated. A lateral film will detect damage in approximately 75% of cervical spine injuries. Conditions that are associated with higher risks for cervical spine damage include neck tenderness, an altered level of consciousness, alcohol intoxication and other signs and symptoms suggestive of spinal damage; such associated conditions may indicate the need for further spinal views. A lateral, antero-posterior and odontoid view will exclude 95% of injuries. A CT of the neck will increase accuracy to 99%. There is less emphasis on a lateral cervical spine being considered as an urgent investigation if the patient has a decreased level of consciousness or severe multi-trauma, as the cervical spine will be considered unstable until definitive cervical spine investigations are complete.

Upright chest x ray: An upright chest x-ray is the next investigation to be performed. Attend to any gas or fluid collections and check for a widened mediastinum. Further investigation is required in the case of a widened mediastinum. Note fractured ribs, lung contusion and heart size.

Pelvic x-ray: Following the chest x-ray and a lateral view of the cervical spine, the only other x-ray that should be obtained early in the patient's management is a pelvic x-ray to exclude fractures that might be sources of substantial blood loss. 'Springing' of the pelvis is a very poor indicator of fractures and probably should no longer be employed. A pelvic x-ray is probably not necessary in a fully conscious patient with no symptoms.

Abdominal examination: A careful examination of the abdomen should be conducted, including palpation of all four quadrants and a pelvic examination if it has not already been performed. Focused abdominal ultrasound or diagnostic peritoneal lavage should be considered at this stage. If the shock cannot be rapidly corrected, or if the bleeding is obvious and is from such a source that it may be life-threatening, surgery should be performed immediately.

Nasogastric (NG) tubes should be used for intubated patients if there is no contraindication, such as the suspicion of a basilar skull fracture, in which case tubes should be placed orally.

A urinary catheter should be inserted if there is no evidence to suggest urethral disruption (e.g. blood at the urethral meatus), no perineal, scrotal or penile injury and no abnormality on examination of the prostate.

Microbiology: Tetanus toxoid and tetanus immune globulin, as well as antibiotics, should be administered if they are clinically indicated.

### Placement

After resuscitation, patients who have sustained severe trauma will follow one of several paths:

- Operating theatre for surgery.
- CT scan.
- Angiography – either aortogram (if there is a widened mediastinum) or pelvic embolisation (for uncontrolled bleeding).
- An intensive care environment: All other investigations and x-rays can be performed in an ICU. In some centres, the initial receiving room or an adjacent area may serve as a site for continuous management, rather than in an ICU.
- General ward (if the patient is stable) or discharge (if there was only minor trauma).

As part of the trauma audit process, the time of transfer from the receiving room to another unit should be recorded and delays should be reviewed.

### Damage-control surgery

Some patients have horrendous injuries and should be considered early for damage-control surgery (see Table 14.5). The aim of the initial surgery is to stop bleeding and prevent contamination. No definitive surgery is done. The patients are then taken to ICU to be warmed and further resuscitated followed by definitive surgery later.

## Continuing management in intensive care

Continuing management in an ICU has the following goals:

- Assessment and continuing resuscitation.
- Co-ordination of all other services and planning for further definitive care.

**Table 14.5.** Criteria for damage control surgery

---

Shock
Hypothermia: temperature $\leq 35\,^{\circ}C$
Non-surgical bleeding: prothrombin time $\geq 16$ seconds, partial thromboplastin time
$\geq 50$ seconds
Acidosis: pH $\leq 7.18$ or worsening base deficit
Massive transfusion or resuscitation: $\geq 10$ units packed red blood cells
Prolonged operation

---

- Secondary examinations for injuries overlooked initially (minor fractures, soft
  tissue damage and nerve injuries can be easily missed during the flurry of initial
  resuscitation).

## Monitoring

A primary, continuing aim during resuscitation is to promote $DO_2$ to the cells (see
Chapter 16) which is the product of adequate oxygen saturation, haemoglobin
and blood flow. Although continued frequent monitoring of skin perfusion, BP,
pulse rate, urine output, chest movement, respiratory rate and colour is essential
in assessing $DO_2$, further monitoring procedures may be needed:

- Arterial blood gases (for assessing oxygenation, ventilation and adequacy of
  circulation).
- CVP (may be of help in assessing blood volume).
- Pulse oximetry.
- PAWP, cardiac output – transthoracic echo cardiography.
- Frequent chest x-rays, biochemistry and haematology tests.
- Tonometry – rarely used now.

## Ventilation and oxygenation

Patients in shock have cellular hypoxia. Frequent determination of blood gases
and pulse oximetry are necessary to assess oxygenation. The possible causes of
acute respiratory failure in this setting include aspiration, lung contusion and
excessive crystalloid transfusion. Nosocomial pneumonia or acute lung injury
(ALI) can develop later.

If the airway is compromised, intubation is necessary. When a patient's ventilation (assessed by clinical appearance and $PaCO_2$) is inadequate, artificial ventilation may be needed. If oxygenation is not adequate with an ordinary face mask,
continuous positive airway pressure (CPAP) delivered by a special mask, by nasal
mask, or via an endotracheal tube (ETT) may be necessary. Where possible, encourage CPAP or pressure-support ventilation (PSV), rather than mandatory
ventilation (with all of its attendant disadvantages) (see Chapter 19).

## Fluid replacement

Peripheral perfusion, arterial BP, pulse rate and urine output remain the most accurate and simple guides to fluid replacement in multitrauma patients. When large amounts of fluid must be used in resuscitation, colloids will cause less peripheral and pulmonary oedema than crystalloids (see Chapter 4). Maintenance fluids are not necessary during the early stages of resuscitation. Titrate the colloid or blood replenishment against intravascular measurements and serial haematocrit values. **Fluid losses often are underestimated, but rarely overestimated**.

Haemoglobin is essential for the oxygen carrying capacity of the blood and it can be monitored in terms of the haemoglobin concentration (maintain at least 10 g/dl) or haematocrit (more then 30%) during active resuscitation.

In addition to coagulation studies and ongoing platelet count, serum potassium and phosphate concentrations should be measured frequently during active resuscitation and replaced as necessary. Hypothermia can severely impair coagulation and must be aggressively corrected.

## Pain relief

Adequate pain relief is crucial after multitrauma. Many limb fractures and chest injuries will lend themselves to local or regional anaesthetic techniques when the patient is stable; otherwise, a continuous opiate infusion titrated against pain will ensure patient comfort (see Chapter 7). Patient controlled analgesia is effective when the patient is co-operative and able.

## Other investigations

When the patient is relatively stable, other investigations may be necessary. Even if a patient appears stable, it is essential that observation and support by trained staff be continued during any procedure or investigation, especially those involving transport.

Cranial CT scan: A cranial CT scan is essential for detecting epidural, subdural and intracerebral haematomas, as well as cerebral oedema and contusions. It is also useful for defining skull and cervical spine fractures. Cranial CT scans should be performed for all patients with neurological impairment or when there are neurological signs of deterioration. This is an essential investigation for all but minor head injuries and is useful for defining the extent of faciomaxillary injuries.

X-rays of long bones: Rarely is it urgent to x-ray the extremities. That should be delayed until the patient has been fully resuscitated. Exceptions would be fractures causing vascular or acute nerve injury and fractures associated with great loss of blood.

Intravenous pyelogram: An IV pyelogram should be obtained for a patient with significant or sustained haematuria or severe abdominal trauma near a kidney or ureter. A single shot of 100 ml of contrast fluid and a plain abdominal film will give adequate information.

Cystogram: A cystogram may be necessary for a patient with haematuria in combination with trauma to the lower abdomen or pelvis. Infuse 150–300 ml of contrast fluid into the bladder through a urinary catheter.

Urethrogram: For a patient suspected of having a urethral tear, a urethrogram requires injection of 30 ml of contrast material gently through the urethral meatus.

CT of abdomen: Abdominal CT is used for assessing the liver, spleen, kidneys, pancreas, retroperitoneal space and free peritoneal fluid.

FAST (Focused abdominal sonography for trauma): FAST is useful for rapid assessment of intra-abdominal free fluid.

The spine: Fractures and dislocations of the spine can result in devastating consequences. After obtaining a lateral cervical x-ray, other views of the cervical and thoracoabdominal spine may be necessary. In these circumstances anterior-posterior and open mouth views are probably indicated. If the patient has further unexplained symptoms or signs, or if the films are not satisfactory, then oblique views, flexion extension views, or CT scan views can also be performed.

Thoracic aortogram: A thoracic aortogram is necessary if rupture of the thoracic aorta is suspected. Suspicion is aroused by features such as a widened mediastinum, obliteration of the aortic knob, apical capping, pleural effusion, opacification of the angle between the aorta and the left pulmonary artery and depression of the left main bronchus to an angle of less than $40°$ with the trachea. Immediate performance of aortography for suspected rupture of the thoracic aorta necessitates a high incidence of investigations whose findings are negative (approximately 80–90%). A thoracic CT scan, even with contrast, is not as accurate as an aortogram in these circumstances. Transoesophageal echocardiography (TOE) is being increasingly used.

## Long-term complications

**The complications in intensive care are minimised by early and aggressive resuscitation.**

A patient who has experienced a period of decreased perfusion related to multitrauma will inevitably sustain some cellular injury, and that is the basis for many of the complications that follow severe trauma. The immune system is affected, predisposing to wound infection and sepsis. Decreased visceral perfusion predisposes to acute stress ulceration, renal failure, hepatic insufficiency, pulmonary insufficiency and MOF (see Chapter 9).

### Acute stress ulceration

Preventive measures should be considered in all cases of multitrauma in the ICU. If early enteral feeding is contraindicated, then treatment with cytoprotective agents, e.g. $H_2$-receptor antagonists should be instituted.

### Acute renal failure

The best protection against renal failure is rapid and efficient resuscitation. Intra-abdominal hypertension should be considered in all at-risk patients and monitored for. Decompressive surgery should be performed if renal function is compromised.

### Wounds

Meticulous surgical debridement of wounds and removal of foreign bodies are the most important steps in preventing wound infection.

Grossly contaminated wounds will become infected with or without the use of antibiotics. These wounds require debridement and avoidance of primary closure.

Maintaining adequate tissue oxygenation and perfusion is more important than prophylactic antibiotics in preventing infection.

Tetanus immunisation is given if necessary.

### Intra-abdominal complications

Always be alert to an intra-abdominal source of infection. Thorough saline washing at the time of laparotomy is important when there has been gut perforation. Intra-abdominal sepsis is a common and often lethal complication after severe injury. Its management is outlined elsewhere.

It may be inappropriate to use primary closure in the presence of contused and ruptured gut, depending on the extent of damage.

Repeated laparotomies are advisable in patients with mesenteric vascular injuries.

### Nutrition (see Chapter 5)

The metabolic responses to trauma are manifested through the neuroendocrine system and include marked protein breakdown. That response can be partially modified by measures such as rapid resuscitation and pain relief. However, the catabolism of trauma is largely obligatory. Enteral feeding should be instituted rapidly if at all possible. The vast majority of patients with severe trauma can tolerate enteral feeding in the early postoperative period. Nasogastric feeding may be initially unsuccessful and other techniques such as nasojejunal feeding or a feeding jejunostomy may provide practical and easy alternatives for facilitating enteral feeding. Parenteral nutrition should only be considered as a last resort and only after the patient has been resuscitated (see Chapter 5).

### Sepsis

Sepsis is a frequent complication of multitrauma, especially in the presence of renal failure. Rapid resuscitation and surgical debridement will decrease the incidence. Prophylactic antibiotics may sometimes be indicated (e.g. intra-abdominal soiling). However, continuing awareness of the possibility of a septic focus and an aggressive search for its source (e.g. intra-abdominal abscess, lung abscess, wound infection) are essential. The use of selective decontamination of the digestive tract (SDD) may decrease the incidence of sepsis among multitrauma patients. Active or passive immune support may play a role in the future.

## Rehabilitation

It is important to counsel relatives and friends early during the management of severe trauma and to be honest about the devastating long-term sequelae, especially if there are head injuries. They should be encouraged to accept the possibility that the healing process may take months or even years, and they should pace themselves accordingly. Patients usually need their greatest support from relatives and friends later during the long and frustrating rehabilitation process, rather than the first few days of resuscitation.

## Fat embolism syndrome

Fat embolism occurs in approximately 90% of patients with long bone fractures. Only 3–4% of those will go on to develop the florid fat embolism syndrome (FES) – severe hypoxia, decreased level of consciousness and petechiae.

### Clinical presentation

There is a wide spectrum of presentation, ranging from mild hypoxia to full-blown FES.

Ninety per cent of patients will develop symptoms within 24 hours of injury, but some can have a latent period up to 72 hours post injury.

The diagnosis is normally made using Gurd's criteria (Table 14.6). One major sign and four minor signs are necessary for a diagnosis of FES.

Respiratory failure: Dyspnoea, tachypnoea and hypoxia are the initial signs. Bilateral infiltrates can be seen on the chest x-ray. Acute lung injury and pulmonary hypertension can develop rapidly in patients with severe FES.

Bronchoalveolar lavage can aid the diagnosis, sensitivity and specificity are increased with serial lavage and > 35% fat-laden macrophages.

Central nervous system: Signs can range from anxiety, irritation and confusion to convulsions and coma (a score of 9 or less on the Glasgow Coma Scale). Exclude other causes (e.g. head injury in trauma). A CT scan may show cerebral oedema. Petechial haemorrhage is common; larger haemorrhages are rare.

Skin and other areas: A petechial rash (axillae, anterior chest or conjunctivae) will appear in 25–50% of patients.

Retinal findings include exudates, haemorrhage and cotton wool spots.

Tachycardia and fever (> 38 °C) are common.

Laboratory findings:

**Table 14.6.** Clinical features of fat embolism

---

Major
1  Petechial rash
2  Respiratory symptoms plus bilateral signs, with positive radiographic changes
3  Cerebral signs unrelated to head injury or any other condition

Minor
1  Tachycardia
2  Pyrexia
3  Retinal changes (fat or petechiae)
4  Urinary changes (anuria, oliguria, fat globules)
5  Sudden drop in haemoglobin
6  Sudden thrombocytopaenia
7  High erythrocyte sedimentation rate
8  Fat globules in the sputum

---

- hypoxaemia, often with a large alveolar-arterial oxygen gradient (see Chapter 17)
- hypocarbia
- decreased haemoglobin
- thrombocytopaenia
- coagulopathy
- hypocalcaemia
- chest x-ray – bilateral infiltrates.

Management: Prophylactic:

- Rapid, expert resuscitation is needed.
- Early immobilisation of fractures reduces the incidence of FES. Early fixation of fractures reduces respiratory complications but may worsen outcome in haemodynamically unstable patients.

**The mainstay of treatment is supportive – there is no definitive treatment**.
Respiratory: The principles of treatment are as for any other form of acute respiratory failure and ALI.
Cardiovascular:

- Maintain oxygen delivery – adequate haemoglobin, cardiac output, and $SaO_2$.
- Right side pressures may be high secondary to pulmonary hypertension.
- Inotropes with or without vasopressors may be required.
- Diuretics can decrease the extravascular water in the lungs.

Central nervous system: Coma in patients with FES usually is completely reversible.

Specific drugs: There is no role for aspirin, dextran, ethyl alcohol or heparin. The place of corticosteroids is not yet clear. Several studies have suggested that prophylactic steroids can benefit high-risk patients, but others have maintained that outcomes are just as good with supportive care only.

Prognosis: The pathophysiology in patients with fat emboli is completely reversible and survival should be 100%. The mortality rate for FES can approach 10%, mainly because of respiratory failure.

# The trauma system and scoring

## The trauma system

It is becoming increasingly recognised that severe trauma should be managed by specialised multidisciplinary units. The expertise needed for dealing with trauma is not ensured simply by putting all the components in one place (intensivists, specialist surgeons, accident and emergency specialists, anaesthetists, rehabilitationists, etc.). A system must be organised around all that expertise and adequate numbers of patients must be available for the team to maintain their skills and for the system to work efficiently. As in the case of cardiac surgery, specialist centres are necessary to concentrate the expertise needed to manage severe trauma. Operational protocols, rapid response multidisciplinary teams and facilities for education, data collection and auditing all must be integral parts of this system if trauma is to be managed effectively. The trauma system need not be a specialised stand-alone unit, but can be integrated into existing tertiary referral centres.

## Trauma scoring

Measurement of the severity of injury is an essential prerequisite for effective trauma care. The trauma system must be monitored and audited. That requires data collection and analysis, which in turn are based on trauma scoring. Trauma scores are also used for triage, prediction of outcome, epidemiology, research and planning of trauma services. Systems of scoring fall into two main patterns: physiological and anatomic.

### Physiological scoring system
Glasgow Coma Scale: The GCS is universally used to classify head injuries.

APACHE II system: The APACHE II system is used to classify patients admitted to ICUs and is based on an acute physiology score, age and chronic health evaluation. This score correlates well with the trauma score and the injury severity score and complements both.

Revised trauma score: The revised trauma score (RTS) is based on a scale of increasing severity from 7.8408 (best prognosis) to 0 (worst prognosis). The trauma score can be used as a component of a triage protocol and used together with other scores for predictive purposes. It is based on three parameters: the GCS, systolic BP and respiratory rate. A cut-off value of less than 4 has been suggested as identifying those individuals requiring care in a trauma centre.

### Anatomic scoring systems

Abbreviated injury scale: The abbreviated injury scale (AIS) was one of the first anatomic scales to be developed and it has been revised several times. The latest is the AIS-90, developed in 1990. The score reflects both the anatomic and pathological results of major trauma. Every injury is coded on the basis of anatomic site, nature and severity. The AIS correlates well with outcomes.

Injury severity score: The injury severity score (ISS) was developed specifically to score major injuries and it expresses a combined score for the most severe injury in each of the three most severely affected areas of the body. The severity is assigned by the AIS and the ISS is expressed on a scale of increasing severity (0–75%). The score is calculated by summing the squares of AIS scores. For example, consider this set of injuries:

| | | |
|---|---|---|
| Abdomen | ruptured spleen | AIS5 |
| Chest | fractured ribs | AIS2 |
| Limbs | fractured femur | AIS3 |

The ISS score will be $5^2 + 2^2 + 3^2 = 25 + 4 + 9 = 38$.

An ISS of 16 or more is taken as defining major trauma and corresponds with an average mortality rate of 10%.

The ISS is used in conjunction with other scores to guide triage and to indicate prognosis and it has been validated for use with penetrating injuries in adults of all ages and for children over the age of 12 years.

### Combined trauma scores

More accurate predictions are often obtained when several scoring techniques are combined. The trauma score, ISS and age are used in combination to form the TRISS method which allows comparison of outcome against a baseline rate while controlling the mix of severities of patients' injuries.

### Outcome comparisons

It is becoming increasingly important to measure one's own trauma practice and compare it with other systems, with a view to identifying weaknesses and attempting to achieve better outcomes. Some tools that help us to compare outcomes are as follows.

Z statistic: The Z statistic is for comparison of outcomes for two population subsets. The Z statistic quantitates the difference between actual and predicted numbers of deaths.

Peer review: Expert reviewers of trauma deaths (working 'blind') are often used to determine whether or not trauma deaths had any preventable components, based on an arbitrary scale. If this tool is tested for interobserver and intraobserver reliability, it can indicate points of possible weaknesses in the system.

Standardised mortality ratio: The standardised mortality ratio (SMR) is the ratio between observed deaths and expected deaths. A SMR below unity indicates a decreased risk of mortality in the sample, whereas an SMR greater than unity indicates increased risk.

# Blunt abdominal trauma

## Diagnosis

### Clinical examination
Clinical examination of the abdomen is mandatory and may reveal signs of external trauma, pain on palpation, guarding, rigidity, distension and so forth. However, such signs sometimes are unreliable in the acute situation and girth measurements are of no value. Immediate laparotomy should be performed in any case in which there is the suspicion of abdominal trauma and haemodynamic instability.

### Chest x-ray
This is necessary when looking for features such as fractured ribs over the spleen (ribs 9, 10 and 11) or liver, pneumoperitoneum or rupture of the diaphragm.

### Diagnostic peritoneal lavage
Diagnostic peritoneal lavage (DPL) is a sensitive test for intraperitoneal blood. It is performed as a sterile procedure in the emergency department by inserting a catheter into the peritoneum just below the umbilicus, or just above the umbilicus in any patient with a fractured pelvis.

Indications: Indications for DPL are equivocal abdominal findings (e.g. where fractured lower ribs or fractured pelvis may obscure findings) or a situation in which there are no clear indications for immediate laparotomy, but the patient

- has unreliable abdominal findings, because of head injury, drugs or paraplegia (or because the patient is paralysed and ventilated)
- faces an anticipated lengthy investigation (e.g. angiography) or surgery for extra-abdominal injuries
- has unexplained blood loss.

Technique for DPL:

1 Decompress the urinary bladder by inserting a urinary catheter.
2 Decompress the stomach by inserting a NG tube.
3 Prepare the abdomen for surgery with antimicrobial solution and drapes.
4 Inject local anaesthetic down to the peritoneum in the midline, one-third the distance from the umbilicus to the symphysis pubis (above the umbilicus where a pelvic fracture is suspected).
5 Vertically incise the skin and subcutaneous tissue down to fascia.
6 Incise the fascia and peritoneum and prevent fascial retraction with clamp.
7 Direct the catheter towards the pelvis.
8 Aspirate, and if frank blood or enteric contents appear, there is urgent need for laparotomy.
9 Infuse warmed isotonic saline at 10 ml/kg (up to 1 L). Gentle agitation will aid mixing and distribution throughout the abdominal cavity.
10 Wait 5–10 minutes and then siphon fluid off by placing the isotonic saline container on the floor.
11 A blood clot or heavily blood-stained fluid is unequivocally positive, as is a red blood cell count of greater than 100 000/ml. Although such findings are uncommon, the fluid should also be examined for white cells, amylase and food particles, with a Gram-stain used to search for bacteria.

Negative findings at lavage rule out significant haemorrhage in the peritoneal cavity. However, they do not rule out retroperitoneal injuries (e.g. duodenum and pancreas). Patients with pelvic fractures can have false-positive findings at lavage, as in approximately 15% of cases blood will leak from the retroperitoneal space into the peritoneum. Angiography may help identify the site of bleeding in these circumstances.

Relative contraindications:

• previous abdominal operations
• morbid obesity
• advanced cirrhosis
• pre-existing coagulopathy
• advanced pregnancy.

## Laparotomy

If hypovolaemia cannot be rapidly controlled and there is no obvious site of bleeding (e.g. external or chest or fractures), there is urgent need for laparotomy.

## CT scan

This has an advantage over DPL because it can detect other intra-abdominal abnormalities, including retroperitoneal haemorrhage. CT scanning is time-consuming and is contraindicated in unstable patients.

## Abdominal ultrasound

In skilled hands, ultrasound is a reliable method for detecting haemoperitoneum and it offers a valuable non-invasive means for investigating blunt abdominal trauma. Free intraperitoneal fluid is best demonstrated in the hepatorenal pouch. Abdominal ultrasound, scintigraphy and CT scan may detect injuries not obvious on DPL, but they cannot substitute for DPL for the detection of intra-abdominal blood.

## Principles of management

### Spleen

The spleen is the most common intra-abdominal organ affected by blunt trauma. About half of all ruptures are associated with fracture of ribs (9–11) on the left side.

There is no place for drainage: Either totally or partially remove the spleen if active, uncontrollable bleeding is suspected.

It is becoming more common to treat splenic trauma conservatively, especially in children. A CT scan is usually obtained and the patient is observed for signs of bleeding. Delayed rupture of the spleen occurs in up to 10% of patients with splenic haematomas.

Patients who undergo total splenectomy have a small risk (<1%) of post-splenectomy sepsis. Encapsulated bacteria such as pneumococci, meningococci and haemophilus are the commonest organisms. Vaccination should be carried out in these patients.

### Liver

The liver is in second place among the intra-abdominal organs most commonly affected by blunt trauma.

Approximately 70% of all liver injuries can be managed conservatively. Others require resection and, in a small percentage, packing to stop the bleeding. The current approach is to perform the minimum surgery necessary to control bleeding.

### Pancreas

Pancreatic injury is relatively rare. However, it is important to mobilise the duodenum and identify the pancreas when performing any laparotomy for trauma. A haematoma around the pancreas at operation should alert the surgeon to the possibility of severe underlying damage.

The amylase concentration is an imprecise diagnostic tool; CT scan is a much better indicator of pancreatic damage.

With blunt trauma, drainage at laparotomy is often sufficient. Duct damage must be surgically repaired early.

### Hollow viscus

The perforation must be repaired early. Liberal peritoneal lavage (10–15 L of warm isotonic saline) should be used at operation.

The bowel may need to be resected and a stoma fashioned.

Adequate drainage and prophylactic antibiotics are necessary for peritoneal soiling.

Repeat laparotomy is advisable after mesenteric vessel injury, in order to assess gut viability.

### Diaphragm

The diaphragm is involved in 4% of all cases of multitrauma and must be surgically repaired.

### Retroperitoneum and pelvis

Pelvic fracture: The diagnosis of a fractured pelvis is made on the basis of an x-ray. 'Springing' of the pelvis is a very unreliable sign and may worsen the injury. There is increasing interest in surgical fixation of pelvic fractures – either external or internal fixation, with or without traction. Stabilisation may be important both for immediate survival (by decreasing the bleeding) and for improvement in long-term functioning. The exact roles of external and internal fixation are not clear at present. Neither is the timing of such procedures. Primary internal fixation may be indicated when laparotomy or bladder repair is being performed in a patient with symphyseal disruption or major vessel laceration.

Retroperitoneal bleed: Bleeding into the retroperitoneum is very common, especially in association with a fractured pelvis and it is best defined by CT scan.

Most retroperitoneal haematomas do not require surgical intervention after blunt trauma, even if discovered at laparotomy. Pelvic retroperitoneal haematoma can result from venous bleeding at fracture sites, disruption of pelvic veins in the posterior pelvic plexus, or disruption of deep pelvic arteries, often distal branches of the internal iliac vessels. Perirenal haematomas and midline haematomas can also occur in the retroperitoneal space.

Although blood loss can be considerable, it usually ceases spontaneously. However, major haemorrhage from this area is frustrating and difficult to treat when life-threatening. Pelvic stabilisation using external pelvic fixation can decrease bleeding and is sometimes lifesaving. In the right hands, interventional radiology and, if necessary, embolisation can achieve excellent results. It should be performed in all cases of proven retroperitoneal haematomas with uncontrollable bleeding. Continuous bleeding can sometimes be from an arterial source rather than venous plexus bleeding. Arterial bleeding is more amenable to surgery than venous bleeding.

## Continuing management in intensive care

Such patients usually have other injuries and require close monitoring of vital signs, continuing resuscitation and further investigation of injuries in many cases.

### Abdominal compartment syndrome

Patients with abdominal trauma may develop increasing intra-abdominal pressures. Such increased pressure will seriously compromise the blood supply to most intra-abdominal organs and can cause renal failure. Girth measurements are of no value in this situation and all patients should have intravesical pressure measurements.

### Intra-abdominal sepsis

Intra-abdominal sepsis and MOF remain major contributors to mortality following severe trauma. Intra-abdominal sepsis is, in fact, usually characterised by the onset of MOF, rather than by localising signs. If suspected, it should be aggressively investigated and treated (see Chapter 9).

## Thoracic injuries

Chest trauma is often associated with trauma at other sites. Resuscitate and monitor these patients as previously outlined for multitrauma and maintain a high index of suspicion regarding other injuries.

In particular, closely monitor for signs of blood loss and respiratory distress.

Surgery is seldom indicated for patients who have sustained blunt chest trauma. The major principle of management is to provide support for the patients while their injuries heal. Most chest injuries are adequately treated with chest drains for air and blood collections, as well as adequate pain relief; but do not hesitate to consider surgery for massive air leak or continuing and significant intrathoracic bleeding.

Conservative management depends on complete pain relief, often in conjunction with manoeuvres to improve oxygenation (e.g. CPAP). If this fails, artificial ventilation may be necessary, especially in the presence of associated injuries.

### Immediate resuscitation

The principles of resuscitation are the same as for multitrauma patients.

#### Airway
Establish a reliable airway.

Breathing: Is there respiratory distress? Look for:

- tachypnoea
- tachycardia
- decreased movement of one side of the chest (the abnormality will always be on that side)
- low oxygen saturation.

Feel for and listen for

- tracheal deviation
- surgical emphysema
- percussion (a large pneumothorax will sound 'hollow')
- breath sounds.

Give all patients 100% oxygen initially.

Rule out the possibility of pneumothorax (simple, tension or open) and haemothorax.

Restore the mechanics of breathing if necessary, by artificial ventilation.

Circulation:

- Rapidly restore the intravascular volume.
- Hypovolaemic shock is by far the most common cardiovascular problem in trauma patients, but one must exclude the possibility of cardiac tamponade, myocardial contusion and infarction.

### Chest x-ray

There is no single investigation which offers more important information than an upright chest film in the presence of chest trauma. Look for:

- pneumothoraces and other examples of extra-alveolar air (EAA), such as sub-cutaneous emphysema, mediastinal emphysema and pneumoperitoneum
- haemothorax
- rib fractures
- lung contusion
- aspiration
- signs associated with a ruptured diaphragm
- widened mediastinum and, more rarely, cardiac tamponade.

**If there is a widened mediastinum or other radiological signs, exclude the possibility of a ruptured thoracic aorta by immediate aortography.**

## Pneumothorax

### Clinical sign

Decreased entry of air and tracheal deviation usually occur with a significant pneumothorax, together with cardiorespiratory collapse, unless it is drained. If the patient is being ventilated and develops a pneumothorax, the ventilatory pressure can suddenly rise and the patient can become hypoxic. A high index of suspicion is essential for patients with multitrauma.

### Management

Open pneumothorax: Cover the pneumothorax immediately with an airtight dressing and insert an intercostal tube but not through the directly damaged part of the chest.

Tension pneumothorax: If the patient is in severe respiratory distress and a pneumothorax is clinically suspected, insert a 12 gauge catheter in the second intercostal space, mid-clavicular line, in order to decompress the air. Follow this with a chest tube in the fifth-sixth intercostal space.

Simple pneumothorax: The rule for all severely injured patients is that a pneumothorax should be drained with a chest tube, no matter how small it is. This is particularly important in the presence of underlying respiratory disease or when a patient is to receive positive-pressure ventilation.

Chest tube: Except in emergency circumstances, insert the chest tube in the fifth or sixth intercostal space, mid-axillary line. It should be a large, straight tube with a blunt plastic tip. Liberal use of local anaesthetic should be followed by an incision of approximately 2 cm; then blunt dissection down to the pleura and insertion of the tube by directing it posteriorly and superiorly toward the apex. Avoid purse string sutures; use simple mattress sutures. Confirm the position of the catheter by chest x-ray and by the presence of bubbling and swinging of the fluid level in the underwater seal. Check the chest x-ray for correct siting of the distal holes within the pleural cavity. Place the underwater seal under the bed during transport. Never clamp an intercostal tube. Suction is often necessary to drain blood and sometimes to drain air. However, suction may exacerbate the air leak. A single tube is usually adequate for air and fluid drainage. Multiple tubes in appropriate positions may be necessary for loculated collections. If a single chamber chest drainage bottle is used to drain chest fluid, it should be changed frequently; otherwise, as the level of fluid rose, the efficiency of drainage would decrease.

## Other manifestations of extra-alveolar air

Whereas a pneumothorax and localised subcutaneous emphysema resulting from a punctured lung are the most common manifestation of EAA, gas can also collect in other sites, leading to conditions such as mediastinal emphysema, pneumoretroperitoneum and pneumoperitoneum. These can occur in association with blunt chest injuries. The mechanism is not necessarily related to puncture of the lung by fractured ribs. It usually involves severe blunt injury against a closed glottis. That causes simultaneous rupture of alveoli at the time of trauma, in a manner similar to a massive Valsalva manoeuvre. Air moves in the adventitia of pulmonary vessels as pulmonary interstitial emphysema to the mediastinum to cause mediastinal emphysema, then up into the neck and over the anterior chest wall to produce subcutaneous emphysema. It can break through the thin mediastinal pleura to cause a pneumothorax, or alongside the oesophagus and aorta to yield pneumoretroperitoneum and pneumoperitoneum. The clinical importance of these phenomena is as follows:

1  Subcutaneous emphysema in the neck, rather than at the site of fractured ribs, may indicate EAA formation by this mechanism, rather than by lung puncture. Subcutaneous emphysema and mediastinal emphysema can also occur in combination with a pneumothorax associated with rupture of the tracheobronchial tree. Rarely, subcutaneous emphysema and mediastinal emphysema can occur after a ruptured oesophagus.
2  The presence of simultaneous subcutaneous emphysema and mediastinal emphysema, simultaneously, without a pneumothorax, points to massive pulmonary interstitial emphysema as the mechanism rather than a punctured lung.
3  Positive-pressure ventilation can predispose to further EAA.
4  Pneumoperitoneum and pneumoretroperitoneum must be differentiated from a ruptured abdominal viscous.
5  Management of EAA formation involves reducing the level of positive-pressure-support. For example, use CPAP rather than intermittent positive-pressure ventilation (IPPV) where possible. Use techniques such as pressure-support in order to reduce the level of positive-pressure.

## Rupture of the tracheobronchial tree

A bronchopleural fistula (BPF) is a communication between the bronchial tree and pleural space, resulting in a massive air leak. Simultaneous rupture of many alveoli can also cause a large air leak.

### Diagnosis
- Presence of a large, continuous leak from the chest tube.
- Persistent pneumothorax, despite chest drains.
- Bronchoscopy – most rupture 1–2 cm from the carina.

## Management

1 Use a large diameter intercostal catheter.
2 Drainage: The catheter either can be attached to an underwater drain or can be connected to suction. Usually a suction level of no more than 20 cmH$_2$O is sufficient to facilitate flow.
3 Ventilatory strategies:
   - Lowest effective tidal volumes, peak inspiratory pressures and positive end-expiratory pressure (PEEP) should be employed to encourage healing of the BPF.
   - High frequency ventilation can encourage decreased ventilatory pressure and healing of the BPF.
   - Independent lung ventilation, using either CPAP or low tidal volumes on the affected side and normal tidal volumes and pressures on the other side, can reduce the leak in a BPF.

Surgery (e.g. bronchial stump stapling or decortication) is sometimes necessary when the leak will not respond to the foregoing measures.

### Haemopneumothorax

The bleeding from a haemopneumothorax usually stops without surgical intervention. Any significant haemothorax (i.e. visible on chest x-ray) should be drained via a large intercostal tube. The same tube can be used to drain both air and blood if a pneumothorax is also present. Blood loss is accurately reflected by the loss from the intercostal tube. Continued bleeding usually indicates arterial loss from an intercostal artery, rather than from the low pressure pulmonary circuit.

Thoracotomy should be considered when the total blood loss is more than 1500 ml or if drainage of blood exceeds 300 ml/h for more than 4 hours.

### Lung contusion

Lung contusion or 'bruised' lung is usually associated with rib fractures, especially a flail chest. In children, contused lung occurs commonly without rib fractures, because a child's rib cage is more flexible.

Lung contusion is usually seen on initial chest x-ray as a patchy infiltrate that typically progresses over the next 24–48 hours before it begins to clear. Lung contusion is invariably associated with hypoxia which can be very severe. The spectrum of severity varies from mild to life-threatening pulmonary oedema. There can be simultaneous alveolar rupture necessitating a ventilatory technique that employs relatively low intrathoracic pressures such as CPAP, in order to avoid further lung damage and EAA formation. Some patients with severe hypoxia and contusion can develop long-term changes in respiratory function and exercise tolerance. The long-term changes probably result from underlying lung damage in combination with high ventilatory pressures.

## Treatment (see the general principles of treating respiratory failure)

The principles of management are as follows:

- Use a face mask with a high concentration of inspired oxygen.
- Use CPAP via a mask if it can be tolerated, provided there are no contraindications such as a fracture of the base of the skull and provided adequate ventilation is possible.
- Maintain circulating volume with colloid or blood, avoiding excessive amounts of crystalloid.
- Use positive-pressure ventilatory techniques such as pressure-support ventilation, if ventilation is inadequate (see Chapter 19).
- Pain relief: Epidural, intrapleural or intercostal nerve blocks will provide excellent pain relief when there are associated rib fractures.

  Monitor progress with:

- Serial chest x-rays (at least daily).
- Serial determinations of arterial blood gases or pulse oximetry.

### Fractured ribs

**Fractured ribs can be a life-threatening condition. The risk increases with age and when the patient is a smoker.**

- Fractured ribs are often associated with severe pain. Pain restricts coughing and breathing, predisposing to sputum retention, atelectasis, pneumonia and respiratory failure.
- Fractured ribs are often associated with underlying lung contusion.
- Fractured ribs can puncture underlying structures.
- Fractured ribs are often difficult to diagnose on initial chest x-ray. As an empirical rule, the actual number of fractured ribs will be double the number seen on chest x-ray.
- The fractures may be simple or multiple or part of a flail chest.
- Fractures of the first and second ribs are associated with higher incidences of damage to the myocardium, major vessels and bronchi.
- Even a small number of simple rib fractures in an elderly patient or in a patient with underlying lung disease can cause life-threatening complications such as hypoventilation, collapse and pneumonia.
  **It is easy to underestimate the seriousness of fractured ribs and flail chest.**

They should be aggressively treated with pain relief, with or without CPAP. These patients tend to look best at admission and to slowly deteriorate, especially those who are old or obese or have underlying lung disease.
- There is little, if any, place for surgical repair of fractured ribs.

Flail chest: Flail chest is caused by fractures in two or more locations on each of three or more adjacent ribs. While the paradoxical movement of the flail segment can interfere with ventilation, the flail segment is more as a marker of underlying severe lung contusion.

Treatment: The thrust of treatment has moved away from stabilisation of rib fractures and mechanical ventilation.

The cornerstone of conservative treatment is *complete pain relief*. Pain relief can be provided by intermittent or continuous doses of narcotics or by regional local anaesthetic techniques such as intercostal nerve block or thoracic epidurals. The choice of techniques will depend on the extent of the rib fractures, the severity of pain and associated injuries and the expertise of the operator.

Complete pain relief often allows adequate spontaneous ventilation. Early assisted ventilation with CPAP or pressure-support ventilation can prevent problems such as lung collapse and pneumonia. A CPAP mask should not be used for patients who have a depressed level of consciousness, facial fractures or base of skull fractures.

Intubation and artificial ventilation are sometimes necessary, especially if there are associated injuries such as head trauma or spinal injuries or when a patient is obese or has grossly unstable rib fractures. Where possible, mask CPAP and complete pain relief should be used, rather than intubation, ventilation and systemic narcotics as the former are associated with fewer complications. Early tracheostomy should be considered in patients with fractured ribs who need intubation, as they usually require at least 2–3 weeks of respiratory support.

## Pleural drainage

Drainage of air or fluid from the pleural space requires an airtight system to maintain the subatmospheric intrapleural pressure. To drain air or fluid, a low resistance tube is needed with a one-way valve (usually underwater). The amount of suction generated is determined by the distance between the pleural cavity and the collection chamber. The lower the chamber, the more suction. However, when air pockets break the continuity of the fluid column, less suction is generated. Thus, in addition to lowering the collection chamber, negative pressure may also be necessary to facilitate air and fluid removal. The collection chamber should always be more than 100 cm below the chest in order to prevent fluid from being sucked up into the chest when large subatmospheric pressures are generated (e.g. during obstructed inspiration). Unless precise flow measurements are used, the amount of suction needed is empirical. Excessive suction can potentiate air leaks.

A small amount of suction (less than $-20 \, cmH_2O$) can help overcome resistance to airflow within the system.

A large diameter chamber (about 20 cm diameter) will maintain the underwater seal with minimum resistance to drainage. The catheter should be placed about 2 cm under the water. If a one bottle system is used there is increasing resistance as the chamber fills as well as difficulty in measuring in the presence of bubbling and foaming. Two, three and four bottle systems will increase safety and efficiency but they are more cumbersome and expensive. Commercial devices that are compact and disposable using two, three or four bottles are beginning to be used in many ICUs (Figures 14.2 and 14.3).

The system is monitored by observing synchronous oscillations. If blockage is suspected, gentle milking of the tube can be performed. The pleural tube should never be clamped and the collection chamber should always be kept below the level of the chest during transport. Consideration should be given to removing the intercostal catheter after bubbling has ceased for more than 12 hours. A chest x-ray is needed after removal of the catheter to exclude accumulation of air or fluid.

## Aspiration

Aspiration should always be considered a possibility especially in association with coma, intoxication and facial fractures.

Aspiration can be distinguished from contusion on the basis of its distribution on chest x-ray, as well as on the basis of the appearance and smell of the tracheal aspirate. Look for radio-opaque foreign bodies (e.g. teeth). Consider bronchoscopy if obstruction by a foreign body is suspected. Respiratory support for aspiration involves the same general principles as for contusion.

## Traumatic rupture of the diaphragm

Rupture of the diaphragm occurs in approximately 5% of cases of blunt trauma to the trunk. The left side is more commonly ruptured than the right which is protected by the liver.

### Presentation
- A ruptured diaphragm is very difficult to detect clinically, particularly if the patient is on positive-pressure ventilation.
- Diminished chest expansion and air entry.
- Tracheal deviation with underlying mediastinal shift.
- Bowel sounds in the chest.

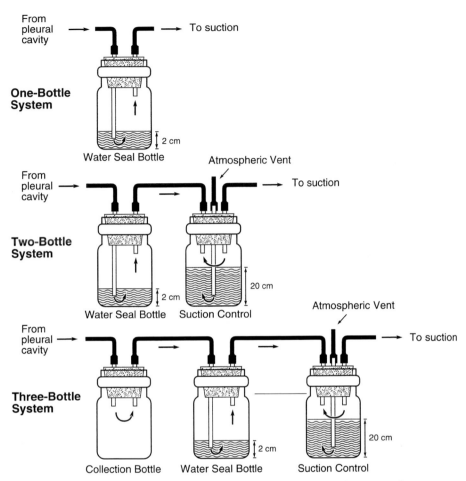

**Figure 14.2.** Pleural drainage systems. The drainage system consists of a water seal, drainage trap, pressure control chamber and connecting tubes. In the case of a single bottle, the water seal also acts as the drainage trap for fluid and air (above). The bottle either is vented to air or has suction attached to it. A two-bottle system contains a bottle that acts as a drainage trap as well as a water seal and a separate bottle for suction control. A three-bottle system has one bottle for drainage, one as a water seal and the third for suction control.

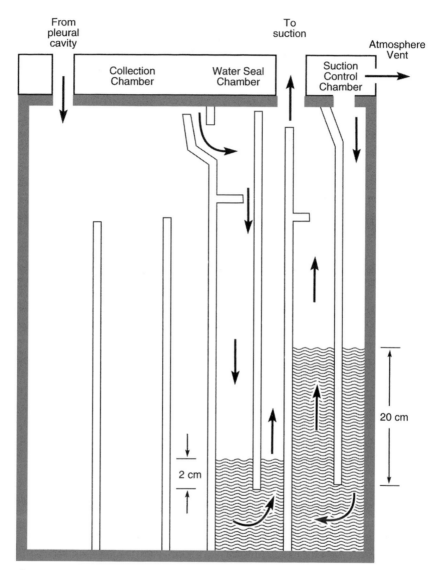

**Figure 14.3.** Commercially available systems can combine the three-bottle setup into one disposable lightweight and transportable package that allows a separate drainage area, underwater seal compartment and suction control compartment (right). Reprinted by permission of Blackwell Scientific Publications Inc. Gilbert, T.B.N., McGrath, B.J., and Soberman, M. Chest tubes: indications, placement management and complications. *Journal of Intensive Care Medicine* 8 (1993): 73–86.

## Investigations

Chest x-ray is by far the most important investigation but can be difficult to interpret. Abnormalities can include:

- elevated left hemidiaphragm
- herniation of abdominal organs
- mediastinal shift
- haemothorax
- atelectasis
- abnormal position of NG tube.

Liver scintigraphy
Ultrasound
CT scan
Laparoscopy/thoracoscopy.

## Management

All diaphragmatic lacerations should be surgically repaired at an early stage because of the risk of herniation of an abdominal viscous.

## Oesophageal trauma

Oesophageal trauma usually is a result of a penetrating injury. Symptoms include pain and dysphagia. Signs include mediastinal air and gastric contents draining from the chest tube. Treatment is surgical. Oesophageal rupture after blunt trauma is rare and usually fatal.

# Cardiac injuries

## Myocardial contusion

Myocardial contusion is associated with blunt anterior chest injuries, especially involving a fractured sternum. The right ventricle lies under the sternum so it is unusual for myocardial contusion to cause haemodynamic compromise.

The contusion can be diagnosed on the basis of serial ECGs, creatinine phosphokinase (CPK) MB fraction levels, troponin I, technetium-99m scanning, ECG gated scintigraphy or echocardiography. None of these is entirely satisfactory either for diagnosis or for demonstrating the extent of the contusion or prognosis. The most promising method for assessment is echocardiography.

Cardiac contusion usually responds to conservative measures. Patients with normal ECGs and normal clinical findings on admission usually do not require monitoring. However, an abnormal admission ECG or an arrhythmia is an indicator for further assessment.

## Penetrating cardiac injuries

### Chest injuries associated with cardiac injuries

- Penetrating wounds that are unlikely, judging from site and direction, to be associated with cardiac injury occurring in patients with no evidence of shock. This grouping comprises approximately 80% of such cases. Treatment includes observation with or without drainage.
- Suspicious chest wounds, usually over the cardiac area, in patients who are hypotensive but who respond well to fluid replacement. Approximately 50% of these patients will deteriorate and need surgical exploration. Monitoring and resuscitation must be carried out while transport is quickly arranged to an institution where facilities for immediate cardiac surgery are available. An ECG should be performed. These account for approximately 15% of all such cases.
- Highly suspicious chest wounds in a small group (approximately 5%) of moribund patients who require immediate thoracotomy to relieve tamponade, rapid fluid resuscitation and internal cardiac massage. Many of these will achieve full recovery if treatment is rapid.

## Pericardial tamponade

Pericardial tamponade usually is associated with penetrating injuries, but can result from severe blunt trauma.

Tamponade rapidly becomes life-threatening by interfering with cardiac function.

Patients with cardiac tamponade classically present with hypotension, distended neck veins and muffled heart sounds. If a patient is also hypovolaemic, the neck veins may not be raised. If the neck veins are raised, consider tension pneumothorax, myocardial contusion and myocardial infarct as alternative diagnoses.

Emergency thoracotomy rather than pericardiocentesis is usually needed, even if the patient appears moribund, as the blood within the pericardium is often clotted. Complications of pericardiocentesis include laceration of the heart and coronary vessels during aspiration.

## Cardiogenic shock

Hypovolaemic shock is by far the most common type of shock associated with trauma. However, cardiogenic shock can occur in some patients (e.g. the elderly) who have myocardial infarction, either as precipitating causes of their accidents or coincidentally.

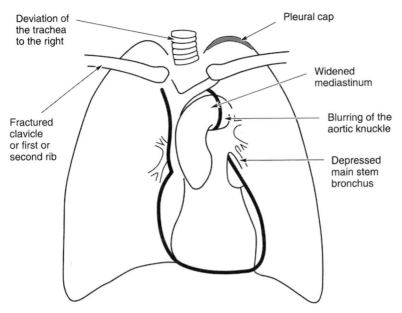

**Figure 14.4.** Radiological signs of a ruptured thoracic aorta.

## Great vessel injury

Great vessel injury is relatively rare after blunt trauma. The diagnosis should be considered in all cases of severe decelerating injuries (e.g. a head-on collision, being thrown from a car or a fall of more than 10 metres). A high index of suspicion is required for this diagnosis and these injuries have serious consequences if they are overlooked.

Most patients with ruptures of the great thoracic vessels die instantly. A survivor will have a contained haematoma and will need rapid management. Half of the surviving patients will die each day if left untreated.

A ruptured thoracic aorta usually is suspected when an upright chest x-ray shows a widened mediastinum and blurring of the aortic knob. Other associated radiological signs (Figure 14.4) include fractures of the first and second ribs, deviation of the trachea to the right and a pleural cap. However, these signs are inconsistent and difficult to interpret on an anterior-posterior x-ray made with the patient supine.

If the mediastinum is seen to be widened on upright chest x-ray, aortography, rather than thoracic CT, is the investigation of choice.

A TOE has also been shown to be useful in the diagnosis of thoracic aortic rupture.

Surgical repair should be performed in specialised centres with cardiopulmonary bypass facilities.

# Spinal injuries

## Injuries of the cervical spine

**An awake, co-operative, asymptomatic patient does not have a cervical spine injury.**

Any patient who has suffered trauma and who has a compromised level of consciousness should be assumed to have injuries of the cervical spine until proved otherwise. Although a high index of suspicion should always be maintained, resuscitation procedures should not be compromised or delayed. Compared with airway obstruction, hypovolaemia and respiratory impairment, spinal injuries are uncommon. If the airway is compromised, intubation has the highest priority, and it can almost always be safely achieved by holding the head and neck in a neutral position during the procedure.

Injuries of the cervical spine are often associated with certain activities (e.g. sporting injuries, diving into a shallow pool) or with severe multitrauma, especially in association with head injuries. Injuries of the cervical spine are found in 5–10% of patients who are unconscious after a fall or a vehicle crash.

One should suspect spinal injury in the presence of the following:

- flaccid areflexia
- localised pain or sensory and motor deficits
- unexplained hypotension, normal pulse rate and peripheral vasodilatation
- diaphragmatic breathing
- absence of anal and bulbocavernosus reflexes
- priapism.

Lateral x-rays of the cervical spine should be obtained for any patient who has sustained severe multitrauma, as soon as the patient is adequately resuscitated. All seven vertebrae must be visualised. Simple antero-posterior and lateral cervical views will exclude most fractures. More sophisticated views may be necessary after resuscitation. When cervical spine damage is suspected in a patient with head injuries, CT views of the cervical spine area in question should be obtained at the same time as a CT view of the head. Subluxation may not be demonstrated on CT scan.

## Management

Spinal immobilisation is the mainstay of treatment
- Hard collar (soft collars are of little value).
- Sandbags on each side of the head, and the head taped to a spine board.
- Manual inline immobilisation, with the head in a neutral position.

Immobilisation helps to reduce fractures and dislocations, correct spinal mis-alignments and decompress the cord and nerve roots. Definitive treatment may involve traction. Surgery is sometimes indicated in unstable fractures in order to facilitate nursing care and reduce delays in mobilisation.

Intubation and ventilation may be required if the cord lesion involves the phrenic nerve C3, C4, C5 or above. Intubation usually can be safely achieved by an experienced operator with an assistant performing manual inline immo-bilisation. Atropine (0.4 mg IV) should be given for persistent bradycardia and inotropic support (e.g. adrenaline infusion is sometimes necessary to correct persistent hypotension. It is important to maintain an adequate perfusion pres-sure in these patients. Overzealous administration of fluids can cause pulmonary oedema.

A urinary catheter and NG tube should be inserted.

Methylprednisolone, 30 mg/kg stat and $5.4 \, mg \cdot kg^{-1} \cdot h^{-1}$ for 23 hours, given within 8 hours of injury, may, in the long-term, help to preserve sensory and motor function, although more research data are needed at this point.

Selective hypothermia, naloxone, hyperosmotic agents and coma treatment have shown equivocal results.

All patients with significant spinal injuries should be transferred to a specialised spinal unit as soon as they have been resuscitated.

## Fractures of the thoracic and lumbar spine

If a thoracic or lumbar spinal injury is suspected, immobilisation must be achieved above and below the site (i.e. head and neck, chest, pelvis and extremities may all need to be immobilised on a spine board). Once resuscitation has been achieved, log roll the patient and assess for pain and a palpable deformity.

### Thoracic spine
The commonest fracture in this region is a wedge fracture from hyperflexion. This fracture is usually stable.

### Lumbar spine
Fractures of the thoracolumbar and lumbar spine are more likely to be unstable than are injuries of the thoracic spine. As the spinal cord terminates at L1-L2, cord lesions at this site can cause a mixture of spinal cord (bladder and bowel signs) and cauda equina signs (sensory deficits in lower limbs).

## Genitourinary trauma

- Genitourinary trauma is commonly associated with pelvic fractures.
- Trauma to the male urethra, bladder and kidneys is relatively common whereas trauma to the ureters is rare.

- A rectal examination should be performed before a urinary catheter is passed.
- Haematuria is a common non-specific sign. Only when the haematuria is significant and prolonged should investigation of the urinary tract be undertaken. An intravenous pyelogram (IVP) probably is worthwhile only if there are more than 30 red blood cells per high power field. The only exception may be haematuria in a patient with severe abdominal trauma in order to determine the state of renal blood flow.
- Urological investigations are time-consuming and only rarely are the injuries immediately life-threatening. They should be delayed until the patient is fully resuscitated.
- An IVP can be achieved with 30% contrast material at 1–2 ml/kg (up to 100 ml), followed by a plain abdominal film within 5–10 minutes. This will show most major abnormalities in the kidney and collecting system. If a kidney is not visualised, selective renal angiography may be indicated. Delayed films and tomography may be needed to further evaluate renal parenchyma and ureters. In the presence of an abnormal IVP, CT is often the next diagnostic step as it is highly sensitive and accurate.

## Kidney trauma

Trauma to the kidneys usually results in contusions or lacerations, which often will heal with conservative management. Persistent haemorrhage or extravasation of urine will require surgery.

## Bladder trauma

Among patients who sustain blunt trauma, bladder rupture is rare when the bladder is empty, usually occurring only when it is full (e.g. after prior alcohol intake), especially in association with fractured pelvic rami or a separated pubic symphysis. Rupture can present as haematuria, positive findings on peritoneal lavage, anuria or even peritonitis.

A retrograde cystogram may be indicated in the presence of haematuria and a fractured pelvis. It can be readily performed by gravity infusion of 150–300 ml of water-soluble contrast material. Antero-posterior, oblique and post-drainage views are necessary to exclude injury. The priority of IVP over cystography hinges on whether upper or lower tract injury is more likely. A CT scan with IV contrast is increasingly being used to evaluate the urinary tract in the presence of pelvic fractures.

## Urethral trauma

Urethral trauma is a rare problem. When it does occur, it is usually in association with severe blunt trauma to the pelvis and perineum. A high riding prostate, blood at the urethral meatus and a scrotal haematoma are contraindications for placing an indwelling bladder catheter. Either a suprapubic cystostomy, if the bladder can be palpated, or urethrogram should be considered.

If the patency of the urethra is in doubt, an urethrogram should be obtained before catheterisation This is achieved by the gentle injection of 30 ml of water-soluble contrast through the urethra via a urinary catheter secured in the meatal fossa by balloon inflation to about 3 ml.

# Penetrating trauma

The early management of a patient who has suffered penetrating trauma is the same as for those with other injuries. The patient should be managed with the same systematic approach in the primary and secondary surveys, as well as for more definitive treatment. Much of this is discussed under specific sections in this chapter (e.g. abdomen, chest, extremities). However, there are specific aspects of penetrating trauma that one should remember during assessment and treatment.

## Penetrating chest injuries

- Lacerations of intrathoracic organs can cause catastrophic blood loss. Emergency thoracotomy rather than trying to maintain the circulation with intravenous fluids may be necessary. The indications for emergency thoracotomy are discussed elsewhere.
- When the positioning of a penetrating foreign object or the entry and exit wounds suggest that the mediastinum has been traversed, exploratory thoracotomy is mandatory, even if the patient is initially stable, as the probability of damage to vital structures is high.
- Pulmonary lacerations are associated with a pneumothorax or haemothorax. Major, life-threatening lacerations are uncommon, representing about 4% of thoracic trauma cases, usually accompanied by haemoptysis or haemopneumothorax with parenchymal haematoma. These patients usually require thoracotomy.
- Cardiac lacerations can result in rapid exsanguination into the pleural space, cardiac tamponade and other injuries, depending on the site of penetration.
- Large vessel penetration presents as massive bleeding in more than 50% of cases. If the damage is intrapericardial, pericardial tamponade may result. Less serious injuries can result in false aneurysms or arteriovenous fistulae. Urgent surgery rather than IV fluid administration is often required.
- A lacerated diaphragm, like rupture of the diaphragm from blunt trauma is a difficult diagnosis to make. Exploratory laparotomy/thoracoscopy may be necessary, especially when the site of penetration raises suspicion that a knife or bullet may have gone through the diaphragm.

## Penetrating abdominal trauma

- Blood loss can be severe. Rapid replacement through large bore cannulae and early cross matching are essential.
- Every entry wound must be noted, particularly when they are multiple. If there are exit wounds in the back, bear in mind the possibility of penetration of abdominal viscera.
- Radiographs may demonstrate missiles or foreign bodies within the body.
- Penetration of the peritoneal cavity may be evident from the location of the entry or exit sites or from radiographic visualisation.
- Stable patients with stab wounds may only require local wound exploration or peritoneal lavage.
- Laparotomy is mandatory if the lavage fluid contains blood or increased amylase.
- Early administration of antibiotics with a wide spectrum, covering anaerobes and gram-negative bacteria and tetanus prophylaxis should be commenced if laparotomy is performed.

## Burns

The initial assessment, management and investigations should be carried out simultaneously, according to the priorities for the particular patient.

### History

It is important to determine the circumstances of the burn.

- Explosions (liquid, steam, fire): Look for other features such as fractures and intra-abdominal bleeding.
- Burning wood, chemicals, plastic: Think of cyanide poisoning and water-soluble gases causing pneumonitis.
- Burns in an enclosed space: Consider carbon monoxide poisoning.

### Initial management

**Secure the airway.**
**Assess and treat respiratory dysfunction.**
**Replace lost fluids.**
**Relieve the patient's pain.**
**Consider escharotomy or fasciotomy.**
**Transfer to a burns centre as soon as the patient is resuscitated.**

## Airway and pulmonary inhalation injuries

Tracheobronchial and pulmonary parenchymal injuries are due to direct effects of heat or chemicals.

Inhalational injuries are seen in about 20% of burn patients and are associated with various factors:

- fire in an enclosed space
- circumferential neck burns
- a period of unconsciousness before rescue (especially in association with drugs, alcohol or head injuries)
- facial burns/singed facial hair
- hoarseness/stridor
- carbonaceous sputum
- dyspnoea, wheezing.

The diagnosis is usually obvious on the basis of history and clinical presentation.

The key to management of these patients is close observation in an environment in which intubation can be achieved rapidly by skilled personnel. If there is evidence of upper airway burn, the patient should be intubated.

Acute upper airway obstruction can suddenly develop, in which case one should intubate and then either artificially ventilate or deliver CPAP. Tracheostomy can be performed safely in burn victims but it may not be technically possible.

All patients suspected of inhalational injuries should have maximum concentrations of inspired oxygen. Chest x-ray and arterial blood gas determinations should be used to assess the severity of the damage. The initial chest x-ray may show nothing abnormal.

Parenchymal lung injury or ALI can be related to the primary injury or, less commonly, can result from overly aggressive fluid resuscitation. Treatment is outlined in Chapter 18.

Carbon monoxide poisoning should always be considered a possibility in burn patients, especially from enclosed spaces. Determine carboxyhaemoglobin levels if in doubt. Symptoms can occur if levels are higher than 15%. Myocardial ischaemia can occur when levels are higher than 25%. A cherry red skin colour is an uncommon and unreliable sign.

## Fluid replacement

The goal of fluid resuscitation is to maintain adequate tissue perfusion without exacerbating the burn oedema. The composition of the resuscitation fluid is less important than is titration of the correct amount for the individual patient's need.

Estimate the percentage of the body burned and the thickness of the burn injury (Figure 14.5). Fluid loss is directly related to the fluid sequestered as a

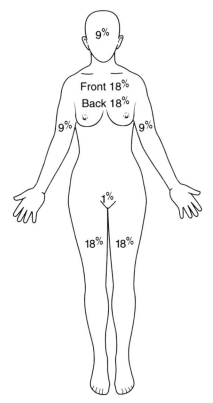

**Figure 14.5.** The 'Rule of nines' for rapid assessment of percentage body burnt. Do not include simple erythema.

result of thermal injury. Little further sequestration of fluid will occur 18–30 hours post-burn.

Intravenous fluid is required if more than 15% of the body is burned.

The choice between colloid and crystalloid solutions is still controversial. Although some of the colloid particles will leak out of the intravascular space in the affected area, colloids may be more efficient in terms of restoring plasma volume and causing less pulmonary and peripheral oedema in the unaffected areas.

Despite the myriad of formulae for fluid replacement, the aim is to maintain organ perfusion. This is best achieved by maintaining urine output at least $0.5 \, \text{ml} \cdot \text{kg}^{-1} \cdot \text{h}^{-1}$ for adults and $1 \, \text{ml} \cdot \text{kg}^{-1} \cdot \text{h}^{-1}$ for children. This will mean giving IV fluid at an approximate 2–4 ml/kg/percentage of body burned (% burn) per day for adults.

## Guidelines

The following is a suggested fluid regimen, assuming that all times are calculated from the moment of injury. Alterations will have to be made according to the patient's clinical status.

Give a balanced salt solution (Ringer's lactate or Hartmann's solution) at 2–4 ml/kg × (% burn)/day. Administer half of the amount in the first 8 hours and the remainder in the next 16 hours. Then give colloid and maintenance fluid as necessary.

Give blood as necessary (usually required if more than 30% of body is burnt).

Intravenous water in the form of dextrose and water may be necessary, in addition to the foregoing requirements as maintenance fluid, in order to prevent hypernatraemia. The amount of water can be empirically titrated against the serum sodium concentration (usually 1–3 L/day).

Remember that the volume necessary to resuscitate patients with burns is dependent on the severity of the burn, age, physiological status and other associated injuries. Resuscitation formula are only guidelines.

## Immediate investigations

Arterial blood gases.
Urea and electrolytes.
Haemoglobin, blood grouping and cross matching.
Chest x-ray.
Carbon monoxide levels.
12-lead ECG.

## Immediate monitoring

Pulse rate and continuous ECG.
Respiratory rate.
Pulse oximetry.
Arterial BP.
Urine output.
Level of consciousness.

## Analgesia

**Intravenous opiates should be given in liberal quantities for this distressing injury.**
An opiate is best given as a continuous IV infusion, titrated against its pain-relieving effects.

## Escharotomy

Immediate escharotomy or fasciotomy is occasionally indicated. Rapid excision of devitalised tissue, combined with early and continuous wound closure with autograft or artificial skin, is essential.

## Nutritional support

Patients with burns have markedly increased metabolic rates, increased rates of glucose production and utilisation, decreased rates of lipid metabolism and increased rates of protein catabolism and anabolism. The principles of nutritional support are the same as outlined for other seriously ill patients (see Chapter 5). Enteral feeding is preferred, where possible, to IV nutrition. Enteral feeding should be initiated within 48 hours of burn injury, utilising feeding tubes until the patient is capable of taking adequate amounts orally. The diet should provide approximately 50% of calories as carbohydrate, 25% as protein and 25% as fat.

**Prophylactic antibiotics and corticosteroids should not be used. Transfer the patient to a specialised burns unit as soon as adequate resuscitation has been achieved.**

## Overall course of burns

Days 1–2
    Resuscitation
    • airway
    • breathing
    • fluids and support of the circulation.
Days 2–5
    Oedema reabsorption
    Increase in urine output with potassium losses
Day 6
    Marked increase in metabolic rate

# Electrical injuries

The damage sustained during electrical injuries is related to various factors:
• Type of current.
• Duration of current flow – the longer the contact, the greater the damage (AC worse than DC because of tetanic effect on muscles).
• Surface area contacted (greater current density in a small area).
• Resistance (more severe damage occurs in areas of high resistance).
• Current (the higher the current, the greater the damage).

- Voltage (anything greater than 40 volts is potentially dangerous).
- Current pathway (related to resistance and voltage).

## Pathophysiology

Electrical injuries are related to primary electrical trauma and electrothermal burns that result from electrical energy being converted to heat as it passes through tissues. Flame burns can also occur if the current ignites clothing or other material.

## Clinical features

Coagulation necrosis: This is the major feature of electrical injuries and it occurs as a result of vessel thrombosis and heat damage. It can result in extensive tissue necrosis, similar to that seen with a crush injury.

Cutaneous wounds: Usually there is a charred entry wound with multiple exit sites.

### Cardiac
- Conduction defects, including ventricular fibrillation (VF), ventricular tachycardia (VT), supraventricular tachycardia (SVT), bundle branch blocks and heart block.
- Myocardial rupture.
- Coronary ischaemia.

### Respiratory
- Upper airway burns.
- Haemopneumothorax.

### Neurological
- Confusion, seizures and loss of consciousness.
- Cerebral haemorrhage, oedema and focal damage.
- Peripheral nerve damage.
- Spinal cord damage.
- Long-term memory and behavioural problems.

### Musculoskeletal
- Tetanic contractions.
- Disruption of muscle cells (release of potassium and CPK).
- Fractures/dislocation of vertebral bodies and other bones as a result of muscle contraction and/or falls.

### Gastrointestinal
- Nausea, vomiting.
- Bleeding.
- Paralytic ileus.
- Perforated bowel.
- Parenchymatous injury (e.g. pancreas, spleen, gall bladder).

### Renal
- Renal failure (albuminuria, haemoglobinuria, myoglobinuria).

### Vascular
- Arterial and venous thrombosis and rupture.
- Haemolysis.
- Microcirculation thrombosis.
- Aneurysm formation.

### Infection
### Cataracts

## Management

### Initial measures
Remove the patient from the source of the current and ensure ABC:

Airway: Secure the airway and, if necessary, intubate.
Breathing: Assist breathing, if necessary.
Circulation: Give external cardiac massage. Defibrillate, if necessary. Begin aggressive fluid replacement.

### Renal function
Renal function deteriorates secondary to hypovolaemia and myoglobinuria. The treatment for the latter is outlined elsewhere.

### Initial investigation and monitoring
Continuous ECG monitoring and pulse oximetry.
Regular monitoring of vital signs (BP, pulse rate, respiratory rate and urine output).
Haemoglobin and haematocrit.
Urea and electrolytes.
Arterial blood gases.
Renal function tests.
Examine for spinal fractures.
Chest x-ray (upright if possible).

## Further management

Assessment, debridement and fasciotomy, if necessary.

Avoid correcting the serum calcium concentration because of the possibility of ectopic calcification.

Tetanus toxoid prophylaxis and IV penicillin as prophylaxis against clostridial infection of open wounds.

# Crush injuries and acute compartment syndrome

## Crush injuries

Although the term 'crush injury' is sometimes used to cover a wide range of pathological changes, from very minor to severe, it is usually reserved for cases at the more severe end of the spectrum. The clinical signs are determined by the extent of the compressed area and the depth and duration of the compression. Such injuries involve both ischaemia and muscle destruction.

## Aetiology

Patient's own weight: (e.g. unconsciousness related to poisoning or long operations). The heavier the patient, the more severe the damage.

External force: use of antishock garments, limbs caught in machinery, injuries resulting from collapse of a building, other traumatic events causing compression and crushing.

## Clinical features

If the injury is severe enough, a crush syndrome will result caused by disintegration of muscle tissue and rhabdomyolysis with influxes of myoglobin, potassium, uric acid and phosphorus into the circulation. All of that results in two main categories of complications:

- Local: There will be variable degrees of pain, swelling and sensory changes.
- Systemic: In more severe cases, hypovolaemia, acute renal failure, severe coagulopathies (including disseminated intravascular coagulation), ALI and shock can all occur.

## Assessment

The extent of both local and systemic damages will require careful monitoring, including regular testing of sensory and motor nerves and assessment of peripheral pulses. Detection of peripheral pulses does not exclude severe crush injury. Direct pressure measurements of muscle compartments may be necessary.

### Treatment
Resuscitation:

- Administer fluids aggressively: hypovolaemia must be rapidly corrected.
- Regular measurements of arterial blood gases and serum sodium, potassium, magnesium, phosphate, creatinine, urea, uric acid and calcium are necessary.
- Serum creatine kinase activities, greater than five times normal, are diagnostic of muscle damage in the absence of other injuries.
- Regular coagulation studies, haemoglobin and platelet counts are necessary.
- Renal function, respiratory function and cardiovascular function should be closely monitored.
- A CT scan of the affected area may demonstrate myonecrosis.

Respiratory failure: ALI should be treated early.

Renal failure: Correction of hypovolaemia is the most important step in the prevention of renal failure. Alkalinisation of the urine may help to prevent renal failure by preventing the myoglobin precipitating in the renal tubules. Aim to keep the urine pH above 6.5 by an infusion of sodium bicarbonate (10–20 mmol/h).

Diuresis: Aim for a urine output > 200 ml/h using isotonic IV fluids. Beware of the exacerbation of hypovolaemia that can occur with the use of diuretics. Dialysis may be necessary if these measures fail. Regularly check serum electrolytes.

Local injury: Excision of dead muscle is not necessarily essential if the wound is closed. Open crush injuries require fasciotomy and immediate radical debridement of dead muscle. Major bleeding is a common complication.

Dead muscle is an excellent medium for infection and sepsis. Amputation should be considered early, especially for a more severely injured limb with skin lacerations.

Fasciotomy should be considered when there is a high compartment pressure or when distal pulses and capillary filling are absent. Because this will convert the wound into an open wound, radical debridement should accompany the fasciotomy. Amputation should be strongly considered in all patients who have sepsis or open wounds in the presence of a severe crush injury. This is because the muscle tissue is already dead in true crush syndrome, as opposed to a simple compartment syndrome.

## Acute compartment syndrome

A compartment syndrome is a condition in which high pressure, within a closed fascial space (muscle compartment), reduces capillary blood perfusion below the level necessary for tissue viability. Permanent loss of function and limb contracture may occur and therefore capillary perfusion should be restored as soon as possible.

## Aetiology

- Fractures (especially of the tibia).
- Contusions.
- Bleeding disorders.
- Burns.
- Trauma.
- Venous obstruction.
- Post-ischaemic swelling after arterial injury or thrombosis.
- Strenuous exercise.
- Prolonged limb compression (e.g. drug or alcohol overdose).
- Tight plaster cast.

### Clinical features: the 5 'P's

Pain: Pain is the most important symptom. It is described as deep and throbbing, with a feeling of unrelenting pressure. The pain is said to be worse on stretching.

Pressure: The compartment is swollen and palpably tense, although palpation offers only a crude indication of pressure.

Paraesthesia: Paraesthesia may also be found.

Paresis: Paresis may also occur independently as a result of nerve and muscle damage.

Peripheral pulses: Capillary refilling and peripheral pulses can be detected in compartment syndrome, even in the presence of severe muscle ischaemia. This should not lead to a false sense of security.

All of these signs and symptoms can occur independently as a result of trauma, and they are difficult to assess in an unconscious patient.

### Measurement of tissue pressure

Because palpation offers only a crude estimation of tissue pressure, and the presence or absence of capillary refilling and peripheral pulses is no guide to the extent of muscle ischaemia, direct measurement of tissue pressure is a more accurate guide to the need for surgical intervention. The principle of such a measurement is a continuous column of fluid from the compartment to a pressure measuring device. Flushing is necessary to guarantee accurate measurements. Devices that can be inserted into the compartment to measure pressure include needles, wicks and slit catheters.

It is suggested that fasciotomies should be performed when the pressure is more than 30 mmHg. In the absence of a pressure measurement, the symptoms and signs previously mentioned can be used as guidelines.

### Treatment

Fasciotomy is the treatment of choice for compartment syndrome. If the muscle appears necrotic, debridement should be carried out and skin incisions not closed. Partial skin closure (if possible, with further debridement) should occur after 3 or 4 days. Other procedures that can reduce pressure, such as fracture reduction or escharotomy, should also be performed.

## Near drowning

The aim of treatment is to re-establish cardiorespiratory function before neurological damage occurs. This is more a function of first aid, rather than intensive care. Rapid initial resuscitation will significantly influence outcome in the ICU.

### Precipitating event

Near drowning incidents often are associated with precipitating causes:

- Epilepsy – obtain a history and determine anticonvulsant levels.
- Alcohol intake – obtain a history and determine the blood alcohol level.
- Spinal cord or head injury – especially in association with diving or surfboard accidents.
- Child abuse – do a skeletal survey.
- Cardiac causes – arrhythmias, acute myocardial infarction.

### Airway

If the patient is unconscious or if there is doubt about the patency of the airway, intubate.

### Respiratory function

People who drown or nearly drown rarely aspirate large amounts of water. At least 10% aspirate no water and probably develop laryngeal spasm – the so-called dry drowning. However, hypoxia is universal in near drowning incidents. In drowning without aspiration, hypoxia results simply from apnoea. When the victim aspirates, the volume and composition of the fluid contributes to the hypoxia. Stomach contents and contaminated water, even in small amounts, can cause severe hypoxia. Pulmonary oedema occurs in both fresh water and salt water drowning and frequently occurs acutely.

Acute lung injury and bronchopneumonia can occur later, usually in association with aspiration.

Management

The standard approach to hypoxia should be used (see Chapter 16).

Principles:

- Use a face mask with a high concentration of inspired oxygen.
- Use CPAP via a mask or tube if it can be tolerated and if ventilation is not a problem.
- Maintain the cardiovascular system with colloid or blood and limit the use of crystalloid fluids.
- Use PSV or IPPV/PEEP if ventilation inadequate.
- Monitor progress:
  Serial chest x-rays (at least daily)
  Serial blood gas determinations and pulse oximetry

## Blood volume and electrolytes

Animal models have shown that fresh water is absorbed into the blood volume causing dilution, haemolysis and electrolyte disturbances, whereas salt water simultaneously decreases the blood volume by osmosis and is absorbed in excessive amounts. However, in clinical practice there is little difference between salt water and fresh water near drowning episodes. Many near drowning victims are hypovolaemic as a result of pulmonary oedema. Colloids should be used for initial resuscitation. Major electrolyte disturbances are not common. Nevertheless, serum osmolality determinations and serum biochemistry tests should be regularly performed.

The cardiovascular system should be monitored by routine measurements of parameters such as arterial BP, pulse rate, peripheral perfusion, arterial pH, serum lactate and urine output and, if necessary, CVP and pulmonary artery catheterisation should be used.

## Hypothermia

The patients are often hypothermic. If a patient's temperature is above 30 °C, allow passive and slow rewarming. Many need catecholamine infusions to maintain the cardiovascular system if the body's core temperature is below 30 °C. Low temperature alone does not indicate an improved chance for good survival. Patients who become hypothermic in water that is near O °C before they go into arrest (primary hypothermia), have a better prognosis than do patients who arrest early in non-icy waters and then become hypothermic (secondary hyperthermia). Treatment of hypothermia is described elsewhere (see Chapter 11).

Deliberate induction of hypothermia as part of treatment is controversial.

## Neurological management

The most important aspect in the management of near drowning victims is maintenance of neurological function. Cerebral oedema and increased intracranial pressure (ICP) usually become evident after 24 hours. Active management of the neurological sequelae (e.g. corticosteroids, barbiturate coma, induced hypothermia) has largely been abandoned. Nevertheless, the basic principles of treating cerebral oedema should be applied if the patient is unconscious (see Chapter 23).

Principles:

- Sit the patient head up (>30° inclination to facilitate venous drainage); however, maintain arterial BP and cerebral perfusion pressure (CPP).
- Keep the head straight, and do not tie the ETT with constricting tapes which could prevent adequate cerebral venous drainage.
- Avoid stimulating procedures or use prior sedation to prevent hypertensive surges in the presence of an increased ICP and damage to the blood–brain barrier.
- Maintain adequate oxygenation; avoid hypercarbia and acidosis.
- Minimise the use of crystalloid solutions – maintain 'euvolaemic dehydration'.
- ICP monitoring can help to increase awareness of the factors that can exacerbate an already elevated ICP. However, it has not, as yet, been shown to influence survival. Sustained intracranial hypertension is a poor prognostic sign.

## Miscellaneous considerations

Coagulopathy: Severe coagulopathy can sometimes occur. Management is described elsewhere.

Renal function: Acute renal failure can occur after near drowning incidents.

**Give no steroids.**

**Give no prophylactic antibiotics.**

**Use routine intensive care:**

Prevention of acute stress ulceration.

Nutrition (see Chapter 5).

Sedation (see Chapter 7).

Prevention of septicaemia (see Chapter 13).

## Prognosis

These patients are classified on the basis of their status on admission to hospital following their rescue:

A: *Awake*, 100% survival.
B: *Blunted level* of consciousness (i.e. obtunded, but can be roused), at least 90% survival. Most deaths are due to cardiorespiratory causes. Patients in this group should recover full neurological function.
C: *Comatose*
Adults: More than 50% survive with variable percentages having some degree of neurological damage and the remainder die.
Children: Fewer than 50% survive neurologically intact; variable percentages of survivors will have some degree of brain damage.

The occurrence of a first gasp within 30 minutes of the initiation of the resuscitation effort and an early resumption of spontaneous respiration are good prognostic indicators, as is neurological responsiveness at the scene of the incident. Very poor prognostic indicators are a submersion duration of greater than 10 minutes and unproductive resuscitation efforts lasting longer than 25 minutes.

Each patient must be assessed individually, especially with regard to body temperature, whether or not neurological improvement occurs, and at what rate it occurs.

## Trauma in obstetric patients

The treatment priorities are the same for multitrauma. However, management of obstetric patients involves special considerations because pregnancy alters the maternal physiology and the foetus is a second potential victim. An obstetrician and paediatric surgeon should be enlisted in most cases.

The uterus is initially protected by the pelvic ring, but it becomes more prone to injury as it enlarges. In the latter part of pregnancy, the uterus is vulnerable to injury and offers little protection to the foetus. Foetal death is much more common than maternal death. Even minor injuries can result in death of the foetus.

There are many physiological changes during pregnancy that can affect the mother's reaction to blood loss and injury. Cardiac output, tidal volume, blood volume and pulse rate are all increased. The gravid uterus can compress the inferior vena cava and severely reduce venous return when the patient is in the supine position – the supine hypotension syndrome.

The uterus is prone to rupture as a result of blunt trauma. Placental abruption occurs in 1–5% of minor injuries and in up to 50% of major injuries and it can occur up to 3 days after the initial trauma. Labour can be precipitated and direct foetal injury can also occur. The foetus must be carefully monitored during this period, for in addition to the danger of abruption, shock and hypoxia in the

## TROUBLESHOOTING

## Trauma patients: the next day

Once patients who have suffered serious multitrauma have been resuscitated and investigated and perhaps undergone surgery, they are usually managed in the ICU. It is then time for a careful review of each case.

### Airway

An early decision may have to be made regarding whether or not a tracheostomy is indicated. This will largely depend on the anticipated length of ventilatory support. As a general rule, if intubation is anticipated for more than 2 weeks, early tracheostomy should be considered.

### Hypoxia

There are many possible causes of hypoxia at this stage, but the most common are post-traumatic ALI, lung contusion, aspiration and fat emboli.

### Fractured ribs and flail chest

If there are significant fractures of ribs or there is a large flail segment, early tracheostomy should be performed, particularly if the patient is aged 50 years or older or has significant chronic underlying lung disease, especially related to smoking. Epidural analgesia should also be considered.

### Hypotension and oliguria

In the early stages of multitrauma, hypotension is related to continued bleeding until proven otherwise. Transfuse and look for the cause – pelvis, chest, abdomen or long bones are the most likely.

### Fever and tachycardia

Nosocomial infection is unusual within the first 48 hours. However, a fever and tachycardia are non-specific and relatively common accompaniments of severe trauma. Consider the possibility of fat emboli. Tachycardia is almost invariable in the first few days following major traum, especially in the young. Exclude obvious causes such as hypovolaemia and pain, but usually it is related to non-specific factors. Early fever and sepsis can also be related to aspiration, a ruptured abdominal viscus or contaminated wounds.

### Delayed abdominal injuries

An overlooked abnormality or its delayed onset can cause features such as an acute abdomen or sepsis (e.g. ruptured viscus) or bleeding and haemoglobin reduction (e.g. ruptured spleen).

### Feeding

A decision must be made whether the patient can tolerate enteral nutrition or whether IV nutrition should be commenced.

## Pain
It is important to provide adequate pain relief for patients who have suffered multitrauma.

## Major fractures and plastic repair
Major fractures and dislocations should be treated early rather than late. Similarly, definite times should be arranged for plastic repair of injuries (e.g. faciomaxillary injury).

## Overlooked bone and soft tissue injuries
It is common to discover previously overlooked small bone fractures and soft tissue injuries (e.g. torn ligaments) up to many weeks after severe multitrauma. If a patient is unconscious, the only hint may be swelling or instability during passive movement. Although such indications may seem minor at the time, they can lead to severe disability.

## Fat emboli
These can cause hypoxia and confusion within 24 hours of fractures.

## Prophylaxis against pulmonary embolism
Low dosage heparin probably should be commenced once active bleeding has ceased.

## Continuing haematuria
Investigate.

## Relatives and friends
It is never too soon to explain to relatives and friends that the patient may be in hospital for weeks or even months, with the possibility of a lengthy rehabilitation period.

mother can cause foetal distress. Immediate delivery is required in the event of foetal distress if the gestation is past 26 weeks.

## Foetal assessment

- Monitor foetal movements.
- Time the uterine contractions.
- Monitor the foetal heart rate (normal 120–160/min).
- Cardiotocographic monitoring should be commenced as soon as possible. Continuous monitoring, rather than intermittent auscultation, is preferable.
- Doppler ultrasound may be useful to determine gestational age and assess foetal well being if the findings from cardiac monitoring are equivocal, as well as to estimate the volume of amniotic fluid if rupture of the amniotic membrane is suspected. However, cardiotocographic monitoring usually is a superior means for assessment.

## TROUBLESHOOTING

## The acute limb

Time is of the essence in assessing and treating an acute limb condition.

### Important history and signs
- pain
- numbness
- temperature changes
- abnormal pulses
- slow capillary return
- crepitus
- cellulitis
- weakness

The examiner must inquire as to the state of the muscles, nerves and distal organs – not simply how the skin appears.

### Major adverse outcomes
Focal death leading to loss of function.
Global death leading to limb loss.
Inflammation and infection that can lead to distant organ dysfunction and even loss of the patient's life.

### Three main entities to consider
Ischaemia (e.g. arterial or graft thrombosis).
Infection (e.g. gas gangrene, diabetic foot).
Compartment compression (e.g. trauma).

### Ischaemia
If it looks ischaemic, it must be considered ischaemic until proven otherwise.
This is a medical emergency, needing rapid restoration of blood flow.
The initial surgery should be definitive.

### Infection
Rapidly spreading necrosis and gas formation may not be obvious simply from skin appearance.
Superficial cellulitis often is a marker of deep suppuration tracking along tendons and fascial planes.
Rapid diagnosis is essential and definitive surgical debridement or amputation must be repeated.
Debridement often must be repeated.

### Compartment syndrome
The term refers to increased pressure within one or more encapsulated compartments of a limb.
The causes include crush syndrome, ischaemia, reperfusion, closed fracture, haematoma and electrical burns.
Unrelieved pressure will result in impaired venous return, impaired arterial inflow, nerve and muscle ischaemia and necrosis.
Decompress rapidly with a fasciotomy.

## Management

The general principles of management are the same as for other patients with multitrauma.

### Airway and breathing

In the latter stages of pregnancy, intubation can be difficult. There may be laryngeal oedema. These patients can rapidly become hypoxic because of a decreased functional residual capacity and increased $VO_2$.

Secure the airway by intubating if necessary. Always give a high concentration of inspired oxygen and immobilise the neck with a rigid collar if there is doubt about the cervical spine.

### Circulation

The foetal circulation is not self-regulating. Uterine blood flow is largely dependent on the systemic BP. Hypovolaemia must be aggressively corrected.

Establish IV access with large cannulae and aggressively infuse fluids in order to reverse any hypovolaemia. Do not hesitate to infuse rapidly cross-matched blood (Rh-negative). Patients should remain in the left lateral decubitus position if possible.

A DPL can be performed using a supraumbilical minilaparotomy.

**Do not hesitate to perform emergency investigations and treatment (e.g. laparotomy) as for any other patient.**

## FURTHER READING

### General aspects of multitrauma

Gupta, K. J., Parr, M. J. A. and Nolan, J. P. General introduction on trauma. In *Pain Management and Regional Anaesthesia in Trauma*, ed. A. D. Rosenberg, C. M. Grande and R. L. Bernstein, pp. 3–28. London: W. B. Saunders, 1999.

Johnstone, R. E. and Graf, D. F. Acute trauma with multiple injuries. *Current Opinion in Anaesthesiology* 14 (2001): 211–15.

Mellor, A. and Smi, N. Fat embolism. *Anaesthesia* 56 (2001): 145–54.

Parr, M. J. A. and Nolan, J. P. Intensive care for trauma patients: the first 24 hours. In *Anaesthesia, Pain, Intensive Care and Emergency Medicine*, ed. A. Gullo, pp. 427–37. Milan: Springer-Verlag, 1999.

Nolan, J. P. and Parr, M. J. A. Aspects of resuscitation in trauma. *British Journal of Anaesthesia* 79 (1997): 226–40.

Pasquale, M., Fabian, T. C. and EAST Ad Hoc Committee on Practice Management Guideline Development. Practice management guidelines for trauma from the eastern association for the surgery of trauma. *Journal of Trauma; Injury, Infection and Critical Care* 44 (1998): 941–57.

### Damage control surgery

Brasel, K. and Weighelt, J. Damage control in trauma surgery. *Current Opinion in Critical Care* 6 (2000): 276–80.

### Thoracic injuries

Cinnella, G. Use of CT scan and transophageal echocardiography in blunt thoracic trauma. *Intensive Care Medicine* 24 (1998): 986–7.

### Cardiac injuries

Feghali, N. T. and Prisant, L. M. Blunt myocardial injury. *Chest* 108 (1995): 1673–7.
Kaye, P. and O'Sullivan, I. Myocardial contusion: emergency investigtion and diagnosis. *Emergency Medicine Journal* 19 (2002): 8–10.
Orliaguest, G., Ferjani, J. and Riou, B. The heart in blunt trauma. *Anesthesiology* 95 (2001): 544–8.

### Burns

Gueugniaud, R.-Y., Carsin, H., Bertin-Maghit, M. and Petit, P. Current advances in the initial management of major thermal burns. *Intensive Care Medicine* 26 (2000): 848–56.

### Crush injuries and acute compartment syndrome

Matsuoka, T., Yoshioka, T., Tanaka, H., Ninomiya, N., Jun, O., Sugimot, H. and Junichiro, Y. Long-term physical outcome of patients who suffered crush syndrome after the 1995 Hanshin-Awaji Earthquake: Prognostic indicators in retrospect. *Journal of Trauma-Injury Infection and Critical Care* 52 (2002): 33–9.

### Electrical injuries

Cydulka, R. K. Electrical injuries: a 30-year review. *Annals of Emergency Medicine* 35 (2000): 634.
Anonymous. Guidelines 2000 for cardiopulmonary resuscitation and emergency cardiovascular care. Part 8: Advanced challenges in resuscitation: section 3: special challenges in ECC. *Circulation* 102 (2000): (Suppl. 8) 1229–52.
Rai, J., Jeschke, M. G., Barrow, R. E. and Herndon, D. N. Electrical injuries: a 30-year review. *Journal of Trauma-Injury Infection and Critical Care* 46 (1999): 933–6.

### Near drowning episodes

Bierens, J. J. L. M., Knape, J. T. A. and Gelissen, H. P. M. M. Drowning. *Current Opinion in Critical Care* 8 (2002): 578–85.

## Trauma in obstetric patients

Baerga-Varela, Y., Zietlow, S. P., Bannon, M. P., Harmsen, W. S. and Ilstrup, D. M. Trauma in pregnancy. *Journal of Trauma-Injury Infection and Critical Care* 46 (1999): 208.

Pak, L. L., Reece, E. A. and Chan, L. Is adverse pregnancy outcome predictable after blunt abdominal trauma? *American Journal of Obstetrics and Gynecology* 179 (1998): 1140–4.

## Pelvic trauma

Incagnoli, P., Viggiano, M. and Carli, P. Priorities in the management of severe pelvic trauma. *Current Opinion in Critical Care* 6 (2000): 401–7.

## Acute limb

Callum, K. and Bradbury, A. Acute limb ischaemia. *British Medical Journal* 320 (2000): 126–35.

## Trauma website

www.swsahs.nsw.gov.au/livtrauma

# 15

# Poisoning

---

- The first priority in the management of poisoning is the initial resuscitation – airway, breathing and circulation.
- Supportive care is the cornerstone of management in the ICU.
- The use of specific antidotes is only rarely lifesaving.
- Self-poisoning often involves multiple drugs, commonly including alcohol.

---

## Initial assessment

The possibility of poisoning should be considered in all unconscious patients. First-line treatment involves securing the airway, giving high-flow oxygen and supporting the patient's breathing and circulation. Examine the patient's whole body carefully for signs of intravenous drug abuse, trauma and pressure areas (Table 15.1). Perform a thorough neurological examination. Smell the patient's breath. The possibility of hypoglycaemia must be considered. Elicit a history from the patient, ambulance officers, friends or relatives. Thiamine (100 mg IM or IV) should be given to all known alcoholic patients in order to treat or prevent Wernicke's encephalopathy.

Most drug overdoses involve multiple drugs.

Although active intervention, such as the use of antidotes, forced alkaline diuresis and dialysis, can sometimes play a crucial role, basic resuscitation measures usually are more important. Our concern in poisoning is to save the patient not the poison!

### Airway

If there is doubt about the patency of the airway, rapidly intubate the patient with preoxygenation and cricoid pressure. As a guideline, patients with Glasgow Coma Scale scores of 9 or less should be intubated. It is dangerous to attempt

**Table 15.1.** The most common toxic syndromes

| | |
|---|---|
| **Anticholinergic syndromes** | |
| Common signs | Delirium with mumbling speech, tachycardia, dry and flushed skin, dilated pupils, myoclonus, slightly elevated temperature, urinary retention and decreased bowel sounds. Seizures and dysrhythmias may occur in severe cases |
| Common causes | Antihistamines, antiparkinson medication, atropine, scopolamine, antispasmodic agents, mydriatic agents, skeletal muscle relaxants and many plants (notably jimson weed and *Amanita muscaria*) |
| **Sympathomimetic syndromes** | |
| Common signs | Delusions, paranoia, tachycardia (or bradycardia if the drug is a pure α-adrenergic agonist), hypertension, hyperpyrexia, diaphoresis, piloerection, mydriasis and hyperreflexia. Seizures, hypotension and dysrhythmias can occur in severe cases |
| Common causes | Cocaine, amphetamines, methamphetamine and its derivatives and over-the-counter decongestants (e.g. phenylpropanolamine, ephedrine and pseudoephedrine). In caffeine and theophylline overdoses, similar findings can occur |
| **Opiate, sedative or ethanol intoxication** | |
| Common signs | Coma, respiratory depression, miosis, hypotension, bradycardia, hypothermia, pulmonary oedema, decreased bowel sounds, hyporeflexia and needle marks. Seizures can occur after overdoses of some narcotics, notably propoxyphene |
| Common causes | Narcotics, barbiturates, benzodiazepines, ethchlorvynol, glutethimide, methprylon, methaqualone, meprobamate, ethanol, clonidine and guanabenz |
| **Cholinergic syndromes** | |
| Common signs | Confusion, central nervous system depression, weakness, salivation, lacrimation, urinary and faecal incontinence, gastrointestinal cramping, emesis, diaphoresis, muscle fasciculations, pulmonary oedema, miosis, bradycardia or tachycardia and seizures |
| Common causes | Organophosphate and carbamate insecticides, physostigmine, edrophonium and some mushrooms |

Reprinted with permission of *New England Journal of Medicine* 326 (1992): 1677–81.

to elicit a gag reflex as the patient may aspirate stomach contents. Paradoxically, further sedation may be needed if the patient is restless or is having a seizure. The patient's level of consciousness and airway patency must be constantly monitored, and intubation must be carried out if there is any doubt. Slow release preparations can cause delayed effects.

## Breathing

Oxygen (at least 30–40%, via a face mask) should be administered to any patient with a compromised level of consciousness. Many drugs (e.g. narcotics, sedatives, tricyclic antidepressants) can cause hypoventilation, hypercarbia and respiratory acidosis.

Monitor the patient's respiratory rate, check arterial blood gases frequently and use pulse oximetry and clinical assessment to determine the need for artificial ventilation with intermittent positive-pressure ventilation (IPPV). Whereas all intubated patients should initially be ventilated, those who are making some spontaneous respiratory effort may be suitable for a change to continuous positive airway pressure (CPAP) or to some partial mode of ventilatory support, such as pressure support ventilation (PSV) or intermittent mandatory ventilation (IMV).

## Circulation

Many of these patients are hypotensive on admission. This can be related to several factors:

- Vasodilatory actions of many drugs (most common).
- Direct cardiac toxicity.
- Hypovolaemia due to decreased fluid intake or fluid loss (e.g. vomiting).

### Hypotension
Hypotension can almost always be reversed with replenishment of intravascular fluid. The fluid must be titrated against cardiovascular measurements – particularly blood pressure and peripheral perfusion. Occasionally large volumes are required. Inotropic support is sometimes needed for resistant hypotension.

### Cardiac problems
Correct hypoxia, acidosis and hypokalaemia, as they predispose to arrhythmias and depress cardiac function.

The poison itself can have a direct cardiodepressant effect (e.g. $\beta$-blockers).

## Investigations and monitoring

Most patients need only monitoring and basic investigations. Initially, frequent (every 15 minutes) monitoring of vital signs, such as pulse rate, BP, respiratory rate and level of consciousness may be required.

Chest x-ray: An x-ray may show signs of aspiration or atelectasis.

ECG: Use initial 12-lead ECG and continuous monitoring if indicated.

Oximetry: Continuous monitoring for hypoxia is necessary.

Routine haematology and biochemistry: Creatinine phosphokinase (CPK), for instance, may be increased because of rhabdomyolysis; theophylline and tricyclic antidepressants can cause hypokalaemia.

Arterial blood gases: Their determination may reveal, for instance, persistent unexplained acidosis due to salicylates, carbon monoxide, methanol and ethylene glycol.

Serum osmolality: When compared with calculated osmolality, the serum osmolality may be helpful in diagnosing poisoning due to methanol or ethylene glycol.

Drugs assays: Urine, blood and gastric contents can be used for drug screening. Early samples of gastric contents (50 ml) and urine (50 ml) should be used for diagnostic and medico-legal purposes. Specific, rapid screening tests are available for drugs such as paracetamol, salicylates, benzodiazepines, opiates and barbiturates. There is also a screening test, based on thin layer chromatography (TLC), that covers about 200 substances. Although blood cannot be used for the TLC screening test, blood samples should be taken to test specifically for other substances including alcohol. Specific serum or plasma concentrations are useful for dealing with the following drugs: paracetamol, iron, salicylates, theophylline, digoxin, anticonvulsant agents, lithium, ethanol, methanol and ethylene glycol.

## Special problems

### Hypothermia

Hypothermia is common after poisoning but it rarely requires active measures. Always measure the central temperature (e.g. rectal or oesophageal). Hypothermia is a marker of increased risk for rhabdomyolysis and aspiration as a result of coma.

Treatment for hypothermia begins with covering the patient with metallic foil or special warming blankets to reduce heat loss. Warm the IV fluids and humidified gas to 37 °C. More active measures are sometimes needed.

### Hyperthermia

Hyperthermia is uncommon and sometimes is associated with tricyclic antidepressants, antipsychotics, antihistamines, amphetamine, cocaine, phencyclidine and salicylates. Hyperthermia must be controlled by aggressive means in order to prevent complications. Fever as a result of infection can, of course, occur (e.g. aspiration).

## Seizures

Seizures can occur as a direct result of the poison and may be difficult to control. Seizures can occur in association with anticonvulsants, phenothiazines, antihistamines, theophylline and tricyclic antidepressants. Seizures can also occur as an indirect result of the poison (e.g. hypoglycaemia, hypoxia or as a result of global ischaemia). Drug or alcohol withdrawal can also precipitate seizures.

Seizures are medical emergencies as they can cause cerebral damage and oedema, hyperthermia, hypoxia and aspiration. The principles of management are listed here but they are discussed in detail elsewhere:

- Intubate and assist ventilation if in doubt about the airway. Initially give IV benzodiazepine. If the seizures are not controlled with benzodiazepines, use IV barbiturates.
- Concurrently given phenytoin (15 mg/kg over 1 h as a loading dose, then 5 mg/kg IV daily as a single dose over 1 h).
- EEG monitoring should be used to assess electrical seizure activity, especially if muscle relaxants are given.

## Rhabdomyolysis

Rhabdomyolysis usually occurs in association with pressure necrosis. It can complicate narcotic and cocaine abuse without coma.
**Always suspect rhabdomyolysis in a patient who is in a prolonged coma.**
Rhabdomyolysis can cause hypovolaemia, shock, hyperkalaemia, hypocalcaemia, acidosis and renal failure. Early, aggressive correction of hypovolaemia and acidosis is essential. Active treatment of hyperkalaemia and renal failure may be necessary. Fasciotomy is sometimes required to relieve compartment pressure and prevent further tissue ischaemia.

## Atelectasis and aspiration

A chest x-ray should be obtained as soon as possible after admission to detect features such as atelectasis and collapse due to hypoventilation or aspiration as a result of coma and depressed reflexes.

## Other general supportive measures

The key to the effective management of a patient who has been poisoned, whether accidentally or deliberately, is meticulous supportive care. Supportive measures are based on the same principles essential for management of all critically ill patients.

- Regular assessment of airway, breathing and circulation.
- Regular turning and pressure care.
- Nasogastric (NG) tube.
- Catheterisation of the bladder.
- Mouth, eye and limb care.
- Prophylactic measures for stress ulceration.

## Precipitating factors and follow up

It is often helpful to obtain psychiatric and/or social worker opinions before a poisoning patient is transferred from the ICU. It is important that the ICU staff present a positive attitude toward these patients. Self-poisoning presents a situation in which it is difficult and frustrating to have to address and face all of the underlying issues, especially the non-medical ones such as poverty, despair, violence and unemployment. Self-poisoning has become medicalised because it is the relatively easy, quantifiable and short-term challenge. After successful resuscitation we often have no option but to place the patient back in the circumstances which precipitated the initial overdose. They may pass through the hands of other professionals such as psychiatrists and social workers, who may have something to offer a minority. It is important to acknowledge the frustration of not being able to address many of the underlying issues which precipitated the overdose and to approach the patient with the dignity and sensitivity that they deserve.

## Active measures

### Decreased drug absorption

The exact role of gastric emptying, gastric lavage and whole gut irrigation, as well as the use of ipecac and charcoal remain controversial.

Any active attempt to empty the stomach is accompanied by the danger of aspiration. The patient must have an intact cough reflex or have a cuffed endotracheal tube (ETT) in place before an attempt is made to aspirate stomach contents.

For patients poisoned by drugs that cause coma and respiratory depression, aggressive removal of the drugs is not warranted. Active gastric emptying of such drugs might give the attending medical staff a sense that they were doing something positive (or punitive in some cases!) but good supportive care is often all that is required.

Active measures to empty the gut should be considered for toxic drugs such as aspirin, colchicine, paraquat, organophosphates, iron, tricyclic antidepressants and paracetamol. Active measures should be avoided in cases involving corrosive chemicals and petroleum products.

## Induced emesis
This technique has been used primarily for small children soon after ingestion of the toxin. However, it seems to be falling out of favour, even for that group. Emesis should not be induced if:

- The child is not fully alert with intact laryngeal reflexes.
- Acid, alkali or petroleum distillates have been ingested.
- More than 3 hours have passed since ingestion.

Ipecac syrup has traditionally been recommended for young children but not for adults in whom sedation and poor drug recovery are problems. Its effectiveness is largely unproven. Paediatric Ipecacuanha mixture (0.12% alkaloids) is usually used: 5 ml for children up to 1 year of age; 10–20 ml for those aged 1–5 years.

## Gastric lavage
The exact role and usefulness of gastric lavage have not been fully established. It should always be considered but not done simply as a routine.

It is probably useful within 4 hours of ingestion and also when one suspects that potentially lethal quantities of a drug have been taken. It can also be useful if slow-release preparations of drugs have been taken. Gastric lavage can be successful for up to 12 hours after ingestion for salicylates, quinidine, tricyclic antidepressants and paracetamol.

Lavage should not be attempted when ingestion of corrosives, caustics, acids or petroleum derivatives is suspected.

Technique: Place the patient in the semiprone position with the head dependent. Insert a special large bore gastric tube to aspirate the stomach. Instil water (1 ml/kg) at body temperature and recover that amount before instilling more. Repeat the cycles until the return water is clear.

## Charcoal
If given early enough, activated charcoal can reduce the gastrointestinal absorption of many drugs including aspirin, paracetamol, phenobarbitone, digoxin, carbamazepine, theophylline and phenytoin. It is of little value for highly charged molecules such as iron, lithium and cyanide or other compounds such as alcohol. There may be the added benefit of clearance from the systemic circulation by 'gastrointestinal dialysis': a concentration gradient for the drug is established between the systemic circulation and the lumen of the gastrointestinal tract. Clearance is thus encouraged from the circulation into the GIT lumen, where it is adsorbed onto the charcoal.

The efficiency of charcoal absorption may be reduced in the presence of shock or impaired gastrointestinal motility. Just as we remain uncertain about many aspects of management after poisoning, the exact role of charcoal has not been established. In practical terms, repeated doses of charcoal do not tend to transit rapidly through the gut.

Technique: Administer activated charcoal at 1 g/kg either orally or through a NG tube. Its action can be enhanced by repeating that dose every 4 hours, especially for drugs that rely on the enterohepatic circulation. Alternatively, continuous NG infusion of charcoal (30–50 g/h) can be used (for paediatric patients, 0.25 g/kg per h). As with adults, there is little evidence for the effectiveness of charcoal in paediatric poisoning. Metoclopramide may speed the gastric emptying of charcoal. Charcoal can be used for long periods after drug ingestion, as it can enhance the clearance of drugs already absorbed. Repeated doses of activated charcoal may decrease the half-lives and increase the clearance of a wide range of drugs, including the following:

- dapsone
- theophylline
- glutethimide
- digoxin
- phenylbutazone
- barbiturates
- quinine
- tricyclic antidepressants
- salicylates
- carbamazepine

### Whole bowel irrigation

Some agents, such as polyethylene glycol electrolyte solutions, can decrease drug absorption by decreasing the time for the drug to transit the gut. Such agents do not act by means of an osmolar effect within the gut. They can be useful for purging intact tablets from the gut (e.g. in cases of iron poisoning). It is a technique suited for conscious patients who have ingested tablets that do not bind well to charcoal and can be identified on a plain radiograph. Because polyethylene will bind to charcoal, the two probably should not be used together.

Technique: These compounds come as commercially available water-soluble powders (e.g. Go-lytely or Colyte) to be dissolved in about 4 L of water. They can be taken orally or delivered via a NG tube. For adults, give the solution at a rate of 1–4 L/h (children 0.5 L/h) and continue until the patient passes clear fluid from the bowel (usually after about 3–5 L) or until the tablets are cleared from the gut.

### Increased drug excretion

These techniques are employed only in specific circumstances.

## Forced alkaline diuresis

Forced alkaline diuresis is a dangerous and unproven technique that is now largely discouraged. It was considered theoretically attractive because it encourages ion trapping in the renal tubules. However, it can result in dehydration, hypokalaemia and pulmonary oedema. Even in acute and severe salicylate poisoning, it has not been shown to improve outcome.

## Faecuresis

Just as we are uncertain about many of the active measures used in the management of poisoning, the effectiveness of giving an osmolar agent is uncertain. Mannitol is sometimes given together with the charcoal. Apart from its uncertain effectiveness, mannitol can lead to hypovolaemia, as a result of its osmolar effect in the gut, as well as hypokalaemia and hypomagnesaemia.

## Haemodialysis

Haemodialysis is effective mainly for low molecular weight drugs that are not effectively bound to plasma proteins and have a small volume of distribution and low rates of spontaneous clearance. It has a limited role, but it can be useful for potentially lethal doses of specific drugs such as lithium, ethylene glycol and salicylates.

Haemodialysis should be considered when these drugs are present at certain high concentrations:

- Salicylates ($>1.2$ g/L initially; $>1.0$ g/L at 6 hours).
- Methanol, ethylene glycol ($>0.5$ g/L).
- Lithium ($>4$ mmol/L).

Haemodialysis can also be useful for the acute acid-base or electrolyte disturbances that accompany poisoning. It is of no benefit for drugs that have large volumes of distribution such as tricyclic antidepressants.

## Haemoperfusion

Haemoperfusion involves passing the patient's blood through a device containing charcoal or adsorbent particles, such as resin columns. The technique has anecdotally been reported to be successful for many drugs but it should be considered only when their concentrations are high:

- Salicylates ($>1.2$ g/L initially; $>1.0$ g/L at 6 hours).
- Theophylline ($>600$ $\mu$mol/L).

Haemoperfusion can also be considered for patients with paraquat poisoning, mushroom poisoning and late presentation paracetamol poisoning. The technique for haemoperfusion is described in the chapter on renal failure.

## Antidotes

Some drugs may require immediate antidotal treatment:

| Drug | Antidote |
|---|---|
| carbon monoxide | oxygen |
| paracetamol | N-acetylcysteine |
| anticholinergics | physostigmine |
| insulin | glucose |
| β-blockers | glucagon/adrenaline |
| organophosphates | atropine and pralidoxime |
| benzodiazepines | flumazenil |
| ethylene glycol | ethanol |
| bromide | sodium chloride |
| calcium channel blockers | calcium |
| cyanide | amyl nitrate, sodium nitrite, sodium thiosulphate |
| heavy metals | chelating agents |
| isoniazid, hydrazine | pyridoxine |
| iron | desferrioxamine |
| | methylene blue |
| narcotics | naloxone |
| warfarin | vitamin K |
| digoxin | digoxin antibody fragments |

For more details, see specific poisons discussed in the next section.

### Immunotherapy
In the future, antibodies to a given drug that can result in inhibition of that drug's action may play an important role. Thus far, immunotherapy has been used for severe digoxin poisoning.

## Some specific poisons

### B-blockers

#### Features
- Common effects include bradycardia, hypotension, peripheral vasospasm, bronchospasm, coma, convulsions and respiratory depression.

#### Management
- Supportive management is recommended.
- Atropine, adrenaline or glucagon infusions may be necessary. Transvenous pacing may also be required. Glucagon is only used if the symptoms are unresponsive to adrenaline. Give glucagon as a bolus at 50 μg/kg IV, up to 10 mg; a maintenance dosage of 2–10 mg/h can be used.

## Carbamazepine

**Carbamazepine can be a particularly dangerous drug in overdose.**

### Features
- Mild ataxia to profound coma.
- Marked depression of brainstem reflexes.
- Convulsions or myoclonic activity.
- Cerebellar dysfunction.
- Marked cardiovascular toxicity, including:
  Tachyarrhythmias and bradyarrhythmias
  ECG: prolonged PR, QRS complex and QT interval
  Conduction disturbances
  Severe hypotension
- Thrombocytopaenia and leucopaenia.
- Pulmonary oedema.
- Anticholinergic effects.

### Management
- The drug has extensive protein-binding capacity (75–85%) and a large volume of distribution (1.5 L/kg), making it relatively inaccessible to active drug elimination.
- Management is mainly supportive:
  Intubation.
  Artificial ventilation.
  Fluid resuscitation.
  Inotropes are often necessary.
  Cardiac pacing may be necessary.
  Seizures must be controlled with aggressive measures.
  Drug removal can be facilitated by multiple doses or even a continuous infusion of activated charcoal via a NG tube. Haemoperfusion with a charcoal column has also been used.

## Carbon monoxide

### Features
- Carbon monoxide displaces oxygen from haemoglobin, myoglobin and the cytochrome system. This causes widespread cellular damage because of decreased oxygen delivery and utilisation.
- A pink colour of the skin is uncommon; cyanosis and skin pallor are more common.
- Carbon monoxide poisoning should be considered a possibility in all patients who have been trapped in a fire.

## Management
- General supportive measures are recommended.
- Give as high a concentration of inspired oxygen as possible (100%, if possible) by a tight-fitting mask or ETT (if necessary) for at least 3 days or longer in symptomatic patients. Remember that pulse oximeters will be misleading because they measure carbon monoxide levels as well as oxygen.
- Many patients have had long-term neuropsychiatric deficits after carbon monoxide poisoning. For that reason, hyperbaric oxygen is now used earlier and more aggressively. Some units use hyperbaric oxygen when the carboxyhaemoglobin concentration is more than 20–30% or when the patient either has lost consciousness at any stage or has neurological deficits or cardiac abnormalities. However, randomised controlled trials have yet to demonstrate a benefit.

### Cocaine

#### Features
- Stimulation of both peripheral and central nervous systems.
- Clinical features include euphoria, agitation, hyperthermia, seizures, confusions, tachycardia and hypertension.
- Cardiac arrhythmias, cerebral haemorrhage, coagulopathy, cerebral oedema and rhabdomyolysis can also occur.

#### Management
- It is important to reduce the psychomotor agitation, using diazepam IV as required.
- Close monitoring and aggressive resuscitation are essential.
- Neuroleptic agents should be avoided.
- β-blockers can result in excessive α activity and hypertension.
- Severe hypertension may require the use of labetalol or sodium nitroprusside.
- A CT scan may be necessary to exclude cerebral haemorrhage.

### Digoxin

#### Features
- Nausea, vomiting, drowsiness and mental confusion.
- ECG: Almost any change is possible, including sinus bradycardia, atrioventricular block, ventricular and atrial ectopics and asystole.

#### Management
- Gastric lavage and support.
- Temporary cardiac pacing and specific treatment of individual arrhythmias may be necessary.
- Treatment is mainly supportive.

- Serum digoxin concentrations will not give a good indication of the severity of digoxin toxicity.
- Digoxin specific antibody fragments are becoming increasingly available. They bind digoxin and hasten its elimination. They should be used for cardiovascular instability secondary to arrhythmias. A recommended regimen is 160 mg as a loading dose, followed by 160 mg as an IV infusion over 7 hours. Alternatively, 6–8 mg/kg repeated over 30–60 minutes can be given. A further dose can be given in cases of incomplete reversal or recurrence of toxicity. Digoxin antibody fragments interfere with digoxin measurements that employ immunoassay techniques.

## Iron salts

### Features

Iron salt poisoning is most severe in young children.

Stage I: Acute gastric disturbances: epigastric pain, nausea, vomiting and haematemesis leading sometimes to necrosis and perforation of the stomach. Rapid pulse and respiratory rate. There may be a symptom-free period for up to 24 hours.

Stage II: Acute encephalopathy: headache, confusion, delirium, convulsions, and coma. Respirations deep and rapid. Cardiovascular collapse may supervene. Hyperglycaemia and leucocytosis.

Stage III: If the patient survives to this stage, acute liver failure may develop, with jaundice, hepatic coma and death.

### Management

- TREATMENT MUST BE RAPID.
- A plain abdominal x-ray will usually demonstrate the number of tablets. Gastric lavage with a large bore tube may facilitate removal of tablets.
- There is little or no place here for activated charcoal as it does not bind iron. Lavage with desferrioxamine 2 g in 1 L of warm water, then leave 10 g in 50 ml in the stomach to chelate the remaining iron in the GIT.
- Whole bowel irrigation with polyethylene glycol electrolyte solution, especially in children, may be useful.
- Desferrioxamine can be given by IV and IM routes. The dosage is the same for both routes and the same for adults and children: a 1 g loading dose, then 500 mg 4-hourly for two doses. Thereafter, 500 mg between 4-hourly and 12-hourly, depending on the severity of poisoning. The total dose should not exceed 6 g in 24 hours. The IV rate should not exceed 15 mg/kg per h.
- Treatment should be continued until serum levels and clinical status are improved.
- If anuria or oliguria supervenes, dialysis should be commenced urgently.

## Lithium

Features
- Polyuria, thirst, vomiting, diarrhoea and agitation.
- In larger doses coma, hypertonia, involuntary movements and convulsions can occur.

Management
- General supportive measures are recommended.
- Correct hypertonicity with 5% dextrose solution.
- Haemodialysis should be considered if there are severe complications or high concentrations of lithium (e.g. > 4 mmol/L).

## Monoamine oxidase inhibitors

Features
- Drug and food interactions can cause headache, fever and hypertensive crises.
- Overdoses usually cause coma, hypotension and, more rarely, convulsions and hyperthermia.

Management
- With drug and food interactions, severe hypertension is the main problem.
- With overdosage, airway control and intravascular fluids to correct the hypotension usually are sufficient.

## Narcotics

Features
- Coma and respiratory depression are the most common presenting signs.
- Look for needle marks, miosis, hypotension, bradycardia, hypothermia, pulmonary oedema, hyporeflexia and decreased bowel sounds.
- Seizures may occur after overdoses of some narcotics (e.g. pethidine and propoxyphene).

Management
- Precautions should be taken against transmission of hepatitis B, C and HIV virus.
- General supportive measures are recommended.
- Intravenous naloxone is a specific antagonist. However, it has a short half-life and coma can recur. Give naloxone 0.8 mg IM followed by naloxone at 0.5 – 2 mg IV. The IM dose has a longer duration of action and coma is less likely to recur, especially if the patient absconds after the IV dose! More may be needed, and

sometimes a naloxone infusion may be required (1–4 mg/h). Less can be used for addicts in whom acute withdrawal can be precipitated. The paediatric dose is 0.1 mg/kg and the infusion 0.01 mg/kg per h.
- There may also be a concurrent infection, rhabdomyolysis, tricuspid valve abnormalities, subacute bacterial endocarditis, pulmonary oedema and problems associated with narcotic withdrawal.

## Organophosphates

### Features
- Symptoms usually appear within 2 hours of exposure.
- Usually there is a distinctive smell around the patient.
- Cholinesterase inhibition causes parasympathetic overactivity, as well as sympathetic, neuromuscular and central neurological abnormalities.
- Signs and symptoms include:

| | |
|---|---|
| salivation | bronchorrhoea |
| bronchospasm | sweating |
| lacrimation | headache |
| restlessness | muscle weakness |
| confusion/convulsions | nausea |
| vomiting | abdominal cramps |
| diarrhoea | bradycardia |
| hypotension | shock |

### Management
- Gastric aspiration and supportive measures.
- Staff should exercise care in handling the aspirate – the odour of the organophosphate usually will be evident in the ICU for many days during management of the patient and it has been implicated in feelings of malaise and headache amongst the staff. Staff should wear gloves, gowns, masks and glasses during the initial management of these patients in order to decrease absorption.
- Atropine should be titrated against signs and symptoms. Aim to maintain the heart rate and reduce pulmonary secretions with a continuous IV infusion or IV increments. Commence with an IV infusion of 5 mg/h and increase as necessary. Very high infusion rates, up to 30 mg/h may be required initially. Glycopyrrolate could be used instead of atropine.
- Pralidoxime will result in specific reactivation of cholinesterase but it needs to be given early (within 24 hours). Dose is 1–2 g IV within 2 minutes. Repeat after 30 minutes if necessary and then give 1–2 g 4-hourly when indicated. Monitor plasma cholinesterase levels until recovery.
- Direct cardiotoxicity has been reported and often inotropic support is necessary.

## Paracetamol

### Features
- No symptoms initially.
- Then anorexia, nausea and vomiting.
- Severe vomiting, abdominal pain and hepatic tenderness on the second day.
- Hepatic toxicity is maximum on days 2–4 and can lead to fulminant liver failure.
- The risk of liver failure is higher in alcoholics, the elderly and patients with anorexia nervosa and underlying liver disease.
- Paracetamol toxicity can also occur with prolonged use for therapeutic reasons.

### Management
- The outcome will be determined by the amount taken and by the time elapsed before effective treatment is provided.
- Use gastric lavage and activated charcoal for patients who present within 4 hours; these may be useful up to 12 hours.
- IV N-acetylcysteine is the treatment of choice for paracetamol poisoning and should be used if:
    More than 10 g has been ingested.
    There is doubt about the amount ingested.
    The plasma concentration of paracetamol, plotted on a semilogarithmic graph against time (Figure 15.1), falls above a line drawn between 1.32 mmol/L (200 mg/L) at 4 hours and 0.33 mmol/L (50 mg/L) at 12 hours after the overdose. A copy of this chart should be in every ICU and emergency department. N-acetylcysteine is very effective up to 8 hours. There is now evidence to suggest that the antidote should be given to all patients, regardless of presentation, even if they have developed fulminant hepatic failure.
- Give N-acetylcysteine, 20% solution, 150 mg/kg in 200 ml of 5% dextrose over 15 minutes initially; then 50 mg/kg in 500 ml of 5% dextrose over 4 hours; finally, 200 mg/kg in 1 L of 5% dextrose over the next 16 hours (total dose 400 mg/kg in 20 hours). Urticaria, bronchospasm or anaphylaxis can occur in up to 10% of patients given N-acetylcysteine, especially asthmatics.
- Patients who ingest large amounts of paracetamol or who present late may develop renal failure (see Chapter 26) or acute hepatic failure (see Chapter 27). Monitoring the prothrombin time (PTT) and its 12-hourly rate of rise is the best marker of hepatic necrosis: peak elevation occurs at 72–96 hours. Treat hypoglycaemia as indicated with dextrose infusion.
- Patients should be transferred to a specialist centre if fulminant hepatic failure is suspected and transplantation considered.

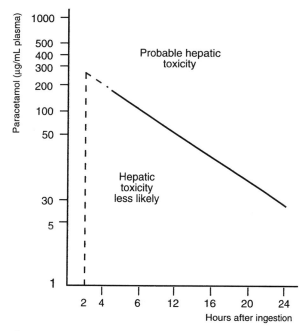

**Figure 15.1.** Toxic concentrations of paracetamol.

## Paraquat

Features

- This potent herbicide causes ulceration of the mucous membranes, nausea, sweating, vomiting, tremors, convulsions and severe pulmonary oedema. Lung fibrosis can occur up to a week after ingestion.
- Cardiovascular collapse and renal failure can also occur.

Management

- General supportive measures.
- Fuller's earth helps adsorb paraquat in the gut. A suspension of 30%, 200–250 ml every 4 hours, should be used until the stools contain Fuller's earth. Activated charcoal can also be given.
- Avoid high oxygen concentration unless it is absolutely necessary, as it can potentiate pulmonary fibrosis. Immediate plasma exchange or haemofiltration may be effective but this remains unproven. Pulse therapy with cyclophosphamide and methylprednisolone may be effective in preventing respiratory complications.

## Salicylates

### Features

- The toxic effects are complex and are related to acid-base disturbances, uncoupling of oxidative phosphorylation and disordered glucose metabolism.
- Initially there will be nausea, vomiting, abdominal pain and tinnitus which can progress to deafness.
- Next will come hyperventilation, flushed skin, sweating and hyperthermia.
- Salicylates have two separate, independent effects on acid-base balance. The first is a respiratory alkalosis as a result of central respiratory stimulation. The second is metabolic acidosis resulting from accumulation of organic acid metabolites and lactate.
- Arterial blood pH is initially normal or raised because of the respiratory alkalosis but metabolic acidosis usually supervenes. This pattern is more common in children.
- Respiratory complications include aspiration pneumonia, pulmonary oedema and acute lung injury (ALI).
- Cardiovascular abnormalities: Mortality is often due to cardiovascular depression which can be unresponsive to treatment. ECG changes include widened QRS complex. Atrioventricular block and ventricular arrhythmias can occur.
- Metabolic disturbances can include hypoglycaemia or hyperglycaemia and hypokalaemia.
- Coagulation disturbances: hypoprothrombinaemia, prolonged bleeding time, thrombocytopaenia and disseminated intravascular coagulopathy (DIC) often causing GIT bleeding.
- More rarely, there may be hyperpyrexia, renal failure and hypoglycaemia.

### Management

- Gastric lavage – within 24 hours of ingestion.
- Administer gastric charcoal.
- Maintain intravascular volume aggressively.
- Glucose infusion if hypoglycaemic.
- Monitor and correct electrolyte disorders.
- Vitamin K may be necessary for hypoprothrombinaemia.
- Marked metabolic acidosis should be corrected with sodium bicarbonate.
- Early determination of the plasma salicylate level is essential:
  Mild toxicity, < 500 mg/L.
  Moderate toxicity, 500–750 mg/L.
  Severe toxicity, > 750 mg/L.
  In children, toxicity can occur at 300 mg/L.
- Although forced alkaline diuresis has largely been abandoned, it is important to give enough fluid to maintain a brisk diuresis.

- Haemodialysis should be considered in cases of moderate or severe toxicity where the levels have not decreased after 2 hours. Dialysis is also indicated for acute renal failure or pulmonary oedema unresponsive to diuretics.
- Other anti-inflammatory agents, such as indomethacin, do not have the same toxic effects of salicylates and treatment is largely supportive.

## Sedatives and neuroleptic drugs

- Barbiturates
- Benzodiazepines
- Glutethimide
- Methaqualone
- Phenothiazines

### Features
- Mainly coma and cardiorespiratory depression.

### Management
- General supportive measures.
- Intubate if there is doubt about the airway.
- Ventilate if there is doubt about breathing.
- IV fluids are commonly needed in large amounts in order to support the circulation (see Chapter 4).
- Benzodiazepine antagonists such as flumazenil (at a dosage of no more than 0.1–0.2 mg/min; 1–2 mg is usually sufficient; the paediatric dose is 5 $\mu$g/kg IV stat, to a total of 40 $\mu$g/kg) can reverse the effects of benzodiazepines and may play a limited role in the management of benzodiazepine poisoning. However, not all the effects of the benzodiazepines are reversed and the relationship between the amount of benzodiazepine ingested and the amount of flumazenil needed to offset the effect is not linear. The half-life of flumazenil is about 1 hour. It can induce acute withdrawal syndromes in patients on long-term benzodiazepines. Flumazenil should not be given to patients who are suspected of taking tricyclic antidepressants or to patients who are having seizures.

## Serotonin syndrome

Combinations of selective serotonin therapeutic inhibitors (SSTIs) or an SSTI plus another drug that works by inhibiting serotonin, e.g. tranadol or the atypical antipsychotics, e.g. olanzapine, may lead to the serotonin syndrome.

- Altered mental state.
- Neuromuscular abnormalities.
- Autonomic dysfunction, e.g. tachycardia, flushing.

Treatment is symptomatic and to stop the offending drugs.

## Overdose
- Secure an airway, ventilate.
- Charcoal.
- Monitor and support central venous system.
- Treat seizures.

Selective serotonin therapeutic inhibitors have a large volume of distribution so dialysis or haemoperfusion is not beneficial.

## Theophylline

### Features
- Nausea, vomiting and abdominal pain.
- Haematemesis, hypotension and tachyarrhythmias.
- Renal failure and rhabdomyolysis.
- Central nervous system excitability and convulsions.
- Hypokalaemia, hyperglycaemia, hypophosphataemia, hypomagnesaemia and hypocalcaemia.
- Acid-base disturbances.
- Leucocytosis.

### Management
- ECG monitoring.
- Gastric lavage with activated charcoal.
- Correction of hypotension with fluid and inotropes if necessary.
- Aggressive measures to control seizures.
- Correction of electrolyte disorders: rapidly correct hypokalaemia as well as phosphate and magnesium levels.
- Determination of electrolyte concentrations at least 4-hourly.
- For serious arrhythmias, propranolol may be useful.
- The plasma concentrations do not correlate well with the clinical severity and therefore the concentrations can serve only as guidelines. Therapeutic levels 80–120 μmol/L.
- Haemoperfusion using a charcoal column should be considered if the serum concentration is high (> 600 μmol/L) or if serious complications occur (e.g. seizures, intractable vomiting, severe metabolic acidosis, renal failure and arrhythmias).

## TROUBLESHOOTING

### Poisoning
Establish control of the airway, breathing and circulation before concentrating on drug removal. Supportive care is all that is required for most patients.

### Airway
Intubate and ventilate if Glasgow Coma Scale (GCS) is less than 9.

### Breathing
Give high-flow oxygen via mask if not intubated. Artificially ventilate if still hypoxic.

### Circulation
Fluid will correct most cases of hypotension. Inotropes are rarely needed.

### Monitoring and investigation
Vital signs such as BP, respiratory rate, temperature, pulse rate and GCS should be measured frequently (e.g. every 15–30 minutes) on admission and then according to progress. Also monitor:
• Blood sugar/electrolytes.
• Arterial blood gases.
• ECG.
• Pulse oximetry.

### Corrections
Correct hypoxia, acidosis and electrolyte disorders.

### Drugs
Identify by direct observations of aspirated tablets. Get a history from witnesses. Conduct a drug screen.

### To decrease absorption
• Use NG aspiration.
• Use lavage if ingestion occurred less than 1 hour earlier.
• Give charcoal, 1 g/kg via NG tube; repeated doses may be indicated.
• Induced vomiting should be considered only for children.

### To increase excretion
Procedures such as faecuresis and haemodialysis are indicated only for specific drugs above certain concentrations.

### Antidotes
Antidotes are available for some drugs.

### Sequelae
The sequelae of poisoning, such as hypothermia, hyperthermia, rhabdomyolysis and seizures, must be recognised early and treated aggressively.

## Tricyclic antidepressants

### Features
Remember the three Cs: coma, convulsions and cardiac arrhythmias.

- Arrhythmias (tachycardia, atrioventricular block and intraventricular conduction disturbances).
- Hypotension.
- Respiratory depression.
- Anticholinergic effects (dry mouth, dilated pupils and urinary retention).

### Management
- Secure the airway and ventilate if necessary.
- Treat seizures aggressively.
- Give intravascular fluids to correct hypotension.
- Correct electrolyte and acid-base disorders.
- Avoid physostigmine as it can worsen convulsions and cardiac effects.
- Arrhythmias:
    Most occur within the first 12 hours.
    May need adrenaline, atropine or temporary pacing for bradyarrhythmias. β-blockers or lignocaine may be useful for tachyarrhythmias and intraventricular conduction disturbances.
    Bicarbonate (1–2 mmol/kg IV) may be useful for conduction delay or ventricular arrhythmias. Titrate to response and arterial pH. Hyperventilation may also be useful.

### FURTHER READING

Kozer, E. and Koren, G. Management of paracetamol overdose. Current controversies. *Drug Safety* 24 (2001): 503–12.

Kerr, G. W. and McGuffie, A. C. Tricyclic antidepressant overdose: a review. *Emergency Medicine Journal* 18 (2001): 236–41.

Mann, J. A current perspective of suicide and attempted suicide. *Annals of Internal Medicine* 136 (2002): 301–11.

Pond, S. M., Lewis-Driver, D. J., Williams, G. M., Green A. C. and Stevenson, N. W. Gastric emptying in acute overdose: a prospective randomised controlled trial. *Medical Journal of Australia* 163 (1995): 345–9.

Trujillo, M. H., Guerrero, M. D., Fragachan, C. and Fernandez, M. A. Pharmacologic antidotes in critical care medicine: a practical guide for drug administration. *Critical Care Medicine* 26 (1998): 377–91.

# Acute respiratory failure

- Oxygen is the first-line drug for acute respiratory failure.
- High concentrations of inspired oxygen almost never depress ventilation in patients with acute respiratory failure.
- Artificial ventilation will improve hypercarbia, but may not improve hypoxia.

## Introduction

This chapter will cover the pathophysiology and general principles of treatment for acute respiratory failure. Specific respiratory conditions will be discussed in Chapter 18.

The respiratory system can be seen as being divided into a gas exchange system (the lungs) and a pump to ventilate that system (the diaphragm). The main functions of the lungs are to take up oxygen and eliminate carbon dioxide ($CO_2$). Oxygen is needed for basic metabolism. Respiratory failure occurs when either gas exchange fails or the pump fails. The classic definitions for the onset of acute respiratory failure that cited exact levels of oxygen and $CO_2$ were inflexible and misleading.

Acute respiratory failure can be divided into failure of oxygenation and/or failure of ventilation leading to hypercarbia (Table 16.1). Although hypoxia and hypercarbia can co-exist, it is helpful for an understanding of acute respiratory failure to look at them separately.

**Table 16.1.** Causes of acute respiratory failure

---

Ventilatory problems
  Airway (e.g. obstruction)
  Neuromuscular pathway
    Brain (e.g. coma from any cause)
    Spinal cord (e.g. poliomyelitis, trauma)
    Nerve (e.g. neuropathies)
    Neuromuscular (e.g. myasthenia gravis)
    Muscular disease (e.g. dystrophies)
  Mechanical system: interference with the bellows action of the ventilatory system (e.g. kyphoscoliosis, obesity, increased intra-abdominal pressure, pneumothorax, pain, flail chest). Exhaustion as a result of lung abnormalities (increased airway resistance and decreased compliance) also represents a failure of the mechanical system.
Gas exchange problem
  Decreased $FiO_2$
  Decreased ventilation (will also cause hypercarbia and hypoxia)
  Diffusion defect
  V/Q mismatch (usually, critically ill patients will have a spectrum of V/Q mismatch and shunting)

---

## Failure of oxygenation

There are four types of cellular hypoxia. They are described in the oxygen carrying capacity equation:

$$\text{Oxygen carrying capacity} = \text{Cardiac output} \times \text{Haemoglobin concentration} \times \text{Saturation of Hb} \times 1.34$$

- Stagnant hypoxia – decreased cardiac output.
- Anaemic hypoxia – decreased haemoglobin.
- Hypoxic hypoxia – decreased oxygen saturation in arterial blood.
- Histotoxic hypoxia – decreased oxygen-binding capacity (1.34 ml of oxygen normally bind to every 1 g of haemoglobin).

While oxygen delivery ($DO_2$) to the tissues can be compromised at all levels, including inadequate cardiac output, anaemia and decreased oxygen-binding capacity, this chapter will concentrate on the principles of oxygen exchange in the lungs, where 'hypoxic hypoxia' occurs.

### Hypoxic hypoxia

Acute respiratory failure is generally associated with hypoxic hypoxia (i.e. there is a problem in getting the oxygen from the inspired gas through the lungs into the

## The oxygen cascade

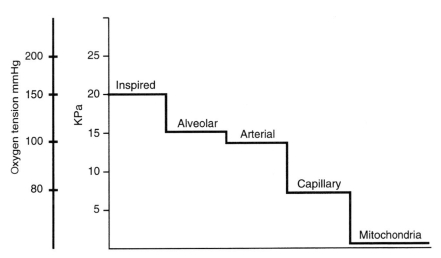

**Figure 16.1.** The oxygen cascade.

capillaries). All causes of hypoxic hypoxia can be related to the oxygen-cascade concept (Figure 16.1).

### Decrease in inspired oxygen

Usually, a decrease in the fraction of inspired oxygen ($FiO_2$) is a problem only at high altitudes or where there is a fault in the gas supply system.

### Alveolar hypoventilation

If the lungs are otherwise normal, hypoxia will occur only with severe hypoventilation. An increase in $FiO_2$ will correct hypoxia in most cases of moderate hypoventilation.

### Diffusion

The term 'diffusion' describes the movement of molecules down a concentration gradient. Diffusion disorders of the lung can occur in diseases such as emphysema. However, diffusion abnormalities play minor roles in most cases of acute respiratory failure.

### Ventilation/perfusion mismatch

Ventilation/perfusion (V/Q) mismatch is the commonest cause of hypoxia in patients with acute respiratory failure. Ventilation and perfusion are well matched in the normal lung. Mismatching affects the exchange of oxygen and $CO_2$, resulting in hypoxia and, to a lesser extent, hypercarbia, as $CO_2$ is a more diffusible gas.

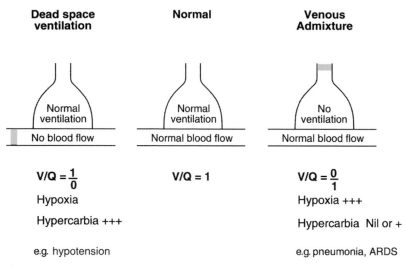

**Figure 16.2.** Ventilation/perfusion (V/Q) matching.

## Shunt

There is some variable degree of true shunting in the presence of acute respiratory failure (i.e. blood and gas do not match at all; Figure 16.2). Most shunting occurs as a result of venous admixture, where capillary blood and alveolar gas do not equilibrate. The larger the shunt, the less responsive it is to added oxygen.

## Other factors

### Increased oxygen consumption (VO$_2$)

Increased consumption of oxygen can contribute to arterial hypoxia. For example, as a result of hypercatabolism or in patients with excessive fever, an increase in peripheral VO$_2$ will decrease the mixed venous levels of oxygen, which, after becoming involved in defective gas exchange in the lungs, will result in arterial hypoxia.

### Oxygen extraction

In order to ensure optimal oxygen extraction, the oxyhaemoglobin curve can be manipulated by encouraging peripheral oxygen unloading. However, the ultimate benefit of such manipulation has not been proved.

### Hypoxic pulmonary vasoconstriction

Alveolar hypoxia causes pulmonary vasoconstriction which can diminish V/Q mismatch (i.e. a decreased amount of blood will perfuse partially ventilated alveoli). Vasodilating drugs such as glycerl trinitrate and calcium channel blockers can inhibit the hypoxic pulmonary vasoconstriction and worsen the hypoxia.

## Effects of hypoxia

Hypoxia causes severe disruptions of cellular function. Central cyanosis is not a reliable sign of hypoxia and more accurate monitoring or measurement is needed in the critically ill. Similarly, signs and symptoms of hypoxia often are late and unpredictable. They can include confusion, irritability, tachypnoea and tachycardia, hypertension eventually leading to bradycardia and hypotension.

The degree of hypoxia can be measured by comparing the $PaO_2$ with the $FiO_2$, by determining the differences between alveolar oxygen and arterial oxygen or by measuring the degree of shunting. Oxygen saturation is continuously monitored in all at-risk patients with a pulse oximeter. This is described in more detail in the section on cardiorespiratory monitoring.

## Failure of ventilation

The commonest cause of hypercarbia is alveolar hypoventilation. Its causes in the ICU include coma and exhaustion secondary to respiratory failure (Table 16.2).

$$PaCO_2 \propto \frac{CO_2 \text{ production}}{\text{Alveolar ventilation}}$$

Alveolar ventilation = Total ventilation − Dead space ventilation

An increase in dead space will decrease alveolar ventilation. Increases in anatomical dead space usually result from the use of artificial airways and ventilatory circuits in the setting of intensive care. Increased physiological dead space usually occurs as a result of a V/Q mismatch.

Hypercarbia usually is associated with hypoventilation (Table 16.3), but it can also result from underperfused alveoli consequent to hypovolaemia and from lung destruction as a result of barotrauma. Increased $CO_2$ production may lead to hypercarbia e.g. as with fever, excessive carbohydrate intake and increased activity.

## Effects of hypercarbia

- Increased respiratory drive.
- Anxiety, restlessness, tachycardia, hypertension and arrhythmias.
- Peripheral vasodilatation.
- Increases in cerebral blood flow and intracranial pressure (ICP).
- Decreased level of consciousness and coma.

**Table 16.2.** Major causes of hypercarbia in intensive care

Decreased $CO_2$ elimination
    There are many causes of hypoventilation (e.g. airway obstruction, drugs, central
        and peripheral nervous disorders)
    Decreased minute volume (e.g. end-stage acute respiratory failure because of
        exhaustion)
    Ventilation perfusion inequality is the commonest cause of hypercarbia in patients
        with chronic lung disease and acute respiratory failure. It is often in association
        with destruction of lung architecture, either chronically (largely as a result of
        smoking-related diseases) or acutely (as a result of pulmonary barotrauma in acute
        respiratory failure)
Excess $CO_2$ production
    This is an uncommon cause of hypercarbia and usually is important only when $CO_2$
        elimination is impaired
    Hyperpyrexia
    Inappropriate carbohydrate load
    Hypercatabolism
    Thyrotoxicosis
Increased dead space
    In the setting of an ICU, increased dead space usually is due to increased equipment
        dead space or decreased pulmonary artery blood flow

- Acute rise in endogenous catecholamines, causing increases in cardiac output and blood pressure (BP).
- Decreased oxygenation by displacing alveolar oxygen.

Carbon dioxide usually is monitored by intermittent sampling of arterial blood gases in the ICU. Capnography can also be used. Monitoring of carbon dioxide is described in the section on cardiorespiratory monitoring.

## Principles of treatment

### Failure of ventilation

Obviously the airway is crucial for respiratory function and it must always be the first consideration in dealing with any respiratory problem. Gas cannot move in and out of the lungs, no matter how efficient they are, if the airway is blocked. Always consider the possibility of a compromised airway and replace the endotracheal tube (ETT) or tracheostomy tube if there is any doubt about its patency.

Treatment and diagnosis of hypoventilation go hand in hand (Table 16.3). If necessary, the airway must be secured and artificial ventilation commenced, while the cause of the ventilatory failure is being determined and treatment selected.

**Table 16.3.** Major causes of hypoventilation in intensive care

Brain
    Drug overdose
    Neurotrauma
    Postoperative anaesthetic depression
    Cardiovascular accident
Spinal Cord
    Poliomyelitis
    Spinal cord trauma
Neuromuscular system
    Myasthenia gravis
    Tetanus
    Organophosphate poisoning
    Neuromuscular blocking drugs
    Peripheral neuritis
    Guillain–Barré syndrome
    Muscular dystrophies
Thorax
    Massive obesity
    Kyphoscoliosis
    Chest trauma and flail chest
    Pneumothorax and pleural effusion
Increased intra-abdominal pressure
Upper airway obstruction
Exhaustion
    Especially in the latter stages of acute respiratory failure as a result of low lung
       compliance or increased resistance

**Hypoxic patients need oxygenation, not necessarily more ventilation.**
Indeed, acute respiratory failure is usually marked by hyperventilation and
hypocarbia in the face of hypoxia. In other words, the patient's existing ventilation usually is more than adequate, especially in the earlier stages. Oxygen
uptake is affected more than $CO_2$ excretion. As the lungs become heavier and
less compliant, the patient has to work harder, and eventually the increased work
will lead to respiratory muscle exhaustion and hypoventilation. The $VO_2$ related
to respiratory work may also be unacceptably high. In the event of hypoventilation or an unacceptable increase in respiratory work, artificial ventilation may
eventually be necessary.

If ventilation is impaired and the $CO_2$ concentration rises, the possible reversible causes should be examined and ruled out; then, if necessary, artificial ventilation should be commenced or increased. Unless the ICP is elevated,
hypercarbia is not as dangerous as hypoxia; this is particularly relevant when
ventilating patients with asthma or chronic airflow limitation (CAL). There is

**Table 16.4.** Principles of treatment for acute respiratory failure

Treat underlying cause
Increase oxygen delivery
    Oxygen
    PEEP
    CPAP
    Fluid treatment
    Artificial ventilation
    Nursing and physiotherapy
    Haemoglobin
    Perfusion
Decrease oxygen consumption
Improve oxygen extraction
Miscellaneous (e.g. bronchoscopy, antibiotics)
Matching $DO_2$ to oxygen consumption

an increasing tendency to accept $PaCO_2$ values higher than 'normal', so long as the arterial pH remains acceptable. Achieving 'normal' $PaCO_2$ values in patients with acute respiratory failure can result in an unacceptably high incidence of complications, such as pulmonary barotrauma.

Ventilation should be achieved at a peak inspiratory pressure (PIP) of less than 35 $cmH_2O$ at a respiratory rate consistent with adequate lung emptying at the end of expiration. The aim of artificial ventilation is to maintain oxygenation at the lowest level of positive intrathoracic pressure.

## Failure of oxygenation (Table 16.4)

Treating hypoventilation with artificial ventilation is relatively straightforward, as compared with managing hypoxia. **The real challenge in patients with acute respiratory failure is to maintain adequate oxygenation.** Management of patients with acute respiratory failure involves the right balance of $FiO_2$, positive end-expiratory pressure (PEEP), sedation, fluid treatment, drugs and positive intrathoracic pressure – all of which involve potential dangers. **Treatment of patients with acute respiratory failure is usually a holding operation while the lungs heal themselves.** Avoidance of any iatrogenic complications of the ventilatory therapy is paramount.

The primary aim in treating acute respiratory failure is to provide more oxygen to the cells, and sometimes to reduce their consumption. The $DO_2$ depends on the following relationship:

$$DO_2 = \text{Cardiac output} \times \text{Hb concentration} \times \text{Oxygen saturation} \times 1.34$$

The following sections will take up each aspect of $DO_2$ in turn, but in clinical practice they must, of course, be considered as complementing and interacting with each other.

For example, more oxygen might be available on each haemoglobin molecule if PEEP were applied to the lungs but the cardiac output might be depressed and therefore oxygen transport would be decreased. Capillary flow might be encouraged because of the fewer numbers of haemoglobin molecules that would result from decreasing the viscosity. However, the oxygen content in the blood would then be decreased. The $DO_2$ requires a balance of many factors and the $DO_2$ equation is one of the most important tools in intensive care.

## Oxygen delivery

### Increased oxygen saturation of haemoglobin (Table 16.5)

Oxygen delivery = Cardiac output × Hb concentration
×**Oxygen saturation** × 1.34

**Oxygen is the first-line drug for hypoxia.** It may have to be delivered via an ETT with artificial ventilation, but in many cases that is not necessary. Many patients with acute respiratory failure are hyperventilating and do not need increased ventilation.

### Complications of oxygen treatment

Carbon dioxide narcosis: Apart from the fact that it can sometimes explode and can support combustion, oxygen is a very safe drug. For some inexplicable reason medical students are taught, and seem to remember forever, that oxygen is a dangerous drug. One almost expects to see it prescribed molecule by molecule like dangerous tablets. Many hypoxic patients, with or without chronic respiratory components in their illnesses, are found behind their masks inhaling 24% oxygen – 3% more than in room air! Oxygen never inhibits breathing in acute respiratory failure and rarely inhibits breathing in acute on chronic respiratory failure. When it does, the onset is slow enough to allow monitoring with pulse oximetry, blood gas analysis and clinical status.

Oxygen toxicity: In the past, fear of oxygen toxicity has been another reason for depriving hypoxic patients of oxygen. High levels of $FiO_2$ oxygen can cause atelectasis, decreased alveolar macrophage activity, decreased ciliary action and, in the long term, lung fibrosis. Oxygen has never been shown to cause lung damage if the $FiO_2$ has been less than 0.5. If at all possible, it should be kept below that level. However, if oxygen is essential for preventing hypoxia, it should not be withheld because of the fear of toxicity. Oxygenation should be carefully

**Table 16.5.** Principles of oxygenation

---

The following guidelines are listed in order of increasing escalation of measures needed
to maintain oxygenation in patients with acute respiratory failure

1   Oxygen

Increase $FiO_2$, but aim to keep below 0.5 with face mask

2   CPAP

CPAP mask or intubation with CPAP at 5–20 $cmH_2O$ CPAP initially, using efficient
circuit $\pm$ PSV or BiPAP

3   Ventilation

Preferably with a technique to maintain spontaneous respiration such as PSV.

Use low tidal volumes ($< 6$ ml/kg) in order to keep the PIP at $< 35$ $cmH_2O$ and the
respiratory rate consistent with adequate $CO_2$ excretion

Use PEEP at sufficiently high levels to keep the lung open at end-expiration

Limit the pressure difference between PEEP and the inspiratory plateau pressures to
avoid 'shear stress' of the lung

Use sedation only if necessary and with continuous sedation to reduce excessive
movement and fighting of the ventilator

4   Fluid therapy

Use minimal crystalloids, while maintaining intravascular volume with colloid or
blood, in all hypoxic patients.

5   Diuretic

Give diuretic in frequent small doses (e.g. 5–10 mg of frusemide initially 4-hourly, or
a continuous IV infusion may help to reduce the lung water). The circulation must
simultaneously be maintained with colloid or blood – the so-called euvolaemic
dehydration.

6   Position

Position the affected lung up in the presence of a unilateral abnormality. Otherwise,
routinely nurse the patient up at an angle of $40^\circ$ or more

7   Give 100% oxygen during endotracheal suctioning

8   Actively cool the patient to reduce severe hyperpyrexia, in combination with sedation
and/or paralysis to prevent shivering

9   LFPPV + $ECCO_2R$ or extracorpeal oxygenation if available

---

Note: See the sections on ventilatory techniques (Chapter 19) for IPPV, PEEP, CPAP,
PSV, BiPAP, IMV, MMV, HFPPV, LFPPV + $ECCO_2R$, reversed I : E ratios and weaning.

monitored (e.g. arterial blood gases, pulse oximetry) with the $FiO_2$ reduced to a
safe level as soon as possible. If the patient has a high shunt fraction increasing
the $FiO_2$ will not have much effect on the $PaO_2$. In that situation, an excessive
$FiO_2$ may be unnecessary and dangerous. On the other hand, hypoxia is definitely
dangerous!

Concentration of inspired oxygen: In view of the conflict between the potential
dangers of oxygen and its essential nature, the amount given will depend on the
amount needed. In acute respiratory failure, keep the $PaO_2$ above 60 mmHg

**Table 16.6.** Approximate oxygen concentrations related to flow rates

| Oxygen flow rate L/min | Approximate FiO$_2$ |
| --- | --- |
| 4 | 0.25–0.35 |
| 6 | 0.30–0.50 |
| 8 | 0.35–0.55 |
| 10 | 0.4 –0.60 |
| 12 | 0.45–0.65 |

(8 kPa) or 90% saturation. That is the critical point at the top of the oxy-haemoglobin dissociation curve. Below that, the curve becomes closer to vertical and saturation of the haemoglobin molecule diminishes rapidly.

Delivery systems (Table 16.6): No mask or catheter device can deliver 100% oxygen, unless it can provide a peak inspiratory flow rate (PIFR) of at least 40 L/min. There are two main types of system for delivering oxygen:

1 Inspired oxygen independent of patient factors (fixed performance masks, e.g. Venturi masks).
2 Inspired oxygen dependent on the patient's respiratory pattern (variable performance masks).

Nasal catheters: The FiO$_2$ is dependent on respiratory rate and tidal volume. As the respiratory rate and tidal volume increases, FiO$_2$ decreases. The nasal catheter (2–6 L/min) functions by filling the nasopharyngeal reservoirs with oxygen which is entrained as the patient inspires. Flow rates higher than 6 L/min offer no advantage for oxygenation and can cause patient discomfort.

Simple oxygen masks: The oxygen flow must be more than 5 L/min in order to avoid carbon dioxide retention. The FiO$_2$ is dependent on respiratory rate and tidal volume. As the respiratory rate and tidal volume increase, FiO$_2$ decreases. The FiO$_2$ varies between 0.35 and 0.50 as the oxygen flow is increased from 5 to 8 L/min.

Venturi oxygen mask: The FiO$_2$ value depends on the degree of entrainment. A variety of entrainment valves provide FiO$_2$ values between 0.24 and something approaching 1.0. The FiO$_2$ may not be independent of respiratory pattern in patients with very high PIFRs.

Reservoir oxygen mask: This mask potentially can provide a FiO$_2$ of 1.0. For efficient operation, the oxygen reservoir should be fully expanded.

If a patient is unable to protect and maintain the airway, or if the patient becomes exhausted, an ETT should be inserted. This will allow efficient delivery of oxygen, and maintenance of PEEP and continuous positive airway pressure (CPAP), as well as artificial ventilation if required.

**Table 16.7.** Positive end-expiratory pressure

| Advantages | Disadvantages |
| --- | --- |
| Improves oxygenation | Decreases venous return |
| Augments intrinsic PEEP levels | Decreases cardiac output |
| Decreases cardiac afterload | Decreases blood flow to extrathoracic organs |
| Recruits alveoli for ventilation | Pulmonary barotrauma |
| | Sedation ± muscle relaxation needed |

Uses

Patients with hypoxia who are artificially ventilated (e.g. atelectasis, pneumonia, ALI)

Practical aspects

Start at 5 cmH$_2$O and do not exceed 20 cmH$_2$O. Give a fluid bolus (200–400 ml) before commencing IPPV + PEEP, in order to prevent hypotension as a result of decreased venous return

### Positive end-expiratory pressure (Table 16.7)

Positive end-expiratory pressure occurs when, instead of allowing airway pressure to return to atmospheric pressure between ventilator breaths, an end-expiratory pressure is applied. The end-expiratory pressure probably prevents collapse of the alveoli, in addition to recruiting non-ventilated alveoli, thus enabling greater numbers to participate in gas exchange and thereby lessening V/Q mismatch.

Optimal PEEP: Although PEEP will improve oxygenation, it may decrease overall oxygen transport by decreasing cardiac output. The increased intrathoracic pressure causes a decrease in venous return, which is usually reversed by the use of intravenous fluids and/or inotropes. Extrathoracic oxygen blood flow is also compromised by PEEP. A combination of decreased cardiac output (blood flow to the organ) and decreased venous return (blood flow from the organ) can markedly reduce blood flow to extrathoracic organs such as the brain, liver and kidneys. The optimal PEEP is the best match between improving the oxygenation and decreasing the oxygen transport due to decreased cardiac output. Another way of expressing the idea of optimal PEEP is that it is the minimal PEEP at which adequate oxygenation is maintained or to keep the maximum volume of lung open at the end of expiration.

Disadvantages of PEEP: The complications of PEEP are the same as those for the increased intrathoracic pressure achieved with artificial ventilation. Barotrauma and decreased cardiac output occur. These are described in more detail elsewhere.

### Continuous positive airway pressure (Table 16.8)

Continuous positive airway pressure is a technique whereby gas is delivered to the airways at a constant pressure, facilitating spontaneous inspiratory effort, as

**Table 16.8.** Continuous positive airway pressure

| Advantages | Disadvantages |
|---|---|
| Improves oxygenation | Potentially has the same |
| Increases lung compliance | disadvantages as PEEP and |
| Decreases work of breathing | artificial ventilation; however, |
| Decreases cardiac preload (may also be a | as levels are lower, the disadvantages |
| disadvantage) | diminish |
| Low intrathoracic pressures | |
| compared with artificial ventilation | |
| Recruits alveoli for ventilation | |

Uses
Hypoxic patients with acute respiratory failure who are spontaneously breathing (e.g. cardiogenic pulmonary oedema, ALI, pneumonia, fat embolism). It may also be useful for acute severe asthma and CAL

Practical aspects
A face mask can be used. The patient needs to be conscious, co-operative, with adequate respiratory drive.

well as providing PEEP. It is a technique used to support spontaneous respiration and to correct hypoxia, not hypoventilation. In many cases of acute respiratory failure, CPAP will increase lung compliance and decrease the work of breathing and thus may eliminate the need for assisted ventilation. It can be delivered by lightweight plastic masks, nasal prongs, ETTs or tracheostomies. A CPAP mask or nasal prongs can be used in a patient who is:

- Conscious and co-operative, with an intact airway.
- Hypoxic, with consistent respiratory drive.

Some masks have an adjustable head strap to prevent leaks. After adequate explanation to the patient they are usually well tolerated. An efficient circuit must be employed. Inefficient CPAP (e.g. inadequate inspiratory flow rates) can cause increased work of breathing and impairment of gas exchange. The increased work of breathing in these systems can be counteracted by increasing inspiratory flow and/or pressure. However, it is may be cheaper and more efficient to use a continuous flow device.

Table 16.9 compares PEEP and CPAP.

## Artificial ventilation

Artificial ventilation will not necessarily improve oxygenation. In some patients it will decrease $DO_2$ by altering the V/Q matching. Matching of ventilation and perfusion is more efficient in spontaneously breathing patients than in those on artificial ventilation. Patients should not necessarily be ventilated for hypoxia unless they are becoming exhausted or unless there is a concurrent abnormality,

**Table 16.9.** Advantages of CPAP compared with IPPV + PEEP

| |
|---|
| Less sedation needed |
| Lower peak inspiratory pressure needed |
| Better oxygenation during spontaneous respiration |
| Less barotrauma |
| Better blood flow to extrathoracic organs |
| Better venous return and cardiac output |
| Better lung lymph drainage |

such as a head injury. Other modalities should be explored first, such as increasing the $FiO_2$ with appropriate oxygen masks or applying CPAP by mask. If ventilation is required, the following guidelines should be used (see Chapter 19 for more details).

Aim to keep the lung expanded with a minimum PIP, using low tidal volumes, even in the presence of higher rather than 'normal' $CO_2$ levels. This concept has been called 'elective hypoventilation' or 'permissive hypercarbia'. The aim is to achieve oxygenation with a minimum of complications resulting from the use of positive-pressure. Some of the techniques that can facilitate positive-pressure ventilation with minimal complications include intermittent mandatory ventilation (IMV), pressure-support ventilation (PSV) and pressure limited, reverse I : E ratio ventilation (see Chapter 19). Conventional intermittent positive-pressure ventilation (IPPV) with PEEP should be avoided in favour of these other modes, where possible.

### Fluid treatment

Poor fluid treatment in intensive care can impair gas exchange: dry lungs are more effective than wet ones.

**The aim of fluid treatment is to keep the interstitial space as dry as possible, while maintaining a normal intravascular volume – so-called euvolaemic dehydration** (see Chapter 4). Thus, the lungs should be kept as dry as possible while not compromising organ perfusion.

There are quite enough causes of increased lung water and acute lung injury (ALI) in the ICU without us contributing to the list by giving excessive salt and water. Irrespective of the colloid osmotic pressure (COP), at least three-quarters of any crystalloid solution is distributed to the interstitial space. Excessive use of crystalloids should be avoided, if possible, in patients with acute respiratory failure.

The pulmonary artery wedge pressure (PAWP) at which lung water will accumulate is lower in patients with acute respiratory failure than in normal patients. Therefore, excessive use of intravascular fluid should also be avoided.

Assessment of lung water is difficult. Currently, the chest x-ray is the best clinical guide to the volume of lung water. There is a good correlation between the extent of lung water and the degree of chest x-ray opacification.

Restrict intake of salt and water: If possible, limit the intake of 'clear' fluids to less than 2000 ml over 24 hours in normal-sized adults with severe respiratory failure. Use non-sodium containing fluids (e.g. 5% dextrose) if the serum sodium concentration is normal, especially if fluids such as colloid (with a high sodium concentration) or blood are being used concurrently. Maintain the intravascular volume and cardiovascular stability with colloids or blood products and inotropes, according to the available cardiovascular measurements.

## Reduction of the lung's interstitial space fluid

Diuretic: Small doses of loop diuretic (e.g. frusemide, 5–10 mg IV, 4-hourly, or the equivalent amount in a continuous IV infusion) may reduce lung water. However, colloid or blood usually will have to be given simultaneously in order to maintain the intravascular volume while depleting the interstitial space with the diuretic. Cations such as potassium, magnesium and hydrogen will become depleted during aggressive diuretic treatment. Their serum levels need to be measured at least once each day (more often for potassium). Meticulous replacement is necessary.

Dialytic modes: Patients on dialysis or haemofiltration can readily have their fluid status altered by increasing or decreasing the ultrafiltration. The fluid removed is the ultrafiltrate of blood – almost the same constituents as interstitial space fluid. Ultrafiltration is a very efficient and convenient way of selectively decreasing the volume of the interstitial fluid. As with diuretic treatment, the intravascular space must be maintained simultaneously with colloid or blood products.

## Nursing and physiotherapy

Positioning of patients: The dependent part of the lung is ventilated and perfused best. Generally speaking, patients with respiratory failure should be sat up, at least 40°, so that perfusion will be directed to the bulk of alveoli at the base of the lung. Nursing in the semirecumbent position also decreases the incidence of aspiration and nosocomial pneumonia. The head down position can cause hypoxia. However, depending on where the pulmonary abnormality is, the patient should be positioned to maximise the matching of ventilation and perfusion (e.g. if the abnormality is more in the left lung, it may help to turn the patient so that the right lung is down). Positioning the patient in the prone position can also improve oxygenation.

Procedures: Nursing procedures can contribute to hypoxia, especially tracheal suctioning. Intratracheal negative pressure can exacerbate pulmonary oedema and will always cause hypoxia. The hypoxia can sometimes be severe and can lead to bradycardia. Intratracheal suctioning should always be preceded by 100% oxygen for 3–5 minutes; its use should be minimised for patients with acute respiratory failure and avoided in those with active pulmonary oedema. With the use of special devices on endotracheal connectors, PEEP and ventilation can be maintained during suction.

Chest physiotherapy: Physiotherapy is aimed mainly at clearing secretions confined to the central airways, in addition to preventing collapse and atelectasis. It cannot modify the course of acute respiratory failure as the abnormality is parenchymatous, rather than in the airways. Care must be exercised in positioning and suctioning patients during physiotherapy as hypoxia can be exacerbated.

### Haemoglobin

Oxygen delivery = Cardiac output × **Haemoglobin concentration** × Oxygen saturation × 1.34

Oxygen is carried on haemoglobin in red blood cells. Each gram of haemoglobin carries 1.34 ml of oxygen. Anaemia is common in the seriously ill, often as a result of coagulopathy and multiple blood tests. The haemoglobin concentration should be kept to at least 10 g/dl in hypoxic patients in order to maintain their oxygen-carrying capacity. However, in a heterogeneous group of patients managed in intensive care, haemoglobins of less than 10 g/dl are tolerated.

### Perfusion

Oxygen delivery = **Cardiac output** × Hb concentration × Oxygen saturation × 1.34

Optimising the saturation on the haemoglobin molecule and ensuring an adequate haemoglobin concentration is of no avail unless there is sufficient blood flow to take the oxygen to the cells. To improve the cardiac output, the following need to be optimum (see also Chapter 21):

- Preload: Titrate the fluid against cardiovascular responses.
- Contractility: Increase the cardiac output and peripheral perfusion with inotropes.
- Afterload: Decreasing the afterload is a manoeuvre used more in patients with primary heart disease than in the seriously ill with multiorgan failure.

Regional blood flow is a function of the perfusing pressure and the resistance to flow. At the tissue level, the factors determining oxygenation are the number of capillaries and the diffusing distance for the gas between the capillary and the

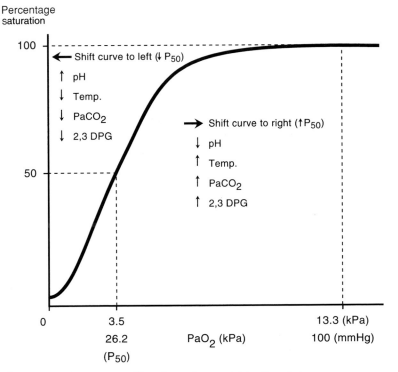

**Figure 16.3.** Factors controlling the oxyhaemoglobin dissociation curve.

cell. Whereas cardiac output and global $DO_2$ are relatively easy to measure and alter, tissue blood flow and $DO_2$ are not amenable to accurate measurement nor are they easily manipulated.

### Combining power of haemoglobin and oxygen

Oxygen delivery = Cardiac output × Haemoglobin concentration
$\qquad$ × Oxygen saturation × 1.34

The factor 1.34 is mentioned for completeness. It is of minor relevance in acute respiratory failure. For each 1 g of haemoglobin, 1.34 ml of oxygen is attached. Occasionally, and in the presence of a normal $PaO_2$, the combining ability is compromised (e.g. carbon monoxide toxicity and cyanide poisoning). Such poisons also affect the ability of the cells to utilise oxygen. The combining power of haemoglobin and oxygen is described by the oxyhaemoglobin dissociation curve (Figure 16.3).

## Oxygen consumption

On the other side of the oxygen equation is consumption. A decrease in the consumption of oxygen should be considered a possibility in severely hypoxic patients when the factors determining $DO_2$ have been optimised and the patient remains hypoxic.

### Temperature

Oxygen consumption will increase markedly with increasing fever. If a patient's oxygenation is marginal, aggressive measures should be taken to treat the cause of fever (e.g. infection, heatstroke, malignant hyperthermia, drugs) and to reduce the fever.

Surface cooling is an efficient method for lowering temperature. It can be achieved by creating a wind tunnel effect, with a fan blowing from the end of the bed and a sheet tightly attached to the upper part of the chest, to avoid corneal drying and ulceration.

Tepid sponging can increase the efficiency of this form of cooling. Sedation with or without muscle relaxation may also have to be employed to stop the shivering response. Shivering increases $VO_2$ greatly. Paracetamol should be used with caution in patients with liver dysfunction. Avoid the use of ice packs for febrile patients as that would simply decrease the skin circulation.

Aim for moderate temperature reduction (e.g. to 38.0 °C) rather than hypothermia. A fever may be necessary for an optimal immune response in the presence of infection.

### Minimising movement

Except for the diaphragm, movement should be discouraged for severely hypoxic patients. Hypoxic confusion sometimes leads to excessive movement at a high oxygen cost. Reassurance and sedation often are the only measures needed. For intractable cases, sedation and induction of paralysis may be necessary. This, of course, means mandatory ventilation, with its own costs. Seizures and excessive muscle movements must be aggressively treated in hypoxic patients.

### Hypercatabolism

Hypercatabolism is often a feature of the seriously ill and is refractory to manipulation, apart from treating the underlying cause. Avoidance of high carbohydrate feeds may help to reduce excessive $CO_2$ production.

## Miscellaneous considerations

The principles of management for patients with acute respiratory failure are based on physiological considerations. Drugs have a limited but well-defined role.

## Drugs

Bronchodilators: Use bronchodilators if there is any evidence of bronchoconstriction.

Antibiotics: Use antibiotics for infections.

Nitric oxide: Nitric oxide is both an endogenous vasodilator and a cellular messenger for the vasodilating actions of nitrates. Inhaled nitric oxide is a selective
pulmonary vasodilator, reducing pulmonary vascular resistance without affecting systemic vascular resistance and improving cardiac output and $DO_2$.
Nitric oxide requires a special delivery system and gas analysis, as metabolites
of nitric oxide, such as nitrogen dioxide ($NO_2$), cause toxicity secondary to
their oxidising effects.

Some trials in adults with ALI, CAL and idiopathic pulmonary hypertension
have shown significant reductions in pulmonary vascular resistance. However,
nitric oxide has not been shown to improve outcome in adults with ALI.

Other drugs: Steroids may be of some benefit in non-resolving ALI. Otherwise
they are associated with higher mortality. Prostacyclin, aprotinin, artificial
surfactant, heparin, thrombolytic agents, indomethacin, imidazole, meclofe-
namate, antioxidants and anti-inflammatory prostanoids have all been tried or
are being tested for treatment of acute respiratory failure with, as yet, equivocal
success.

## Extracorporeal gas exchange

If all else fails, some form of extracorporeal support could be considered. While
extracorporeal membrane oxygenation (ECMO) is rarely used today, more recent
variations combining low frequency positive-pressure ventilation (LFPPV) and
extracorporeal $CO_2$ removal (ECCO$_2$R), have proved to be successful in some
cases of severe acute respiratory failure: carbon dioxide is eliminated through
an extracorporeal circuit, while oxygenation is achieved using oxygen insufflated
directly into the trachea. Two to three artificial breaths each minute are delivered
with pressures limited to less than 35 cmH$_2$O.

## Matching oxygen delivery and consumption

The $DO_2$ is the amount of oxygen delivered to the body tissues and usually it is well
matched to metabolic requirements. Under basal conditions, $VO_2$ is about 25%
of $DO_2$, yielding an oxygen extraction ratio of 0.25. Decreases in $DO_2$ are usually
matched by increases in the oxygen extraction ratio, allowing the $VO_2$ to remain
constant. However, once oxygen extraction is maximum, further decreases in $DO_2$
will be matched by parallel decreases in $VO_2$ – the so-called supply dependence
(Figure 16.4). This critical point is reached when tissue extraction cannot increase
enough to compensate for the reduction in $DO_2$. The critical value is the same

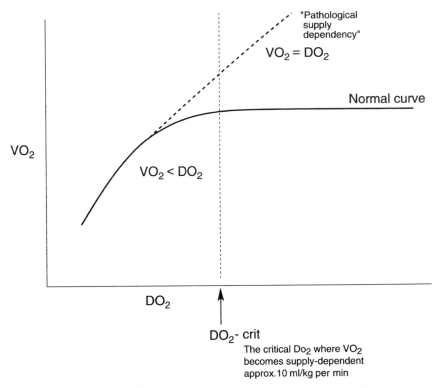

**Figure 16.4.** Relationship between oxygen consumption and oxygen supply.

whether the reduced $DO_2$ results from lowering the haemoglobin or decreasing the oxygen concentration in inspired air. The critical level at which this occurs in animal models is about 8–10 ml · kg$^{-1}$ · min$^{-1}$. When an oxygen debt occurs, anaerobic metabolism produces lactic acid. If the condition goes uncorrected, tissue hypoxia will occur, eventually leading to cellular damage and death.

In the presence of certain conditions, such as septic shock, ALI and multiple trauma, there will be increases in $VO_2$.

Some conditions such as sepsis may also be characterised by an impairment in oxygen extraction. This can result from arteriovenous shunting, capillary obstruction due to microemboli or localised disseminated intravascular coagulation, capillary compression due to excessive peripheral oedema, primary cellular dysfunction or a maldistribution of perfusion, with over-supply of oxygen to some tissues and under-supply to others. Vasomotor reactivity could also be impaired by the release of vasoactive agents in precapillary sphincters and arterioles.

The ideal rate of $DO_2$ is difficult to define for the seriously ill. Whereas it is easy to recommend that we provide $DO_2$ adequate to meet the demand, measurements of demand usually require intensive and time-consuming monitoring, with all of its disadvantages. Moreover, it is difficult to draw conclusions about cellular oxygen supply from $VO_2$, as this is not necessarily the same as actual cellular requirements. In addition, interpretation of absolute whole body $VO_2$ values is complicated by the fluctuations that can occur with the patient's activities such as positioning, independent of real changes in consumption.

Whether critically ill patients benefit from manipulating their $DO_2$, and maybe therefore their $VO_2$, is now slightly clearer. There is good evidence that optimising the haemodynamic parameters preoperatively in patients who are having major surgery improves their outcome.

Once the patients are critically ill, aiming for supranormal haemodynamic values – cardiac index greater than 4.5 $L/m^2$ body surface area and $DO_2$ greater than 650 ml/min per $m^2$ – does not improve outcome in sepsis or in a mixed group of critically ill patients. One study showed an increase in morbidity associated with the manoeuvres necessary to achieve increased $PO_2$.

**In the critically ill, we probably should aim for at least normal $DO_2$, as this has been demonstrated to reduce the incidence of organ failure and to improve patient outcome.** Thus, a patient should have adequate fluid resuscitation, a saturation of at least 90% and a haemoglobin of at least 10 g/dl. Inotropes and vasopressors may also be necessary. Thus, the emphasis probably should be more on $DO_2$, and away from consumption, which currently is beset by many problems with interpretation.

## TROUBLESHOOTING

### Sudden onset of hypoxia

Observe for chest movement.

Hand ventilate the patient on 100% oxygen.

Check the delivery of oxygen system (ventilator/circuit/artificial airway).

Listen for breath sounds and pathological breath sounds (e.g. pneumothorax, bronchospasm, acute lung collapse or aspiration).

Ensure that any chest drains are not blocked.

If hypoxia does not resolve quickly with 100% oxygen, then intubate the patient if that has not already been done.

Pass catheter down artificial airway to check for patency and if any doubt replace it.

Immediately obtain a chest x-ray.

Treat according to the underlying abnormality (e.g. titrate PEEP for pulmonary oedema, drain pneumothorax).

## TROUBLESHOOTING

### Hypoxia: where to go when the patient is already on 100% oxygen

Often there is little more that one can do for these patients but here are some suggestions for fine-tuning:

Check ventilator, gas delivery, lines, etc.

Reassess the chest x-ray and physical examination in order to exclude a reversible component (e.g. collapse, effusion or loculated pneumothorax).

Position – change the patient's position in order to match ventilation with perfusion more effectively. This may involve placing the more seriously affected lung uppermost or sitting them up at an angle of 40° or more if the abnormality is equally distributed. Turning the patient to the prone position will often result in temporary improvement.

The PEEP should be adjusted to optimise $DO_2$.

One should consider decreasing the patient's $VO_2$ (e.g. cooling or sedation).

Coughing and 'fighting' the ventilator can exacerbate hypoxia. Muscle relaxants can help to reduce $VO_2$ in these patients.

Fluids should be used carefully. The intravascular volume should be maintained with colloid or blood and excessive use of crystalloid infusion avoided. Small amounts of diuretic may help to reduce lung water. Similarly, increased fluid removal during dialysis may improve oxygenation.

Trial and error with different ventilatory techniques may improve oxygenation. For example:

- Increased spontaneous breathing will sometimes improve oxygenation.
- Reverse the I : E ratio to 3 : 1 or 4 : 1 with PEEP at 5 $cmH_2O$ and pressure limited to less than 40 $cmH_2O$.
- Decrease inspiratory flow rates to avoid excessive PIP and pulmonary barotraumas.
- Use differential ventilation in cases of unilateral lung disease.

Extracorporeal techniques may benefit some patients in this group.

### FURTHER READING

Appendini, L. About the relevance of dynamic intrinsic PEEP (PEEPi, dyn) measurements. *Intensive Care Medicine* 25 (1999): 252–4.

Galley, H. F. (ed.) *Critical Care Focus. 2 Respiratory Failure.* London: BMJ Books, 1999.

Gattinoni, L., Brazzi, L., Pelosi, P., Latini, R., Tognoni, G., Pesenti, A., Fumagalli, R. and the $SvO_2$ Collaborative Group. A trial of goal-orientated hemodynamic therapy in critically ill patients. *New England Journal of Medicine* 333 (1995): 1025–32.

Marras, T., Herridge, M. and Mehta, S. Corticosteroid therapy in acute respiratory distress syndrome. *Intensive Care Medicine* 25 (1999): 1191–3.

Pelosi, P. and Gattinoni, L. Respiratory mechanics in ARDS: a siren for physicians? *Intensive Care Medicine* 26 (2000): 653–6.

Roussos, C. and Zakynthinos, S. Fatigue of the respiratory muscles. *Intensive Care Medicine* 22 (1996): 134–55.

Siegemund, M., van Bommel, J. and Ince, C. Assessment of regional tissue oxygenation. *Intensive Care Medicine* 25 (1999): 1044–60.

Singh, S., Wort, J. and Evans, T. W. Inhaled nitric oxide in ARDS: modulator of lung injury? *Intensive Care Medicine* 25 (1999): 1024–6.

Ware, L. B. and Matthay, M. A. The acute respiratory distress syndrome. *New England Journal of Medicine* 342 (2000): 1334–49.

# 17

# Interpretation of the portable chest film

> - The chest x-ray is one of the most useful tools for assessing seriously ill patients and x-rays should be taken at least once daily on all patients.
> - A routine for assessing radiographs should be developed and followed in every case so that nothing will be missed.
> - All plain chest radiographs should be taken with the patient sitting erect, unless there is an absolute contraindication.

The portable antero-posterior (AP) chest film is one of the most useful tools in critical care medicine. It is a mandatory supplement to the examination of the respiratory system. A chest x-ray should be obtained at least daily, in addition to x-rays following intubation or placement of an intrathoracic line and in response to sudden changes in the patient's clinical state such as fever, hypoxia or increased ventilatory pressures.

There is an art to interpreting chest x-rays in the ICU. These patients often are unconscious and difficult to position, they usually cannot co-operate in breath holding and they can move during the exposure, causing blurring. Also, the AP projection magnifies the heart and mediastinum making interpretation of those regions difficult.

Although it may be tempting to take a chest x-ray with the patient supine, it is crucial that one gain the co-operation of both nursing and radiology staff so that the film can be exposed with the patient sitting erect. Air–fluid interfaces can only be visualised accurately with the patient erect. Moreover, pneumothoraces, the distribution of pulmonary vessels and lung oedema, can be interpreted more accurately when the patient is erect (Table 17.1).

A CT is sometimes useful, especially for abnormalities around the lung bases, for differentiating between effusions and intrapulmonary abnormalities, for localising loculated pneumothoraces and for documenting chronic changes following an acute insult such as acute lung injury.

**Table 17.1.** Differences between an erect and supine chest x-ray

| | |
|---|---|
| 1 Air | A pneumothroax may not be seen in the apex. |
| | Air will accumulate anteriorly and is not easily seen. |
| 2 Blood | Haemothoraces will not accumulate near the diaphragm. They will be seen as a 'veil' across the whole lung field. |
| 3 Blood vessels | Gravity affects the amount of blood in the various zones of the lung. In a supine film the zones are horizontally distributed not vertically. |
| 4 Mediastinum | May look widened on a supine film. In a trauma patient, an erect chest x-ray or a CT scan should be used to rule out ruptured aorta. |

## A routine for interpretation

A routine should be established and followed assiduously in every case in order to avoid overlooking anything important. With practice, a chest film can be rapidly interpreted. The nursing staff and others involved in the care of patients, such as physiotherapists, should also be trained in interpretation and be made aware of the most important findings on each patient's chest x-ray. The following is a suggested routine:

1 Determine the patient's name and the date.
2 Check whether the patient was erect or supine, AP or posterior-anterior.

The next four steps involve assessing the quality of the film, in order to distinguish between real abnormalities and artefacts. Features that must be assessed include position, exposure, movement and expansion:

3 Position: Check that the film is centred. The spinous processes of the thoracic vertebrae should be midway between the heads of the clavicles. If the film is not centred, the mediastinal anatomy can be distorted.
4 Exposure: The fourth thoracic vertebral body should just be visible behind the mediastinum. Overexposure can cause underestimation of pulmonary abnormalities, whereas underexposure can result in overestimation of pulmonary abnormalities. Sometimes over-exposure is necessary (e.g. to detect fractured ribs).
5 Movement: Check for sharpness. If respiratory motion occurs during the exposure, or if exposure times are long, blurring can occur. This can simulate early pulmonary oedema. The thicker the chest wall, the greater the chances of movement artefact, because of the longer exposure time needed to penetrate the tissue.
6 Expansion: This must be assessed in comparison with previous radiographs. If expansion is not taken into account, an abnormality can falsely appear to be

Right border                                     Left border

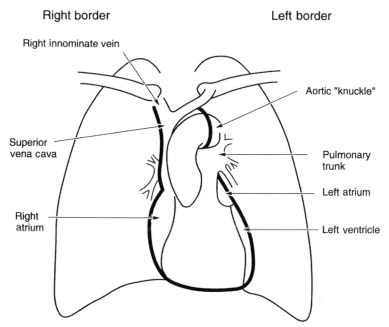

Right innominate vein

Superior
vena cava

Right
atrium

Aortic "knuckle"

Pulmonary
trunk

Left atrium

Left ventricle

**Figure 17.1.** Diagrammatic representation of the chest, showing the left and right mediastinal borders. Reprinted by permission of Blackwell Scientific Publications, Inc. Ellis, H. and Feldman, S. *Anatomy for Anaesthetists*, 6th edn. p 86. Oxford: Blackwell Scientific, 1993.

improving or worsening. Expansion should be to the fifth anterior rib or the ninth rib posteriorly.

The next four steps involve looking at the abnormality.

7  Tubes and lines: Check the positioning of the lines and hardware and any complications associated with its insertion.
8  Lung fields: Check the trachea and compare one lung to the other. Inspect around the hilum and apex, then laterally and then over the diaphragm.
9  Heart and mediastinum: Check for features such as the size and shape of the cardiac silhouette, hilar lymphadenopathy and signs of pulmonary hypertension (Figure 17.1).
10  Soft tissues and bones: Soft tissue features such as subcutaneous emphysema, peripheral oedema and obesity can be seen on chest films. Sometimes fractures outside the thoracic cage, such as the jaw and humerus, can also be detected on a chest film. Even more subtle features, such as the superimposition of the head in the mediastinum, indicating a semiconscious patient, can offer clues useful to a trained observer.

Any interpretation of a film will be limited without clinical data and previous radiographs.

## Tubes and catheters

### Endotracheal tube (ETT), nasotracheal tube and tracheostomies

- Correct placement of every tracheal intubation should be checked by a chest film. The tip of the tube should be at least 2 cm above the carina and the cuff should be at least 2 cm distal to the vocal cords to allow for the considerable movement (up to 2 cm) that can occur during flexion and extension of the head.

### Nasogastric (NG) tube

- Check to see that the tube is below the diaphragm and within the stomach and is not curled in the pharynx or oesophagus. Rarely, the NG tube can accidentally be placed in the trachea, pushed through lung tissue and appear to be below the diaphragm. The NG tube must cross the diaphragm in the midline to be in the stomach. A pneumothorax is common if the NG tube is pushed distally into the lung.

### Central venous catheters

- A chest film should be obtained immediately after placement to confirm correct positioning and to check for iatrogenic complications such as bleeding or pneumothoraces.
- The tip should be located beyond all peripheral valves and in the superior vena cava, not within the right atrium. This corresponds to the aortic knuckle or T4 on an upright chest x-ray. Bleeding as a result of puncturing large central veins during insertion, characteristically produces an opacity over the apex of the lung or widening of the upper mediastinum.
- The catheter tip can perforate a vessel and move extravascularly over time. Evidence for this will be seen on a chest x-ray as a pleural effusion due to misplaced intravenous fluid. If misplacement is suspected, aspirate from the distal limb for confirmation.

### Pulmonary artery catheters

- These catheters are associated with the same complications described for central lines, as well as potentially more dangerous developments such as pulmonary embolism, infarction or haemorrhage as a result of vessel rupture. These complications in the face of doubtful benefits has meant a decrease in the use of PA catheters.

- The position of the tip of the catheter may help in interpreting readings of wedge pressure. Ideally, it should be directed toward the base of the lung in the so-called West zones 3 or 4 and should be no more than 2–3 cm beyond the heart border. Excessive coiling of the catheter in the heart can predispose to migration and wedging of the catheter.

## Transvenous pacemakers
- Depending on where the catheter is inserted, there can be complications similar to those seen with central line placement.
- The tip of the pacemaker should be positioned at the apex of the right ventricle, wedged between the trabeculae carneae to ensure stability as well as direct contact with the endocardium.

## Pleural drains
- Assess the effectiveness of air and/or fluid drainage after insertion.
- A radio-opaque strip demonstrating the commencement of side holes can help to guarantee that the catheter is placed within the pleural cavity, not in the soft tissues of the chest wall. Check that all the side holes are within the pleural cavity.
- The chest film should allow one to rule out the possibility of complications such as local lung damage.

## Differentiating intrapulmonary pathology

The lung appears to react in much the same fashion to many different insults, at least from a radiological point of view. There are no absolute radiological patterns that would allow one to distinguish among pathological processes such as cardiogenic pulmonary oedema, aspiration, ALI, pneumonia and fat embolism. The reading of the chest film must be tempered by clinical findings, together with knowledge of the time periods for onset and disappearance of shadows resulting from the natural history of the disease process and treatment.

Moreover, accurate assessment of pulmonary abnormalities is dependent on the volume of air in the lungs. For example, a large tidal volume or a high level of positive end-expiratory pressure (PEEP), may make the abnormality appear less severe.

### Pulmonary oedema

Chest radiography is, at present, the best technique in terms of availability, reproducibility, non-invasiveness, practicality and cost, for assessing the presence and extent of pulmonary oedema. The technique is as sensitive as the double

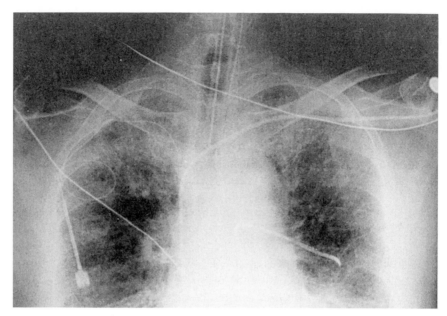

**Figure 17.2.** Patient with cardiogenic pulmonary oedema and bilateral basal collapse, with right side subclavian central venous catheter, left side subclavian pulmonary artery catheter and ETT. Note that the intrapulmonary opacity is difficult to distinguish from other pulmonary abnormalities such as ALI (Figure 17.3).

indicator dilution technique for measuring extravascular lung water (EVLW) and can detect EVLW increases as small as 10%.

## Cardiogenic pulmonary oedema (Figure 17.2)
- Classical findings (Figure 17.2) include the following:
    Spectrum of changes from pulmonary venous congestion to widespread alveolar shadowing
    Blurring of hilar vessels
    Upper lobe blood diversion
    Diffuse micronoduli
    Central or bats wing distribution of lung water
    Interstitial oedema (fluid in fissure, Kerley B lines and peribronchial cuffing)
    Alveolar oedema (homogeneous opacification with air bronchograms)
    Cardiomegaly
    Pleural effusions.
- The pulmonary artery wedge pressure (PAWP) correlates well with changes:
    PAWP < 12 mmHg: normal appearance
    PAWP = 12–22 mmHg: dilatation of peripheral vessels and interstitial oedema.
    PAWP > 22 mmHg: alveolar oedema.

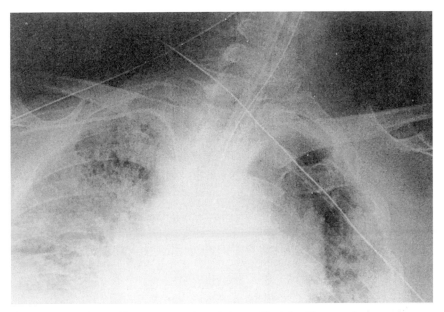

**Figure 17.3.** Patient with severe acute lung injury, with right side central venous subclavian catheter, ETT, NG tube and ECG leads. Note that the intrapulmonary opacities are difficult to distinguish from those in Figure 17.2.

- Movement by the patient can cause blurring on the film, which can simulate early pulmonary oedema.
- A patient with normal lungs may have radiographic signs that mimic pulmonary oedema if a supine AP film is taken (e.g. upper lobe blood diversion and peribronchial cuffing). Chest films should be taken upright if at all possible.
- Abnormalities of lung parenchyma and the integrity of the vascular bed will affect the distribution of pulmonary oedema. It is very common, for example, to see atypical patterns of pulmonary oedema in the presence of chronic lung disease.

## Acute lung injury
- Acute lung injury is a form of pulmonary oedema. It may be difficult to distinguish radiologically from other intrapulmonary abnormalities such as aspiration, cardiogenic pulmonary oedema and pneumonia (Figure 17.3). It must therefore be differentiated on clinical grounds (see Chapter 18).
- The radiographic findings can vary from mild changes to a 'white-out' of both lung fields.
- Radiological signs usually can be detected within 24–36 hours of the precipitating insult and include a perihilar haze, interstitial oedema and alveolar filling.

- Classical findings include
  Air bronchograms.
  Increased lung opacification distributed relatively equally over central and peripheral regions.
  Enlargement of right ventricle and main pulmonary arteries is sometimes seen.
- Changes that occur later, and possibly as a result of ventilatory pressures, rather than the disease process include cavitation and fibrosis. These changes can take many months to resolve.

## Pneumonia

- Pneumonia is a clinical pathological condition with no definite radiological appearance to differentiate it from other intrapulmonary abnormalities. The radiograph is a helpful adjunct to the diagnosis.
- Lung opacification may be lobar or widespread. The so-called atypical pneumonias are usually associated with widespread and discrete opacifications that can become confluent as the disease progresses.
- Often air bronchograms will be associated with the opacification.
- Although the opacification associated with cardiogenic and non-cardiogenic pulmonary oedema can be difficult to distinguish from that seen with pneumonia, bronchial breathing is more commonly associated with pneumonia, presumably because consolidation leads to a more dense area around the airways than does oedema.
- Radiological changes classically do not become detectable until after the first clinical signs and symptoms, and there is a similar delay before radiological signs of improvement can be seen in the recovery stage.
- Apart from showing lobar consolidation, a chest film is more a tool to follow the course of treatment rather than a specific diagnostic indicator.

## Aspiration

The sequelae of aspiration will depend on the type of material aspirated, its volume and distribution, and the host's reaction to the aspirated material. The radiological features can vary from localised shadowing to a bilateral whiteout.

### Foreign body – particulate matter
- The distribution will depend on the position of the patient at the time of aspiration. It is common to aspirate into the right main bronchus.
- Radio-opaque material can be directly visualised.
- Atelectasis, air trapping or mediastinal shift may be seen.

### Infected material
- Consolidation occurs slowly over 5–7 days, often accompanied by pleural exudate and it may take weeks to clear.
- Cavitation may occur at a later stage.

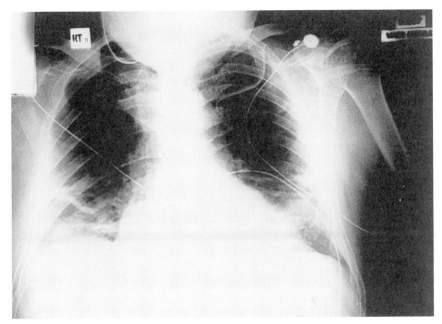

**Figure 17.4.** Patient with severe pancreatitis with bilateral basal collapse and reduced lung volumes. Note that the head is dipping onto the mediastinum. This is usually an indication of exhaustion or a decreased level of consciousness and is a strong predictor of imminent intubation.

## Liquid aspiration

- A wide spectrum of radiological changes can be seen, depending on the nature and volume of the aspirated liquid.
- The distribution is usually bilateral.
- Severe damage can occur; for example, aspiration of gastric acid can result in ALI.

## Smoke inhalation and toxic gases

- A wide range of damage is possible.
- Focal or patchy alveolar filling can occur within a few hours.

## Atelectasis and collapse

- 'Collapse' usually refers to a lobe or lung, whereas atelectasis affects a smaller subunit (Figure 17.4).
- Radiological signs include the shadow of the collapsed portion of lung and displacement of other structures to take up space normally occupied by that collapsed lung, including crowding of lung markings in the collapsed area, separation of lung markings in the non-involved area, elevation of a hemidiaphragm and mediastinal shift.

### Pulmonary embolism

- Radiography is not an accurate method for diagnosing pulmonary emboli.
- Non-specific signs include focal redistribution of blood flow, pulmonary infarction, atelectasis, pleural effusion and an elevated hemidiaphragm.

### Pleural effusion

- Blunting of the costophrenic angle is commonly seen when the effusion is small.
- On an upright film, the effusion classically forms a homogeneous density at the base of the lung, with a meniscus extending laterally through which lung markings can sometimes be seen.
- On a supine film, the fluid is usually seen to be distributed evenly over the whole pleural space, causing a 'veiling' effect through which lung markings can be seen.
- Effusions can also become loculated anywhere in the pleural space.
- More accurate definition of the effusion can be obtained by the use of ultrasound or CT scanning.

### Abdominal pathology affecting the chest x-ray

- A chest x-ray can be an excellent reflection of intra-abdominal abnormalities in intensive care (e.g. intra-abdominal sepsis causing ALI).
- An intra-abdominal mass effect can cause elevation of the diaphragm and atelectasis. Abdominal pain can also cause atelectasis. Basal effusions can occur postoperatively or as a result of sub-diaphragmatic infection.
- Gastric dilatation commonly accompanies resuscitation efforts involving the use of a mask.
- Pneumoperitoneum can result from recent laparotomy, from a ruptured intra-abdominal viscous or from pulmonary barotrauma.

### Extra-alveolar air (EAA)

- Excessive alveolar pressure can cause distension and rupture. The air will travel from the ruptured alveoli along the vascular sheaths towards the mediastinum as pulmonary interstitial emphysema (PIE). This is difficult to detect radiologically but it can be seen as a generalised, irregular, radiolucent mottling, especially in the perihilar region and sometimes as cysts.
- Under continuing pressure, the EAA can then produce mediastinal emphysema. The gas can then move into the tissue planes of the neck and possibly elsewhere over the chest, as subcutaneous emphysema.
- Under further pressure, the EAA can burst through the thin mediastinal pleura causing pneumothorax and even into the abdomen, causing pneumoretroperitoneum and pneumoperitoneum.

### TROUBLESHOOTING

## Hypoxia without significant chest x-ray shadowing

### Non-respiratory problems
- Compromised airway (consider the possibility of a blocked airway).
- Problems with the oxygen delivery system or ventilatory malfunction.
- High oxygen consumption (e.g. hyperthermia).
- Intracardiac shunt.

### Respiratory Problems
- Pulmonary emboli.
- Asthma.
- Chronic lung disease.
- Early stage of the pathology, where radiological changes are not yet obvious (e.g. pneumonia).

## Chest trauma

For both blunt trauma and penetrating trauma, an upright chest x-ray should be among the first investigations ordered. The features to be looked for include the following:

Pneumothoraces EAA: These often are due to penetration of lung tissue by fractured ribs but they can also occur as a result of blunt injury.

Haemothorax: Haemothorax often accompanies other abnormalities such as pneumothoraces, lung contusion and rib fractures. If it can be seen on the chest radiograph, then there will be at least 500 ml in the pleural cavity and it should be actively drained.

Contusion: Contusion represents oedema or haemorrhage into alveoli as a result of blunt trauma. It is usually obvious within the first 24 hours and begins clearing after 2–3 days, with total resolution by 1–2 weeks. However, with severe contusion, it may be several weeks before resolution begins.

Fractured ribs: Rib fractures often are seen together with lung contusion and should be documented, especially for purposes of pain relief. Remember it is difficult to image all rib fractures and often there are more than can be seen on the chest x-ray: As a general rule, there are approximately twice as many fractured ribs as can be seen on the chest film.

Other possible features: Diaphragmatic rupture, signs of oesophageal trauma, pericardial tamponade, a widened mediastinum suggesting large vessel injury and tracheobronchial tears are all rarer, but serious, complications. Further investigations such as angiography, CT scan, bronchoscopy or oesophagoscopy may also be necessary.

## TROUBLESHOOTING

### Interpreting non-specific opacities on the chest x-ray

Determine that the opacity is genuine (i.e. not a result of movement, underexposure or rotation). Rule out the possibility of other opacities such as pleural abnormalities and soft tissue abnormalities (usually extend outside the chest wall).

Parenchymal or intrapulmonary opacities in ICU patients usually are due to oedema, blood or infection. Other causes, such as carcinoma, are rare.

#### Oedema

There can be cardiogenic and non-cardiogenic (ALI) pulmonary oedema, as well as fluid overload.

- Interstitial oedema.
    - Fluid in fissures.
    - Pleural effusions.
    - Kerley B lines.
    - Peribronchial cuffing.
- Alveolar oedema.
    - Confluent homogenous opacities that are usually bilateral.
    - Air bronchograms.
- Cardiogenic pulmonary oedema.
    - Large heart and increases in size and density of hilar vessels.
    - PCWP > 20 mmHg.
    - Perihilar distribution and upper lobe diversion.
- Non-cardiogenic pulmonary oedema.
    - Small heart (normal).
    - Peripheral and generalised distribution.
    - PAWP < 20 mmHg.

The patient's history and clinical signs are essential for distinguishing between cardiogenic and non-cardiogenic pulmonary oedema, and the chest x-ray is a helpful adjunct to the diagnosis.

#### Blood

Pulmonary haemorrhage can, for example, occur as a result of:

- Trauma (contusion).
- Ruptured pulmonary vessel, as a complication of using a pulmonary artery catheter.

Features:
- Sudden onset.
- No air bronchograms.
- Confluent and discrete opacity.

#### Infection

Pneumonia
Features:

- Air bronchograms with bronchial breathing.
- Slow radiological onset and resolution.
- Spectrum from lobar to bronchopneumonia.
- Usually accompanied by clinical signs of infection.

## FURTHER READING

Brainsky, A., Fletcher, R. H., Glick, H. A., Lanken, P. N., Williams, S. V. and Kundel, H. L. Routine portable chest radiographs in the medical intensive care unit: Effects and costs. *Critical Care Medicine* 25 (1997): 801–5.

Desai, S. R. and Hansell, D. M. Lung imaging in the adult respiratory distress syndrome: current practice and new insights. *Intensive Care Medicine* 23 (1997): 7–15.

Ellis, H. and Feldman, S. *Anatomy for Anaesthetists*, 6th edn. Oxford: Blackwell, 1993.

Winer-Muram, H. T., Rubin, S. A., Miniati, M. and Ellis, J. V. Guidelines for reading and interpreting chest radiographs in patients receiving mechanical ventilation. *Chest* 102 (1992): 565S-70S.

# 18

# Specific respiratory problems

## Cardiogenic pulmonary oedema

Cardiogenic pulmonary oedema is usually seen in the setting of acute left ventricular failure (LVF) in association with ischaemic heart disease (IHD).

Cardiogenic pulmonary oedema as an accompaniment to LVF can result from conditions such as acute myocardial infarction (AMI), arrhythmias, cardiac tamponade and valvular abnormalities. However, no specific cause is obvious in the majority of cases. This is especially true with paroxysmal nocturnal dyspnoea or 'flash' pulmonary oedema. The oedema presents acutely, often at night, with the patient suddenly waking up breathless. These patients typically are old, with histories of IHD and hypertension. Many of these patients have normal systolic function and it is thought that the cause of the pulmonary oedema is left ventricular diastolic dysfunction. The precipitating event may be silent myocardial ischaemia. Patients with acute cardiogenic pulmonary oedema often have accompanying tachycardia, hypertension and hypoxia which in turn will increase left ventricular dysfunction and exacerbate the pulmonary oedema. Moreover, the increased work of breathing and the increased inspiratory effort can, in themselves, further exacerbate the oedema (Figure 18.1).

### Investigations, diagnosis and monitoring

- The history and examination should strongly suggest the diagnosis.
- Chest x-ray will demonstrate Kerley B lines; thickened fissures; peribronchial cuffing; increased vessel diameter and upper lobe diversion, a perihilar bat wing appearance, pleural effusions and intrapulmonary shadowing often with cardiomegaly.
- Examine 12-lead ECG to exclude ischaemia, AMI, etc.
- Measure arterial blood gases to determine extent of gas exchange abnormality and acidosis.
- Cardiac enzymes to exclude AMI.

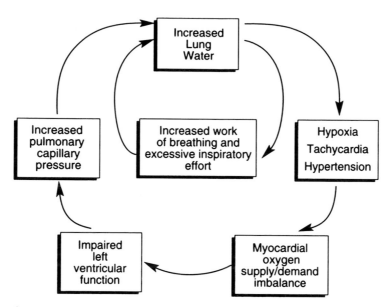

**Figure 18.1.** Factors exacerbating cardiogenic pulmonary oedema.

- Monitor vital signs (e.g. arterial BP, pulse rate, respiratory rate and urine output).
- Continue ECG monitoring.
- Monitor with pulse oximetry.
- Urgent cardiac ultrasound for diagnostic reasons and assessment of severity.

## Features

- A history of dyspnoea and orthopnoea usually when sitting upright and tachypnoea with an obvious increase in the work of breathing.
- Often sweaty with increased pulse rate and BP.
- Crepitations, wheeze and, in severe cases, pink frothy sputum.
- Signs of cardiac failure, such as cardiomegaly, third heart sound and elevated jugular venous pressure.

## Management

Resuscitation: Control the airway, maintain a high fraction of inspired oxygen ($FiO_2$) and support the breathing and circulation where necessary.

Reversible causes: Reverse any contributing cause (e.g. arrhythmia, hypertension, myocardial ischaemia, cardiac tamponade).

Position: Sit the patient up if possible.

Non-invasive continuous positive airway pressure (CPAP) or biphasic positive airway pressure (BiPAP) have revolutionised the management of cardiogenic pulmonary oedema. It can be delivered by a face mask, helmet or cuffed endotracheal tube (ETT) and is a very effective and easily applied measure for controlling pulmonary oedema. Continuous positive airway pressure or BiPAP improve oxygenation, and increase lung compliance, thus making it easier for the patient to breathe. The increased intrathoracic pressure as a result of CPAP also decreases the preload and afterload, improving left ventricular function, increasing cardiac output and relieving the pulmonary oedema. By improving the work of breathing and decreasing inspiratory effort, CPAP can limit the formation of further oedema. Continuous positive airway pressure has been shown to rapidly correct hypoxia and reduce tachypnoea and hypertension, all of which can worsen left ventricular diastolic dysfunction.

Diuretic: A diuretic (e.g. frusemide, 20 mg IV, if not already on a diuretic and 40 mg IV otherwise) will cause immediate venodilatation and eventually will reduce lung water. More diuretic may be necessary, but use it judiciously as excessive diuresis can cause hypovolaemia and cardiovascular impairment.

Vasodilatation: Use vasodilating drugs slowly and carefully and only if the arterial BP is normal or high for that patient. Use a drug such as nitroglycerine with mainly venodilating effects in order to decrease preload. Where hypertension is of prime concern, a drug with both venous and arterial effects such as sodium nitroprusside, could be used.

Narcotic: Give morphine in increments of 2 mg IV, titrated slowly over 2 minutes to reduce dyspnoea, to decrease anxiety and to contribute to vasodilatation.

Inotropic agents: An IV inotropic agent such as dobutamine may also be beneficial in cases of severe pulmonary oedema. However, beware of increases in pulse rate and arterial BP, both of which will increase myocardial oxygen demand and adversely affect left ventricular function. If hypotension occurs, secondary to, for example, an AMI, a vasopressor agent such as adrenaline or noradrenaline may be required.

Intubation and ventilation: Intubation and ventilation with positive end-expiratory pressure (PEEP) can be a last resort but usually that can be avoided by the use of CPAP.

Intravascular volume: Hypovolaemia, paradoxically, can be a problem in the management of pulmonary oedema. It is related to fluid losses from the lung capillaries and aggressive use of diuretics and it can be exacerbated by the inappropriate use of vasodilators. Because these patients often need higher preload than usual for optimum ventricular function, they can become hypotensive and oliguric, requiring fluid resuscitation in order to correct the hypovolaemia. Because of the delicate balance between pulmonary oedema and hypovolaemia in these patients, a series of fluid challenges may assist in determining the ideal intravascular volume.

## Acute respiratory distress syndrome (ARDS) and acute lung injury (ALI)

Since its initial description in 1967, there probably has been more written about this particular syndrome than about any other in intensive care medicine. Precise definitions are difficult because of the huge spectrum of the syndrome. It is loosely defined as hypoxia in the right clinical circumstances, with a normal or low left atrial pressure – or so-called non-cardiogenic pulmonary oedema. It is characterised by diffuse alveolar infiltrates on chest x-ray, dyspnoea, tachypnoea, decreased compliance, increased shunting, severe hypoxia and an increase in lung water. Acute respiratory distress syndrome is not so much a specific disease, but rather the sum of the lung's general response to critical illness.

### Aetiology

There probably are several distinct ARDS states, each with its own initiating cause but all ending in a common pulmonary response.

The term 'ARDS' is often used synonymously with 'acute respiratory failure' (see Chapter 16) and is usually a complication of another disease process such as sepsis or multiorgan failure (MOF). In fact, ARDS probably represents one manifestation of a generalised inflammatory process leading to endothelial cell injury and eventually MOF, rather than being a disease in its own right. It has many causes which are usually divided according to the origin of the insult (Figure 18.2). These insults are believed to lead to a final common pathway by damaging the alveolar–capillary interface, this damage, in turn, causing fluid to leak into the interstitial space and/or flooding of alveoli with protein-rich fluid.

Insults via the airway (e.g. aspiration of acidic gastric contents, smoke inhalation, near drowning incidents).

Insults via the circulation (e.g. septicaemia, shock, MOF, fat embolism, amniotic fluid embolism and pancreatitis).

Direct insults (e.g. pulmonary contusion).

Combination insults (e.g. pneumonitis, such as bacterial or viral pneumonia).

Despite extensive research, the exact cause of the alveolar–capillary membrane damage is uncertain. Leucocytes, platelets, microemboli, neurogenic influences and mediators such as prostaglandins, oxygen radicals, complement, leucotrienes, activated neutrophils and alveolar macrophages have all been implicated (Table 18.1). The process usually is widespread and often affects capillary beds other than the lungs. Whether the lungs initiate this process or are simply among the organs involved as part of MOF is unknown. Conclusions in this area are difficult because animal models do not necessarily reflect what happens clinically.

**Table 18.1.** Possible contributory factors in acute respiratory distress syndrome

Complement system
Oxidants
Proteases (elastase)
Endotoxin
Cytokines (e.g. tumour necrosis factor, endothelin)
Lipid mediators: leucotrienes, eicosanoids, platelet-activating factor
Growth factors
Coagulation system
Metalloproteinases, protocollagen
Kallikreins (Kinins)
Fragment D

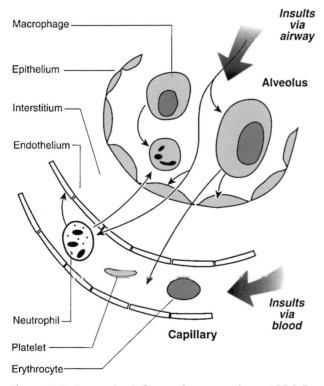

**Figure 18.2.** Factors that influence the progression to ARDS. Reprinted by permission. Repine, J.E. Scientific perspectives on adult respiratory distress syndrome. *Lancet* 339 (1992): 466–9.

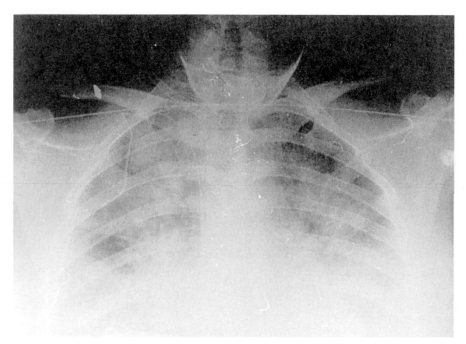

**Figure 18.3.** Severe ARDS secondary to sepsis.

## Measurement of pulmonary oedema

Chest x-ray: The chest x-ray remains the reference point for estimating lung water and its indications usually correlate very well with those from more sophisticated and expensive techniques such as double indicator dilution.

There are characteristic chest x-ray findings in patients with ARDS (Figure 18.3).

- Normal pulmonary vascular pattern.
- Absence of septal (Kerley's) lines.
- Air bronchograms.
- Infrequent perivascular cuffing.
- Normal heart size.

Computerised tomography (CT): A CT scan offers a more accurate way of quantifying lung water than chest x-ray. However, it is limited by its expense and the difficulties of transporting critically ill patients.

Magnetic resonance imaging (MRI): Nuclear magnetic resonance imaging (MRI) of protons in water permits quantification of lung water. The problem of motion during breathing can be overcome by 'gating'. However, the technique is still expensive and cumbersome in its application.

Double indicator dilution: The correlation between lung water measurement with the indicator technique and autopsy measured lung water is good. The double indicator dilution technique relies on heat as the diffusible indicator and uses a pulmonary artery catheter. It is more expensive and more complex than the method of chest x-ray and thus far it has not been demonstrated to be more accurate.

## Features and management

Only the main features of ARDS will be discussed here. The principles of management for this syndrome are summarised in tables and are discussed in detail in Chapter 16.

1 Gas exchange abnormalities: Hypoxia is due to a mismatch between perfusion and ventilation. This is mainly due to perfusion of non-ventilated or under-ventilated alveoli, which in turn is caused by atelectasis or alveolar flooding.

Failure of carbon dioxide ($CO_2$) exchange is also due to a mismatch between perfusion and ventilation, mainly as a result of ventilation of unperfused alveoli, which in turn is a consequence of vascular obstruction. Hypercarbia occurs only during end-stage ARDS. Initially a patient will compensate by hyperventilation.

2 Pulmonary hypertension: Pulmonary hypertension develops early in ARDS and is a result of vasoconstriction and vascular occlusion. Nitric oxide, a selective pulmonary vasodilator, may be useful.

3 Decreased pulmonary compliance: An increase in lung water results in increased lung stiffness, tachypnoea, diffuse intrapulmonary shadowing seen on chest x-ray, decreased airway calibre and a marked increase in the work of breathing.

Adult respiratory distress syndrome often accompanies MOF of various causes. Often it is difficult to distinguish between pneumonia and ARDS on clinical grounds and chest x-ray. The features of the two entities overlap.

Although cardiac function is usually normal in patients with ARDS, the amount of fluid that collects in the lungs in ARDS patients is a function of the pulmonary hydrostatic pressure, which is related to left atrial filling pressure and the degree of capillary leak. Thus, intravascular volume replacement should not be excessive. Crystalloids will be distributed mainly to the interstitial space (ISS), independent of the left atrial filling pressure and so the use of large amounts of crystalloids should be avoided in patients with ARDS (see Chapter 4).

The rate of accumulation of extravascular fluid in ARDS patients is related to gravity, structural compression from within the lung and the underlying alveolar–capillary membrane leak. The improvement in gas exchange with the use of artificial ventilatory techniques is probably related to the number of recruitable alveoli that initially were not involved in gas exchange because of oedema or atelectasis. Alveoli that are involved in a consolidation process, such as pneumonia, are less amenable to recruitment. Thus, intermittent positive-pressure ventilation (IPPV), PEEP and CPAP may be less effective in patients with pneumonia than in those with ARDS and cardiogenic pulmonary oedema.

There is usually a peripheral defect in oxygen utilisation associated with ARDS. This may be due to the widespread nature of microvascular permeability, as a result of the primary disease process or as a result of inappropriate fluid replacement causing interstitial oedema.

The pathophysiological changes seen with ARDS can vary over time. Initially there will be hypoxia, dyspnoea and tachypnoea, with little in the way of changes visible on chest x-ray. That will be followed by the classic changes seen on chest x-ray, with worsening hypoxia. That state can worsen, with more dense and more extensive changes appearing on the chest x-ray, accompanied by clinical deterioration. After approximately 10 days, long-term changes, such as fibrosis, can supervene and cause long-term respiratory disability.

There is active research in a number of areas having to do with modifying the mediators of lung damage. Possible mediators include neutrophil proteases, oxygen radicals, lipid peroxides, plasma proteolytic enzymes, lypoxygenase products, platelet activating factor, free fatty acids and cytokines. Although that research is to be encouraged, the final common pathway (if there is one in ARDS) has not been found. The use of a single drug acting via one mediator may be of little benefit. If there is to be a pharmacological cure for ARDS, the answer may be in finding a 'cocktail' of modulators, rather than a single one. The principles of management for ARDS are the same no matter what the cause and they are discussed in detail elsewhere (see Chapter 16). The principal challenge is to address the underlying problem.

### Outcome

The outcome for a patient with ARDS will depend on its cause (e.g. when ARDS is associated with prolonged MOF, the mortality is high). Abnormal pulmonary function is found in approximately 40% of survivors 6 months after recovery from ARDS, but by 1 year lung function usually will return to normal. Thoracic CT scans will reveal extensive fibrosis in many of these patients. Those changes will slowly resolve with time.

## Pneumonia

Pneumonia can be defined as an inflammatory process in which the host reacts to uncontrolled multiplication of pathogenic organisms in the distal airways and alveoli of the lung.

Pneumonia does not encompass inflammation of the large airways – a condition that results in production of sputum and bronchitis. Most intubated and many non-intubated patients in an ICU will eventually develop bronchitis or colonisation of the airways. This is important when interpreting sputum cultures because detection of organisms in sputum is very common in an ICU. However, that does not signify pneumonia and even if pneumonia coincidentally exists, the organisms grown in the sputum usually bear no relationship to the organisms causing the pneumonia, especially in the case of nosocomial pneumonia.

## Features

Lung consolidation: Air in the alveoli is replaced by exudate and cellular material leading to the following manifestations.

- Radiological opacities – presenting either a picture typical of consolidation or an interstitial pattern or a combination of the two (Figure 18.4).
- Bronchial breath sounds on auscultation.
- Non-compliant lungs.
- Impaired gas exchange – hypoxia, hyperventilation and hypocarbia until exhaustion supervenes at which time hypercarbia will occur.

Classically, primary pneumonia is associated with one or more of these features:

- fever
- cough
- sputum production (change in colour and increased viscosity)
- dyspnoea
- pleuritic pain
- tachypnoea
- malaise
- tachycardia
- widespread rales and bronchial breath sounds
- cyanosis and other features of hypoxia.

## Primary pneumonia (community acquired)

Pneumonia remains a leading infectious cause of death in the developed world. Patients with pneumonia who require admission to intensive care still have a high mortality rate.

Infection of lung tissue results in intrapulmonary shunting, impaired distribution of ventilation and decreased lung compliance, in addition to the systemic effects that result from the infection. The features are listed above.

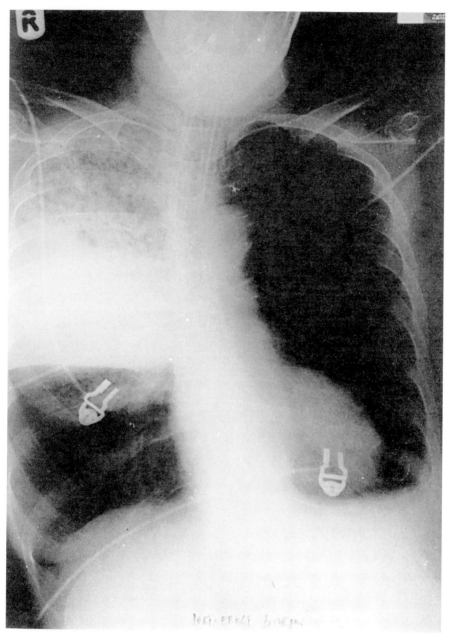

**Figure 18.4.** Right upper zone lobar pneumonia.

The typical history for community-acquired pneumonia is acute onset of fever, with chills and rigors, associated with dyspnoea, tachypnoea and a productive cough. The so-called atypical pneumonias include those caused by *Mycoplasma pneumoniae, Legionella* spp., *Chlamydia* spp., *Coxiella burnettii, Pneumocystis carinii* and viruses. The pneumonias in this group are typified by extrapulmonary features, diagnoses made primarily by serologic methods, and failure to respond to conventional antibiotics. For that reason, in patients with severe pneumonias of unknown origin, erythromycin is usually included as first-line treatment.

## Investigations and diagnosis

The history and examination should strongly suggest a diagnosis of pneumonia:

Chest x-ray: demonstrates the distribution, extent, and complications (e.g. abscess, effusion) associated with the pneumonia.
Blood count: leucocytosis.
Arterial blood gases: demonstrates extent of impaired gas exchange.

### Isolation of the organism

This can be difficult, and often no organism can be isolated, especially if antibiotics have been commenced. Common organisms causing primary pneumonia include:

*Streptococcus pneumoniae*
*Mycoplasma pneumoniae*
*Legionella* spp.
*Staphylococcus aureus*
*Haemophilus influenzae*
Viruses (particularly influenza A)

Less common organisms include:

*Chlamydia psittaci*
*Streptococcus* (other species)
*Coxiella burnetti*
Coliforms
*Pneumocystis carinii*
*Chlamydia pneumoniae*

Despite thorough screening, in almost one-third of cases no organism can be found.
Sputum:

- Obtain a good sputum specimen. Salivary specimens are useless and will be discarded by the microbiological laboratory.

- Gram stain: Look for polymorphonucleocytes (PMN) and a heavy and pure population of bacteria as evidence for microbiological pathogenicity.
- Culture for bacteria (e.g. pneumococcus and *Haemophilus*).
- Special tests are only required in certain situations such as special stains and cultures for fungi, acid-fast bacilli (AFB) and cultures to exclude tuberculosis (TB) or direct fluorescent antibodies (DFA) for *Pneumocystis* and *Legionella*.

Bacteria in the sputum do not necessarily equate with infection of the lower respiratory tract, even in patients with pneumonias such as the more typical pneumococcal pneumonia. If the sputum has an abundance of PMN and a pure growth of bacteria, it is more likely to be pathogenic.

Blood cultures: Blood cultures are mandatory because pneumonia is an infection of the lung parenchyma and organisms are isolated in blood in about 30% of cases of pneumococcal pneumonia and at much lower rates for other types of pneumonia. Positive findings from blood cultures are strongly predictive of infection with the isolated bacteria.

Serology:

Paired sera must be tested for antibodies to

*Mycoplasma pneumoniae*
*Legionella* spp. (Legionnaires' disease) – may take up to 6 weeks to seroconvert
*Coxiella burnetti*
Viruses
*Chlamydia psittaci* (psittacosis)

*Legionella*: The laboratory diagnosis of legionellosis is based on isolation of the organisms, seroconversion and direct detection by fluorescent antibody techniques or DNA probes. Direct immunofluorescence of the sputum, bronchial washings or pleural fluid has a sensitivity of less than 80%. While serum or indirect fluorescent antibody is commonly employed, some patients never seroconvert.

*Mycoplasma*: The laboratory diagnosis of *Mycoplasma* pneumonia is generally retrospective and based on serologic evidence of infection. It is a slow growing and fastidious organism that is difficult to culture. A DNA probe test for *Mycoplasma pneumonia* is now available. Cold agglutinins are demonstrated in over 50% of cases but that is not a specific test. Positive tests for IgM are present in up to 90% of patients at presentation.

*Chlamydia pneumoniae*: Although the diagnosis can be made serologically and by isolation from respiratory samples in cell culture, specific confirmation reagents are not yet commercially available.

More invasive techniques for isolation and culture of micro-organisms are discussed in the section on nosocomial pneumonia.

## Treatment

Antimicrobial treatment is usually commenced on clinical grounds before an organism is isolated. Even after extensive investigation, up to 60% of micro-organisms remain undetected. These cases are often called 'viral pneumonia', without any evidence to support the diagnosis. The term 'viral pneumonia' should be reserved for cases where a viral cause is actually demonstrated.

Oxygen: The $FIO_2$ should be adjusted according to frequent assessment of oxygenation via arterial blood gases or pulse oximetry.

Fluids: The intravascular volume must be aggressively resuscitated while not overloading the ISS with excessive crystalloids.

Ventilatory support: Ventilatory support may be necessary but is not as effective in patients with pneumonia as in those with pulmonary oedema, probably because there are fewer recruitable alveoli. Because of the dangers of positive-pressure ventilation, spontaneous respiration with CPAP should be encouraged before mandatory ventilation is utilised. The most appropriate ventilatory techniques are discussed in detail elsewhere.

Physiotherapy: Physiotherapy is of little value in the acute stage of pneumonia.

## Features and specific antimicrobials

*Streptococcus pneumonia*: This is the most common causative organism, accounting for more than 50% of all community-acquired pneumonias. These patients usually are systemically ill and present early. Approximately half of them will have a positive sputum culture.
Treatment:

- benzylpenicillin, $2–3 \times 10^6$ units 6-hourly
  *or*
- for those with true penicillin allergy, ceftriaxone 1–2 g IV once daily
  *or*
- cefotaxime, 1 g IV 8-hourly.

*Haemophilus influenzae*: This is relatively uncommon and often is associated with bronchitis in patients with chronic airflow limitation (CAL).
Treatment:

- ampicillin, 1–2 gm IV 6-hourly
  *plus*
- ceftriaxone, 1–2 g IV daily
  *or*
- cefotaxime, 1 g IV 8-hourly.

*Legionella species*: Legionnaires' disease often presents as severe progressive pneumonia and it can be associated with a wide variety of other manifestations that often precede pulmonary involvement. The presence of several of the following features should suggest the diagnosis:

- Prodromal flu-like illness, with dry cough, myalgia, rigors, watery diarrhoea, dyspnoea, malaise or headache.

- Renal failure, myoglobinuria and a high level of creatinine phosphokinase (CPK).
- Hyponatraemia and hypophosphataemia.
- Central nervous system involvement (headache, confusion, disorientation, stupor, seizures and coma).
- Myocarditis (tachycardia and bradycardia).
- Very high fever (> 39 °C).

Isolation of this organism is very difficult. The diagnosis can be confirmed by detection of an antibody rise in paired sera or by a rapid DFA test on sputum or bronchial washings. Some patients never seroconvert. If in doubt, commence treatment on clinical grounds. There are more than 30 species of *Legionella* and therefore it may not be detected even with the use of paired sera, which can test only the more common varieties. *Legionella* is discussed in more detail elsewhere. Treatment:

- erythromycin 4 g IV daily in divided doses for 3 weeks (because of the danger of thrombophlebitis use a central line)
  *and/or*
- rifampicin up to 600 mg IV daily in divided doses for severe cases
  *or*
- ciprofloxacin 200 mg IV 8-hourly.

*Mycoplasma pneumoniae*: General symptoms such as fever, malaise and headache precede the chest symptoms by 1 to 5 days. A chest x-ray will show patchy opacities, often in only one lobe. Cough and radiographic changes can persist for weeks if there is no treatment. Death is rare. Extrapulmonary manifestations include erythema multiforme, Stevens–Johnson syndrome, myocarditis, anorexia, nausea, vomiting, hepatitis, thrombocytopaenia, coagulopathy and meningoencephalitis. Treatment:

- erythromycin, 1 g IV 6-hourly (a 2-week course may be needed for eradication and should be recommenced in cases of relapse).

## Other organisms that should be considered in case of primary pneumonia

### Viruses
*Klebsiella pneumoniae* (in older or alcoholic patients).
Miliary tuberculosis (in debilitated or alcoholic patients).
*Coxiella burnetii* (Q fever in abattoir workers or people working on farms).
*Pneumocystis carinii* (in patients suspected of having AIDS or in other immunocompromised patients).

*Chlamydia psittaci* (associated with exposure to pet birds especially if the pets are ill or have died).

## No definite organism

Usually, no definite cause is determined. A regimen that will cover most cases of primary pneumonia is as follows:

- erythromycin 1 g IV 6-hourly
  *plus either*
- cefotaxime 1 g IV 8-hourly
  *or*
- ceftriaxone 1 g IV daily
  *or*
- benzylpenicillin 1.2 g IV 4–6-hourly
  *plus*
- gentamicin 5–7 mg/kg IV daily.
  If psittacosis is suspected, add:
- rolytetracycline 275 mg daily.

## Nosocomial pneumonia

Dealing with nosocomial or hospital-acquired pneumonia is not as straightforward as treating primary pneumonia.

- The diagnosis is very difficult to make.
- There are many possible causative organisms.
- The causative organism is difficult to isolate.

While there is a lack of general agreement on such fundamental issues as how to define nosocomial pneumonia, it is even more difficult, perhaps even impossible, to reach consensus on basic information such as incidence, treatment and outcome.

## Diagnosis

The diagnosis of pneumonia is usually made on the basis of a combination of some of the following criteria. However, in the setting of the seriously ill each of these has inadequacies.

- Fever or hypothermia: Fever is common in patients in an ICU for a great variety of reasons.
- Leucocytosis or leucopaenia: These are both very common features in seriously ill patients and may not even indicate infection.

- Purulent secretions: These are almost a universal finding in seriously ill patients, especially intubated patients, and often indicate bronchitis or colonisation, not pneumonia.
- New or progressive infiltrations seen on chest x-ray: Progressive infiltrates seen on chest x-ray are common in the seriously ill and often are related to other lung abnormalities such as ARDS or aspiration. The onset and persistence (for at least 24 hours) of a new infiltrate seen on a good quality chest x-ray are suggestive of nosocomial infection. A CT scan of the thorax often can help to define intrapulmonary abnormalities.

The diagnosis is likely if all four of these criteria are met and probable if three are met.

Nosocomial pneumonia by itself often is not accompanied by the systemic features of sepsis (e.g. hypotension, decreased level of consciousness, jaundice, renal failure).

### Pathogenic organism

Because of the difficulty in making a clinical diagnosis of nosocomial pneumonia, the key is to find a definite pathogenic organism.

**Colonisation of the airways, especially with gram-negative organisms, is a feature of many patients in ICU. This usually does not indicate pneumonia. In fact, in the setting of the seriously ill, there is little correlation between the organisms isolated from sputum and the presence or absence of pneumonia.** Organisms such as pseudomonads, *Acinetobacter*, fungi and methicillin-resistant staphylococci are common colonisers in intubated patients. Their continuing presence is facilitated by indiscriminate use of antimicrobials.

The source of such an organism may be related to aspiration of oropharyngeal secretions. Gastric contents made alkaline in order to prevent stress ulceration will encourage bacterial overgrowth and may be a source of oropharyngeal organisms which are then aspirated.

### Isolation of organisms

Tracheobronchial secretions: There are great discrepancies between organisms in the sputum and pathogens in the lower respiratory tract. Concurrent antibiotic treatment further complicates this picture. Conventional sputum cultures are very unreliable for intubated patients. To be of any use, the sputum must be induced and must not be contaminated with saliva. If there is a pure growth accompanied by polymorphonucleocytes, the significance of pathogenicity is increased.

Blood cultures: Positive finds from blood cultures offer proof of pneumonia but the findings are positive in fewer than 20% of patients with nosocomial pneumonia.

Immunologic methods: The delay inherent in obtaining positive results from paired sera makes that method unsuitable for assisting in rapid therapeutic

**Table 18.2.** Protective specimen brush technique

1　High dosage nebulised lignocaine, 10–15 ml of 4% solution, until gag reflex is abolished in non-intubated patients.
2　In intubated patients, sedation and a short-acting paralytic agent are recommended.
3　Do not inject lignocaine through the suction channel of the FOB or the ETT.
4　Position the FOB close to the orifice of the study area with new or increased infiltrate on chest x-ray.
5　Advance the PSB catheter 3 cm out of the FOB to avoid collection of pooled secretions on the catheter's tip.
6　Advance the inner cannula to eject the distal carbon wax plug into a large airway.
7　Advance the catheter into the desired subsegment.
8　Advance the brush and wedge it into a peripheral position; gently rotate it several times. If purulent secretions are visualised, rotate the brush into them.
9　Retract the brush into the inner cannula and the inner cannula into the outer cannula and remove them from the bronchoscope.
10　The distal portions of the outer and inner cannulae must be separately and sequentially wiped clean with 70% alcohol, cut with sterile scissors and discarded.
11　Advance the brush out and sever it with a sterile wire clipper into a container with 1 ml of saline solution or Ringer's lactate solution to avoid drying and rapid loss of bacteria.
12　Submit for quantitative culture within 15 minutes.

Reprinted by permission. Meduri, G. U. Ventilator associated pneumonia in patients with respiratory failure. A diagnostic approach. *Chest* 97 (1990): 1208–19.

decisions. Immediate antigen or antibody tests seem to offer a lot of promise for the future, but thus far they are of limited use for nosocomial pneumonia.

Bronchoscopy: Samples obtained by suction through a fibreoptic bronchoscopy (FOB) are usually contaminated by upper airway organisms. Techniques that use protected specimen brushes (PSB) are expensive and complicated but provide more accurate results (Table 18.2). In order to get the ideal specimen that will allow one to distinguish between colonisation and infection, the bronchoscope must be guided to the appropriate area and the specimen must be protected from contamination if it is to yield quantitative cultures that can meet validated diagnostic thresholds. Both the sensitivity and specificity of PSB techniques have ranged between 60% and 100%. Some of the limitations of PSB techniques are unreliability when a patient is already being treated with antibiotics, the limited area of the lung that can be sampled and the delay in processing the microbial cultures. The use of bronchoalveolar lavage (BAL) combined with PSB techniques may add diagnostic accuracy.

Bronchoalveolar lavage: Bronchoalveolar lavage is lavage of a lung subsegment using 100–200 ml of physiologic solution through a FOB wedged in an airway.

The BAL provides sampling of a larger amount of lung tissue than does the PSB technique, but it is subject to the same risk of contamination. The BAL is an accurate technique for diagnosing pneumonia caused by organisms that do not colonise the upper airway and it has largely replaced open lung biopsy for diagnosis of opportunistic infections in the immunocompromised patient. The main complication of BAL is hypoxia during the procedure and also there is the possibility of translocating toxins or organisms during the procedure. The best results are obtained when patients are not already receiving antimicrobials.

Protected BAL: Protected BAL involves selecting a sampling area using a FOB, based on the chest x-ray appearance. A transbronchoscopic balloon-tipped catheter is advanced into the segment, the balloon is inflated with 1.5 ml of air to occlude the bronchial lumen and aspiration is performed with 30 ml aliquots of sterile saline solution. The specimen obtained is then centrifuged, cultured and examined with Gram and Giemsa stains. Protected BAL has higher specificity and sensitivity than other current techniques.

Transbronchial biopsy: Biopsy not only is helpful for isolating bacteria but also is useful for viruses and fungi and for differentiating between non-infective lesions (e.g. carcinoma, Wegeners granulomatosis) and infective lung lesions. The complications of biopsy can include pneumothorax.

Transthoracic needle aspiration: Aspiration offers the advantage of allowing one to identify parenchymal infections that are solid, but is associated with high incidences of pulmonary bleeding and pneumothorax, especially in artificially ventilated patients.

Open lung biopsy: Open lung biopsy is the most accurate method for achieving a definite histological or microbiological diagnosis. It is crucial that obviously affected lung be biopsied for isolation of microbes. This technique is very invasive and entails a far higher risk of complications than do the other procedures.

The false-negative rates and the overall success for any of these diagnostic techniques cannot be assessed yet, as there is no gold standard technique for diagnosing nosocomial pneumonia and even post-mortem examination involves potential sources of error.

The simple techniques are unreliable and the more reliable techniques are complicated.

## Organisms
The most common isolates are gram-negative organisms such as

*Pseudomonas aeruginosa.*
*Enterobacter* spp.
*Klebsiella* spp.
*Escherichia coli*
*Serratia* spp.
*Proteus* spp.

*Acinetobacter*
*Haemophilus influenzae*

Less common organisms include:

*Staphylococcus aureus*
*Streptococcus pneumoniae*
Anaerobic bacteria
Fungi.

Immunosuppressed hosts: In patients with cellular and humoral immunosuppression, one also must consider:
*Pneumocystis carinii* (especially in association with AIDS and after organ transplantation).
Cytomegalovirus (CMV) (especially after organ transplantation).
*Aspergillus* spp. (especially in patients with leukaemia).
*Cryptococcus neoformans* (especially in patients with lymphomas).

### Acute lung injury and pneumonia
Pneumonia and ALI overlap considerably in the seriously ill. They are impossible to distinguish without isolation of a specific organism. Patients with pneumonia can develop features of ALI. The diagnostic criteria for ARDS and nosocomial pneumonia are so non-specific that they are often considered together. This causes confusion, especially when considering antimicrobial treatment.

## Treatment

### Preventative treatment
- Prevent airway colonisation by judicious use of parenteral antibiotics (sound indications and for limited periods).
- Use of local antibiotics in the oropharynx and stomach may decrease the incidence of nosocomial pneumonia.
- The use of sucralfate rather than $H_2$-receptor antagonists or antacids, to prevent stress ulceration may decrease the incidence of colonisation and nosocomial pneumonia.
- Minimise instrumentation and intubation of the upper airways.
- Attempt to preserve the cough reflex, where possible, and limit the time a patient is intubated and ventilated.
- Prevent aspiration past ETT cuffs by clearing pharyngeal secretions and maintaining cuff pressure.
- Maintain patients sitting upright at more than $40^\circ$ to prevent aspiration.
- Use meticulously sterile technique for endotracheal suction.
- Strictly enforce hand washing between any two procedures.
- Maintain the integrity of the gastrointestinal mucosa.

### Definitive treatment

**Treatment is largely based on empirical use of antibiotics – a best-guess approach.** While we are all taught that the choice of the appropriate antibiotic combination must be based on the isolated bacteria, it is uncommon to isolate a definitive microbe. One of the most difficult decisions in intensive care is to choose the initial antibiotic treatment for suspected nosocomial pneumonia – not only which antibiotics, but whether or not any antibiotic at all should be commenced. The diagnosis is almost impossible to make with certainty and the organism, if any, is rarely found. It is further complicated by the fact that gram-negative pneumonia does not respond rapidly to antibiotic treatment and therefore it is difficult to judge the success of the selected antibiotic on clinical grounds. On the other hand, the mortality remains high and it is a bold intensivist who can resist the temptation to use antibiotics. The incidence of nosocomial pneumonia and survival patterns have not been in any way affected by the influx of the latest and most expensive broad-spectrum antibiotics. The following combinations of antibiotics are given as guidelines. Close microbiological surveillance and liaison with the microbiology department are essential in order to define the particular spectrum of organisms in an individual ICU.

### Initial treatment

- aminoglycoside (e.g. gentamicin 5 to 7 mg/kg IV daily)
  *plus either*
- ticarcillin/clavulanate 3 g IV 4–6-hourly
  *or*
- ceftazidime 1 g IV 8-hourly.
  *or*
- imipenem 500 mg IV 6-hourly
  *or*
- meropenum 500 mg IV 8-hourly
  *or*
- ciproflaxacin 200 mg IV 8-hourly.

When *Pseudomonas aeruginosa* is suspected, a combination of an aminoglycoside and piperacillin or ciprofloxacin is usually selected. Imipenem is also used as a broad-spectrum alternative when an organism has not been isolated. If aspiration is suspected, clindamycin plus an aminoglycoside can be used. If *Staphylococcus aureus* is suspected, vancomycin should be used. *Legionella* spp. can also cause nosocomial pneumonia.

Further antibiotic strategy will depend on clinical response and isolation of organisms. If there is no improvement within 3 days, consideration should be given to reinvestigation and either ceasing the antibiotics or changing them.

**Table 18.3.** Some causes of pulmonary infiltrates
in immunosuppressed patients

Infective
  Bacterial
    *Staphylococcus aureus*
    Coliforms
    *Legionella* spp.
    *Nocardia*
  Protozoans
    *Pneumocystis carinii*
  Fungi
    Aspergillus
    *Cryptococcus*
    *Candida*
  Viruses
    CMV
    Herpes simplex
    Herpes zoster
Non-infective causes
  Pulmonary oedema
  ARDS
  Cytotoxic drug injury
  Radiation infiltration
  Pulmonary haemorrhage

## Outcome

The outcome figures for nosocomial pneumonia depend on the difficult issue of
the accuracy of the initial diagnosis and, as there currently is no gold standard
for diagnosis, outcome figures must be viewed with caution. Various studies have
cited mortality figures ranging from 40% to 90%.

### Strategy in immunocompromised patients with pulmonary infiltrates (Table 18.3)

Routine tests: Conduct a full examination and routine investigations including
extensive sputum and blood cultures.

Drugs: Exclude the possibility of drug-related causes (e.g. bleomycin).

Transtracheal aspiration: This procedure may be useful for bacterial isolation.

Bronchoalveolar lavage: Use 150–200 ml of normal saline in 30-ml aliquots
with the FOB wedged in an appropriate subsegmental bronchus. Conduct a microscopic examination of the centrifuged sample for bacteria, fungi, mycobacteria and *Pneumocystis carinii*. Direct immunofluorescent antibody staining for

*Legionella* and CMV. As BAL can cause hypoxia, close monitoring during the procedure is necessary.

Endobronchial brushing:

- The incidence of barotrauma is significant.
- Sensitivity is approximately 75% for fungi and *Pneumocystis carinii.*
- The use of a PSB culture will facilitate the diagnosis in cases of bacterial pneumonia.

Transbronchial biopsy:

- With fluoroscopic guidance, taking three specimens will yield tissue in up to 95% of cases.
- There are risks for pneumothorax (about 10%) and haemorrhage (about 20%).
- Examine the tissue as in open lung biopsy.

Open lung biopsy:

- The diagnostic yield is at least 90%.
- Yields will largely depend on the quality of the laboratory technique, not the size of the specimen.
- Pleural leak for more than 3 days occurs in 10–25% of cases.
- Use direct examination for bacteria, mycobacteria, fungi, *Pneumocystis carinii* and CMV. Use direct immunofluorescent antibody for *Legionella* and CMV. Examine cultures for bacteria, mycobacteria fungi and viruses.

Empirical approach: A broad-spectrum, best-guess antibiotic regime is usually undertaken where adequate examination facilities are not available or when treatment cannot be delayed. Consultation with a clinical microbiologist or infectious diseases physician should be sought.

## Aspiration

Aspiration occurs most often in patients with decreased levels of consciousness (e.g. head injury, epilepsy, recent operation) who have impaired cough and gag reflexes. The sequelae of aspiration into the lungs will depend on the type of material aspirated, its volume, its distribution within the lungs and the patient's reactions to the aspirated material.

### Foreign body or particulate matter

A foreign body often will lodge in the right main bronchus. Such material often can be visualised radiologically if it is radio-opaque (e.g. a tooth). Otherwise, the sequelae from the aspirated material can be visualised (e.g. atelectasis, air trapping, mediastinal shift or local hyperinflation; Figure 18.5).

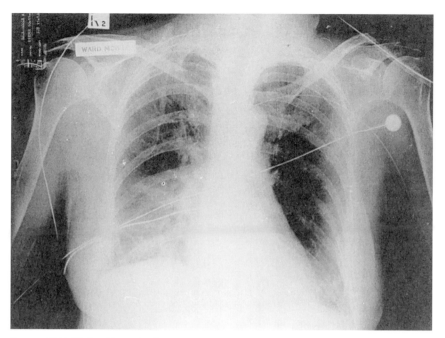

**Figure 18.5.** Right side aspiration.

Treatment: In order to prevent long-term complications such as chronic in-fection, the obstructing material should be removed under direct vision or by lavage.

### Aspiration pneumonitis

Acute lung injury after the inhalation of regurgitated gastric contents. Classically described as Mendelson's syndrome after a series of patients who aspirated during obstetric anaesthesia.

A pH less than 2.5 and a volume aspirated of greater than 0.3 ml/kg will cause a severe chemical burn to the trachobronchial tree. The patient's signs and symptoms can be mild to severe with dyspnoea, wheeze, tachypnoea and hypoxia.

Treatment: Broad-spectrum antibiotics should be used only if the symptoms fail to resolve after 48 hours. Cover for anaerobes is not required. Corticosteroids should not be used. If the gastric acid is likely to be sterile, i.e. the patient is nor-mally conscious, does not have a small bowel obstruction and not on drugs which decrease the stomach's hydrogen ion concentration – protein pump inhibitors, antacids or $H_2$ receptor antagonists – then antibiotics are not required and the patient should be treated symptomatically.

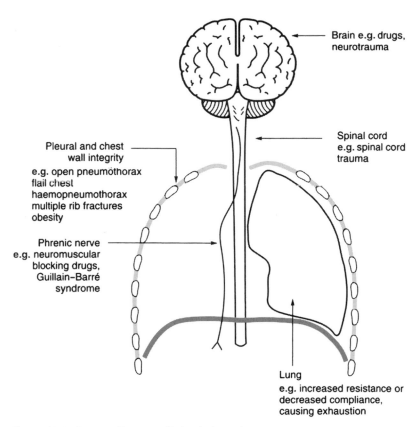

**Figure 18.6.** Causes of hypoventilation in intensive care.

## Aspiration pneumonia

This develops after the aspiration of colonised oropharyngeal secretions. This is often unwitnessed and the diagnosis is made with a new infiltrate on the chest x-ray in a characteristic lung segment in a susceptible person (e.g. decreased level of consciousness).

Critically ill patients are at high risk as they are often nursed lying down, have nasogastric tubes in and have GIT paresis. Nursing patients upright will minimise aspiration pneumonia occurrence.

Treatment: Antibiotics should definitely be used for aspiration pneumonia. Antibiotics with gram-negative activity such as third-generation cephalosporins or fluoroquinolones and piperacillin should be used. Anaerobic cover is not usually required but should be used in patients with evidence of lung abscess on chest x-ray.

# Hypoventilation

The causes of hypoventilation are shown in Figure 18.6 and the specific disorders of neuromuscular function that can affect the respiratory system are listed in Table 18.4. The most common cause of hypoventilation and hypercarbia is related to the current approach to artificial ventilation. In order to avoid overinflation of alveoli and pulmonary barotrauma, tidal volumes are reduced and the peak inspiratory pressures (PIP) are limited to less than 30–40 cmH$_2$O. This strategy is called elective hypoventilation or permissive hypercarbia. Hypoventilation in these circumstances is an acceptable trade-off in order to limit lung damage.

## Management

Treatment and diagnosis go hand in hand. The specific treatment for hypoventilation will depend on the cause, as discussed in Chapter 16.

The airway must be secured and ventilation commenced (if necessary), while the cause of the ventilatory failure is being determined. Ventilation should be commenced with a tidal volume of no more than 7 ml/kg, at a respiratory rate designed to reduce CO$_2$ levels slowly, especially if there is evidence of subacute or chronic hypercarbia. The aim of ventilation is to maintain oxygenation at the lowest level of positive intrathoracic pressure, keeping the PaCO$_2$ and arterial pH within reasonable limits – it is not necessary to achieve a so-called normal PaCO$_2$.

# Upper airways obstruction in adults

Acute upper airways obstruction is a medical emergency. The common causes are outlined in Table 18.5.

## Management

The specific management will depend on the cause, but in general terms, the principles are as follows:

Basic airway manoeuvres: In non-intubated patients, the following should be employed:

- head tilt
- chin lift
- jaw thrust
- suction
- oxygen.

**Table 18.4.** Disorders of respiratory neuromuscular function

| Level | Examples | Clinical characteristics |
|---|---|---|
| Upper motor neurone | Hemiplegia<br>Quadriplegia<br>Extrapyramidal disorders | Weakness<br>Hyper-reflexia<br>Increased muscle tone<br>Perhaps sensory and<br>  autonomic changes |
| Lower motor neurone | Poliomyelitis | Weakness<br>Atrophy<br>Flaccidity<br>Hyper-reflexia<br>Fasciculations<br>Bulbar involvement<br>No sensory changes |
| Peripheral neurones | Guillain–Barré syndrome<br>Acute intermittent porphyria<br>Diphtheria<br>Lyme disease<br>Toxins (e.g. lead)<br>Critical illness polyneuropathy | Weakness<br>Flaccidity<br>Hyporeflexia<br>Bulbar involvement<br>Sensory and autonomic<br>  changes |
| Myoneural junction | Myasthenia gravis<br>Botulism<br>Organophosphate poisoning | Fluctuating weakness<br>Fatigability<br>Ocular and bulbar<br>  involvements<br>Normal reflexes<br>No sensory changes |
| Muscle | Muscular dystrophies<br>Polymyositis | Weakness<br>Normal reflexes<br>No sensory or autonomic<br>  changes |

Reprinted by permission of Kelly, B. T. and Luce, J. M. The diagnosis and management of neuromuscular diseases causing respiratory failure. *Chest* 99 (1991): 1485–94.

Obstructed artificial airway: Ensure that the artificial airway is not obstructed: Pass a suction catheter, or, if there is any doubt, immediately remove the tube and replace it with another. With very viscous secretions, the suction catheter may pass through with relative ease and totally occlude on withdrawal.

Underlying abnormality: Where possible, correct the underlying abnormality (e.g. remove foreign body, drain haematoma, treat infection).

Endotracheal intubation: If necessary, endotracheal intubation should be performed. This can be achieved by a variety of techniques according to the clinical circumstances and skills of the operator: direct laryngoscopy with IV

**Table 18.5.** Common causes of upper airway obstruction in adults.

Compromised airway secondary to decreased level of consciousness
Obstructed ETT or tracheostomy tube
Postoperative obstruction secondary to neck surgery or haematoma (e.g. carotid artery
    surgery, thyroidectomy)
Trauma
Foreign body
Inhalation injury and oedema
Complications of artificial airways (e.g. post-extubation oedema)
Adult epiglottitis
Severe tonsillitis or pharyngitis
Acute on chronic obstruction (e.g. laryngeal tumour)
Anaphylaxis and laryngeal oedema

or gaseous anaesthetic induction, fibreoptic laryngoscopy, rigid bronchoscopy or blind nasal intubation. If those measures fail, emergency cricothyroidotomy, tracheostomy or insertion of minitracheostomy tube may have to be performed.

## Postoperative chest complications

Many patients are admitted to the ICU for postoperative management, including ventilation. These patients often have chest complications.

- Microatelectasis and infection.
- Collapse secondary to hypoventilation, sputum retention and intra-abdominal abnormalities.
- Interstitial oedema because of excessive perioperative fluid.
- Hypoventilation.
- Aspiration.
- Pleural effusion.
- Pulmonary emboli.
- Acute or chronic lung problems.

Pre-existing lung disease, age, body status and the site of operation will all affect the incidence and severity of complications.

### Some aspects of management

It is assumed that appropriate oxygen treatment and monitoring will be undertaken.

## Preoperative assessment and preparation

Careful assessment of cardiorespiratory function is essential. Physiotherapy, especially in patients with pre-existing chronic lung disease may be required as part of the preparation for surgery.

## Patient position and mobilisation

Where possible, the patient should be sat up, in order to improve oxygenation and minimise basal collapse. As soon as possible they should be sat up out of bed and mobilised at the earliest stage.

## Physiotherapy

Incentive spirometry, encouragement of coughing and aggressive physiotherapy are useful for clearing secretions and preventing atelectasis. These manoeuvres, combined with adequate pain relief to facilitate breathing, are particularly valuable in patients with CAL.

## Continuous positive airway pressure

Continuous positive airway pressure, via a mask or nasal prongs, is excellent for postoperative hypoxia and may prevent atelectasis. It can be used either continuously or intermittently (e.g. 10 minutes every hour). It may be necessary to deliver continuous CPAP through an ETT or tracheostomy tube when a prolonged postoperative course is anticipated (e.g. obese patients with CAL and upper abdominal wounds).

## Fluid replacement

Rational fluid treatment is necessary – excessive amounts of crystalloid fluid should be avoided (see Chapter 16).

## Pain relief

Pain relief is of paramount importance, particularly after abdominal and thoracic procedures. This is most efficiently achieved with regional or local analgesia. Otherwise, liberal and efficient use of narcotics should be employed. Paradoxically, adequate pain relief with an appropriate dose of narcotic may enhance ventilation, rather than depress it. The right dose of narcotic must be achieved – a fine line balancing the advantages of achieving pain relief and facilitating coughing and breathing against the disadvantages of respiratory depression. Use of horizontal, rather than vertical, abdominal surgical incisions and injection of the wound with local anaesthetics at the end of the operation can reduce pain and improve respiratory function.

For the analgesic regime see Chapter 7.

## Minitracheostomy

Temporary use of a 'minitracheostomy' tube inserted through the cricothyroid membrane with frequent tracheal suction, may be helpful in patients with sputum

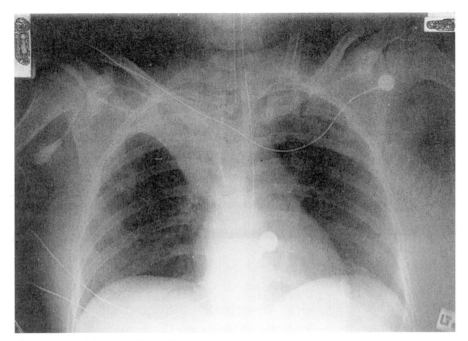

**Figure 18.7.** Right upper lobe collapse.

retention, lung collapse and failure to cough adequately. It can be particularly useful in patients with CAL.

### Artificial ventilation

The indications for postoperative ventilation have not been precisely defined. However, it is common practice to ventilate patients overnight or for several hours after major or prolonged surgery (e.g. cardiothoracic surgery, major vascular surgery, emergency abdominal surgery). It has the advantage of providing adequate ventilation in the face of post-anaesthetic drug effects, ensuring adequate pain relief without compromising ventilation and facilitating tracheal toilet. However, positive-pressure ventilation also has disadvantages and spontaneous ventilation, with adequate pain relief and oxygenation, should be established as soon as possible.

## Atelectasis and collapse

Atelectasis can vary from microatelectasis of a small part of the lung to collapse of a lobe or even a whole lung. It is a common occurrence in intensive care. Atelectasis should be looked for each day on routine chest radiography in all seriously ill patients, whether ventilated or spontaneously breathing (Figure 18.7).

## Radiological features

Features include opacification of lung parenchyma distal to the occluded airway, as well as displacement of structures such as the diaphragm, trachea, mediastinum and other structures within the affected lung. The extent of collapse in lung bases can often be difficult to see on chest x-ray. Auscultation often helps.

## Aetiology

The cause of atelectasis in intensive care is related to regional hypoventilation and retained or viscous sputum as a result of poor diaphragmatic movement. It is often secondary hypoventilation resulting from a decreased level of consciousness or pain. Despite reflex hypoxic vasoconstriction within the collapsed area of lung, some hypoxia will result and secondary infection can occur within the atelectatic area.

## Management

### Preventative

Aggressive physiotherapy is necessary for all at-risk patients. Meticulous regular care for the airway with regular tracheal suction is required, especially in intubated patients. Early mobilisation and total pain relief are also useful in preventing lung collapse.

### Definitive management

Microatelectasis: Physiotherapy, adequate pain relief and deep breathing, incentive spirometry and minitracheostomy are useful.

Collapsed lung lobe: Collapse of a lung lobe or a major lung unit is usually as the result of sputum retention. This should respond to appropriate physiotherapy manoeuvres such as placing the patient with the collapsed lung unit up, and positioning them 30° head down, while simultaneously and aggressively percussing the chest. If the patient has an artificial airway and is being 'bagged', it is advantageous to conduct these manoeuvres with the patient's respiratory cycle being held in full inspiration. Occasionally bronchoscopic intervention with lavage and suction is necessary (Figures 18.8 and 18.9).

## Fibreoptic bronchoscopy in intensive care

In addition to being used for diagnostic purposes such as tumour biopsy and sputum collection, the FOB is useful for visualising and removing airway obstructions such as sputum plugs.

A special membrane in the ETT connector through which the FOB is inserted, is available for use with intubated patients.

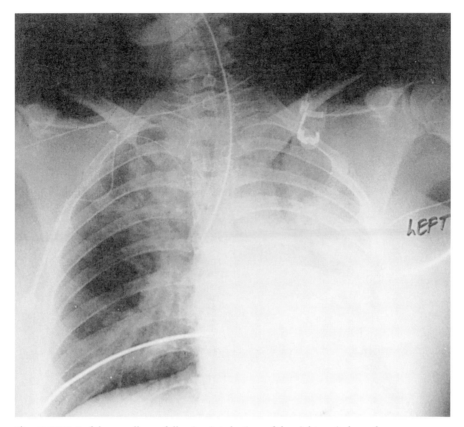

**Figure 18.8.** Left lung collapse following intubation of the right main bronchus.

Precautions: It is advisable to have an additional clinician solely to moni-tor the patient during bronchoscopy, especially if the patient is intubated and ventilated.

- Preoxygenate with 100% oxygen for 5 minutes and use 100% oxygen during the procedure as patients often are hypoxic to begin with.
- Use 4% lignocaine solution to anaesthetise the airway in order to avoid paralysing the patient.
- Cease the use of PEEP as the FOB creates a PEEP effect within the lumen of the artificial airway.
- Monitor the inspiratory ventilator pressures closely.
- Aspirate for short periods, monitor the patient's oxygenation and vital signs (e.g. pulse rate, BP, pulse oximetry) and observe for signs of pulmonary barotrauma. A post-bronchoscopy chest x-ray is necessary, both to look for complications and to observe the benefits of the procedure.

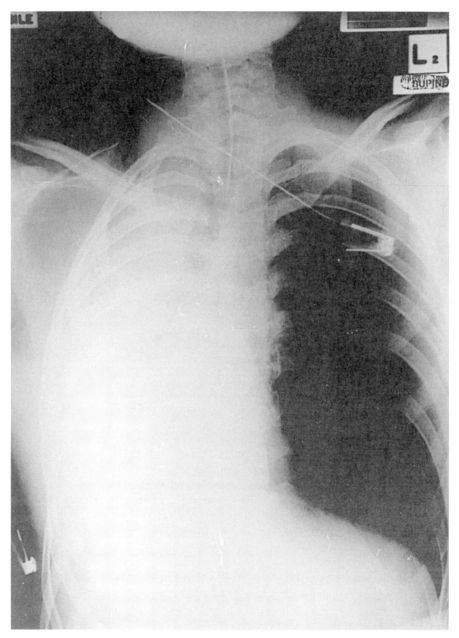

**Figure 18.9.** Right lung collapse. Note mediastinal shift.

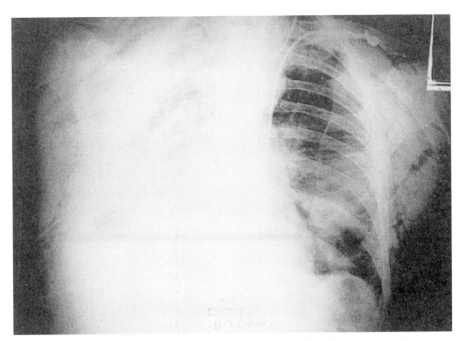

**Figure 18.10.** Predominately unilateral lung abnormalities with right side consolidation. Note the evidence of pulmonary barotrauma, probably as a result of excessive total volume into the remaining normal lung tissue.

## Unilateral lung pathology

Severe, predominantly unilateral lung abnormalities are rare, but they can cause hypoxia resistant to conventional respiratory support (Figure 18.10). If positive-pressure is applied to these patients, it will cause overinflation of the unaffected lung and diversion of pulmonary blood flow to the affected lung. Increasing the PEEP in these circumstances may paradoxically worsen the hypoxia.

### Management

Correct any reversible abnormalities in the affected lung by means of physiotherapy or bronchoscopy if collapse is suspected.

These patients can be nursed laterally with the affected lung uppermost to maximise pulmonary blood flow to the unaffected lung. This can, of course, be done only for limited periods of time and may cause infected contents from the uppermost lung to drain into the lower (normal) lung.

If these measures fail and the hypoxia is severe, independent lung ventilation may be indicated.

### Technique of independent lung ventilation

Intubate using a plastic endobronchial tube (EBT) with suitable cuffs for long-term use. These patients can be very hypoxic and a meticulous intubation technique is necessary. These patients must be heavily sedated to allow adequate controlled ventilation in cases of selective lung ventilation.

The unaffected lung should be ventilated with a normal tidal volume for one lung (250–350 ml), minimal PEEP and appropriate $FiO_2$.

The affected lung can be connected either to CPAP or a separate source of ventilation. It is not necessary to synchronise the two ventilators. Higher levels of PEEP should be applied to the affected lung and a tidal volume and rate should be used to minimise the PIP and maintain oxygenation. Alternatively, a constant pressure (CPAP) can be applied to the affected lung in order to improve oxygenation without the dangers of high peak pressures. High frequency ventilation has also been applied to the affected lung using an EBT.

### Indications for selective lung ventilation

This technique should be restricted to patients with severe intrapulmonary abnormalities such as aspiration, pulmonary oedema, ALI or pneumonia that is predominately unilateral and unresponsive to conventional treatment. It can also be used for unilateral persistent air leaks and bronchopulmonary fistulae, as well as for cases of unilateral collapse resistant to normal manoeuvres.

## Acute severe asthma

'Acute severe asthma' is now preferred to the term 'status asthmaticus', and it describes asthma that over a short period of time becomes increasingly severe and does not respond to usual treatment. The pathogenesis is uncertain.

### Clinical features and assessment
- History of asthma.
- Altered level of consciousness.
- Silent chest on auscultation.
- Difficulty completing sentences without a pause for breath.
- Tachypnoea.
- Serial measurements demonstrating a decrease in peak expiratory flow rates (PEFR) or forced expiratory volume in 1 second ($FEV_1$).
- Pulse rate $>110$ beats/min and bradycardia as hypoxia supervenes.
- Arterial BP is usually raised.
- Pulses paradoxus $>10$ mmHg.

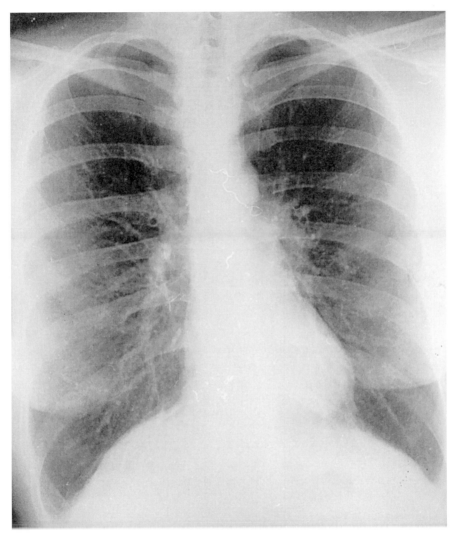

**Figure 18.11.** Acute severe asthma. Note overdistended lung fields.

- Use a chest x-ray to determine the degree of hyperinflation and to rule out infection and pneumothoraces (Figure 18.11).
- Cyanosis or severe hypoxia. Hypoxaemia is invariable and may paradoxically worsen with the use of bronchodilators.
- $PaCO_2$: Hypocarbia occurs initially, and as the patient's condition worsens, the $PaCO_2$ rises.
- Low arterial pH.

**Table 18.6.** Management of acute severe asthma

---

Reassurance
Oxygen Initially 100% and then as according to oximetry
Bronchodilators
   Nebulised β2-agonist: Give continuous nebulised drug if necessary
   Intravenous β2-agonist: Give if nebulised drug is unsuccessful
   $+/-$
   adrenaline
   $+/-$
   aminophylline
Corticosteroids
Fluids
CPAP
Artificial ventilation
   Preload with intravascular fluid
   100% oxygen initially
   Monitor cardiorespiratory system closely
   Avoid cardiovascular depression with drugs
   Elective hypoventilation
   Keep PIP $< 50$ cmH$_2$O
Other measures
   Chest compression
   Extracorporeal oxygenation
   Other drugs, such as
      ketamine
      halothane
      ether
      magnesium

---

- Subjective impressions: increased work of breathing, sweating and distress, with exhaustion eventually supervening.
- No single index has yet been developed that could accurately predict the severity of asthma.

## Management (Table 18.6)

It is not surprising, given that the pathophysiology of acute asthma is poorly understood, that there are many controversies about its management.

### Preventative management
Certain asthmatic patients are particularly at risk from sudden deterioration and death:

- Those with childhood onset asthma that has continued for over 20 years.
- Women over 45 years of age.
- Those with chronic persistent asthma with remission periods of less than 3 months.
- Those with a history of previous life-threatening asthmatic episodes.
- Those with night attacks and early morning deterioration in lung function.
- Those recently discharged from hospital after an episode of acute asthma.

The ICU staff must carefully instruct these patients (as well as their relatives and attending physicians) regarding the particular regimen suitable for the individual patient. These patients need to understand how to monitor the disease, preferably with an individual peakflow meter, and how to avert attacks. In severe cases, and after lack of success with conventional nebulised bronchodilators, the relatives can be instructed in how to deliver 0.5 mg of adrenaline subcutaneously (SC). There must be a sound plan already in place for rapid referral to a specialist centre with advanced facilities for intensive care.

## Definitive management

Oxygen: All patients should receive the maximum $FiO_2$ that can be delivered by face mask if there is no element of chronic obstructive lung disease. Oxygen does not depress ventilation in patients with acute severe asthma.

Fluids: If a patient is unable to tolerate oral fluids, give 2–3 L of IV fluids over 24 hours for adults. There is no firm evidence that excess IV fluid will decrease the incidence of viscous sputum.

Steroids: Hydrocortisone (100 mg IV 6-hourly) or methylprednisolone (40–125 mg IV 6-hourly) is recommended. Because the effectiveness of steroids becomes maximum after 6–8 hours, their role in immediate resuscitation is limited. Nevertheless, asthma is primarily an inflammatory disease of the airways, rather than a bronchoconstrictive disease and therefore anti-inflammatory drugs such as steroids are essential to reverse the underlying problem.

$\beta_2$-agonists: Controversy surrounds the use of bronchodilators for patients with acute severe asthma: the choice of drug, the dosage, the route of administration and the timing. $\beta_2$-agonists such as salbutamol (2.5–10 mg nebulised) are the first-line drugs and are effective for reducing life-threatening bronchoconstriction for most patients. Other $\beta_2$-agonists such as terbutaline, rimiterol, fenoterol and reproterol can also be used. Increasingly, higher doses of nebulised $\beta_2$-agonists are being recommended for acute episodes in order to preclude the need for intubation and ventilation. Under controlled circumstances, continuous administration of nebulised $\beta_2$-agonists should be used, when necessary, or until unacceptable side effects occur (e.g. serious tachycardia or arrhythmias). Although IV administration of $\beta_2$-agonists may be no more effective than the nebulised form, the IV route should be used for acute severe asthma when the patient has difficulty in breathing and adequate delivery cannot be ensured. Aerosol delivery is particularly unpredictable in intubated patients, as much of it becomes deposited on the ETT. The IV dosage for salbutamol is 5–10 μg/kg slowly over 15 minutes as a loading dose if there has been no previous salbutamol, then 5–20 μg/min in adults titrated against the severity of asthma.

Anticholinergic bronchodilators: Ipratropium bromide (500 μg nebulised) may provide a small additional benefit when used with $\beta_2$-agonists.

Aminophylline: Intravenous aminophylline is usually used when high dosages of β2-agonists have not been effective. There is little evidence, however, that it improves bronchodilatation and it has toxic side effects such as arrhythmias, agitation and seizures. Patients must be monitored with a continuous ECG display and potassium levels must be checked regularly. Many facilities no longer recommend the use of aminophylline for acute severe asthma. One must question patients about prior use of slow-release oral theophylline and decrease the initial aminophylline IV dose accordingly. Serum potassium concentrations must be determined immediately as chronic theophylline use will decrease serum and total body potassium levels, and acute IV use will decrease the serum potassium further. Hypokalaemia predisposes to arrhythmias.

The aminophylline dosage is initially 6 mg/kg as a loading dose over 30 minutes; then 0.2–0.9 mg/kg per h if the patient is not already on theophylline. Otherwise, 2–3 mg/kg as a loading dose. The pharmacodynamics of aminophylline are complicated. Aim to keep plasma concentrations of 10–20 mg/L.

Adrenaline: Adrenaline has been used successfully for many years in the form of a subcutaneous (SC) injection. The action of IV adrenaline, however, is more rapid and more reliable. As is the case for most drugs, the role of IV adrenaline in treating patients with acute severe asthma is as yet unclear, but a trial of adrenaline may allow one to avoid intubation and ventilation. It can be used immediately after nebulised $\beta_2$-agonist has been determined a failure and may in fact work by decreasing inflammation in the bronchioles through its α action and vasoconstriction rather than by adding extra β-agonist effect.

The dosage of adrenaline should be 5–10 ml of a 1:10 000 solution IV over 5–10 minutes, repeated as necessary.

All patients should be monitored with continuous ECG display.

If a patient is stable after the initial dose of adrenaline, a continuous infusion at 1–20 μg/min should be commenced and titrated against the patient's symptoms. This can be achieved by diluting 5 mg of adrenaline in 100 ml of isotonic saline and empirically titrating it against a clinical effect.

Paradoxically, BP and pulse rate usually will decrease with the use of adrenaline as the patient's condition improves. If the BP rises, if serious arrhythmias occur or if the patient's condition is rapidly deteriorating, alternative treatment must be considered. Vomiting may be observed during the adrenaline infusion.

Frequent checks of serum potassium concentration should be made because adrenaline, aminophylline and $\beta_2$-agonists can cause hypokalaemia and predispose to cardiac arrhythmias.

Acute severe asthma seems to run a time course of approximately 24–48 hours. Do not abruptly cease administration of adrenaline, as sudden exacerbations of asthma can occur even after 24 hours. Gradually wean the patient from adrenaline and be prepared to increase the infusion rate if deterioration occurs during the weaning process.

Antibiotics: Antibiotics are rarely indicated for acute severe asthma. Use of these agents should be restricted to patients with bacteriologically proven infection or infiltrates on chest x-ray.

Physiotherapy: Physiotherapy is useful in the recovery phase, when patients begin clearing mucous plugs. Intubated patients need aggressive physiotherapy in order to avoid atelectasis and lung collapse.

## Ventilatory support

### Continuous positive airway pressure/BiPAP

When considering ventilatory support, use CPAP or BiPAP via a face mask initially. Commence at low levels of CPAP initially (e.g. 5 cmH$_2$O) and increase in 2 cmH$_2$O increments according to the patient's level of response; the patient is often the best judge. Sometimes increasing levels of inspiratory support with BiPAP may avoid intubation and ventilation.

## Artificial ventilation

Artificial ventilation is a procedure of last resort and should be used only if medications fail. Asthmatic patients present a difficult ventilatory challenge. Gas has to be forced in under pressure to an already overdistended chest and then has to escape passively through occluded airways (Figure 18.12). Serious complications of ventilation are common in these circumstances. The decision to ventilate is a clinical one, based on the patient's degree of exhaustion and the relative improvement with more conservative measures.

### Approach

Attitude: Reassure the patient and explain what will happen.

Oxygenation: Preoxygenate with 100% oxygen.

Intravascular volume: Preload the patient rapidly with 500 ml of colloid. During spontaneous breathing, these patients have a very negative intrathoracic pressure and venous return is enhanced. When positive-pressure ventilation is commenced, intrathoracic pressures increase and venous return is severely impaired. Moreover, such patients often are dehydrated as a result of decreased oral intake,

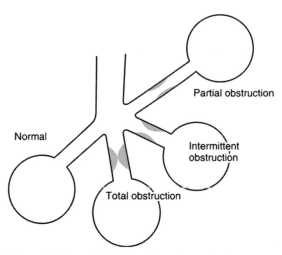

**Figure 18.12.** Model of alveoli in asthma. The heterogeneous population of alveoli in asthmatic lungs means that positive-pressure ventilation may overdistend the normal population, underventilate the occluded alveoli and perhaps cause gas trapping in others.

excessive sweating and tachypnoea. Be prepared to infuse more fluid according to the cardiovascular response to positive-pressure ventilation.

Induction agent: Use an agent which will cause minimal cardiovascular depression (e.g. a small amount of anaesthetic induction agent or benzodiazepine plus narcotic), as well as a rapidly acting muscle relaxant to ensure adequate conditions for rapid sequence intubation. Use cricoid pressure during intubation in order to prevent aspiration.

Pressure-support: Ideally patients should be breathing spontaneously not heavily sedated on pressure-support ventilation (PSV).

Intermittent positive-pressure ventilation: Some patients will not tolerate PSV and ventilation will need to be controlled.

Sedation: Maintain sedation (e.g. midazolam and morphine) as a continuous IV infusion. Although morphine may release histamine, it is probably safe to use for sedation.

Muscle relaxation: Asthma is one of the few occasions where a muscle relaxant may be indicated for facilitating ventilation (e.g. vecuronium 8 mg initial dose, then an infusion of 5–10 mg/h) to prevent fighting against the ventilator and increasing the already high inspiratory pressures.

Oxygenation: Maintain with appropriate $FiO_2$ according to frequent determinations of blood gases and pulse oximetry.

Ventilator modes: Do not overventilate or aim for 'normal' $PaCO_2$. Electively hypoventilate and tolerate high $PaCO_2$ (keep $PaCO_2$ < 90 mmHg [12 kPa] and pH > 7.2 [63 mmol/L H$^+$]) in order to avoid high ventilatory pressures, barotrauma and cardiovascular depression.

Each patient will need individual settings to maintain adequate oxygenation without overdistension of alveoli. As an initial setting, use:

- a 1 : 1 inspiratory: expiratory ratio
- a low tidal volume (usually less than 400 ml).

Increase the ventilation by increasing the respiratory rate, but with an expiratory pause sufficient to allow for adequate lung emptying and to prevent 'stacking' of gas within the lung after each inspiration.

A slow inspiratory flow rate is optimal for low inspiratory pressures, but may not be sufficient for the delivery of an adequate tidal volume. Reduce the inspiratory flow rate to as low a level as is compatible with adequate ventilation.

Keep PIPs less than 50 cmH$_2$O if at all possible.

Chest x-ray: Inspect the patient and examine the chest x-ray for evidence of subcutaneous emphysema or mediastinal emphysema. This indicates extensive alveolar rupture and a high likelihood of pneumothorax formation; inform the staff, and have an intercostal catheter available, but do not insert it prophylactically.

## Other possible measures

- Ketamine (20–40 μg/kg per min) may be useful for asthma that is unresponsive to other measures.
- Magnesium sulphate (1.2 g in 50 ml of isotonic saline IV over 20 minutes) has been reported to improve peak flow rates.
- Halothane has been used as a last resort in ventilated patients with severe asthma. Care must be exercised to avoid cardiovascular depression and increased intracranial pressure. Ether, isoflurane and enflurane have also been used.
- Manual chest compression during expiration may be needed in a minority of artificially ventilated patients in order to assist expiratory gas flow.

## Chronic airflow limitation (CAL)

Airflow can be limited because of narrowing of the airways or diminished elastic recoil in the lung. The clinical manifestations of these have been believed to be chronic bronchitis and emphysema respectively. That may well be an inaccurate oversimplification. It is probably better to think of both diseases as forming part of the spectrum known as CAL, characterised by cough, dyspnoea, sputum production, airflow limitation and impaired gas exchange. The lesions associated with CAL include

**Table 18.7.** Management of chronic airflow limitation in intensive care

---

Consider carefully what intensive care can offer in terms of the reversible components of the presentation, especially when contemplating ventilation

Give oxygen

Correct any reversible component (e.g. drain a pneumothorax, treat infection)

Reduce the work of breathing (e.g. reduce sputum formation and bronchoconstriction)

Begin a trial of drug treatment (e.g. inhaled β2-agonists and corticosteroids)

Reduce pain after surgery, and encourage early mobilisation

Use chest physiotherapy

Begin a trial of CPAP or BiPAP with non-invasive mask ventilation

Consider mechanical ventilation

---

Acinus: emphysema

Bronchi: Smooth muscle hyperplasia

Mucous gland enlargement

Bronchioles: narrowing and obliteration; mucous plugging

Inflammation

Fibrosis

One or another of these lesions may dominate but the usual picture is that the lesions occur in diverse combinations to varying degrees of severity. The reasons for such large variations among patients is unclear.

Many patients admitted to intensive care, for whatever reason, will have some degree of CAL as smoking remains prevalent in many communities. For these patients gas exchange will be compromised and artificial ventilation will be associated with more complications. Some of these patients will be admitted primarily for an acute exacerbation of CAL. The most important decision in the management of these patients is whether or not to admit them to the ICU. The expensive resources in the ICU may have little to offer patients with severe limitations of respiratory reserve that result from advanced CAL.

The admission policy will depend on the severity of the chronic component and the presence of an acute and reversible component. A careful history will usually elicit a patient's previous exercise tolerance and quality of life. There may be little or no acute component and, in fact, the so-called deterioration may represent end-stage disease, at which point a diagnosis of 'dying' should be considered.

## Management (Table 18.7)

### Oxygen

There are certain individuals with severe CAL who are sensitive to even small increases in inspired oxygen concentration. For some reason, every medical student seems to remember that oxygen is dangerous in these circumstances and therefore it is often delivered in only meagre and insubstantial amounts to all hypoxic patients. Oxygen-sensitive patients are rare and yet our obsession with the potential danger from oxygen is responsible for widespread 'elective' hypoxia in hospitalised patients throughout the world.

In these days of readily available determinations of blood gases, these rare individuals can be recognised and their inspired oxygen can be titrated carefully, whilst the remainder can survive in much safer circumstances with appropriate oxygenation. Oxygen is essential for optimal alveolar function and also helps to reduce pulmonary vasoconstriction and hypertension.

## Correct any reversible components
Because the respiratory reserves of patients with CAL are minimal, reversing even small components of the disease can be beneficial. For example, even small pneumothoraces should be drained. The work of breathing can be decreased by decreasing secretions and bronchoconstriction or by treating infection.

## Drugs
The role of drugs in treating CAL is uncertain and depends on the degree of destruction of the lung architecture. There has been little evaluation of the role of drugs in treating acute exacerbations of CAL. Often the only way to determine their effectiveness is to try one or more drugs and evaluate their clinical effectiveness in each individual patient. Corticosteroids are sometimes helpful. Bronchodilators can be useful. Aerosol or IV β2-adrenergic agents are more effective than IV aminophylline in the acute situation.

Inhaled β2-agonists: The β2-agonists have not been well evaluated regarding dosage and effectiveness in treating CAL, but they are worth a trial.

Anticholinergic drugs: Nebulised ipratropium has bronchodilatory effects and may reduce the volume of sputum.

Theophylline: Their role in treating CAL is not clear. Nevertheless, many patients are on long-term theophylline therapy.

Corticosteroids: Corticosteroids may be worth a trial in patients with acute exacerbations of CAL.

## Surgery
Thoracic or abdominal surgery, or even the insult of minor surgery, can reduce what little respiratory reserve is left in these patients causing rapid deterioration in respiration function. This can be minimised by the following measures.

Pain relief: Provide adequate pain relief, especially local or regional analgesia perioperatively, in order to encourage breathing and coughing and avoid sputum retention.

Perioperative physiotherapy.

Nasotracheal suction: Use nasotracheal suction or minitracheostomy to facilitate sputum clearance.

Incentive spirometry: Incentive spirometry and early mobilisation also helps.

Low-dose heparin: Prophylactic use of low-dosage heparin can minimise the risk of thromboembolic phenomena.

### Cardiac failure

Cardiac failure, with pulmonary and peripheral oedema, often can supervene in patients with CAL. It may be part of a primary process or secondary to right ventricular failure. The diagnosis is not easy and interpretation of pulmonary oedema on a chest x-ray can be difficult because of distorted vascular markings and lung architecture.

Cardiac failure in these circumstances can be managed by cautious diuresis, β2-agonist (e.g. salbutamol) and occasionally left and right side afterload reduction with nitroglycerine.

### Lung volume reduction surgery

Early studies show that if the patient survived the surgery their quality of life improved but not their longevity.

### Non-invasive ventilation

Dynamic hyperinflation of the lung is common in patients with CAL. The expiratory time is reduced to the point where complete exhalation cannot occur before the next inspiratory cycle is initiated. This leads to gas trapping at the end of expiration, also known as breath-stacking, occult PEEP, 'auto' PEEP or 'intrinsic' PEEP ($PEEP_i$). The level of $PEEP_i$ may not be the same for each breath, nor can it be accurately predicted for each patient. It depends on factors such as lung compliance and resistance for any given airway diameter, inspiratory flow and respiratory rate.

Intrinsic PEEP increases the work of breathing by acting as an inspiratory threshold load. Continuous positive airway pressure can counterbalance the effects of $PEEP_i$ and will reduce the work of breathing, as well as the sensation of dyspnoea. A well-designed CPAP circuit is essential. The level of CPAP should be titrated against the subjective improvement in the patient's response (usually 5–10 $cmH_2O$). The level of applied PEEP should be less than the patient's PEEP. Check the chest x-ray to assess the level of hyperinflation.

BiPAP is an extension of the concept of CPAP but provides adjustable inspiratory support as well as CPAP. Both BiPAP and CPAP are delivered in the first instance in a non-invasive fashion with the use of either face or nasal masks. BiPAP and CPAP delivered non-invasively have become the first-line ventilator support mode for patients with CAL.

### Mechanical ventilation

Artificial ventilation should be avoided, if at all possible, because of several considerations.

**Table 18.8.** Degrees of severity for pulmonary embolism

| Severity grade | Haemodynamic disturbance | Oxygenation | Clinical symptoms |
|---|---|---|---|
| I | Absent | Normal | Short-lasting |
| II | Mild | Normal | Moderate but persisting |
| III | Moderate | Abnormal | Severe |
| IV | Severe | Very abnormal | Shock |

- Coughing reflex and clearing of secretions are reduced.
- Lung architecture is already disrupted and would be prone to further damage by positive airway pressure.
- Patients with CAL are notoriously difficult to wean from artificial ventilation.
- Unless there is a significant acute respiratory component, the prospect for long-term survival of these patients is poor.

Approach to ventilation: Do not aim for 'normal' concentrations of blood gases. These patients often are severely hypoxic and hypercarbic at their best. Keep the $PaCO_2$ at the patient's normal level. Encourage spontaneous breathing and titrate the number of mechanical breaths against the patient's requirements. 'Pressure assist' or pressure-support during inspiration may also help weaning. Avoid excessive use of sedation or muscle relaxants as that would prolong the already difficult weaning process. Tracheostomy may be needed if weaning from ventilation is delayed. An early introduction of enteral nutrition is important.

## Pulmonary embolism

### Incidence in ICU

The exact incidence of deep venous thrombosis (DVT) and pulmonary embolism (PE) is unknown and probably depends on factors such as age, the nature of underlying disease and co morbidities. Critically ill patients are more likely to develop DVT than other patients.

### Pathophysiology

Pulmonary emboli are usually multiple. Acute obstruction of the pulmonary arterial tree will result in V/Q abnormalities, hypoxia and circulatory failure. Severe disturbances occur in about 10% of patients with PE (Table 18.8).

#### Diagnosis
Finding the source of the PE can be a frustrating and often futile exercise. Femoral and iliac veins can be the sources of multiple emboli and further investigation may be necessary in those circumstances.

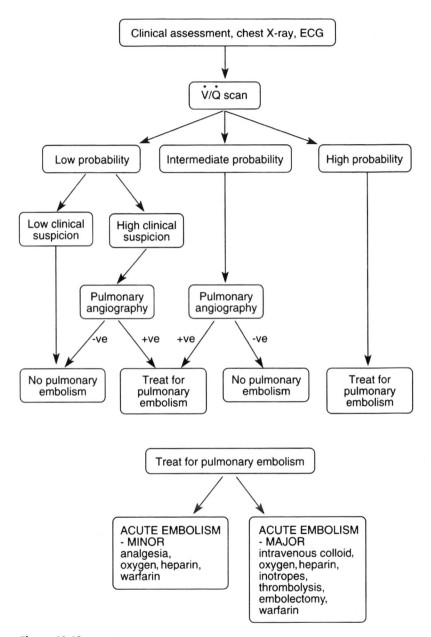

**Figure 18.13.**

Pulmonary embolus is easily misdiagnosed. No single symptom or combination of symptoms is diagnostic. The classic clinical signs (dyspnoea, haemoptysis and pleuritic chest pain) are uncommon. Determinations of arterial blood gases and serum enzymes show no consistent pattern on which a firm diagnosis could be made. However, a decrease in the platelet count is highly suggestive of a PE. D-dimer is not a useful test in the critically ill as there are many other causes for an elevation.

There will be positive findings from chest x-ray in about 50% of patients (e.g. pulmonary haemorrhage or infarction, raised hemidiaphragm, atelectasis, oligaemia or pleural effusion). However, those features can accompany many illnesses in intensive care.

More than 50% of patients with PE will have normal ECG patterns. Abnormal findings such as right side heart strain are frequently transient, delayed or non-specific.

Transoeophageal echocardiography can demonstrate obvious right ventricular strain and persistent pulmonary hypertension in cases of significant emboli. It can also be used to monitor therapy.

When the findings from a perfusion lung scan are normal, the possibility of significant PE can almost be entirely excluded. However, in the presence of pre-existing lung abnormalities, lung scans can be very misleading.

Spiral CT with contrast is replacing pulmonary angiography as the gold standard investigation. The timing of the dye injection and scans is critical to get good quality pictures. This technique is best suited to identify PE in the proximal pulmonary vascular tree.

Pulmonary angiography is invasive and has complications. However, it is much better at detecting distal pulmonary emboli than spiral CT.

## Management

Most patients who survive the first 30 minutes following PE will live, unless a further embolism occurs (Figure 18.13).

### Prophylaxis
Low dosage heparin has been demonstrated to decrease the incidence of DVT and PE in seriously ill medical patients. A reduced incidence has also been shown in postoperative patients and trauma patients. Graded compression stockings and sequential compression devices may reduce the incidence of DVT. They are efficacious in patients undergoing surgery.

### Supportive
Oxygen: Supplemental oxygen is almost always required.

Continuous positive airway pressure: CPAP can improve gas exchange in patients with PE.

Fluid: Expansion of the intravascular volume to correct hypotension is necessary (see p.   ). If that fails, inotropes should be used.

Inotropes: As in other forms of circulatory failure, finding the most suitable inotrope is a matter of trial and error.

- Dobutamine can be used initially for mild haemodynamic disturbances as it increases cardiac output and reduces pulmonary vascular resistance.
- Adrenaline or noradrenaline: Inotropes with vasoconstrictor activity are often used for more severe haemodynamic disturbances in order to maintain arterial BP and vital organ perfusion.

## Definitive management

Heparin: Heparin will not dissolve an existing clot; it only prevents extension. It can be given as an intermittent bolus every 4–6 hours or, preferably, via a continuous IV infusion. The dosage can be selected empirically (e.g. 1000 units/h) or can be determined on the basis of tests such as the activated partial thromboplastin time (which should be about twice the control level), the clotting time or the thrombin time or a combination of all three. In the case of proven PE, heparin is usually given for 7–10 days, followed by a change to an oral anticoagulant for 3–6 months, with an overlap period of approximately 5 days when both drugs are given.

Thrombolytics: Thrombolytics should be given to patients with sustained hypotension, shock or acute right ventricular failure (RVF) and those with obstruction to more than 50% of their pulmonary circulation. Heparin probably should be administered before and after the thrombolytic agent.

Streptokinase: A bolus dose of 1 million units over 30 minutes probably will be sufficient. However, some authorities recommend 100 000–200 000 units hourly for 24 hours.

Allergic reactions occur in about 5% of patients. Most are mild and can be minimised by giving hydrocortisone (100 mg IV) before the infusion. The possibility of an anaphylactic reaction should be anticipated and must be treated rapidly.

Urokinase: A dose of 15 000 units/kg probably will be sufficient. Urokinase is as effective as streptokinase and appears to be non-antigenic in humans. However, it is expensive and is not available in all countries.

Recombinant tissue plasminogen activator (rt-PA): A dose of 50 mg IV, repeated if necessary, has been used successfully in initial trials for PE.

Contraindications and complications:

- History of stroke, seizure or other intracranial disease.
- Recent major gastrointestinal bleeding.
- Trauma or major surgery within 10 days.
- Persistant hypertension or history of poorly controlled hypertension.

- Unexplained anaemia, thrombocytopaenia or elevated prothrombin time.
- During pregnancy and the puerperium.

If bleeding occurs, the infusion should be stopped (the half-life of these agents is no more than 20 minutes) and fresh frozen plasma should be given.

Emergency pulmonary embolectomy: If thrombolytic treatment is contraindicated or is unsuccessful, there may be a place for embolectomy.

Embolectomy should be considered in all cases of severe PE (e.g. patients with more than 50% occlusion of the pulmonary arteries and patients with continuing circulatory shock, hypotension or RVF that has not responded 1 hour after the onset of PE or after thrombolytic treatment).

Interruption of the inferior vena cava: The use of various techniques such as clips, filters and umbrellas can be considered after failure of anticoagulant therapy in the less severely ill, as well as for recurring cases of PE or when anticoagulation is considered hazardous.

## Obstructive sleep apnoea

Obstructive sleep apnoea is defined as the absence of airflow lasting for at least 10 seconds and occurring more than 30 times during a 7-hour sleep. Sleep apnoea syndrome is divided into three groups:

Obstructive: where airflow ceases despite continuation of abdominal and thoracic inspiratory movements.
Central: where cessation of airflow is accompanied by cessation of respiratory efforts.
Mixed: obstructive and central.

Obstructive sleep apnoea is by far the most common form, affecting 1–4% of the adult population.

### Clinical features

- Snoring (cardinal symptom).
- Excessive daytime sleepiness (cardinal symptom).
- Psychosocial problems and deterioration of intellectual function.
- Early morning headache.
- Arterial hypertension.
- Severe nocturnal hypoxia.
- Right side heart failure and pulmonary hypertension.
- Polycythaemia.
- Obesity, hypothyroidism, acromegaly.
- Short, thick neck, retrognathia, nasal obstruction and oropharyngeal mass.
- Often associated with excessive alcohol intake.

## Diagnosis

Obtain a clinical history from patient and spouse. Night sleep studies are needed to confirm the diagnosis and determine the method and urgency of treatment. Certain features are documented during sleep studies:

- Continuous pulse oximetry and pulse rate recovery.
- Continuous ECG.
- Continuous electromyogram of the diaphragm.
- Continuous oronasal airflow measurement (thermistor or pressure transducer).
- Continuous sleep state recording (EEG or electro-oculogram).
- Continuous measurement of chest wall and abdominal motions (inductive plethysmography).
- Continuous recording of room noise.
- Cardiorespiratory investigation to determine extent of impairment.

## Treatment

### General
- The patient must lose weight.
- The patient must abstain from alcohol and cigarettes.
- One must either rule out the presence of hypothyroidism and acromegaly or else treat those conditions.

### Drugs
Naloxone, acetazolamide, medroxyprogesterone, theophylline, strychnine and nicotine have all been tried, with little benefit, in patients with sleep apnoea.

### Surgery
Anatomical obstruction: Surgical correction of any anatomical obstruction (e.g. nasal polyps, septal deviation, enlarged tonsils and adenoids) may cure some patients.

Uvulopalatopharyngoplasty: This procedure is designed to increase the cross-sectional area of the airway. The results are unpredictable.

Tracheostomy: Tracheostomy should be considered in serious cases where other measures have failed.

### Nasal CPAP
The principle of nasal CPAP is to provide a pressure at the collapsible segment of the upper airway that will be sufficient to counteract negative inspiratory pressures. The simplest system involves a blower, delivering air via a nasal mask. The system must have minimal inspiratory resistance during respiration. This form of treatment is becoming increasingly used for obstructive sleep apnoea.

**TROUBLESHOOTING**

## Haemoptysis in intensive care

Determine that there has been no iatrogenic trauma to upper airways as a result of the use of suction catheters, ETT, etc.

Vasculitis – Wegener's granulomatosis or Behçet's disease.

Complication of tracheostomy.

Complication of thoracic surgery.

Blunt and penetrating trauma can cause bleeding.

A pulmonary artery catheter can rupture a pulmonary vessel.

Look for pulmonary embolism or infarct.

Bronchiectasis.

Look for bleeding from carcinoma.

An infection such as TB can result in bleeding as it erodes into pulmonary vessels.

Pulmonary oedema or long-standing mitral valve disease can result in haemoptysis.

Check coagulation/platelets.

## FURTHER READING

### Upper airways obstruction

Weiler, N., Eberle, B. and Heinrichs, W. The laryngeal mask airway: routine, risk, or rescue? *Intensive Care Medicine* 25 (1999): 761–2.

### Cardiogenic pulmonary oedema

Pang, D. M. B., Keenan, S. P., Cook. D. J. and Sibbald, W. J. The effective of positive-pressure airway support on mortality and the need for intubation in cardiogenic pulmonary edema. A systematic review. *Chest* 114 (1998): 1185–92.

Yan, A. T., Bradley, T., Douglas, M. D. and Liu, P. P. The role of continuous positive airway pressure in treatment of congenitive heart failure. *Chest* 120 (2001): 1675–85.

### Adult respiratory distress syndrome

Garber, B. G., Hebert, P. C., Yelle, J-D., Hodder, R. V. and McGowan, J. Adult respiratory distress syndrome: a systematic overview of incidence and risk factors. *Critical Care Medicine* 24 (1996): 687–95.

Marini, J. J. and Evans, T. W. Round table conference: acute lung injury. 15th–17th March 1997, Brussels, Belgium. *Intensive Care Medicine* 24 (1998): 878–83.

Tobin, M. J. Advances in mechanical ventilation. *New England Journal of Medicine* 344 (2001): 1986–96.

Ware, L. B. and Matthay, M. A. The acute respiratory distress syndrome. *New England Journal of Medicine* 342 (2000): 1334–49.

## Pneumonia

Anonymous (1996). Hospital-acquired pneumonia in adults: diagnosis, assessment of severity, initial antimicrobial therapy, and preventative strategies: a consensus statement. *American Journal of Respiratory and Critical Care Medicine* 153 (1996): 1711–25.

Young, P. J. and Ridley, S. A. Ventilator-associated pneumonia. Diagnosis, pathogenesis and prevention. *Anaesthesia* 54 (1999): 1183–97.

## Aspiration

Marik, P. E. Primary care: aspiration pneumonitis and aspiration pneumonia. *New England Journal of Medicine* 344 (2001): 665–71.

## Acute severe asthma

Bauer, T. T. and Torres, A. Aerolized $\beta_2$-agonists in the intensive care unit: just do it. *Intensive Care Medicine* 27 (2001): 3–5.

Peigang, Y. and Marini, J. J. Ventilation of patients with asthma and chronic obstructive pulmonary disease. *Current Opinion in Critical Care* 8 (2002): 70–6.

## Chronic airflow limitation

American Thoracic Society. Inpatient management of COPD. *American Journal of Respiratory and Critical Care Medicine* 152 (1995): S97–106.

Gladwin, M. and Pierson, D. J. Mechanical ventilation of the patient with severe chronic obstructive pulmonary disease. *Intensive Care Medicine* 24 (1998): 898–910.

Maggiore, S. M. Lung volume reduction for patients with severe COPD. *Intensive Care Medicine* 25 (1999): 1319–22.

Stoller, J. K. Acute exacerbations of chronic obstructive pulmonary disease. *New England Journal of Medicine* 346 (2002): 988–94.

## Pulmonary embolism

Goldhaber, S. Z. Pulmonary embolism. *New England Journal of Medicine* 339 (1998): 93–104.

Goldhaber, S. Z. Echocardiography in the management of pulmonary embolism. *Annals of Internal Medicine* 136 (2002): (Suppl.) 691–700.

## Obstructive sleep apnoea

Turkington, P. M. and Elliott, M.W. Rationale for the use of non-invasive ventilation in chronic ventilatory failure. *Thorax* 55 (2000): 417–23.

# 19

# Ventilatory techniques

- There will be an optimum ventilatory mode for each patient at each stage of that patient's disease.
- Because of the many serious disadvantages of positive-pressure ventilation, spontaneous respiration should be encouraged as soon as possible following acute respiratory failure.
- Ventilating the seriously ill depends more on the operator than the machine.
- Weaning is a dynamic and continuous process that begins the moment a patient is artificially ventilated.
- Oxygenation takes precedence over the need for optimal ventilation and carbon dioxide ($CO_2$) levels – 'permissive hypercarbia' or 'elective hypoventilation' forms the basis of artificially ventilating patients in intensive care in order to reduce lung damage.

## Intermittent positive-pressure ventilation

The lungs are designed to be inflated by the creation of negative intrapleural pressure. Early artificial ventilators such as the iron lung followed that sound physiological method and created a vacuum around the chest to cause air flow.

The use of positive-pressure ventilation became widespread in the early 1950s and its use has, in many ways, defined the practice of intensive care medicine. Intermittent positive-pressure ventilation (IPPV) is the commonest form of positive-pressure-support used in intensive care. A certain tidal volume is delivered at a set rate to maintain a minute volume consistent with $CO_2$ elimination, while oxygenation is determined mainly by the fraction of inspired oxygen ($FiO_2$).

### Main indications for IPPV

1 Failure of ventilation (e.g. caused by neuromuscular diseases such as tetanus or Guillain–Barré syndrome or resulting from neuromuscular blocking drugs).

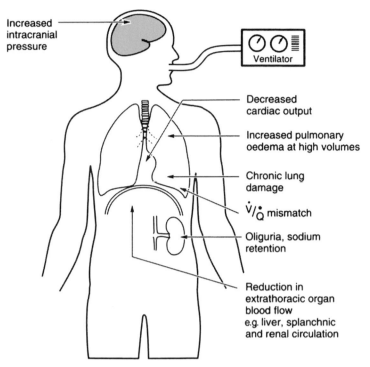

Increased intracranial pressure

Ventilator

Decreased cardiac output

Increased pulmonary oedema at high volumes

Chronic lung damage

$\dot{V}/\dot{Q}$ mismatch

Oliguria, sodium retention

Reduction in extrathoracic organ blood flow e.g. liver, splanchnic and renal circulation

**Figure 19.1.** Complications of positive intrathoracic pressure.

2  To facilitate $CO_2$ excretion.
3  To facilitate the delivery of oxygen.
4  To reduce the work of breathing in patients with cardiorespiratory failure (e.g. the later stages of acute respiratory failure).

## Complications of positive intrathoracic pressure

The adverse effects of positive intrathoracic pressure (ITP) are principally due to cardiovascular impairment and the direct effect of pressure on lung tissue (Figure 19.1).

### Pulmonary effects of positive-pressure ventilation

When positive-pressure ventilation was first employed on a wide scale in the early 1950s, machines would simulate normal tidal volumes and rates. If the lungs were otherwise normal and the inflationary pressures were relatively low, lung damage due to positive-pressure would be minimal. However, as the practice of

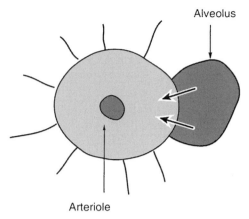

Alveolus

Arteriole

**Figure 19.2.** Origin of extra-alveolar air. Air under pressure moves from overdistended alveoli into the adventitia of pulmonary arterioles and venules. It moves along the adventitia toward the mediastinum as pulmonary interstitial emphysema (PIE).

ventilating patients with underlying lung disease became widespread, pulmonary barotrauma (lung damage secondary to excessive pressure), causing alveolar overdistension became an increasing problem.

The incidence of barotrauma increased even further with the advent of volume cycled ventilators and the use of high levels of positive end-expiratory pressure (PEEP). Modern ventilators guaranteed the delivery of a preset tidal volume, independent of the compliance or resistance of the lungs. This results in non-ventilation of some alveoli and overdistension of other, often normal alveoli. It is not only high pressures that can damage lung tissue; high tidal volumes and alveolar overdistension can also result in rupture. In fact, excessive volumes are probably more important than excessive pressures in causing alveolar overdistension and rupture – resulting in volutrauma rather than barotrauma. Alveolar overdistension also causes increased permeability pulmonary oedema. Ironically, that is often the problem for which the patient is being ventilated.

Gas from ruptured alveoli forms pulmonary interstitial emphysema (PIE), which travels in the adventitia of the pulmonary vessels (Figure 19.2). The gas bubbles coalesce along large vessels and migrate centrally to form mediastinal emphysema (ME). With further development of PIE and ME, the gas can burst through the mediastinal pleura to form pneumothoraces or can track along the fascia in the neck to form subcutaneous emphysema (SE) (Figure 19.3). Pneumothoraces and SE can occur together or independently in this setting. With increasing pressure, gas can track along the aorta and oesophagus to form pneumoretroperitoneum, pneumoperitoneum and even air embolism (Figure 19.4). It is important to recognise the presence of extra-alveolar gas, either clinically or on x-ray. Mediastinal emphysema can, for example, collect under tension in

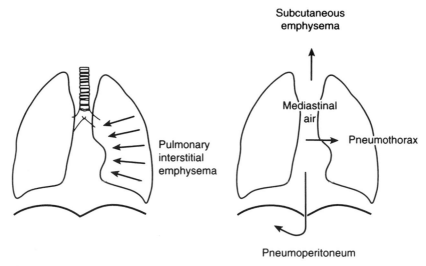

**Figure 19.3.** Forms of pulmonary barotrauma. Extra-alveolar air moves as pulmonary interstitial emphysema to form mediastinal emphysema. From there, under continued pressure, it can form subcutaneous emphysema, pneumothoraces, pneumoretroperitoneum and pneumoperitoneum. Reprinted by permission of W.B. Saunders. Hillman, K. Pulmonary barotrauma. *Clinical Anaesthesiology* 3 (1985): 877–98.

the mediastinum and cause cardiac tamponade. Both SE and ME are indicators of imminent risk for pneumothorax formation unless ventilatory pressures and volumes can be reduced. Gas from a ruptured viscus must be differentiated from pneumoperitoneum and pneumoretroperitoneum.

The incidence of pulmonary barotrauma can be reduced by limiting peak inspiratory pressures (PIP) to less than 35 cmH$_2$O, by reducing tidal volumes to 5–10 ml/kg and by being more concerned with adequate oxygenation, rather than 'normal' arterial pressure of CO$_2$. The lungs are delicate structures that can easily be damaged by pressure and overdistension. Pulmonary barotrauma can also result in chronic lung damage or bronchopulmonary dysplasia as a result of rupture of the terminal airways and alveoli. Ventilatory techniques that can limit the adverse effects of excessive pressure are increasingly being used and they are discussed in the next section of this chapter.

Relative hypoxia can also paradoxically occur when artificial ventilation is commenced. This is because of an exacerbation of mismatching in ventilation ($\dot{V}$) and perfusion ($\dot{Q}$). The upper zones of the lung are preferentially ventilated compared with the lower zones, whereas spontaneous respiration favours lower zone ventilation. Pulmonary blood flow can be decreased as a result of positive-pressure exacerbating $\dot{V}/\dot{Q}$ distribution abnormalities.

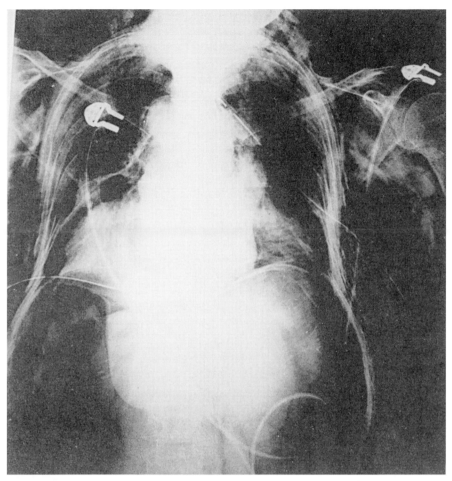

**Figure 19.4.** Pulmonary barotrauma, with massive extra-alveolar air formation, including mediastinal emphysema, subcutaneous emphysema, bilateral pneumothoraces (treated with intercostal catheters) and pneumoperitoneum.

## Cardiovascular effects of positive-pressure ventilation

Applying positive pressure to the lungs decreases venous return which in turn decreases cardiac output and blood pressure, unless the body naturally compensates or there is a clinical intervention such as fluid infusion or inotrope administration. In addition to decreased arterial blood pressure secondary to decreased cardiac output, there is decreased venous return from extrathoracic organs. This is due to the fact that ITP is impeding venous return. Decreased cerebral venous return can increase intracranial pressure (ICP), especially when the pressure is already abnormally high. As part of the body's normal responses to increased ITP and decreased venous return, there is also a tendency for sodium and water retention.

## Positive end-expiratory pressure

Positive end-expiratory pressure is used for maintaining functional residual capacity (FRC) and improving oxygenation. Adding PEEP to IPPV will improve oxygenation, probably by recruiting non-ventilated alveoli and by keeping alveoli open at the end of expiration. This results in more alveoli being available for oxygenation through the whole respiratory cycle. The PEEP may also help to redistribute blood flow to ventilated alveoli.

The amount of PEEP needed to achieve optimum oxygenation usually varies between 5–20 $cmH_2O$ but pressures of up to 30 $cmH_2O$ have been used. Because of the dangers associated with PEEP, there is an increasing tendency to use lower levels. However, higher PEEP levels may sometimes be necessary to decrease shearing forces associated with tidal volume excursions. A high PEEP level associated with a relatively low PIP in some circumstances will result in a relatively low mean airway pressure and tidal volume in association with minimal shearing forces and lung damage.

### Optimal peep
The optimal level of PEEP is the airway pressure at which oxygen transport (the product of cardiac output and arterial oxygen content) is maximal. Because PEEP decreases cardiac output and venous return to the heart, the compromise between improved oxygenation and reduced cardiac output is a matter of trial and error. Moreover, PEEP increases the PIP, which is associated with increased pulmonary barotrauma and other complications. These adverse effects must be considered when determining the optimum PEEP. Because in determining the optimal PEEP one must take all of these factors into account it is, at best, an empirical estimate. Maximum alveolar recruitment should be aimed for while simultaneously avoiding alveolar overdistension and barotrauma. This is difficult because of the widespread heterogeneity throughout the lungs. The optimal PEEP probably is the lowest at which adequate oxygen delivery ($DO_2$) can be achieved.

## Choosing the right ventilatory mode

In attempts to improve gas exchange while avoiding the disadvantages of high ITP and alveolar overdistension, forms of ventilatory support other than IPPV and PEEP are increasingly being used (Figure 19.5). Many of these newer modes are

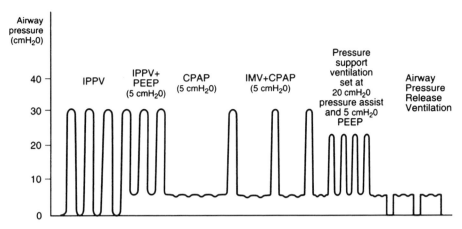

**Figure 19.5.** Different ventilatory modes. IPPV, intermittent positive-pressure ventilation; PEEP, positive end-expiratory pressure; IMV, intermittent mandatory ventilation; CPAP, continuous positive airway pressure.

incorporated into the ventilators being used in intensive care. They can provide many more ways of delivering a tidal volume under pressure. Efficient spontaneous respiration is an essential requirement for successful use of continuous positive airway pressure (CPAP), intermittent mandatory ventilation (IMV) and PSV. Modern ventilators can sense a spontaneous breath and rapidly respond with adequate flow rates. As soon as artificial ventilation is commenced, one should begin planning a weaning strategy that will encourage spontaneous respiration.

The aim of ventilatory assistance has increasingly come to involve guaranteeing adequate oxygenation at safe pressures while tolerating hypercarbia. Hypercarbia, by itself, may not be as harmful as was once thought. Hypercarbia causes peripheral vasodilatation, increases endogenous catecholamine release and will decrease the arterial pH. Relative contraindications to hypercarbia include intracranial abnormalities and cardiac arrhythmias. The rate of change of the $PaCO_2$ is as important as its absolute value. Sudden increases or decreases should be avoided. Where there is no definite contraindication to hypercarbia, oxygenation should be achieved at the lowest PIP. Another way of looking at this aim is to limit the expansion of the lung during any single tidal volume. To achieve that, the difference between the level of end-expiratory pressure and PIP should be minimised. Ideally, that can be achieved with CPAP.

It is very difficult to clinically assess and compare different ventilatory modes. No large trial has shown one technique to be more effective than another. As is true for many aspects of intensive care medicine, **there probably is a best ventilatory technique for a particular patient at a particular time and it is more likely to be found by trial and error than to be by revealed by dogma.** Moreover,

**Table 19.1.** Guidelines to artificial ventilation in intensive care

---

Use conventional IPPV when a patient has neuromuscular disease, when a patient has
been given excessive sedation or neuromuscular blocking agents, or when the lung
compliance or resistance problem is so severe that the patient cannot ventilate
adequately.

When a patient requires assisted ventilation, commence when possible with pressure
assist ± IMV. Then commence the weaning process to CPAP as aggressively as you
would wean a patient off inotropes. First wean to spontaneous respiration, then reduce
the pressure support.

Encourage spontaneous breathing modes such as CPAP, pressure assist or IMV and
accept a higher than normal $PaCO_2$ – permissive hypercarbia. Keep PIP $< 35$ cmH$_2$O.

Maintain PEEP, usually between 5 and 15 cmH$_2$O.

Maintain minimal difference between PIP and PEEP in order to maximise alveolar
recruitment and reduce shearing forces within the lung. Ensure flow rate is high
enough for spontaneous breathing modes.

Check the patient, ventilator and circuit in an attempt to reduce the work of breathing
and facilitate spontaneous respiration.

---

the decision to choose one technique over another should depend on the skill of
the driver rather than on the flashiness of the machine (Table 19.1).

## Continuous positive airway pressure

Continuous positive airway pressure is more than spontaneous breathing with
PEEP. Inspiration is also facilitated by a constant pressure source (Figure 19.5).
Perfect CPAP is achieved when airway pressure is constant throughout the respiratory cycle. This results in minimal work of breathing, increased lung compliance
and improved oxygenation, without the disadvantages of excessive inspiratory
pressure associated with IPPV.

Continuous positive airway pressure addresses the main problem of acute respiratory failure: Oxygenation, as opposed to ventilation. Most patients with
early acute respiratory failure are typically hyperventilating and hypocarbic.
The failure of ventilation becomes increasingly evident as the work of breathing
increases, eventually leading to exhaustion. Often that can be avoided by employing CPAP early in the course of the disease. This increases lung compliance and
decreases the work of breathing which, in turn, prevents reduced lung volumes
and lung collapse.

It must be stressed that for CPAP to function efficiently as a form of respiratory support, the circuit must provide almost constant positive pressure during
both inspiration and expiration, with minimal negative pressure swings during
inspiration. The drop in pressure on inspiration is proportional to the work of

breathing. Currently, many simple continuous flow circuits with an appropriate reservoir bag or a Venturi device offer more efficient CPAP than that available from more expensive and sophisticated ventilators. This is because of the limitations of demand valves used in most ventilators. The work of breathing with a demand valve often is considerably greater than that needed with a continuous flow system.

## Intermittent mandatory ventilation

Intermittent mandatory ventilation provides a spectrum of ventilatory support between total artificial ventilation, on the one hand, and CPAP or total spontaneous ventilation, on the other (Figure 19.5). Mandatory breaths are synchronised with the patient's efforts in most ventilators.

Intermittent mandatory ventilation combines conventional IPPV, which delivers a tidal volume at a predetermined frequency, with gas under pressure for spontaneous breathing. The number of mandatory ventilated breaths that the patient receives is titrated against the need for those breaths, as determined by arterial blood gases and clinical assessment. In between the predetermined mandatory breaths, the patient spontaneously breathes. Intermittent mandatory ventilation is an ideal weaning mode, as the number of mandatory breaths can be reduced according to the patient's need. It is important, however, to reduce the tidal volumes of the mandatory breaths in order to reduce lung damage.

## Mandatory minute volume

Mandatory minute volume (MMV) ensures a predetermined minute volume whether it is composed of spontaneous or mechanical breaths. The major disadvantage of MMV is that the set minute volume may be reached by various inadequate respiratory patterns (e.g. a minute volume of 6 L could be made up of four large breaths of 1.5 L each or 40 breaths at 150 ml each). This problem may be partially overcome by being programmed to disregard breaths below a certain tidal volume. However, IMV may be more useful than MMV, as it guarantees a minimal mechanically delivered tidal volume as well as a minute volume.

## Pressure-support ventilation (inspiratory assist)

This mode is available on most ventilators. Each spontaneous breath is sensed and assisted by a preset amount of positive pressure (Figure 19.5 and Table 19.2). It can be used in two ways. Firstly, low levels (2–10 cmH$_2$O pressure) of 'pressure assist' are needed to overcome the high inherent work of breathing in ventilators during spontaneous respiration. Secondly, high levels (5–50 cmH$_2$O) of assist can be used as a ventilatory mode in its own right. In other words, when the pressure

**Table 19.2.** Respiratory disease models and ventilatory strategies

| Disease | Underlying pathophysiology | PEEP | Inspiratory support |
|---|---|---|---|
| Asthma | Varying proportion of normal or partially and totally obstructed alveoli | Small amount (2–5 cmH$_2$O) may be advantageous | CPAP may reduce work of breathing but IPPV is often necessary, limiting PIP with varying levels of hypercarbia |
| Cardiogenic pulmonary oedema/ALI | Varying proportion of alveoli flood with fluid. Many potentially recruitable alveoli | Usual levels of 5–15 cmH$_2$O | CPAP or Pressure-support/assist modes often successful |
| Severe pneumonia | Varying proportion of densely consolidated alveoli: few potentially recruitable alveoli | Excessive PEEP levels may simply overdistend normal alveoli. Usually <10 cmH$_2$O. | CPAP often not successful. Assisted positive pressure ventilation usually needed. Beware of overdistending normal alveoli causing barotrauma |

assist is set higher than the PEEP level, a form of positive-pressure ventilation occurs. It is, in fact, patient-triggered, pressure-limited IPPV. When the assist level is the same as the PEEP level, it becomes CPAP. Obviously the patient must have an adequate spontaneous respiratory rate for this mode to be successful.

The tidal volume delivered will depend on the preset level of pressure as well as the underlying lung compliance and resistance. This can result in variable tidal volumes and variable rates of $CO_2$ excretion.

Gradually decreasing the level of preset inspiratory pressure in the assist mode will add another dimension to weaning.

### Inverse ratio ventilation

The normal spontaneous inspiration: expiration (I:E) ratio is approximately 1 : 2. By changing I : E ratio to 3 : 1 or even 4 : 1, improvement in oxygenation at a lower mean airway pressure can be achieved, probably by gas trapping and a PEEP effect in the alveoli. The technique of reverse I : E ratio pressure-limited ventilation with small values of PEEP has been used successfully in patients with acute severe respiratory failure. It should be avoided in patients with acute asthma and used with caution in patients with chronic airways disease or in any respiratory disease in which expiration may be delayed. Inverse ratio ventilation is available on many modern ventilators, as well as any ventilator with separate inspiratory and expiratory timing. As is the case for all ventilatory modes, its exact clinical role is not known but when IMV and pressure-support have failed, it may give better ventilation for lower mean airway pressure than can conventional IPPV and PEEP. A patient will require heavy sedation with or without muscle relaxants for this technique to be successful.

## Airway-pressure-release ventilation

This technique involves CPAP with intermittent releases of pressure (Figure 19.5). The intermittent release of pressure from the CPAP level is equivalent to expiration with passive exhalation of gas. The lungs are then reinflated to the CPAP level according to preset timing in combination with a special valve. The degree of ventilatory assistance provided by airway-pressure-release ventilation will be determined by the frequency and duration of pressure release, the CPAP level, the pressure-release level, the patient's lung and thoracic compliance and the flow resistance in the patient's airways and in the pressure-release valve. This technique may offer improved gas exchange with lower mean ITP.

## High frequency positive-pressure ventilation

High frequency positive-pressure ventilation (HFPPV) is a controversial technique that uses small tidal volumes delivered at rapid rates. There are three main types:

- HFPPV 60–120/min.
- High frequency jet ventilation (HFJV) at 60–300/min.
- High frequency oscillation (HFO) at 300–1800/min.

Despite enormous interest in this area, its clinical application in adults is currently limited to the use with bronchopleural fistulae, as well as rare cases in which other modes have failed. Currently, the equipment is complicated, the parameters are not easily monitored and the gases difficult to humidify.

## Recruitment and sighing

Recruitment of alveoli occurs during the whole of inspiration. There is little evidence about the best way of maximising recruitment of alveoli, while at the same time minimising overdistension and rupture of the alveoli. The population of alveoli within diseased lungs are very heterogeneous – some 'fast' or normal alveoli, opening within a fraction of a second, others taking up to 30 seconds and some not being recruitable at all.

De-recruitment is an expiratory phenomenon which is impeded by the length of expiratory time and the amount of expiratory pressure (PEEP).

The optimum level of PEEP, like the optimum ventilatory mode is extremely variable among different patients with different disease states and within the same patient at different times in their illness. The best PEEP may be the one which results in the best $PaO_2/FiO_2$, but this may be at the expense of alveoli overdistension and possible rupture. Suboptimal levels of PEEP result in alveolar collapse and hypoxia but, of course, less overtension and rupture.

Remember in cases of increased chest wall stiffness, such as in obesity or raised intra-abdominal pressure, an increased amount of inspiratory pressure is required to overcome the chest wall stiffness. This increased pressure is not present at the alveolar level resulting in lack of alveolar recruitment and an increased tendency to collapse during expiration. Higher inspiratory pressures and PEEP levels or recruitment manoeuvres may be advantageous for these patients.

There is evidence, especially when using low tidal volumes and low PEEP levels, that alveolar collapse occurs and that regular recruitment manoeuvres may help to open them.

Suggested recruitment manoeuvre: 35–50 cmH$_2$O held for 20–40 seconds.

The beneficial effect (improved oxygenation and lung compliance) of these manoeuvres may last for up to 30 minutes. Similarly sighs, in the same circumstances, may aid alveolar recruitment. Sighs involve increasing the volume or pressure applied to the lungs for 2 or 3 breaths approximately every half-an-hour. A sigh may involve transiently increasing the PEEP level; delivering a controlled inspiration during CPAP; or adding an increased plateau pressure for 2–3 seconds during pressure-limited ventilation.

The disadvantages of recruitment manoeuvres and sighs are the same as for any other ventilatory manoeuvre involving high pressures or volumes: firstly, there may be adverse haemodynamic effects, especially in the presence of hypovolaemia; secondly, alveolar rupture may occur. Like most other aspects of artificial ventilation, there are no strict guidelines as to the indications for these manoeuvres. Perhaps carefully applying these strategies, while at the same time looking for an improvement in oxygenation, is the best way of monitoring the effectiveness of recruitment and sighing.

## Inspiratory waveforms

Although many ventilators provide inspiratory waveform options such as square waves and accelerating or decelerating waves, none has been shown to have a distinct advantage over others in clinical practice. Moreover, the waveforms are generated within the ventilator and become modified in the ventilator tubing, the artificial airway and the patient's own airway.

## Negative pressure ventilation

Interest is being rekindled in this area as the adverse effects of positive-pressure ventilation are increasingly being realised. However, the machinery is expensive and cumbersome and, as yet, is not well suited to many critically ill patients.

## Non-invasive ventilation and BiPAP

Non-invasive positive-pressure ventilation (NIPPV) using a mask has been used successfully in patients with neuromuscular weakness (e.g. Duchennes muscular dystrophy) and restrictive chest wall defects and has become a popular mode for patients with chronic airflow limitation (CAL). Mask ventilation has also been used with some success for patients with acute lung injuries (ALI). One of two modes is commonly used: either pressure-support ventilation or patient-triggered volume-limited IPPV. Non-invasive positive-pressure ventilation is commonly used with bilevel positive airway pressure (BiPAP) which simply supports spontaneous respiration with adjustable levels of PEEP and inspiratory pressures. Non-invasive positive-pressure ventilation appears to reduce the incidence of intubation and positive-pressure ventilation in CAL but not in ALI.

## Proportional assist ventilation

Unlike other forms of assisted ventilation, proportional assist ventilation applies inspiratory pressure according to the patient's effort rather than being preset. The more effort the patient applies the greater the inspiratory assist. It may be viewed as an extra set of respiratory muscles responding to the patient's needs. Flow rate and/or volume are used by the ventilator to determine the level of inspiratory assist.

## Extracorporeal techniques

When conventional ventilation fails to oxygenate adequately or to remove $CO_2$, extracorporeal techniques are sometimes used. Because they are expensive and time-consuming with a high incidence of complications, we need good evidence that extracorporeal techniques make a difference in outcomes. Initial trials using extracorporeal oxygenation failed to show any difference in outcomes. However, the technique is still used in patients with potentially reversible disease when all else has failed. Variations include the following:

### Low frequency positive-pressure ventilation with extracorporeal removal of $CO_2$

This technique is designed to protect the lung from the adverse effects of pressure by insufflating oxygen at low pressures, ventilating at very low rates and removing

$CO_2$ by an extracorporeal circuit. The results in patients with severe respiratory failure have been impressive but the technique requires a high level of expertise, expensive equipment and manpower.

### Independent lung ventilation

## Adjusting the ventilator

Familiarise yourself with the particular ventilator used in your own ICU. Read the instruction manual; use it and discuss it. **Then read the instruction manual again.**

### Basic principles

Guarantee ventilation: Watch the patient's chest movements initially, not the machine.

$FiO_2$ and PEEP level: Set levels to achieve optimal oxygenation. Where possible, keep the PEEP below 10 $cmH_2O$ and the $FiO_2$ below 0.5 cm $H_2O$.

Inspiratory pressure: Wherever possible, reduce the PIP to less than 35 $cmH_2O$.

Monitor: Both the low and high pressure alarms should be set in order to minimise barotrauma and warn of disconnection.

### Portable ventilators

Transport of the seriously ill ventilated patient is increasingly necessary both between hospitals and within a hospital. The oxygen-powered, fluid-logic-controlled, portable ventilators are ideally suited for this purpose. However, they are not suitable for spontaneous respiration and a separate circuit and one-way valve should be incorporated for that purpose.

## Weaning

Weaning is the process of gradually reducing a patient's dependence on ventilatory support. Because of the detrimental effects of artificial ventilation and positive intrathoracic pressure, patients should not be ventilated for any longer than is necessary.

Traditionally, weaning did not commence until the original disease process had been reversed and the $FiO_2$ and PEEP levels were low. Moreover, there had been an obsession with predicting which patients would be capable of being weaned. That is no longer necessary.

With increasing dependence on alternative modes of ventilation, weaning has now become a continual and dynamic process. In contrast with the former pattern of sedating, paralysing and taking over the patient's ventilatory function

**Table 19.3.** Optimising weaning

Provide reassurance and explanation
Limit unnecessary sedation
Treat any underlying disease and correct any reversible problems (e.g. drain pleural
    effusions)
Optimise cardiac function
Use maximum diameter for artificial airways
Increase trigger sensitivity
Adjust inspiratory support
Use high flow rates or large, compliant reservoir bags
Suction and attempt to reduce airway secretions
Place patient in upright posture when possible
Limit the length and weight of ventilator tubing
Limit $CO_2$ production (e.g. fever)
Correct electrolyte and acid-base disorders
Relieve pain
Reverse bronchospasm
Try to facilitate adequate sleep
Ensure nutritional support

totally, various ventilatory modes have been developed that encourage spontaneous breathing and are appropriate for a particular patient at a particular time
in a given illness. A general approach (Table 19.3) is to correct as many of the
reversible abnormalities as possible (e.g. electrolytes and fluid status), choose a
ventilatory circuit and mode that will require minimal work for spontaneous
breathing and then to give it a go! In other words, continually adjust the ventilatory mode and settings to the patient's needs. The number of breaths and pressure
assistance should be continually reduced, weaning the patient in the same way
we continually wean from inotropes (i.e. based on regular patient assessments).

## Patient assessment during weaning

Vital signs: Signs such as respiratory rate, tidal volume, oxygen saturation levels,
pulse rate, colour and BP must all be monitored carefully during weaning.
Patient appearance: Monitoring the clinical appearance of the patient is a useful
way of assessing the success of weaning. Signs of increased work of breathing
include tachypnoea, sweating, increased use of accessory muscles, obvious distress
and unco-ordinated respiration. Trained nursing and medical staff in intensive
care can recognise these signs at an early stage and adjust the weaning process
accordingly.

    Arterial $CO_2$: Monitoring the partial pressure of arterial $CO_2$ is another way
of assessing weaning. There are many reasons why the $PaCO_2$ can be higher than
normal in the seriously ill and as long as the arterial pH is above a certain limit
(e.g. hydrogen-ion concentration < 63 nmol/L or pH > 7.2), a high $PaCO_2$ is not

necessarily unacceptable. During weaning, the PaCO2 will transiently rise, until the patient readjusts to levels of $PaCO_2$ and pH which determine respiratory rate. Patience and tolerating higher levels of $PaCO_2$ is required.

## Weaning sequence

One should aim for the following as soon as possible:

1 Wean the patient from controlled ventilation to spontaneous breathing – CPAP or pressure support ventilation.
2 Wean $FiO_2$ levels to less than 0.5.
3 Wean PEEP levels (not below 5 $cmH_2O$).

## Techniques for weaning

### Intermittent mandatory ventilation

Intermittent mandatory ventilation provides a natural basis for weaning. Patients should be encouraged to breathe spontaneously on CPAP during acute respiratory failure. When that is not possible, the number of mandatory breaths from the ventilator should be adjusted according to need. Similarly, and whenever possible, the number of mandatory breaths should be decreased in the same way that inotropes are increased or decreased to support cardiovascular function.

### Pressure-support ventilation

By gradually decreasing the preset amount of patient triggered positive-pressure-support, another dimension to weaning is possible. Many modern ventilators have this mode as well as IMV and the two usually are used together to facilitate weaning.

### T-piece system

Weaning with a T-piece system involves alternating between breathing sponta-neously through a T-piece circuit and using mandatory ventilation. The time period for each will vary according to the patient's condition. This all or none technique has been largely superseded by IMV and pressure-support ventilation. Unlike IMV, a T-piece circuit does not have the flexibility for a specific amount of controlled ventilatory support to be tailored for each patient.

## The work of breathing

The work of breathing must be minimised if there is to be success in weaning. It may even be possible to avoid the use of ventilation if the work of breathing can be reduced. Many of the newer modes of ventilatory support can specifically decrease the work of breathing (e.g. CPAP and pressure-support ventilation), so that mandatory IPPV can be avoided. The work of breathing is related to the pressure generated by the respiratory muscles when displacing a volume of gas.

## Measuring the work of breathing

It is very difficult to get accurate measurements of the work of breathing in intensive care. The current techniques are complicated and require sophisticated technology. In clinical practice, patient observation is often used. If the work of breathing is excessive, the patient will look distressed, sweaty and tachypnoeic with excessive use of the accessory muscles of respiration. If the patient is being ventilated or is on CPAP, the initial drop in inspiratory pressure necessary to achieve a spontaneous breath will correlate well with the work of breathing. A high negative pressure means increased work of breathing.

## Clinical aspects of the work of breathing

To minimise the work of breathing, meticulous attention must be paid to the various patient and equipment-related determinants. It is not simply a matter of increasing the pressure support or maintaining IPPV in order to 'rest the patient'. Often ventilation can be avoided or weaning facilitated by meticulously examining every component that may be contributing to increase the work of breathing.

### Patient determinants

1 Airway (resistive forces)

Secretions: Even minimal secretions can reduce the airway diameter and increase the work of breathing. Regularly perform airway suction and physiotherapy.

Bronchospasm: A decreased airway diameter is a crucial factor in causing increased resistance and increased work of breathing. Bronchospasm must be reversed with bronchodilators.

2 Chest wall and lung compliance (elastic forces)

Treat any underlying disease (ALI, pneumonia, atelectasis) that decreases lung compliance. Sit the patient upright in order to increase compliance. Aggressively drain air pockets or pleural effusions.

3 Minute volume and $CO_2$ production

The major determinant of the work of breathing is the minute volume. This can be reduced by decreasing physiological and anatomic dead space. Excessive $CO_2$ production can cause increased minute volume and should be limited by reducing fever and perhaps reducing the carbohydrate intake. Shivering, inotropes, agitation, seizures, myoclonus and any other causes of excessive muscle activity can also increase $CO_2$ production.

4 Expiratory work

Increasingly it is being realised that expiration requires work in certain pathological conditions (e.g. asthma) and in all patients who are intubated and connected to breathing systems.

Resistance can be reduced by minimising airway secretions and bronchospasm, as well as by reducing the length and increasing the diameter of artificial airways and circuits. Some PEEP valves (e.g. mushroom and scissor valves) have high expiratory resistance. The PEEP levels should be increased when intrinsic PEEP is suspected.

## Equipment determinants

1  Artificial airway

The single most important equipment-related determinant of the work of breathing is the diameter of the artificial airway. A tube with the largest possible diameter should be employed. For this reason, orotracheal tubes and tracheostomy tubes have distinct advantages over nasotracheal tubes in spontaneously breathing patients. The larger the diameter of the tube, the less the resistance. Tracheostomy tubes of 8 mm for females and 9 mm for males will significantly reduce the work of breathing, as compared with tubes that are even one size smaller. The length of the tube and an absence of built-up secretions are also important. Similarly, kinks should be avoided, angles minimised and large connectors should be used.

2  Circuit and humidifier

An increased length of tubing will cause increased resistance. Humidifiers with inspiratory underwater baffles should be avoided and condenser humidifiers changed regularly.

3  CPAP devices

A continuous flow device usually will decrease the work of breathing, as compared with the demand valve systems incorporated into modern ventilators. Large compliant reservoir bags are more effective than small non-compliant ones and whereas flow rates in the ventilator can decrease the work of breathing, turbulence can result if the flow is too high, thus increasing the work of breathing.

4  Ventilators

Techniques such as pressure-support were developed to decrease the inherently high work of breathing with demand valve systems. The demand valve should be adjusted to maximum sensitivity and the peak inspiratory flow rate (PIFR) needs to be high (at least four times the minute volume, i.e. 50 L/min) or to just exceed the patient's PIFR. A minimum amount of PEEP (3–5 cmH$_2$O) and pressure-support (5 cmH$_2$O) should be used for all spontaneously breathing patients supported by a ventilator.

## Humidification

Whenever the nose and mouth are bypassed, inspired gases should be humidified and heated artificially. The following are minimum requirements for humidification.

Water content: The 'absolute' or maximum humidity at a temperature of 37 °C is 44 mg/L; this is achieved with normal nose breathing. For artificial ventilation, it is suggested that gases have a water content of at least between 30–40 mg/L and be heated to 37 °C in order to protect ciliary function.

Resistance: For spontaneous respiration, resistance should be minimal ($< 3$ $cmH_2O \cdot L^{-1} \cdot s^{-1}$ [$< 0.29 \, kPa \cdot L^{-1} \cdot s^{-1}$]).

Safety alarms: Alarms are needed as protection against overheating and over-hydration in hot water bath humidifiers.

## Condenser humidifiers

A condenser humidifier consists of a tube containing material that conserves heat and water from the patient's expiratory efforts.

Advantages:

- simple
- safe
- disposable.

Disadvantages:

- inefficient humidification with high flow rates and high $FiO_2$
- increased dead space
- risk of infection
- increased risk of endotracheal tube occlusion
- resistance can increase with use.

Their main disadvantage – inefficient humidification – makes condenser humidifiers suitable only for short-term artificial ventilation such as intraoperatively. The place of condenser humidifiers in the ICU has not been precisely determined. Because of the increased dead space and resistance, as well as the increased tendency for occlusion, they should be avoided during any long-term ventilatory mode that employs spontaneous breathing.

## Hot water bath humidifiers

These devices provide the most common form of humidification in the ICU. Inspired gas passes over the water surface before delivery to the patient. Modifications can include increasing the surface area by using coils of absorbing paper and using heated delivery lines to prevent condensation.

The temperatures of the water bath and heating wires should be adjusted to achieve a delivery temperature of close to 37 °C.

Disadvantages:

Infection: The water reservoir and tubing should be changed every 24–48 hours. Only sterile water should be used.

## TROUBLESHOOTING

### Fighting the ventilator

Is the problem with the patient or with the ventilator?
Observe for air entry.
Take the patient off the ventilator and 'bag' the patient.

### Patient

Listen for air entry.
Exclude blocked artificial airway and remove tube if in doubt.
Exclude the possibility of hypoxia and hypercarbia.
Check the chest x-ray.
Often a ventilated patient will be 'distressed' because of the increased work of breathing
associated with the underlying lung disease: decreased lung compliance (e.g. ALI,
pneumonia) or increased resistance (e.g. asthma).
Check arterial pH – acidosis of any origin is a very strong driver of ventilation.
Consider providing reassurance, relieving pain or increasing the sedation only after
excluding other causes.

### Ventilator

Check the ventilator function while 'bagging' the patient.
Check the circuit, including the humidifier (especially if using a heat and moisture
humidifier, which can develop increased resistance over time).
Eliminate sources of increased work when the patient is spontaneously breathing.
Check the airway diameter and the length of the artificial airway. Ideally, adult
males should have, as a minimum, a 9-mm diameter tube and adult women an
8-mm tube.
CPAP systems: Spontaneous breathing systems should have minimal respiratory
pressure swings.
Check that the ventilator settings match the patient's needs. For instance, one may
need to
increase tidal volume
increase pressure support
decrease trigger threshold
increase flow rate
increase number of breaths on IMV.

Overheating: Adequate alarm and safety devices should be employed to prevent
overheating and hyperpyrexia.
Inadequate humidification: Flow rates for fully humidified gas as high as 60 L/min
can be achieved with some of the more modern humidifiers. If higher flows are
required, a dual system of gas delivery using two humidifiers may be necessary.

## FURTHER READING

### General

Bersten, A. D. A simple bedside approach to measurement of respiratory mechanics in critically ill patients. *Critical Care and Resuscitation* 1 (1999): 74–84.

Marini, J. J. Recruitment maneuvers to achieve an "open lung" – Whether and how? *Critical Care Medicine* 29 (2001): 1647–8.

Pinsky, M. R. The hemodynamic consequences of mechanical ventilation: an evolving story. *Intensive Care Medicine* 23 (1997): 493–503.

Tobin, M. J. Advances in mechanical ventilation. *New England Journal of Medicine* 344 (2001): 1986–96.

### Complications of positive intrathoracic pressure

International Consensus Conferences in Intensive Care Medicine. Ventilatory-associated lung injury in ARDS. Official conference report cosponsored by the American Thoracic Society, the European Society of Intensive Care Medicine and the Societe de Reanimation de Langue Francaise and approved by the ATS Board of Directors. *Intensive Care Medicine* 25 (1999): 1444–52.

Dos Santos, C. C. and Slutsky, A. S. Mechanotransduction, ventilatory-induced lung injury and multiple organ dysfunction syndrome. *Intensive Care Medicine* 26 (2000): 638–42.

### Modes of ventilation

Evans, T. W. Organised jointly by the American Thoracic Society, the European Respiratory Society, the European Society of Intensive Care Medicine, and the Siociete de Reanimation de Langue Francaise and approved by the ATS Board of Directors, December 2000. International consensus conferences in intensive care medicine: non-invasive positive-pressure ventilation in acute respiratory failure. *Intensive Care Medicine* 27 (2001): 166–78.

The Acute Respiratory Distress Syndrome Network. Ventilation with lower tidal volumes as compared with traditional tidal volumes for acute lung injury and the acute respiratory distress syndrome. *New England Journal of Medicine* 342 (2000): 1301–8.

Keenan, S. P., Kernerman, P. D., Cook, D. J., Martin, C. M., McCormack, D. and Sibbald, W. J. Effect of noninvasive positive-pressure ventilation on mortality in patients admitted with acute respiratory failure: a meta-analysis. *Critical Care Medicine* 25 (1997): 1685–92.

Keogh, B. F. and Bateman, C. J. Lung protective ventilatory strategies – will these prevail in the next millennium? *British Journal of Anaesthesia* 83 (1999): 829–32.

Kuhlen, R. and Rossaint, R. Proportional assist ventilation. *Intensive Care Medicine* 25 (1999): 1021–3.

Suter, P. M. Let us recruit the lung and keep an open mind. Editorial. *Intensive Care Medicine* 26 (2000): 491–2.

## Weaning

Esteban, A. and Alia, I. Clinical management of weaning from mechanical ventilation. *Intensive Care Medicine* 24 (1998): 999–1008.

## Work of breathing

French, C. J. Work of breathing measurement in the critically ill patient. *Anaesthesia and Intensive Care* 27 (1999): 561–73.

## Humidification

William, R., Rankin, N., Smith, T., Galler, D. and Seakins, P. Relationship between the humidity and temperature of inspired gas and the function of the airway mucosa. *Critical Care Medicine* 24 (1996): 1920–9.

# 20

# Cardiorespiratory monitoring

- There is no single value for any physiological variable that can be said to be the normal value. Measurements should be interpreted more in terms of being adequate or inadequate.
- Trends are more important than single values.
- Continuous monitoring of oxygenation is indispensable in intensive care.
- It is important to understand the limitations of sophisticated invasive monitoring and the value of clinical observations and simple monitoring.

The heart and lungs together are responsible for pumping oxygenated blood to the tissues. The process of monitoring the effectiveness of oxygenation cannot be broken apart and divided between the cardiovascular and respiratory systems.

Although intensive care medicine traditionally has been associated with sophisticated, expensive and invasive techniques, that orientation is now being critically examined. There is a trend toward simpler, continuous monitoring techniques that are non-invasive.

It is important to display physiological variables clearly and to interpret their significance accurately. A single flowchart will facilitate documentation and interpretation. However, such information can reflect only an instant in time. Continuous displays of measurements such as ECG, pulse oximetry and intravascular pressures are often employed to track the more useful information revealed by trend data.

Current techniques for cardiorespiratory monitoring often are limited to global and relatively crude measurements. The obsession in the 1970s with generating numbers derived from the pulmonary artery catheter has been largely superseded by the desire to achieve continuous, non-invasive monitoring. However, even the new devices designed for that purpose usually have been limited to measurements of global functions such as arterial oxygen saturation, blood pressure and expired partial pressure of carbon dioxide. More complex and more invasive measurements such as determining the relationship between oxygen delivery ($DO_2$) and

**Table 20.1.** Non-invasive and invasive cardiorespiratory monitoring

---

Non-invasive cardiorespiratory monitoring
    Pulse rate and rhythm
    Blood pressure
    Peripheral perfusion
    Temperature (core/peripheral difference)
    Urine output
    Echocardiography
    Non-invasive cardiac output
    Radionuclide imaging
    Respiratory rate and character
    Tidal volume
    Pulse oximetry
    Capnography
    Chest radiograph
    Fluid balance
Invasive cardiorespiratory monitoring
    Central venous pressure
    Arterial pressure monitoring
    Pulmonary artery catheterisation
    Pulmonary artery pressure
    PAWP
    Cardiac output
    Oxygen consumption
    Oxygen delivery
    Mixed venous oximetry
    Lung water

---

oxygen consumption ($VO_2$), are difficult to perform, prone to inaccuracies and hard to interpret and at best they tell us about the whole body, rather than the status of individual tissues. It is to be hoped that the next major breakthrough in monitoring will bring us practical, reliable, inexpensive, non-invasive means to achieve continuous monitoring of cardiorespiratory function at the tissue or cellular level (Table 20.1).

## Non-invasive monitoring

### Heart rate and rhythm

Although it can be affected by many factors in the seriously ill, the heart rate remains a valuable source of information and a parameter that is easy to measure. Most seriously ill patients are connected to an ECG monitor with a continuously displayed ECG trace, with alarms to detect the extremes of heart rate. In addition to heart rate, ECG monitoring can detect arrhythmias and pacemaker functioning and ST-segment analysis can reveal myocardial ischaemia.

## Blood pressure

Vital organs depend on autoregulation for their blood flow. The kidney, heart and brain need effective driving pressures across their vascular beds for adequate perfusion. Non-invasive and invasive techniques for measuring BP correlate well. There are increasing numbers of automatic devices that can display non-invasively measured BP.

## Peripheral/core temperature difference

The relative 'coolness' of distal limbs can serve as a rapid and useful guide to peripheral perfusion. Measuring the central temperature and comparing it with the measured peripheral temperature (e.g. temperature of the big toe) probably is not necessary. Estimating the degree of coolness of the periphery (e.g. toes, feet, lower half of the leg) can give an empirical impression of circulatory status. The difference between peripheral and central temperatures cannot be used to discriminate among cardiac failure, hypovolaemia and other forms of cardiovascular failure and cannot be quantified.

## Urine output

The kidney is very sensitive to changes in BP and flow. Hourly measurements of urine output can give an excellent reflection of general tissue perfusion. This method loses some of its value in the presence of drugs such as diuretics, glycosuria or when renal function is compromised.

## Respiratory rate and type of breathing

Simple measurements or observations of respiratory rate and type of breathing can provide information about the disease process, as well as the effects of drugs and lung mechanics.

## Tidal volume

Tidal volume is relatively easy to measure in a spontaneously breathing, intubated patient. Most ventilators have mechanisms for measuring and displaying tidal volume and minute volume. However, even more important than tidal volume or minute volume is the end product of effective ventilation: adequate gas exchange.

## Chest radiograph (see Chapter 17)

The chest x-ray provides important clinical information that cannot be elicited by physical examination and should be obtained at least once each day for most seriously ill patients. Additional x-rays will be needed following intubation and central line placement. The radiography should be performed whenever possible, with the patient sitting upright so that abnormal fluid and air collections can be seen. The chest x-ray can allow for effective monitoring of fluid status, as lung water content will correlate reasonably well with chest x-ray density.

## Fluid balance

Fluid balance has some bearing on intravascular fluid status, but there are many better and more direct measurements. Although fluid balance can give an excellent indication of the fluid losses from certain sites (e.g. nasogastric (NG) contents and wounds), the net figure measured every 24 hours is misleading as there are many 'unseen' inputs and outputs that are not measured (e.g. water of oxidation, insensible losses). Furthermore, a single net figure cannot indicate which of the body's fluid spaces are depleted, nor what fluid should be used for replenishment (see Chapter 4).

## Tissue perfusion

Doppler laser devices for measuring blood flow in the skin may become more widely employed. Currently, we estimate general tissue perfusion on the basis of parameters such as urine output and peripheral skin temperature.

Transcutaneous $PO_2$ monitoring can also provide an early and accurate non-invasive indicator of the adequacy of $DO_2$ to the skin.

## Tissue pH and $CO_2$ levels

The presence of compensated shock is difficult to detect with global measurements of variables such as BP, and pulse rate, cardiac output, $VO_2$ and $DO_2$. Moreover, compensated shock can result in ischaemia of organs such as the gastrointestinal tract (GIT). The GIT is selectively impaired in patients who are in shock. It is one of the first organs affected and one of the last to be restored by resuscitation. Measurement of GIT perfusion is therefore important and can be estimated on the basis of the intramural pH (pHi) or more accurately, gastric tonometer derived gastric arterial $CO_2$ difference. The tonometer consists of a catheter with a Silastic balloon at its tip which is introduced into the stomach. The balloon is filled with saline and allowed to equilibrate with luminal $PCO_2$, which is assumed to be the same as $PCO_2$ of the superficial mucosa. Determination of the arterial bicarbonate concentration will allow calculation of the pHi using the

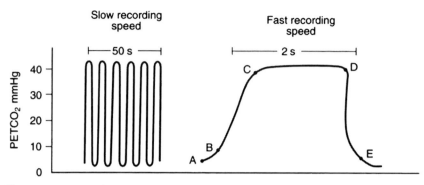

**Figure 20.1.** Normal capnogram.

Henderson–Hasselbalch equation. This measurement reflects splanchnic tissue oxygenation and is an indirect and early estimate of global tissue oxygenation.

## Capnography

A capnometer measures the concentration of $CO_2$, usually by infrared analysis. A device that continuously records and displays $CO_2$ concentrations as a waveform is a capnograph (Figure 20.1). Capnography is the study of the shape of the curve that shows the changing concentrations of $CO_2$ in expired gas. The end-tidal $CO_2$ ($ETCO_2$) will depend on the amount produced by the body and on the adequacy of transport to and across the lungs.

Potential uses of capnography in intensive care:

- At intubation, a normal $ETCO_2$ can help confirm tracheal placement of the ETT.
- End-tidal $CO_2$ monitoring can warn of sudden changes in the breathing system because of leaks, disconnections or obstruction.
- Capnography can give an indication of the efficiency of the weaning process.
- Capnography can provide information about hypoventilation and hyperventilation, apnoea and periodic breathing.
- Carbon dioxide elimination and physiological dead space can be measured by measuring the $CO_2$ fraction in mixed expired gases. This can give an indication of metabolic activity.
- A reduction in cardiac output will be accompanied by a reduction in expired $CO_2$. This can result from any form of shock. Air embolism or blockage of the pulmonary capillaries due to any cause can also decrease expired $CO_2$. Mixed venous $CO_2$ is more dependent on changes in alveolar ventilation than on cardiac output. A difference between the concentrations of arterial $CO_2$ and mixed venous $CO_2$ is most likely to be produced by low cardiac output. Tissue hypoxia can be assumed when this difference exceeds 10 ml/dl.

**Table 20.2.** Application of transoesophageal echocardiography

Continuous intraoperative monitoring (e.g. myocardial ischaemia, adequacy of
  surgical repair)
Thoracic aortic pathology (e.g. dissection, aneurysm)
Valvular function (particularly the mitral valve)
Excluding infective endocarditis and its complications
Intracardiac masses (e.g. thrombi, tumours)
Coronary artery disease
Congenital heart disease
Information on cardiac contractility, filling status and output can be used

There are limitations to capnography with regard to the predictability of the
correlation between $ETCO_2$ and $PaCO_2$. The difference between arterial $PaCO_2$
and $ETCO_2$ is due to alveolar dead space. In patients with respiratory failure or
rapidly changing cardiovascular conditions, that correlation is even less reliable.
Although capnography theoretically should have many uses in the ICU, it has not
universally replaced intermittent arterial $PCO_2$ monitoring in the way that pulse
oximetry has come to be used as a continuous form of oxygenation monitoring.

## Pulse oximetry

Pulse oximetry is discussed in detail elsewhere.

## Echocardiography

Echocardiography is increasingly being used to assess cardiac function (Table
20.2). It can be used to diagnose abnormalities of structure (e.g. valves, pericardial
effusions) as well as to assess functioning by directly revealing wall movement and
defining the chamber dimensions throughout the cardiac cycle, thereby allowing
estimation of the ejection fraction. The technique also can be used to diagnose
pulmonary embolism, valvular infections and aortic dissection. Its use in the
ICU has been limited because of the distortion of ultrasound waves passing
through air and bone. In up to 30% of seriously ill patients, hyperinflated
lungs due to underlying abnormalities or secondary to ventilation can cause
inadequate images. The use of transoesophageal echocardiography (TOE) gives
a much cleaner image of the heart and offers real time bedside diagnosis and
monitoring of a variety of structural and functional abnormalities of the heart.
It provides information on cardiac contractility, filling status and output.

## Non-invasive determination of cardiac output

There are many techniques for non-invasive determination of cardiac output. One
technique employs Doppler ultrasonic velocimetry in conjunction with ultrasonic

**Table 20.3.** Some limitations of cardiorespiratory measurements and monitoring

*Haemoglobin saturation*
Only measured saturations should be used when calculating the shunt equation and $DO_2$ and
  $VO_2$ as there can be large differences between measured and calculated oxygen saturation

*Arterial pressure*
Direct monitoring is more accurate then indirect pressure measurement
The femoral artery is the best site for accurate pressure measurements
Short, non-compliant catheters and extension tubing should be used
Avoid bubbles and clots in the system

*Atrial pressures*
With the patient supine, mid-axillary line is the standard site for atrial pressure measurement
The pulmonary artery waveform display is necessary to detect inadvertent wedging and
  overwedging and to visualise respiratory variations
End-expiratory readings should be used
The PAWP measurements should be from a proximal branch of the pulmonary artery in a West
  zone III part of the lung
Remember the limitations of PAWP as representative of left ventricular end-diastolic volume or
  lung capillary pressure

*Cardiac output*
The temperature difference between injectate and blood temperature should be maximal
Standardise injections to end expiration

echo imaging of the ascending aorta in order to determine stroke volume. The
product of stroke volume and heart rate is then used to determine cardiac output.
All of these measurements are non-invasive. However, this technique involves
many assumptions and has inherent inaccuracies and, as yet, there is no universal
agreement on its correlation with more established techniques.

# Invasive monitoring

## Monitoring of arterial blood pressure

Direct measurement of arterial pressure is common in the ICU, both for continuous monitoring and for blood sampling. It is therefore little trouble to connect a
transducer and monitor the arterial BP continuously. Directly measured arterial
pressure may vary from that measured indirectly. Both techniques have inherent
inaccuracies and, as with most measurements, the trend should be looked at,
rather than an absolute reading (Table 20.3).

Arterial catheters: The modified Allen test is rarely used now to assess collateral
flow before insertion of a catheter. Usually a catheter will be inserted into the radial
artery, but the dorsalis pedis, brachial, axillary and femoral arteries can also be
used. There does not appear to be a higher incidence of infection with femoral

artery cannulation. If there are no signs of infection, the catheter does not need to be changed routinely.

The main complication of arterial catheterisation is thrombosis. It is common, but it rarely causes serious morbidity. The catheters should be removed immediately if there are any signs of ischaemia. Complications such as emboli, haemorrhage, infection and inadvertent injection of drugs are much rarer. Very small amounts of air can travel retrogradely into cerebral vessels and so great care must be exercised, especially during flushing.

## Central venous pressure

In most cases, a seriously ill patient will have a line inserted into a central vein to facilitate drug and fluid infusion. As with arterial monitoring, the central venous line can also be used for pressure monitoring.

The normal central venous pressure (CVP) is normally 0–8 mmHg (0–1.1 kPa), but there are many possible causes of right-side heart dysfunction and high pulmonary artery pressure in the critically ill. This can mean that the 'normal' CVP is high. **A high CVP may be a reflection of pulmonary abnormality, high pulmonary artery pressure or high ventilatory pressure, rather than a reflection of cardiac dysfunction or intravascular volume disturbance**. Moreover, the CVP can be high, normal, or low in the presence of hypovolaemia. Trends, rather than single readings, must be looked at. Right atrial pressure often is not a reflection of left atrial pressure in the seriously ill.

A catheter can be inserted from the cubital fossa or directly from the thorax via the subclavian or internal jugular vein. The femoral vein can also be used. Complications of central venous cannulation can include pneumothorax, arterial puncture, haemothorax, nerve damage, air embolism, catheter embolism, cardiac perforation and tamponade, venous thrombosis and embolism, as well as infection. These complications are common, but serious complications occur in fewer than 2% of these patients and death is extremely uncommon.

A chest x-ray should always be performed after insertion of a central catheter to check for positioning and complications (e.g. pneumothorax and mediastinal bleeding). The tip should lie outside the boundaries of the pericardial sac, in any large vein above or below the heart. The carina is a valuable and simple anatomical landmark for correct placement. If infection is suspected, the catheter should be removed, the skin site should be swabbed and material adhering to the tip or intradermal section should be cultured. Two sets of peripheral blood cultures should be taken.

## Pulmonary artery catheter

No other instrument is so strongly associated with the practice of intensive care medicine as the flow-directed pulmonary artery (PA) catheter. To 'Swan' a patient, or put in a 'Ganz', has become one of the hallmarks of our specialty. It became an impressive and unusual skill amongst those practising in the ICU. The mystique became exaggerated because of the enormous number of figures and amount of data that could be generated from a few measurements. Such abundant figures often served to complicate a simple picture. The catheter itself was probably overused. As in the case of many innovations in medicine, we are now critically redefining the role of the PA catheter. It is expensive and needs complicated machinery to support it; it also requires valuable labour time to insert it and maintain it. That, of course, could be justified if it could be shown to significantly affect patient outcomes. Unfortunately, this has never been demonstrated. Furthermore, measurements of parameters such as pulmonary artery wedge pressure (PAWP) may be of limited value in the critically ill, and many of the derived variables such as pulmonary vascular resistance may be meaningless.

Indications: The indications for insertion of a PA catheter have not been defined. The rates at which PA catheters are used vary for different ICUs and between different countries. Some physicians insert them whenever a central line is needed; others never use them. We await studies demonstrating the usefulness of PA catheters and detailing the precise indications for their use.

There are two situations in which a PA catheter may prove useful:

1  Where there is difficulty with fluid replacement, especially in patients in whom cardiac function is also compromised, this is particularly important in patients with pulmonary oedema and renal failure.
2  Where oxygen supply and demand needs to be more precisely defined.

Complications: The complications of a PA catheter can include all the complications associated with insertion of central venous catheters (see p.   ), as well as arrhythmias (usually terminated by withdrawal), bundle branch block, pulmonary infarction, pulmonary artery rupture and knotting, and damage to the endocardial structures of the heart.

The risks begin to outweigh the potential benefits after 48 hours and the catheter should be removed as soon as possible after this time.

## Pulmonary artery wedge pressure

The PA catheter is inserted in the same way as a central venous catheter. A distal balloon is inflated to facilitate its passage through the right side of the heart into the pulmonary artery (Figure 20.2). When the balloon is wedged in a small branch of the pulmonary artery, the distal lumen should be measuring a pressure that is a reflection of the left atrial pressure, assuming that there is a continuous column of fluid from the tip of the catheter to the left atrium. This assumption may be affected by factors such as alveolar pressure and the zone of the lung where the tip resides. The catheter tip should be placed in zone III of the lung, confirmed

**Table 20.4.** Conditions that can result in discrepancies between PAWP and left ventricular end-diastolic pressure

Mitral valvular disease
Aortic incompetence
IPPV + PEEP
Increased intrathoracic pressure from any cause
Left to right intracardiac shunt
Increased pulmonary artery resistance
Tachycardia
Chronic airflow limitation
Catheter not placed in West zone III
Non-compliant left ventricle
Reduced pulmonary vasculature (e.g. pulmonary embolism or pneumonectomy)

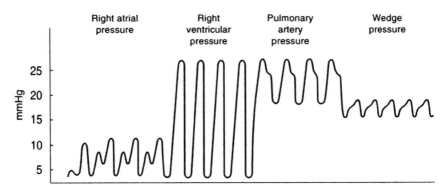

**Figure 20.2.** Waveforms generated by a PA catheter as it is floated into the pulmonary artery.

by a chest x-ray showing the tip below the left atrium. Alternatively, one can be reasonably sure of correct positioning if the PAWP reading is not markedly affected by a sudden increase or decrease in positive end-expiratory pressure (PEEP). Even when the catheter is correctly positioned, it can be difficult to assess left ventricular preload by PAWP. This is particularly the case in the critically ill where the relationship between end-diastolic pressure and volume (compliance) is non-linear (Table 20.4 and Table 20.5). As a guideline, however, a PAWP of more than 18 mmHg will be associated with increased lung water in patients with cardiogenic pulmonary oedema. In ALI, the accumulation of lung water will increase as the PAWP increases. However, reduction of preload can lead to decreased cardiac output and generalised ischaemia, especially renal insufficiency in the critically ill. Often, therefore, an increase in lung water will be accepted as the price for adequate tissue perfusion.

**Table 20.5.** Assumptions in the measurement of PAWP

| |
|---|
| Left ventricular end-diastolic volume |
|   ↓   LV compliance normal |
| Left ventricular end-diastolic pressure |
|   ↓   Normal mitral valve |
| Left atrial pressure |
|   ↓   Normal airway pressure |
| Pulmonary artery wedge pressure |
|   ↓   Normal pulmonary vascular resistance |
| Pulmonary artery diastolic pressure |
|   ↓   Right side of heart equals left side |
| Central venous pressure |

## Cardiac output

The cardiac output is usually measured by the thermodilution method, using a PA catheter with a thermistor near the tip. A known volume of fluid is injected near the right atrium and the blood flow is calculated from the temperature drop sensed by the thermistor in the PA after mixing has occurred. The cardiac output or index can be used as a prognostic indicator and guide to treatment. The adequacy of cardiac output must be judged in light of whether or not $DO_2$ is adequate. Sepsis and trauma are commonly associated with a high cardiac output. It is better to avoid thinking in terms of a 'normal' cardiac output – it is either adequate or inadequate for $DO_2$ (Table 20.6).

## Mixed venous oxygen saturation

The mixed venous oxygen saturation ($SvO_2$) can be measured intermittently as a sample taken from the PA catheter, or continuously by a modified PA catheter with a sensing device at its tip. The $SvO_2$ reflects the status of oxygen supply and consumption (Table 20.7). The oxygen supply is dependent on cardiac output, haemoglobin concentration and arterial oxygen concentration. The demand side of the equation depends on cellular extraction of oxygen. Normal $SvO_2$ is approximately 60–80%. A decreasing $SvO_2$ indicates that the demand is becoming greater than the supply.

When the compensatory mechanism for matching oxygen demand and supply are exhausted, at approximately 40% of normal levels, lactic acidosis is likely to occur. A sudden significant decrease in $SvO_2$ (10–20%) indicates that an urgent clinical review is necessary. An increase in $SvO_2$ indicates that arterial oxygen supply has increased or that demand has decreased (e.g. hypothermia, paralysis, sedation); septic shock can also be associated with an increase in $SvO_2$ because of decreased tissue oxygen extraction. This may paradoxically occur in the presence

**Table 20.6.** Some measured and calculated haemodynamic variables with normal ranges

| Parameter | Measurement | Normal |
|---|---|---|
| Systemic BP (mean) | Direct | 120/80 (mean 95) mmHg (15.9/10.6 (12.5) kPa) |
| Pulmonary artery pressure (mean) (PAP) | Direct | 20/10 (mean 13) mmHg (2.6/1.3 kPa) |
| Heart rate (HR) | Direct | $80 \pm 10$ beats/min |
| PAWP | Direct | $10 \pm 2$ mmHg ($1.3 \pm 0.3$ kPa) |
| CVP | Direct | 0–8 mmHg (0–1.1 kPa) |
| Cardiac index (CI) | Direct | $3.0 \pm 0.5 \; \text{L} \cdot \text{min}^{-1} \cdot \text{m}^{-2}$ |
| Stroke volume index | CI/HR $\times$ 1000 | $40 \pm 7 \; \text{ml} \cdot \text{beat}^{-1} \cdot \text{m}^{-2}$ |
| Systemic vascular resistance index (SVRI) | $\dfrac{\text{MAP}^a - \text{CVP}}{\text{CI}} \times 80 \, \text{dyn-s} \cdot \text{cm}^{-5}$ | $1760 - 2600 \; \text{dyn-s} \cdot \text{cm}^{-5} \cdot \text{m}^2$ |
| Pulmonary vascular resistance index (PVRI) | $\dfrac{\text{PAP} - \text{PAWP}}{\text{CI}} \times 80 \, \text{dyn-s} \cdot \text{cm}^{-5}$ | $45 - 225 \; \text{dyn-s} \cdot \text{cm}^{-5} \cdot \text{m}^2$ |
| $O_2$ consumption ($VO_2$) | Direct, or CI $\times$ ($CaO_2 - CvO_2$) $\times$ 10 | $100 - 170 \; \text{ml} \cdot \text{min}^{-1} \cdot \text{m}^2$ |
| $O_2$ delivery | CI $\times$ ($CaO_2$) $\times$ 10 | $520 - 720 \; \text{ml} \cdot \text{min}^{-1} \cdot \text{m}^2$ |
| $O_2$ extraction | ($CaO_2 - CvO_2$)/$CaO_2$ | $22 - 30\%$ |

**Table 20.7.** Mixed venous oxygen saturation

$SvO_2$ describes the adequacy of oxygen delivery relative to oxygen consumption
Major determinants
 $O_2$ consumption
 Cardiac output
Normal values
 $SvO_2$, 60–80%
 $PvO_2$, 33–55 mmHg (4.4–7.3 kPa)

of hypotension. Despite its theoretical advantages, the clinical indications for $SvO_2$ monitoring are far from clearly defined.

## Dual oximetry

Dual oximetry consists in simultaneous measurements of arterial oxygenation using pulse oximetry and mixed venous oximetry measured with a modified PA catheter. Dual oximetry provides real time values for arterial and $SvO_2$. When the oxygen supply is estimated by pulse oximetry, variations in $SvO_2$ can be more easily interpreted as either decreases in oxygen supply or increases in oxygen demand.

## Oxygen consumption and delivery

Sequential measurements of cardiac output, $VO_2$ and $DO_2$ will reveal the point at which further increases in cardiac output will not increase $VO_2$ or $DO_2$. Simultaneous measurements of oxygen extraction will identify patients who have a failure in oxygen utilisation such as occurs in severe sepsis. This concept is discussed in more detail in Chapter 13.

## Lactate

When $DO_2$ fails to match $VO_2$, anaerobic metabolism occurs, and lactate is generated. However, the relationship between serum lactate and tissue oxygenation in the seriously ill is complex.

## Monitoring of gas exchange

### Carbon dioxide

Carbon dioxide levels are determined by $CO_2$ production and elimination and offer a reflection of the adequacy of ventilation. The partial pressure of $CO_2$ in arterial blood ($PaCO_2$) can be measured by intermittent sampling of arterial blood gases. End-tidal expired $CO_2$, which is a reflection of alveolar $CO_2$, can be continuously measured and displayed using capnography. Tissue $CO_2$ levels can be continuously monitored with transcutaneous electrodes. Monitoring of ventilatory function is considered elsewhere.

### Oxygenation

One of the prime aims of intensive care medicine is to provide adequate oxygenation to cells. To monitor the efficiency and adequacy of oxygenation, we first need to measure the inspired oxygen concentration, expressed as a fraction ($FiO_2$) or percentage (Table 20.8). This is then compared with the oxygenation of arterial blood expressed as a partial pressure ($PaO_2$) or concentration ($CaO_2$). Normal $PaO_2/FiO_2$ values are 500–600 mmHg (66.7–80 kPa). In severe respiratory failure, values can fall as low as 40–50 mmHg (5.3–6.7 kPa). The amount of oxygen used by tissues can then be estimated by comparing the arterial oxygen concentration and the mixed venous oxygen concentration ($PvO_2$ or $CvO_2$). The lungs are

**Table 20.8.** Oxygen measurements

| | |
|---|---|
| $FiO_2$ | Fraction of inspired oxygen |
| $PiO_2$ | Partial pressure of inspired oxygen: $(760 - 47) \times FiO_2$ mmHg |
| | $((101 \times 3 - 6.2) \times FiO_2$ kPa) |
| $PAO_2$ | Partial pressure of oxygen in the alveoli: $PAO_2 = PIO_2 - PaCO_2/RQ$ |
| $PaO_2$ | Partial pressure of oxygen, arterial |
| $SaO_2$ | Oxygen saturation of haemoglobin (Hb) |
| $CaO_2$ | Oxygen content $= $ (Hb concentration) $\times$ (% saturation) $\times$ 1.34 |
| $(A\text{-}a)DO_2$ | Alveolar-arterial oxygen gradient: $PAO_2 - PaO_2$; normal value, |
| | 15−35 mmHg (0.13−4.7 kPa) |
| $PaO_2/FiO_2$ | Similar information as $(A\text{-}a)DO_2$, but results are in the direction opposite |
| | to $(A\text{-}a)DO_2$ |
| $SvO_2$ | Mixed venous oxygen saturation |
| $PvO_2$ | Partial pressure of oxygen; mixed venous blood |
| | Venous admixture or shunt |
| $\dot{Q}S/\dot{Q}T$ | $\dfrac{\dot{Q}S}{\dot{Q}T} = \dfrac{Cc'O_2 - CaO_2}{CcO_2 - C\bar{v}O_2}$ |
| | content For practical purposes, $Cc'O_2 = CAO_2$ |
| Lactate | Adequacy of oxygen consumption relative to $O_2$ demand |
| pHi | Intramucosal pH (measures tissue oxygenation) |
| RQ | Respiratory quotient |

responsible for efficient oxygenation and their efficiency can be expressed as the alveolar–arterial oxygen difference in partial pressures of oxygen ($PAO_2$–$PaO_2$) or the percentage of venous admixture or shunt (QS/QT). The normal $P(A–a)O_2$ is $< 50$ mmHg (6.6 kPa), breathing 100% oxygen. In the most severe forms of respiratory failure, values can be as high as 550 mmHg (73.1 kPa). The percentage of venous admixture or shunting is normally less than 10%. Inadequate oxygenation causes cells to undergo anaerobic metabolism and produce lactate. Lactate can therefore be a measure of inadequate oxygenation.

Oxygenation can be monitored by intermittent sampling of arterial blood gases, measuring $PaO_2$ and comparing it to $FiO_2$. The frequency of blood gas sampling may need to be increased in hypoxic patients. Continuous monitoring of tissue oxygenation would be more appropriate in those circumstances. Continuous tissue oximetry (pulse oximetry) to measure oxygen saturation is a simple, relatively inexpensive and accurate way to monitor peripheral saturation. Although pulse oximeters are subject to some shortcomings, they provide a convenient and reliable way to monitor oxygenation and they are now almost mandatory for all hypoxic patients.

The $PvO_2$ can be monitored continuously with specially adapted PA catheters.

**Table 20.9.** Factors that may interfere with oximeter accuracy

---

*False high O$_2$ saturation levels*
Elevated methaemoglobin
Elevated carboxyhaemoglobin
Hypothermia
Ambient light

*False low O$_2$ saturation levels*
Skin pigment
Elevated serum lipids
Nail polish
Ambient light

*Poor signal detection*
Motion
Poor peripheral perfusion
Hypothermia
Malposition

---

## Oxygen monitoring

Monitoring inspired oxygen concentration: The concentration of inspired oxygen can be estimated from the gas flow rates or measured directly in the delivery tubing. Too much or too little oxygen will cause tissue damage.

Monitoring oxygen tension: Oxygen tension is measured by polarographic electrodes either in vitro using intermittent arterial blood gas samples or in vivo by continuous intravascular or transcutaneous techniques.

Oxygen saturation monitoring (pulse oximetry): The relationship between the saturation of oxygen on haemoglobin (SaO$_2$) and the oxygen tension (PaO$_2$) is expressed by the oxyhaemoglobin dissociation curve. Saturation can be measured invasively using an arterial blood gas sample or non-invasively using pulse oximetry. Both methods use the principles of spectrophotometry. The non-invasive technique is the standard technique for continuous monitoring of oxygenation in the ICU. Pulse oximeters have lightweight, accurate and reliable skin sensors. However, they may not adequately detect arterial waveforms when tissue perfusion is inadequate. Moreover, pulse oximeters cannot determine other forms of haemoglobin, such as carboxyhaemoglobin or methaemoglobin, which, if present, will result in an overestimation. Pulse oximeters can also be affected by skin pigmentation, jaundice, dyes and pigments, external light sources and anaemia (Table 20.9). Another major disadvantage is that the accuracy of pulse oximeters is ± 3–5%, which can result in large errors on the flat part of the oxyhaemoglobin dissociation curve. Thus, levels going from a PaO$_2$ of 60 mmHg (8 kPa) (90% saturation) to a PaO$_2$ of 100 mmHg (13.3 kPa) (98% saturation), represents only an 8% difference in saturation. Therefore, within the normal range of oxygenation, pulse oximeters can be relatively inaccurate. Moreover, saturation levels below 80% also have limitations and care should be taken with their interpretation. This may be related to the difficulty in calibrating and developing algorithms below this saturation level. Until better calibration algorithms are available, oximeters should be considered unreliable at levels below 70%.

**Continuous monitoring of oxygenation in intensive care is as common and as indispensable as the continuous ECG.**

## FURTHER READING

Chapman, M. V., Mythen, M. G., Webb, A. R. and Vincent, J. L. Report from the meeting: Gastrointestinal Tonometry: State of the Art. 22nd–23rd May 1998, London, UK. *Intensive Care Medicine* 26 (2000): 613–22.

Connors, A. F., Jnr., Speroff, T., Dawson, N. V., Thomas, C., Harrell, F. E. Jnr., Wagner, D., Desbiens, N., Goldman, L., Wu, A. W., Califf, R. M., Fulkerson, W. J. Jnr., Vidaillet, H., Broste, S., Bellamy, P., Lynn, J. and Knaus, W. A. for the SUPPORT Investigators. The effectiveness of right heart catheterization in the initial care of critically ill patients. *Journal of the American Medical Association* 276 (1996): 889–97.

Dueck, R. Noninvasive cardiac output monitoring. *Chest* 120 (2001): 339–41.

Groenveld, A. B. J. and Kolkman, J. J. Factors affecting gastrointestinal luminal $PCO_2$ tonometry. *Intensive Care Medicine* 25 (1999): 249–51.

Hatfield, A. and Bodenham, A. Ultrasound: an emerging role in anaesthesia and intensive care. *British Journal of Anaesthesia* 83 (1999): 789–800.

Napolitano, L. M. Capnography in critical care: accurate assessment of ARDS therapy? *Critical Care Medicine* 27 (1999): 862–3.

Polelaert, J., Schmidt, C. and Colardyn, F. Transoesphageal echocardiography in the critically ill. *Anaesthesia* 53 (1998): 55–68.

Shoemaker, W. C., Belzberg, H., Gutierrez G., Taylor, D. E. and Brown, S. D. Recent advances in invasive and non-invasive monitoring. *New Horizons* 4 (1996): 393–4.

# 21

# Acute cardiovascular failure

- Continuous correction of the intravascular volume is one of the most important manoeuvres in intensive care.
- Inotropes and vasopressors should be titrated against desired effects – there is a right combination at a right dose for each patient at different times during their illness.
- Early signs of poor peripheral perfusion must be rapidly and aggressively corrected.

This chapter will discuss the general principles of treating acute cardiovascular failure. Specific problems (e.g. cardiogenic shock) are discussed elsewhere.

## Pathophysiology

Acute cardiovascular failure occurs when there is insufficient blood flow to meet tissue demands. Either the heart is inefficient or the vascular tree fails to deliver the blood effectively to the tissues. This can be due to a primary heart problem (e.g. valvular rupture) or can be secondary to a systemic process (e.g. septic shock) (Table 21.1).

### Cardiac output

Cardiac output = Heart rate × Stroke volume

### Stroke volume

Stroke volume is dependent on preload, afterload and contractility.

Preload: Preload is a measure of the end-diastolic length of muscle fibres prior to contraction. It is usually estimated on the basis of ventricular filling pressures.

**Table 21.1.** Causes of acute cardiovascular failure

Common causes
    Endocardial: acute valvular insufficiency
    Myocardial: ischaemia, infarction, arrhythmias, heart block, cardiomyopathy
    Pericardial: tamponade, aortic dissection
    Outside the heart: pulmonary embolus, pulmonary hypertension secondary to acute
        respiratory disease
Secondary causes
    Other disease processes, sepsis, poisoning, phaeochromocytoma

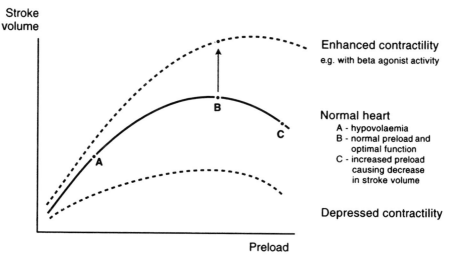

**Figure 21.1.** The Frank– Starling curve for cardiac function.

Optimising the preload is the first therapeutic manoeuvre in acute cardiovascular system (CVS) failure. Initially the heart is very responsive to preload, but during late CVS failure an increase in preload will not increase cardiac output (Figure 21.1).

Afterload: Afterload is the force that impedes or opposes ventricular contraction. For a normal heart, impedance to ejection is due mainly to systemic vascular resistance (SVR). In many forms of acute CVS failure SVR will be high because both stimulation of the sympathetic nervous system and the presence of angiotensin II will be causing vasoconstriction. A high SVR may maintain blood pressure, but is not advantageous to flow.

Contractility: Contractility is a measure of the change in the force of contraction over a given time period; contractility is independent of preload and afterload. It is difficult to estimate in the clinical situation – cardiac echo provides an accurate estimation.

## Heart rate

When the stroke volume cannot be increased because of a diseased myocardium, the heart rate must increase to maintain cardiac output. However, an increased heart rate will lead to a decreased diastolic filling of the coronary arteries and therefore to a decrease in the oxygen supply to an already stressed myocardium.

Because an increase in heart rate often is a compensatory mechanism, pharmacological intervention to lower the heart rate may also lower cardiac output.

## Myocardial oxygen balance

An imbalance between myocardial oxygen supply ($MDO_2$) and myocardial oxygen demand ($MVO_2$) can impair ventricular performance:

$$MDO_2 = (\text{coronary blood flow}) \times (\text{Hb concentration}) \times (\%\ \text{saturation}) \times 1.34$$

Determinants of coronary blood flow:

- aortic diastolic pressure
- heart rate
- myocardial extravascular compression

Major determinants of $MVO_2$:

- heart rate
- preload
- afterload
- contractility.

Note that the heart rate is involved in determining both supply and demand.

The lower limit of coronary autoregulation is 40–70 mmHg; subendocardial ischaemia will occur below that value.

The balance $MVO_2/MDO_2$ can be important. For instance, dobutamine will increase cardiac output (increase $MDO_2$) but will also increase heart rate and contractility which increases $MVO_2$.

Vasodilators will off-load the heart and increase cardiac output, but will also decrease diastolic pressure and thus decrease $MDO_2$.

## Blood pressure

The BP is critical for maintenance of an effective driving pressure across the vascular beds. It is a function of cardiac output and SVR:

$$\text{Blood pressure} = \text{Cardiac output} \times \text{SVR}$$

Cardiac output and BP should not be thought of in terms of normal or abnormal. A better concept is their adequacy or inadequacy to maintain end-organ function.

The amount of pressure or flow (cardiac output) required must be determined on an individual patient basis. For example, if a patient was previously hypertensive, then the autoregulation curve for the kidneys will be shifted to the right and a higher mean arterial pressure (MAP) will be needed to maintain renal function.

## Types of heart failure

### Forward versus backwards

These are old terms, but they are sometimes useful. Forward failure and backward failure can occur simultaneously in a given patient (cardiogenic shock), but often one form of failure predominates.

Forward failure: The major problem is decreased cardiac output with oliguria, confusion and hypotension.

Backward failure: The main problems are increased pressure and volume 'behind' the failing cardiac chamber, leading to pulmonary oedema, increased jugular venous pressure (JVP), hepatomegaly and peripheral oedema.

### Systolic versus diastolic

Systolic failure: This is failure of the pump. Forward failure and backward failure are examples of this.

Diastolic failure: Approximately one-third of patients with acute heart failure will show normal systolic function on echocardiography. Diastolic failure is failure of the ventricle to relax and allow filling: Left ventricular end-diastolic pressure (LVEDP) will be high but left ventricular end-diastolic volume (LVEDV) will be reduced, the ejection fraction will be increased and cardiac output may be normal.

Diastolic dysfunction can be difficult to define with a pulmonary artery catheter, which is used to measure pressures, not volumes; echocardiography is more useful in defining diastolic dysfunction. Because treatment for systolic and diastolic dysfunction can be quite different, estimations of their separate functions are important.

### Right versus left

Right side heart failure: Right side heart failure features high right side pressures, slightly lower or equal left side pressures and normal findings on chest x-ray.

Left side heart failure: Left side heart failure involves both forward failure and backward failure as described earlier.

## Autonomic nervous system

The sympathetic nervous system (SNS) is important because of its physiological control over the CVS and because many of the pharmacological agents used in treating diseases are designed to manipulate various parameters via the SNS

## Myocardial receptors

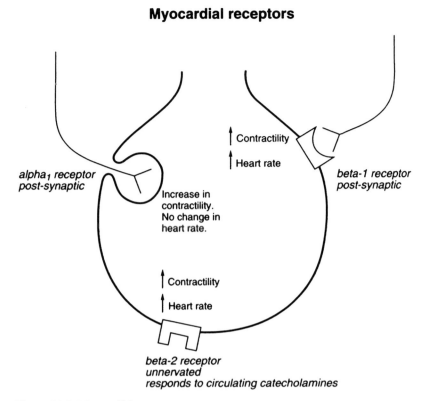

**Figure 21.2.** Myocardial receptors.

(Figures 21.2 and 21.3). In a patient with acute heart failure, the SNS is activated by hypotension and angiotensin II to produce tachycardia, vasoconstriction and increased contractility.

The classic model of the SNS may not apply in the presence of disease states and the actions of the SNS may be different during acute disease than during a chronic disease. Therefore, selection of vasoactive drugs remains empirical, by trial and error, with various combinations often being needed.

## Treatment of acute cardiovascular failure

### Clinical presentation

The signs and symptoms at presentation will depend on the underlying cause (e.g. a patient with mitral valve rupture will present with rapid onset pulmonary oedema). Ischaemia or infarction can have a slow onset, with initial dyspnoea and pain (Table 21.1). The LVEDV and LVEDP will rise, the heart rate will increase and the stroke volume will decrease. The cardiac output will be largely unchanged.

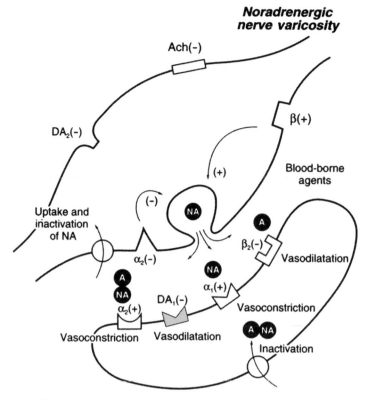

**Figure 21.3.** Interactions between the adrenergic nervous system and circulating catecholamines on smooth and cardiac muscle.

As the left ventricle fails, dyspnoea, tachypnoea, tachycardia, hypotension, confusion and oliguria will appear along with poorly perfused peripheries. These correspond to a further increase in left ventricular volume, a decrease in stroke volume and a decrease in cardiac output (Table 21.2). Optimising background chronic heart failure is important especially when acute heart failure is as a result of decompensating chronic heart failure (Table 21.3).

## Management

### Reversible causes

Reverse any immediately reversible causes of cardiovascular failure such as arrhythmias, pericardial tamponade, hypovolaemia, pulmonary embolism, coronary artery occlusion or valvular disease (Table 21.4).

**Table 21.2.** Differences between acute and chronic heart failure

Retention of sodium and water is a feature of chronic heart failure, not acute heart failure

Patients with acute heart failure are normovolaemic or relatively hypovolaemic, as a result of increases in hydrostatic pressure causing acute intravascular fluid loss, whereas patients with chronic heart failure are hypervolaemic, as a result of salt and water retention

Cardiomegaly occurs in patients with chronic heart failure, but not necessarily those with acute heart failure

Acute pump failure can expose the pulmonary circulation to sudden increases in pressure, resulting in severe pulmonary oedema

These differences are important because treatment strategies such as the use of digoxin and diuretics may have little place in the treatment of acute heart failure as opposed to chronic congestive heart failure

**Table 21.3.** Drug therapy optimising chronic heart failure

ACE inhibitor: or II-receptor antagonist if intolerant of ACE inhibitor

β-blocker: add to ACE inhibitor when condition is stable but patient remains symptomatic in a community, not hospital setting

Spironolactone: if persistent heart failure

Diuretic: only if evidence of fluid overload

Digoxin: if persistent severe symptoms

Anticoagulation or antiplatelet agents if indicated

## Optimising the preload

The most common cause of transient hypotension and inadequate tissue perfusion in the seriously ill is hypovolaemia (e.g. rewarming after surgery, vasodilatation secondary to sepsis, fluid loss as a result of polyuria or other occult fluid losses). The effect of hypovolaemia on BP will be exacerbated by high intrathoracic pressures, secondary to ventilatory support, that will decrease venous return and cardiac output.

Fluid challenge: Give fluid or blood (depending on haemoglobin concentration) as a bolus of 200–500 ml immediately. Assess responses. A further bolus or constant infusion (50–300 ml/h) may be required.

Fluid replenishment should be charted on an hourly basis with intermittent boluses as necessary, modified frequently according to the intravascular measurements of blood volume: e.g. pulse rate, urine output, BP, cardiac output, CVP, pulmonary artery wedge pressure (PAWP) and peripheral perfusion. Fluid such as colloid or blood is preferable to crystalloids when titrating against intravascular measurements as less volume is needed and they cause less peripheral

**Table 21.4.** Principles of treatment for acute cardiovascular failure

1  Reverse any immediately reversible causes (e.g. tamponade, arrhythmias, pulmonary embolism, occluded coronary arteries, bleeding, valvular disease)
2  Fluid challenge: If hypovolaemia is suspected, give 200–500 ml of intravenous fluid or blood (depending on the haemoglobin concentration).
   Depending on the responses of intravascular measurements (e.g. pulse rate, BP, urine output, CVP, PAWP, peripheral perfusion), commence infusion 50–200 ml/h and adjust frequently
3  Inotropes and vasopressor: After the intravascular volume has been replenished, catecholamine support may be needed
   There will be a best drug combination at the best dosage for each patient at any given stage of their illness
   A therapeutic challenge must be given, and its efficacy must be assessed by cardiovascular measurements (e.g. cardiac output, BP, preload measurements, serum lactate, mixed venous oxygen saturation, urine output) taken before and after the drug challenge
   The correct dosage of inotrope or vasopressor must be assessed clinically at the bedside, often on a minute-to-minute basis
4  Vasodilatation
   Afterload reduction is sometimes useful for heart failure or hypertension
5  Other measures (e.g. pacemakers, IABP)

and pulmonary oedema (see Chapter 4). Seriously ill patients often require large amounts of intravascular fluid.

The patient's preload is best judged on the basis of the response to a fluid load, rather than on the basis of a single reading, such as right (CVP) or left (PAWP) atrial pressure.

Following a fluid challenge, there may be clues that the patient's preload could be further optimised:

- A minimal change or no change in PAWP.
- An increase in cardiac output.
- Improvements in terms of BP and urine output.
- A decrease in heart rate.

Conversely, there may be clues that no more preload will be beneficial:

- High PAWP ($> 20$ mmHg).
- Decreased $SaO_2$ (may mean alveolar flooding).
- No change in cardiac output.

If preload is optimised, but the haemodynamics still have not improved, then inotropes and vasopressors will be required to increase cardiac output and BP.

**Table 21.5.** Selectivity of catecholamines for adrenergic receptors

| Catecholamine | $\alpha_1$ | $\alpha_2$ | $\beta_1$ | $\beta_2$ | DA |
|---|---|---|---|---|---|
| Adrenaline | ++ | ++ | +++ | +++ | 0 |
| Noradrenaline | +++ | +++ | +++ | + | 0 |
| Isoprenaline | 0 | 0 | +++ | +++ | 0 |
| Dopamine | 0 to +++ | + | ++ to +++ | +++ | +++ |
| Dobutamine | 0 to + | 0 | +++ | + | 0 |
| Dopexamine | 0 | 0 to + | +++ | + | |

DA, dopaminergic receptor.
Reproduced with permission, from Zanltsky, A., and Chernow, B. Catecholamines, sympathomimetics. In Chernow, B. and Lak, C.R. (eds) *The Pharmacologic Approach to the Critically Ill Patient.* Baltimore: Williams and Williams, 1983.

## Inotropes and vasopressors

Inotropes increase contractility, whereas vasopressors increase SVR by increasing peripheral vasoconstriction. Most exogenous catecholamines will increase both inotropic activity in the heart and vasoconstriction in the peripheral vasculature (Table 21.5).

Factors affecting the choice of an inotrope or vasopressor:

- The chosen end point against which the drug will be titrated (e.g. heart rate, cardiac output, BP, peripheral perfusion).
- The underlying disease state.
- The variability of responses according to age.
- Fashion: Pharmaceutical companies can exert enormous pressure on physicians. Many clinicians have been conditioned to use the latest and most expensive drugs (e.g. dopexamine and dobutamine, instead of older and cheaper drugs such as adrenaline and noradrenaline).
- The exact actions of most drugs on the heart and vessels in humans are uncertain, even when in a state of good health. Most experimental work has been performed on animals. However, differences in the autonomic nervous systems of the various species make any comparison difficult.
- Catecholamines have varying dose-dependent effects that are even more unpredictable in disease states.
- Adrenergic desensitisation or downregulation of adrenoceptors can occur in disease states.

Therefore, any drug should be empirically tested at a certain dosage in a particular patient at a particular time during the disease. Specific end-points should be used as guidelines to efficacy, with either the dosage being adjusted accordingly or the drug changed. There have been few controlled clinical trials comparing catecholamines for efficacy in seriously ill patients.

**Table 21.6.** Difficulty interpreting arterial lactate as a sign of circulatory failure

---

Some tissues metabolise lactate (liver, kidneys, heart)

Other tissues produce lactate (e.g. skeletal muscle, brain, gut, erythrocytes)

Lactate synthesis may occur under conditions of normal $DO_2$ when rate of glucose or glycogen metabolism exceeds oxidative capacity of mitrochondria (e.g. during administration of catecholamines)

Acidosis encourages lactate uptake by cells and alkalosis encourages decreased cellular uptake

Causes other than tissue hypoxia are implicated in sepsis (e.g. intracellular metabolic blocks)

Normal arterial lactate does not necessarily mean adequate oxygenation of all organs

---

**The choice between inotropes/vasopressors is more dependent on the clinical circumstances of the patient than on the pharmaceutical characteristics of the drug.**

**One of the primary goals in treating the seriously ill is to correct hypotension.** The dangers of hypotension probably have been underestimated. This is related to attention being focused on flow assessment rather than pressure, as well as an obsession with decreasing the afterload in an attempt to increase cardiac output. This focus overlooks the fact that vital organ perfusion is critically dependent on an adequate pressure.

**Inotropes are like fluids – a challenge should be given and the response measured and evaluated.** There appears to be a point of maximum effect from inotrope infusions, above which increasing the dosage will have little impact. There is little evidence of any linear response to dosage changes in the seriously ill.

Interpreting acid-base data as a marker of adequate or inadequate resuscitation or cardiac output is not straightforward (Table 21.6).

## Practical guidelines to inotrope/vasopressor choice

If a patient's BP is relatively normal and there is a primary problem with oxygen delivery ($DO_2$) after a fluid challenge has failed, then a drug that will primarily increase the cardiac output such as dobutamine, with or without low dosage dopamine, may be appropriate. If the arterial BP is low, despite an adequate preload, drugs such as adrenaline or noradrenaline may offer useful combinations of first choice. Despite the theoretical danger of excessive vasoconstriction as a result of vasopressors, the increased BP often increases, rather than decreases peripheral perfusion to the skin, kidneys and other organs.

## Inotropes/vasopressors (Table 21.7)

Dobutamine will increase cardiac output when filling pressures are normal or high, with little change in BP. Although predominantly a selective $\beta_1$-agonist,

**Table 21.7.** Infusion rates for drugs acting on the cardiovascular system

| Drug | Concentration | Rates and comments |
|---|---|---|
| Dopamine | 200–800 mg/500 ml | $6$–$15\ \mu g \cdot kg^{-1} \cdot min^{-1}$ (mainly $\beta$ effects) $> 15\ \mu g \cdot kg^{-1} \cdot min^{-1}$ (increasingly $\alpha$ effects) |
| | 200 mg/ 50 ml (in syringe pump) | $< 50\ \mu g \cdot kg^{-1} \cdot min^{-1}$ is often needed for severe sepsis; as the effects are predominantly $\alpha$ in this dosage range, it may be better to use adrenaline or noradrenaline |
| Dobutamine | 250–500 mg/500 ml 250 mg/ 50 ml (in syringe pump) | $2.5$–$10\ \mu g \cdot kg^{-1} \cdot min^{-1}$ |
| Noradrenaline | 4–20 mg/500 ml | Noradrenaline should be titrated against the patient's response |
| | 2 mg/50 ml (in syringe pump) | This is extremely variable and can be as high as 15 mg/h in severe sepsis; commence at $0.5\ \mu g \cdot kg^{-1} \cdot min^{-1}$ (approximately 2 mg/h). |
| Adrenaline | 5–20 mg in 500 ml | Adrenaline should be titrated against the patient's response |
| | 4 mg in 50 ml (in syringe pump) | This is extremely variable; as much as 20 mg/h may be necessary for severe sepsis; commence $0.5\ \mu g \cdot kg^{-1} \cdot min^{-1}$ (approximately 2 mg/h) |
| Isoprenaline | 2–4 mg in 500 ml | $0.02$–$0.10\ \mu g \cdot kg^{-1} \cdot min^{-1}$. |
| | 2 mg/50 ml (in syringe pump) | Titrate against heart rate for complete heart block; adrenaline is probably a better drug. |
| Phentolamine | 50 mg/500 ml | Commence at 0.1 mg/min, increasing every 5 min, to a maximum of 2 mg/min; as the major effect is on peripheral resistance, its main use is for hypertension. |
| Sodium nitroprusside | 50 mg/500 ml | Commence at $0.5\ \mu g \cdot kg^{-1} \cdot min^{-1}$, increasing every 5 min by $0.2\ \mu g \cdot kg^{-1} \cdot min^{-1}$, up to a maximum of $8\ \mu g \cdot kg^{-1} \cdot min^{-1}$; avoid excess drug during prolonged administration |
| | More concentrated solutions can be used in higher doses | Thiocyanate levels must be kept lower than 10 mg/dl |
| Nitroglycerine | 50–100 mg/500 ml | Commence at 400 $\mu$g/h, and increase by 400 $\mu$g every 5 minutes; its major effect is on venous capacitance; headache can be a problem with higher dosages |
| Milrinone | 10 mg in 50 ml | Loading dose 50 $\mu$g/kg; maintenance dosage $0.3$–$0.75\ \mu g \cdot kg.^{-1} \cdot min^{-1}$ |
| Dopexamine | 50 mg in 50 ml | $0.5$–$10\ \mu g \cdot kg^{-1} \cdot min^{-1}$; vasodilatation and inotropy; reflex tachycardia may be a problem |
| Vasopressin | 50 units in 50 ml | $0.04$ – $0.10$ units/minute via a central vein |

dobutamine also has $\beta_2$ activity that causes peripheral vasodilatation and possibly hypotension. Dobutamine is associated with tachycardia, which in patients with ischaemic heart disease can cause myocardial ischaemia. Dobutamine can be useful to match $DO_2$ with oxygen consumption ($VO_2$).

Dopamine has a wide spectrum of actions ranging from dopaminergic at low dosages to $\beta$ and $\alpha$ effects as the dosage increases. At higher dosages, its actions can simulate those of other drugs, such as dobutamine or adrenaline, depending on the proportions of its $\alpha$ and $\beta$ action (Table 21.5).

Adrenaline is cheap and has a wide spectrum of $\beta_1$, $\beta_2$ and $\alpha$ action. It increases cardiac output and BP.

Noradrenaline has a spectrum similar to that of adrenaline, but is more efficient for increasing the BP through its predominant $\alpha$ effects. It has less $\beta$ action than adrenaline. It is useful in patients with septic shock.

Isoprenaline has pure $\beta$ effect only. Classically it has been used to increase the heart rate during bradycardias. However, it also decreases coronary perfusion by $\beta_2$ vasodilatation. Adrenaline probably is a better drug.

Dopexamine is a synthetic analogue of dopamine, with the theoretical advantage of having dopaminergic activity without $\alpha$ effects. Care must be taken not to compromise the myocardial oxygen balance, because by decreasing myocardial perfusion pressure, dopexamine will increase the oxygen demand and lower its supply.

Phosphodiesterase inhibitors: These drugs act at a cellular level to inhibit phosphodiesterase, resulting in an increased concentration of cyclic adenosine monophosphate. Theoretically these drugs are inotropes and vasodilators, but their predominant action is vasodilatation. The exact roles for this group of drugs in acute heart failure are yet to be defined. There are two types of compound in this group of drugs: the imidazole derivatives and the bipyridine derivatives. The bipyridine derivatives include amrinone and milrinone. Amrinone causes potent vasodilatation of the systemic and pulmonary arterial and venous beds. It also has mild inotropic effects. Amrinone may be effective in treating right-side heart failure, as it off-loads the right ventricle and increases right ventricular contractility. Currently it is usually used in combination with other inotropes and vasopressors. Hypotension and reflex tachycardia can occur if amrinone is used by itself. It has a long elimination half-life that is further prolonged in patients with renal failure. Milrinone is about 15 times as potent as amrinone and has a similar pharmacological profile.

The imidazole derivatives are the other group of phosphodiesterase inhibitors. They include enoximone and piroximone. They have actions similar to those of amrinone and milrinone and also are best used in combination with a drug such as adrenaline in order to enhance stroke volume. The duration of action of the imidazole derivatives is much longer than that for the bipyridine derivatives. It has been suggested that enoximone may be more effective than dobutamine for overcoming the condition of a β-blocked heart, but the therapeutic roles for these drugs still are far from clear.

Vasopressin: Antidiuretic hormone (ADH) acting via vasopressin receptors is a powerful vasoconstrictor when given in high doses. It has similar actions to adrenaline with a half-life of 10–20 minutes. It is used as a second-line drug in cardiac arrest and as an infusion in severe sepsis refractory to catecholamines, dose 1–10 units/h.

**Afterload reduction is important when fine-tuning single organ failure. In acute multiorgan failure it is often not possible.**

**Occasionally when very high doses of inotropes are ceased, especially in septic patients, there is minimal change in BP, indicating a problem in receptor responsiveness. 'Industrial' doses of inotropes needed to sustain a fading BP are associated with a poor prognosis.**

## Vasodilatation

A decrease in resistance to left ventricular ejection will increase the stroke volume. This is particularly important in patients with pure heart failure characterised by low cardiac output and high SVR. Vasodilators can act predominantly on the arterial circulation, decreasing the afterload, or on the venous circulation, decreasing the preload. A lower preload is particularly important in a patient with cardiogenic pulmonary oedema.

The major factor limiting the use of vasodilators is hypotension which results in decreased rather than increased perfusion.

**Afterload reduction is more of an obsession of cardiologists dealing with the fine-tuning of single organ heart failure.**

Vasodilating drugs:

Sodium nitroprusside: Sodium nitroprusside causes arterial and venous dilatation.

Phentolamine: Phentolamine is an α-receptor antagonist that acts mainly on the arterial circulation.

Nitroglycerine: Nitroglycerine acts mainly on the venous circulation with arterial effects at higher dosages.

Phosphodiesterase inhibitors: Vasodilators should be carefully titrated against whatever effect is required (e.g. cardiac output). The dosage should be increased incrementally while not allowing the BP to fall rapidly below the patient's normal pressure range.

## Diuretics

Diuretics are useful for chronic heart failure and acute left ventricular failure. They should not be used in patients with right-side heart failure and diastolic dysfunction, as a high preload is necessary to maintain cardiac output.

**TROUBLESHOOTING**

### Inotrope selection

The best inotrope combination and dosage will vary (sometimes rapidly) according to the patient's condition. Avoid belonging to the school of single inotrope use. Use different combinations and dosages according to desired effects.

What is the problem?

  Pressure (e.g. hypotension).

  Flow (decreased cardiac output).

  $DO_2/VO_2$ mismatch.

Is there anything correctable?

  E.g. cardiac tamponade, arrhythmia.

Have you optimised the preload?

## Other forms of support

### Cardiac pacing

Cardiac pacing is used infrequently in the ICU as compared with coronary care units.

  Indications:

Bradyarrhythmias:

- Profound bradycardia (with symptoms).
- Sinus arrest (with symptoms).
- Complete atrioventricular block (with slow escape rhythm).
- Tachyarrhythmias
- Termination of supraventricular or ventricular tachycardias resistant to drug treatment, by overdrive pacing, is an alternative to cardioversion.

Although most temporary pacemakers are inserted transvenously, the oesophageal and percutaneous routes are also used.

Percutaneous pacing pads are placed on the anteroposterior chest, much as for defibrillation, and the output is increased until cardiac pacing is achieved. Because a high output is necessary to pace the heart through the thick chest wall, synchronous stimulation of skeletal muscle can occur. High levels of discomfort and pain often accompany percutaneous pacing. It should be a temporary measure while waiting for transvenous pacing.

### Intra-aortic balloon pump

The intra-aortic balloon pump (IABP) improves the myocardial oxygen supply by diastolic augmentation of aortic pressure and reduces the afterload by a sudden deflation of the balloon during systole. The balloon is timed to inflate just after the dicrotic notch of the arterial pressure trace and is deflated by triggering from

## TROUBLESHOOTING

### Features of main inotropes

Dopamine
- Mimics dobutamine when used at medium dosages and adrenaline at higher doses.

Adrenaline
- Increases BP.
- Guarantees perfusion pressure for vital organs, sometimes at the expense of tissue perfusion.
- Despite the theory, ventricular arrhythmias and oliguria are uncommon complications.
- A good all-purpose inotrope, especially when there is decreased BP (e.g. sepsis).

Noradrenaline
- Similar to adrenaline, but with greater peripheral vasoconstrictor effects.
- Useful for refractory hypotension, especially in patients with sepsis.

Dobutamine
- Increases cardiac output and $DO_2$.
- Blood pressure: no change or decreased.
- Used mainly to increase $DO_2$ in patients with a normal BP.

Isoprenaline
- Similar to dobutamine, but causes marked tachycardia.
- Very little used in the ICU.

Dopexamine
- Dopamine without the vasoconstriction.
- Inotrope and vasodilator.

Amrinone/Milrinone
- Mild inotrope, mainly a vasodilator.
- Used to off-load the heart when BP is adequate.

the R wave of the ECG or from the arterial pressure waveform. The IABP can be inserted either percutaneously or as a formal surgical procedure.

The question of who benefits from use of the IABP has few clear-cut answers. The technique provides short-term benefits for post myocardial infarction patients with acute ventricular septal defects or mitral valve insufficiency, as well as for post-cardiac surgery patients. Thus far, patients with cardiogenic and septic shock have shown no long-term benefits from use of the IABP. The best use of the IABP is as a bridge to transplantation or coronary artery grafting.

## Ventricular assist devices

These are either roller or centrifugal pumps that assist ventricular output. Their main uses are before or after cardiac transplantation and to wean patients off cardiopulmonary bypass. Their complications are many (e.g. bleeding, coagulopathy, infection).

## FURTHER READING

Gunn, S. R. and Pinsky, M. R. Implications of arterial pressure variation in patients in the intensive care unit. *Current Opinion in Critical Care* 7 (2001): 212–17.

Kellum, J. A. and Pinsky, M. R. Use of vasopressor agents in critically ill patients. *Current Opinion in Critical Care* 8 (2002): 236–41.

Millane, T., Gibson, G., Gibbs, C. R. and Lip, G. Y. H. Clinical review: ABC of heart failure. Acute and chronic management strategies. *British Medical Journal* 320 (2000): 559–62.

Rudis, M. I., Basha, M. A. and Zarowitz, B. J. Is it time to reposition vasopressors and inotropes in sepsis? *Critical Care Medicine* 24 (1996): 525–37.

Schmidt, H. B., Werdan, K. and Muller-Werdan, U. Autonomic dysfunction in the ICU patient. *Current Opinion in Critical Care* 7 (2001): 314–22.

Sibbald, W. J., Messmer, K. and Fink, M. P. Roundtable conference on tissue oxygenation in acute medicine. Brussels, Belgium, 14–16 March 1998. *Intensive Care Medicine* 26 (2000): 780–91.

# 22

# Specific cardiovascular problems

---

- The best antiarrhythmic is adequate coronary perfusion.
- Atrial fibrillation (AF) is common in sepsis.
- Sinus tachycardia is common in the first 72 hours following severe trauma even in the absence of hypovolaemia, sepsis and pain.
- Avoid correcting long-standing hypertension in intensive care.

---

## Arrhythmias

Cardiac arrhythmias are common in the ICU. The causes, predisposing factors, clinical significance and management strategies for arrhythmias in the ICU are often different from those for patients with primary cardiac disease in the more classical setting of coronary care units (CCUs). This section will concentrate on arrhythmia management only as it relates to the ICU (Table 22.1).

Arrhythmias in the ICU can be classified into two categories:

- Some arrhythmias result from irritant effects on a previously normal heart. They are usually supraventricular. Management is dependent on identification and alteration of the predisposing factors such as hypoxia, hypokalaemia, sepsis, central-line irritation and inadvertent boluses of concentrated drugs through central lines.
- Arrhythmias in the second grouping occur as a result of myocardial ischaemia caused by an imbalance between oxygen supply and oxygen demand. These arrhythmias are the same as those seen commonly in patients with primary heart disease. These arrhythmias can be either supraventricular or ventricular in origin.

**Table 22.1.** Aetiology of arrhythmias in the ICU

---

Common factors in the seriously ill
    Hypokalaemia
    Hypomagnesaemia
    Acidosis
    Hypoxia
    Sepsis, pancreatitis, multitrauma, MOF
    Pro-arrhythmic effects of antiarrhythmic drugs (e.g. digoxin)
    Inotropic drugs (inadvertent purges of adrenaline)
    Irritation from central line or pulmonary artery catheter
    Microshock

Underlying patient factors
    Coronary artery disease
    Congenital heart disease
    Valvular heart disease
    Hyperthyroidism
    Hypothyroidism
    Phaeochromocytoma

---

## Initial management of arrhythmias

### Resuscitation

If the cardiovascular system is severely compromised, immediate cardiopulmonary resuscitation (CPR) and cardioversion should be instituted.

### Cardioversion

Cardioversion is the treatment of choice in the presence of haemodynamic compromise due to a tachyarrhythmia, whether it is supraventricular or ventricular (Table 22.2). Energy levels given here are for conventional monophasic waveform shocks. Defibrillation with biphasic waveforms requires less energy and the energy level does not increase with further shocks.

| | |
|---|---|
| Ventricular fibrillation (VF) | 200–360 J |
| Ventricular tachycardia (VT) | 100–360 J |
| Supraventricular tachycardia (SVT) | 20–200 J |
| Atrial flutter | 50–200 J |
| Atrial fibrillation (AF) | 100–200 J |

Cardioversion itself can cause VF, sinus arrest or increased atrio-ventricular (AV) node block. Patients who are receiving drugs that block conduction across the AV node (e.g. digoxin, calcium channel blockers, β-blockers) can develop sinus arrest after cardioversion. Synchronous DC cardioversion for supraventricular arrhythmias decreases the risk of inducing ventricular tachyarrhythmias.

**Table 22.2.** Elective cardioversion

1 Give nothing orally for at least 4 hours.
2 Have IV cannulae in situ.
3 Use sedative/anaesthetic drugs with minimal cardiovascular depressant activities.
4 Select synchronous mode for cardioversion, apart from VF or very rapid SVT and VT.
5 Select lower range energy levels initially and increase if unsuccessful.

Contraindication: Dislodgement of an intracardiac mural thrombus can occur, particularly if the rhythm disturbance has been present > 48 hours or an unknown time. If the need for cardioversion is urgent, TOE should be performed to exclude a thrombus. Anticoagulation with heparin precardioversion and then for 4 weeks post-cardioversion is recommended. If a cardiac thrombus is present cardioversion will need to follow 3 weeks of anticoagulation.

## Cardiac pacing

Cardiac pacing is especially useful for bradyarrhythmias in the presence of cardiovascular instability. For example:

- Complete AV block, with slow escape rhythm.
- Profound sinus bradycardia.
- Sinus arrest.

Cardiopulmonary resuscitation may be necessary to support the circulation before the pacing device is inserted. Drug treatment may also be useful for bradyarrhythmias. Temporary transcutaneous pacing should be used if drugs do not increase the heart rate and perfusion.

## Correct an underlying cause

Potassium is particularly important. Hypokalaemia is common in the seriously ill and it should be aggressively corrected. Hypokalaemia is a potent cause of ventricular and supraventricular arrhythmias. Keep the serum potassium on the higher side of normal (i.e. > 4.0 mmol/L). Other electrolytes, including magnesium, should also be measured frequently and corrected.

Oxygen delivery to the myocardium: Maintain adequate oxygen delivery ($DO_2$) to the heart by attention to the following parameters:

- Coronary perfusion pressure (diastolic pressure minus right atrial pressure).
- Haemoglobin concentration.
- Oxygen saturation.
- Coronary blood flow.

Tachycardia decreases myocardial oxygen supply and increases demand.

Central lines: Closely monitor the insertion of pulmonary artery catheters. Any central line within the heart can cause mechanical irritability and arrhythmias.

**Table 22.3.** Treatment of arrhythmias

| Arrhythmia | Diagnostic hints | Treatment | Additional comments |
|---|---|---|---|
| Ventricular premature beats | Irregular, broad complex ventricular beats | Nil if haemodynamically stable. Monitor | Often occurs with right side heart catheterisation and reperfusion after thrombolysis |
| Ventricular tachycardia | Broad complex tachycardia Evidence of AV dissociation clinically on ECG | Cardioversion. Amiodorone 150 mg IV bolus, Lignocaine 0.5–0.75 mg/kg IV | Often due to myocardial ischaemia. Reverse abnormalities such as hypokalaemia |
| Ventricular fibrillation | Irregular broad complex tachycardia. No discrete QRS morphology. Cardiorespiratory arrest | Cardioversion, CPR and adrenaline | Terminal event unless treated. Usually due to myocardial infarction |
| Torsades des Pointes | Polymorphic QRS complexes that change in amplitude and cycle length. QT interval > 0.60 second | Remove underlying causes. Cardioversion. β-blockers for congenital prolonged QT syndrome. Magnesium | Due to prolonged QT syndrome (congenital, hypokalaemia, hypomagnesaemia, antiarrhythmics, phenothiazines, antidepressants, erythromycin, cisapride) |
| Multifocal atrial tachycardia | Discrete P waves of variable morphology and variable P-R interval | Treat underlying cause. Often resistant to cardioversion | Associated with pulmonary disease, particularly chronic lung disease |
| Paroxysmal supraventricular tachycardia | Narrow complex tachycardia. P waves often inverted or retrograde. Carotid sinus massage may cause reversion | As for atrial flutter | Common accompaniment of sepsis. History of Wolf–Parkinson–White syndrome contraindicates drugs that block AV conduction (β-blockers, digoxin, calcium-channel blockers and adenosine). Often resistant to cardioversion and digoxin in the ICU |

| | | | |
|---|---|---|---|
| AV junctional tachycardia | Narrow complex tachycardia. No P waves or retrograde P waves. Rate slowed with carotid sinus massage | Exclude digoxin toxicity. Atrial pacing. Amiodarone, β-blocker, calcium-channel blocker | Cardioversion should not be attempted. Often occurs after AMI and cardiac surgery |
| Atrial flutter | Flutter waves II, III, aVF. Regular R:R interval, often at 150 bpm, indicating 2:1 AV block | Cardioversion. Preserved heart function – calcium-channel blockers, β-blockers. EF < 40%, digoxin, diltiazem, amiodarone | Ventricular rate > 140 bpm needs urgent reversion either with IV treatment or cardioversion |
| Atrial fibrillation | Irregular R-R interval, with no discrete P waves | Aim to slow ventricular response rather than convert to sinus rhythm. Use drugs as for atrial flutter | Common accompaniment of sepsis. If rhythm present > 48 hours do not cardiovert without checking for intracardiac thrombus |
| Sinus bradycardia | Sinus rate of < 60 bpm | Correct hypoxia. Atropine 0.3–0.6 mg. Adrenaline 0.1 mg increments IV. Pacemaker | Commonly associated with hypoxia in ICU. Check for drugs that impair AV conduction. Manifestation of sick-sinus syndrome and increased ICP, may be normal in athletes |
| Sinus arrest | Prolonged pause between P waves. Usually reverts spontaneously | Treatment not usually necessary. Stop digoxin. Pacemaker | Usually due to excessive vasovagal stimulation. Check digoxin level |

Boluses of arrhythmogenic drugs: Arrhythmias can be caused by boluses of the many potent and concentrated drugs delivered to seriously ill patients. Check the delivery device and protocols for flushing central lines. The dead space in delivery tubing may contain concentrations of drug.

Microshocks: The measures taken to ensure electrical safety in modern ICUs makes the likelihood of microshocks rare.

## Specific treatment for arrhythmias (Tables 22.3 and 22.4)

### Sinus tachycardia

Sinus tachycardia is very common in intensive care and almost always is a physiological response to underlying disease (e.g. fever, pain, sepsis). It is also a common accompaniment of severe trauma, even when hypovolaemia is corrected and pain relieved. Treatment should be directed at the underlying cause, not the arrhythmia.

### Atrial fibrillation

Atrial fibrillation (AF) tends to be a very common accompaniment of any severe illness, especially sepsis, but also pneumonia, pancreatitis, multitrauma and multiorgan failure. Hypovolaemia and sepsis can precipitate AF in the seriously ill. Potentially correctable factors include atrial distension, hypoxia, electrolyte abnormalities, thyrotoxicosis and drug side effects.

Cardioversion is usually not successful in this setting. The main aim of treatment is rate control. Reversion to sinus rhythm is unlikely while the patient remains critically ill. Digoxin, intravenous β-blocker, intravenous calcium channel blockers or amiodarone can be used. These patients invariably have compromised cardiovascular function as a result of the underlying disease and the arrhythmia should be treated as soon as possible.

If the patient remains in AF for more than 48 hours then anticoagulation should be considered. This should be a priority if the patient is likely to revert to sinus rhythm spontaneously or with drugs. Transoesophageal echocardiography (TOE) should be done before elective cardioversion.

Amiodarone:

- Emergency dose: 300 mg IV, rapidly.
- Otherwise infuse 5 mg/kg IV over 1 hour in a dilute solution of 250 ml of 5% dextrose. Repeat 4–6-hourly if required.
- Then, 1200 mg/24 h infusion.

Amiodarone can cause AV block, sick sinus syndrome and hypotension in the short term. Other side effects include corneal deposits, skin photosensitivity, hyper- and hypothyroidism and pulmonary interstitial fibrosis.

Sotalol: Sotalol is a non-selective β-blocker and a class III antiarrhythmic agent. Its dose should be 0.5–1.5 mg/kg over 10 minutes, repeated after 6 hours.

Ibutilide: Ibutilide is a unique class III agent which is effective in reverting AF to sinus rhythm. Dose: 1 mg IV over 10 minutes with a repeat dose 10 minutes later if needed.

Digitalisation: Patients with acute rapid AF can be digitalised in order to reduce the ventricular response rate. Check the potassium level, it should be greater than 4.0 mmol/L.

- Loading dose: Give digoxin at 0.5–1.0 mg IV over 20 minutes or 0.25 mg IV every 2 hours. Total dose should be no more than 1.5 mg in 24 hours.
- Maintenance dosage: 0.25 mg IV daily, modified according to regularly measured levels, especially in the presence of compromised renal and hepatic function.

Verapamil: Verapamil can be used together with digitalisation to control rapid AF. Both drugs block AV conduction. Because of verapamil's tendency to cause hypotension, amiodarone is more commonly used.

- Bolus: Give boluses of 1 mg IV each minute, up to a total of 10 mg or until there is a satisfactory response in heart rate or hypotension prevents further drug use.
- Infusion: If repeated boluses of verapamil are needed, an infusion through a central venous line can be used at a rate of 5–20 mg/h to maintain the heart rate between 80 and 110 beats/min.

In some patients, this will induce reversion to sinus rhythm and it will control the ventricular response in others.

If the heart rate remains stable for more than 3 hours with verapamil treatment at less than 5 mg/h, an attempt to discontinue the infusion can be made.

Verapamil should be used cautiously in patients with compromised left ventricular function. Always commence with small doses and monitor the cardiovascular system carefully.

## Supraventricular tachycardia (SVT)

Like AF, SVT is a common accompaniment of severe illness in intensive care and it does not necessarily indicate underlying primary heart disease. Predisposing factors include sepsis, MOF and hypovolaemia. The SVT can be exacerbated by electrolyte disorders such as hypokalaemia and hypomagnesaemia.

Cardioversion often is not successful in this setting. If the cardiovascular system is compromised, then cardioversion should be attempted initially (20–200 J). Otherwise, attempt to reverse any predisposing factors and control the rate with drugs.

Adenosine: Rapid incremental IV boluses of 6 and 12 mg are successful in reverting SVT in over 90% of cases. The half-life is very short (< 2 seconds) and side effects few: transient dyspnoea, flushing and chest pain. Contraindications

**Table 22.4.** Drugs used to treat antiarrhythmias

| Drug | Indication | IV dose | Complications | Interactions |
|---|---|---|---|---|
| Lignocaine | VT<br>VF<br>Second line drug | 0.5–0.75 mg/kg over 1–2 minutes. Dose may be repeated at 20 minute intervals up to a total dose of 300 mg | Convulsions.<br>Allergy.<br>Cardiovascular system collapse with bradycardia | Anticonvulsants may increase hepatic metabolism. Additive cardiodepressant effect with phenytoin |
| Amiodarone | Narrow or broad complex tachycardias | 5 mg/kg over 1 hour in 250 ml of 5% dextrose. Followed by repeat infusions of 1200 mg/24 hours for up to 7 days or until oral treatment can be started | Hypotension.<br>Long-term use leads to corneal deposits, photosensitivity, thyroid disorders, interstitial pneumonitis, hepatoxicity, nausea and vomiting | Long half-life. Potentiates bradycardia with calcium-channel blockers and β-blockers |
| Sotalol | Narrow or broad complex tachycardias. AF and flutter | 0.5–1.5 mg/kg over 10 minutes. May be repeated after 6 hours | Pure β-blocker.<br>Hypotension, bradycardia, cardiac failure | Prolongs QT interval; therefore should not be given with drugs that prolong QT interval (quinidine, disopyramide). |
| Adenosine | Cardioversion of narrow complex tachycardia. Diagnosis of wide complex tachycardia | 6 and 12 mg by rapid IV injection via large peripheral vein | Avoid in those with asthma. Avoid in those with Wolf-Parkinson-White syndrome. Transient flushing, chest discomfort and dyspnoea. | Dipyridamole blocks cellular uptake and thereby increases adenosine levels |

| Drug | Indication | Dose | Adverse effects | Comments |
|---|---|---|---|---|
| Ibutilide | AF<br>Atrial flutter | 1 mg over 10 minutes.<br>A second dose may be given 10 minutes after the first | Prolongs QT and may cause torsades des pointes | Should be avoided with drugs that prolong QT interval (quinidine, disopyramide) |
| Verapamil | Cardioversion of narrow complex tachycardia.<br>Slowing of ventricular rate in AF | 1 mg/min up to 20 mg | Hypotension.<br>Acceleration of ventricular response rate in pre-excitation syndrome | A-V node block with β-blockers.<br>Asystole with cardioversion.<br>Decreased sensitivity with hypokalaemia |
| Digoxin | As for verapamil | 0.5–1.0 mg IV over 30 minutes; or 0.25 mg IV every 2 hours, to a total dose of no more than 1.5 mg in 24 hours | Virtually any arrhythmia.<br>Acceleration of ventricular response rate in pre-excitation syndrome. | Calcium-channel blockers and amiodarone will increase digoxin levels.<br>Caution in those with renal dysfunction |
| Procainamide | PAT[a]<br>AF<br>VT | 7–10 mg/kg at a rate no greater than 50 mg/min to a toal dose of 1000 mg | Hypotension.<br>Widening of QRS complex.<br>Prolonged PR interval.<br>Hypersensitivity | Contraindicated in patients with AV block and torsades des pointes |

[a] Paroxysmal atrial tachycardia.

**Table 22.5.** Broad complex tachyarrhythmias

| | |
|---|---|
| 90% of broad complex tachycardias are VT. | |
| SVT | VT |
| No AV dissociation | AV dissociation |
| Regular P waves may be seen | P waves may be seen marching through ventricular complexes |
| Previous ECG with bundle branch block | Previously normal ECG |
| No fusion or capture beats | Fusion and capture beats may be evident |
| QRS width < 0.14 second | QRS width > 0.14 second |
| No concordance in V$_1$–V$_6$ | Concordance in V$_1$–V$_6$ |
| Same axis compared with previous ECG without arrhythmia | Different axis compared with previous ECG without arrhythmia |

include AF with ventricular pre-excitation, patients with asthma and those taking dipyridamole.

Verapamil: The use of verapamil is discussed elsewhere.

Digoxin: Digoxin treatment is discussed elsewhere.

Procainamide: Give 7–19 mg/kg IV over 10 minutes, followed by an infusion of 1–4 mg/min.

Cardiac pacing: Overdrive atrial pacing may be necessary for patients in whom drugs and cardioversion have been ineffective.

## Ventricular tachycardia and fibrillation

These are uncommon arrhythmias in seriously ill patients in the ICU, as opposed to patients with primary ischaemic heart disease. Rapid defibrillation improves outcomes. For VT and VF treatment protocols, see Chapter 10.

## Broad complex tachyarrhythmias of uncertain origin

In some patients there may be little clinical or ECG evidence to differentiate VT from SVT with aberrant conduction. More than 90% of cases will be VT. When in doubt, treat the arrhythmias as VT and refer the patients electively for electrophysiological studies at a later date (Table 22.5). Immediate treatment: Follow the VT/VF protocol (see Chapter 10).

1  Attempt rapid defibrillation, commencing at 200 J and increasing to 360 J, if the patient is haemodynamically compromised.
2  Perform CPR and give adrenaline 1 mg every 3 minutes.
3  Amiodorone 300 mg IV rapidly and 1200 mg/24 h IV infusion.

4 Procainamide (7–10 mg IV over 10 minutes, followed by an infusion at 1–4 mg/min) may be effective whether the wide-complex tachycardia is ventricular or supraventricular. It will not affect VT.

5 Adenosine, as rapid boluses at 0.05 mg/kg IV, is a relatively safe antiarrhythmic that can be used in these circumstances and may be successful in correcting SVT.

6 Although IV verapamil is highly effective in terminating SVT, its use should be avoided in patients who have a broad complex tachyarrhythmia of unclear cause.

### Some complications of antiarrhythmic drugs

Combinations of antiarrhythmics can be dangerous, as drug interactions can occur. It is better to give one drug to its limit of safety and attempt cardioversion should this fail.

With the exception of amiodarone and digoxin, all antiarrhythmics are negatively inotropic and, when given intravenously, may cause hypotension.

All antiarrhythmics have pro-arrhythmic properties. Drugs such as quinidine, flecainide, encainide, digoxin, amiodarone, calcium-channel antagonists and β-blockers can either exacerbate existing arrhythmias or cause new ones. The risk of pro-arrhythmia is increased in patients with abnormal hearts, electrolyte abnormalities, during the initial treatment with the drug and the use of multiple drugs.

## Right ventricular failure

The function of the right ventricle is an important consideration in the seriously ill. For example, both underlying lung disease and artificial ventilation can cause right ventricular strain.

Right ventricular failure can be difficult to diagnose. Its features include an elevated jugular venous pressure (JVP) with a positive Kussmaul sign, hepatic congestion, sacral and lower limb oedema, right ventricular heave and a loud $P_2$ on auscultation. Haemodynamic monitoring will reveal the classical combination of low pulmonary artery wedge pressure (PAWP) and high central venous pressure (CVP). However, this is often not seen in the ICU, especially after the patient has been resuscitated with IV fluids. The chest x-ray will show clear lung fields. A dilated, poorly functioning right ventricle will be seen on TOE.

Acute increases in pulmonary artery pressure as a result of various lung disorders can lead to increases in right ventricular afterload, right ventricular volume, right ventricular wall stress and oxygen consumption ($VO_2$) (Table 22.6). High pulmonary artery pressures can cause ballooning of the right ventricle, which in turn can cause a paradoxical right-to-left septal shift – the so-called internal

**Table 22.6.** Situations in which right ventricular dysfunction may occur in intensive care

Acute on chronic lung disease
Pulmonary embolism
Acute respiratory failure causing pulmonary hypertension (e.g. ALI, pneumonia,
    aspiration, asthma, pneumothorax)
Right ventricular infarction, especially in association with inferior infarction
Positive end-expiratory pressure and ventilation
Cardiac contusion

tamponade effect or ventricular interdependence, which can in turn compromise left ventricular output.

## Clinical approach to right ventricular dysfunction

Correct the correctable: Keep the patient well oxygenated to prevent or minimise hypoxic pulmonary vasoconstriction (HPV). Treat any underlying condition, such as acute lung injury (ALI), pulmonary embolism, myocardial ischaemia/infarction or infection, in an attempt to reduce pulmonary artery pressure and right ventricular work.

Increase right ventricular preload: The first response to most acute episodes of hypotension in the ICU should be to increase the preload with colloid or blood. Increasing the preload of the right ventricle will similarly improve right ventricular function in many cases. This is an important manoeuvre, especially in the presence of right ventricular infarction. Drugs that can reduce right ventricular preload (diuretics, vasodilators) should be avoided. However, over-distending the right ventricle can cause decreased coronary blood supply and severely impair filling of the left ventricle.

Decrease right ventricular afterload: Although the option of decreasing the right ventricular afterload sounds attractive, it has certain disadvantages. Firstly, achieving pulmonary vasodilatation with agents such as sodium nitroprusside, hydralazine, or prostacyclin does not address the underlying lung parenchymal abnormality and may over-ride the hypoxic vasoconstrictive response, worsening the hypoxia. Secondly, it may decrease systemic blood pressure and therefore coronary perfusion pressure. Because of increased wall tension, the right ventricle is particularly sensitive to decreased coronary perfusion pressure. Nitric oxide may decrease pulmonary artery pressure and simultaneously improve hypoxia.

Inotropes and vasopressors: Both adrenaline and noradrenaline have both been shown to improve coronary blood flow and right ventricular contractility. This can be particularly important for the acute right ventricular load associated with pulmonary embolism.

# Severe hypertension

## Aetiology

Hypertensive crises are most commonly seen in ICUs in the following settings:-

- Post-operation (e.g. post-cardiac bypass, vascular surgery, or with any prolonged surgery, and in association with inadequate analgesia).
- Paradoxical hypertension or a labile BP often occurs in association with hypovolaemia, particularly in previously hypertensive patients or in association with patients suffering from autonomic disorders. It seems that the brittle cardiovascular system associated with such conditions over-reacts to intravascular volume depletion.
- Iatrogenic (due to inadvertent administration of a vasopressor or flushing of a central line with a fluid containing a vasopressor agent).
- Hypertension is often seen in association with acute cardiorespiratory events such as pulmonary oedema, acute severe asthma, angina pectoris or myocardial infarction.
- Hypertension secondary to increased intracranial pressure (ICP) accompanying any intracerebral catastrophe.
- In association with poisoning or abuse of illicit drugs (e.g. amphetamines, monoamine oxidase inhibitors, cocaine (see Chapter 15).
- In association with diseases such as renal dysfunction, phaeochromocytoma, thyrotoxicosis and pre-eclampsia.
- Autonomic disorders such as poliomyelitis, tetanus and Guillain–Barré syndrome.
- Primary hypertension (not commonly seen now because of improved long-term antihypertensive control). It is occasionally seen as a rebound phenomenon after clonidine or β-blocker withdrawal or in non-compliant patients.

## Management

### Clinical evaluation

Determine the duration of hypertension, the history of onset of the present crisis and the patient's current drug therapy.

Determine target organ involvement via history and physical examination, paying particular attention to the optic fundi, central nervous systems, renal function and cardiorespiratory system (Table 22.7). Initial investigations should include 12-lead ECG, chest x-ray, biochemistry, urinalysis, full blood count and CT scan if the patient is confused or if there are focal neurological signs.

### General measures

Confirm BP reading – check cuffs, transducers and other measuring equipment.

**Table 22.7.** Treatment recommendations in hypertensive emergencies

| Condition | Recommended treatment | Drugs to avoid |
|---|---|---|
| Aortic dissection | β-blocker, metoprolol, vasodilator, SNP, trimethaphan | Diazoxide |
| Eclampsia | Hydralazine, magnesium, Labetalol, calcium-channel blockers | ACE inhibitors |
| Cerebrovascular accident | None – no evidence that hypertension has an adverse outcome in the acute phase. Diastolic < 120 mmHg | |
| Intracerebral and subarachnoid haemorrhage | No treatment unless diastolic BP >120 mmHg | SNP – may increase ICP |
| | Systolic BP > 200 mmHg. Labetolol | Clonidine may cause drowsiness |
| Increased sympathetic activity – e.g. cocaine, amphetamines, autonomic drug function | Calcium-channel blockers SNP. Phentolamine. | β-blockers result in unopposed α action and vasoconstriction |
| Acute pulmonary oedema | Nitroglycerine Nitroprusside | β-blockers |
| Acute myocardial ischaemia | Nitroglycerine. Labetolol, esmolol. Calcium-channel blockers | Diazoxide |

Measure the BP in all limbs.

Decide whether the hypertension is a true emergency (e.g. in association with pre-eclampsia or aortic dissection) or whether it can be controlled electively (e.g. longstanding hypertension with minimal acute effects on target organs). It is the presence or absence of acute or progressive target organ dysfunction that will determine whether or not immediate treatment of the hypertension is required, not the absolute value of the BP.

Reverse the reversible (e.g. alleviate postoperative pain, reduce anxiety, check gas exchange and exclude the possibility of a full bladder or inadvertent vasopressor infusion). It is important always to check for hypovolaemia as a paradoxical cause of hypertension.

## Approach to severe hypertension
**Longstanding severe hypertension must be treated slowly and smoothly.**

The organs most at risk from hypertension are the heart, kidney and brain. They are autoregulated at a high baseline pressure in patients with longstanding

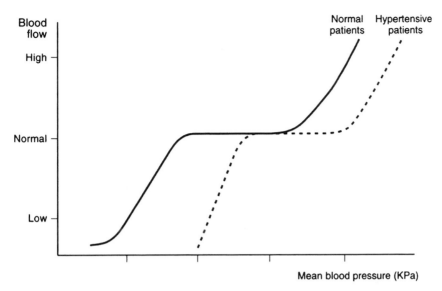

**Figure 22.1.** Autoregulation in normal and hypertensive patients.

hypertension (Figure 22.1). Organ autoregulation will adjust to a lower arterial pressure at a slow rate. The pressure must be monitored carefully during this adjustment stage. **The arterial pressure should be reduced slowly over 3–4 days in order to prevent relative hypotension and ischaemia in organs normally accustomed to high pressure.** The aim of immediate treatment is to reduce the diastolic BP by 10–15% over minutes to hours, depending on the nature of the emergency and to reduce the mean pressure by no more than 30% in the first 24 hours, especially if hypertension has been longstanding.

Continuous monitoring of arterial pressure and cardiac, renal and cerebral functions is mandatory.

Correct the hypovolaemia that often accompanies severe hypertension because of sodium and water losses. The circulation will become angiotensin-dependent in these circumstances. **It is important not to use diuretics or inhibitors of angiotensin-converting enzyme (ACE) initially, as dangerous levels of hypotension can result.**

## Drug usage in severe hypertension

Administer small doses of antihypertensive drugs while closely monitoring arterial pressure, pulse rate, cardiac, renal and cerebral functions. It is not possible to predict the critical diastolic pressure at which coronary perfusion will be compromised in any given individual. Thus, the arterial pressure should be lowered in a gentle fashion in order to avoid myocardial ischaemia.

Short-acting drugs should be used initially, in order to prevent prolonged hypotension.

There is no single drug of choice for severe hypertension. At present, the most commonly employed agents are as follows:

Sodium nitroprusside (SNP) – give a continuous IV infusion (50 mg/50 ml), commencing at 5 μg/min and going up to a maximum of 500 μg/min ($0.5–10$ μg · $kg^{-1}$ · $min^{-1}$), slowly and smoothly, in order to avoid precipitous decreases in arterial pressure. Measure plasma thiocyanate and look for unexplained metabolic acidosis in cases of prolonged high dosage infusion. Use SNP cautiously in patients with hypertensive encephalopathy, as it can cause a rise in ICP.

Nitroglycerine: Nitroglycerine at 5–100 μg/min as an IV infusion may be useful in hypertensive patients with acute left ventricular failure, acute coronary insufficiency and postoperative hypertension. Remember that nitroglycerine has its main vasodilatory action on the venous circulation, not the arterial circulation, and therefore will not have a major effect on severe hypertension.

Hydralazine: Give 0.1 mg/kg IV and repeat at 15-minute intervals. In order to prevent BP fluctuations, it may be preferable to use an IV infusion of 1.5–5 μg · $kg^{-1}$ · $min^{-1}$.

Labetalol: Labetalol is a combined α and β-blocker. Use an IV bolus of 20–80 mg every 5–10 minutes, up to 300 mg; or IV infusion commencing at 10 mg/h titrating against patient response. Exercise caution in patients with heart failure or phaeochromocytoma.

Inhibitors of ACE: These drug inhibitors can cause profound vasodilatation and sudden hypotension when used in patients with longstanding hypertension. They should be used for long-term control of hypertension, not as a first-line treatment. They should not be used in pregnancy.

- Captopril: It has been suggested that 6.25 mg can be given as an initial oral dose. However, when there is doubt, give one-quarter that dose and observe the response. Gradually increase the dosage, according to the patient's responses, at intervals of 8 hours or 12 hours.
- Enalapril: Similarly, an initial dose of 2.5 mg orally has been suggested. This can also cause severe hypotension. If in doubt, give one-quarter of that dose as a maximum and observe the response; then continue with the 0.6-mg doses once or twice daily and increase the dosage as necessary.

Phentolamine: IV bolus of 5–10 mg every 5–15 minutes or IV infusion (5–500 μg/min). Along with SNP, it is the drug of first choice for treating a severe adrenergic storm and may have advantages over SNP for patients with encephalopathy as it does not increase cerebral blood flow. Phentolamine use is often associated with compensatory tachycardia.

β-blockers: Mainly used as adjunct therapy initially. Avoid or use carefully in phaeochromocytoma and acute heart failure. Esmolol is a short-acting β blocker which has advantages in critically ill patients. Initially 0.5 mg/kg then an infusion at 25–100 $\mu$g $\cdot$ kg$^{-1}$ $\cdot$ min$^{-1}$.

Diazoxide: Diazoxide is an arteriolar dilator. It can be unpredictable when used in a bolus dose and may cause increases in heart rate. Suggested dose is 50–100 mg bolus IV injection within 30 s, every 5–15 min, up to 600 mg, until the desired effect is achieved.

Clonidine: Clonidine is a central $\alpha_2$ agonist. It can cause sedation. Give either orally or intravenously. The oral dose is 0.1 mg every 20 minutes. Intravenously it can cause an initial increase in BP, 75–150 $\mu$g as a bolus.

Nifedipine: Nifedipine should not be given orally in hypertensive emergencies as it can cause sudden decreases in BP. Intravenous drugs are initially preferred.

## Hypertensive encephalopathy

Hypertensive encephalopathy is a rare but serious sequela of severe hypertension. The ICP is raised in these circumstances. Many antihypertensive drugs (such as nitroprusside and hydralazine) cause a further rise in the ICP by causing cerebral vasodilatation.

A slow infusion of an $\alpha$-blocker such as phentolamine or labetalol may be best employed initially.

## Further treatment of hypertension

Avoid fluid retention as arterial pressure falls with the gradual introduction of diuretics.

Aim for monotherapy, although 2–3 drugs in combination are occasionally necessary.

Reconsider a secondary cause of hypertension (e.g. phaeochromocytoma, renal artery stenosis) if arterial pressure remains resistant to treatment.

## Acute coronary syndromes

Acute coronary syndromes encompass unstable angina and ST segment elevation and non-ST segment elevation myocardial infarctions.

Ischaemic heart disease is very common in the Western world, especially in the older population (Figure 22.2). Many seriously ill patients being treated in ICUs probably have concurrent coronary artery disease. Cardiac ischaemia or acute myocardial infarction (AMI) potentially can complicate the clinical course of many patients being managed in the ICU. This text will not deal exhaustively with the management of myocardial ischaemia or AMI. There are many good journal articles covering this area. However, because coronary artery disease is so common in our community, some aspects of its presentation and management in the seriously ill will be discussed here (Table 22.8).

**Table 22.8.** Diagnosis of myocardial infarction

| | |
|---|---|
| Definition | Ischaemic symptoms with raised cardiac enzyme concentration to greater than twice normal |
| ECG | ST segment elevation > 1mm in relevant leads (STEMI). |
| | ST segment depression with twice normal cardiac enzyme concentration (non-STEMI). |
| | New left bundle branch block |
| | A pre-existing left bundle branch block makes ECG diagnosis of AMI difficult |
| Cardiac enzymes | CK-MB isoenzyme activity |
| | > 4% of CK level |
| | elevation after 6 hours, peak activity 10–30 hours. |
| | Troponin T or I. |
| | The presence in the serum of cardiac troponin T or I indicates myocardial damage. Serum marker of choice in acute coronary syndromes |
| Echocardiography: | Identifies segmental wall motion abnormalities consistent with AMI. |
| Radio-isotope imaging | Technetium pyrophosphate imaging or 'hot spot' scan can help to identify acute damage secondary to AMI |

## Clinical features of acute coronary syndromes in intensive care

- If conscious, the patient may complain of typical chest pain. However, perioperative infarctions often are silent.
- Typical changes on 12-lead ECG.
- A new bundle branch block.
- Increase in cardiac enzymes – troponin or creatinine kinase – MB fraction (CK-MB).
- ST segment elevation or depression on continuous ECG monitoring.
- Sudden onset of ventricular arrhythmia (e.g. VT or VF).
- Sudden changes in arterial BP (hypotension or hypertension).
- Any change in heart rate (sinus tachycardia caused by increased pain and anxiety or sinus bradycardia due to intracardiac conduction delays).
- Increasing requirements for analgesia or sedation.
- Onset of cardiogenic shock (hypotension and decreased peripheral perfusion.
- Sudden onset of pulmonary oedema.

## Diagnosis of acute myocardial infarction

- Maintain a high index of clinical suspicion.
- 12-lead ECG changes. Remember that the classic changes of ST-segment elevation myocardial infarction (STEMI) may not occur for up to 24 hours and may

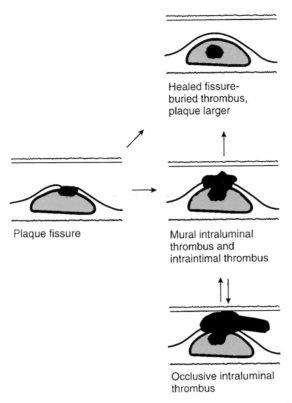

Healed fissure-
buried thrombus,
plaque larger

Plaque fissure

Mural intraluminal
thrombus and
intraintimal thrombus

Occlusive intraluminal
thrombus

**Figure 22.2.** Pathophysiology of ischaemic heart disease. Plaque fissuring is probably responsible for many of the manifestations of ischaemic heart disease.
The plaque fissure can heal (top) or can go on to form thrombosis that partially occludes the coronary artery (middle), causing symptoms of unstable angina. Complete obstruction (bottom) can also occur, resulting in total occlusion and myocardial infarction if there is no collateral flow.
Reprinted by permission of the American Heart Association. Fuster, V., Stein, B., Ambrose, J.A., Badmion, L., Badmion, J.J. and Chesebro, J.H. Atherosclerotic plaque rupture and thrombosis. *Circulation* 82 (Suppl. II) (1990): 1147–59.

be non-specific. ST-segment depression or T-wave inversion in five or more ECG leads also has adverse prognostic implications.

- Cardiac enzymes: There may be other explanations for many of these enzyme elevations in the seriously ill; what is required for diagnostic purposes is a rise in the specific cardiac enzymes, CPK-MB or troponin levels (Table 22.8).
- Echocardiography may demonstrate abnormal wall motion typical of AMI.

**Table 22.9.** Approach to thrombolytic treatment of acute myocardial infarction

---

1 Aspirin 150 mg/day
2 Streptokinase, 1.5 million units over 30–60 minutes
  *then*
  Aspirin, 75 mg
  +
  Heparin, 12 500 units SC twice daily after 24 hours
3 If there is streptokinase allergy or exposure to streptokinase between 5 days and 1
    year previously:
  Recombinant tissue plasminogen activator (rt-PA), 100 mg as follows:
  15 mg IV stat,
  *then*
  0.75 mg/kg as an infusion over 30 minutes
  *then*
  0.5 mg/kg as an infusion over 1 hour
  *then*
  aspirin 75 mg
  Full heparinisation IV after rTPA infusion, bolus of heparin 60 units/kg (maximum
    4000 units) followed by an infusion of 12 units/kg/h max 1000 units/h). Keep
    APPT 50–70 s in the first 48 h
4 Reteplase (mutant of rTPA) with a longer half-life. Two 10 mg boluses given 30
    minutes apart as well as full heparinisation

---

## Treatment of acute myocardial infarction

The aim of treatment is to open the offending coronary artery. Although there are many contraindications in critically ill patients, angiography, angioplasty or acute revascularation surgery should be considered particularly if the patient is at high risk of an adverse myocardial outcome and younger than 75 years old.

Thrombolytics, anticoagulants, aspirin and antiplatelet drugs (e.g. glycoprotein IIb/IIIa inhibitors) have all been shown to be useful in patients with myocardial infarction (Table 22.9) but the seriously ill often have contraindications to their use (Table 22.10). Treatment should take the following factors into account:

- Size of AMI: The extent of the ECG changes, the size of the cardiac enzyme changes, and echocardiography can give an indication of infarction size.
- Extent of physiological compromise (e.g. degree of hypotension).
- Coagulation profile: Measure the baseline prothrombin time, activated partial thromboplastin time and platelet count.
- Presence of major bleeding predisposition (e.g. recent surgery).
- Presence of major intravascular lines (remember that it is better to insert these prior to administration of thrombolytic agents).

**Table 22.10.** Thrombolytic therapy

Indications:
  Patient presenting within 12 hours of clinical symptoms suggestive of a myocardial
    infarction
  ECG: ST elevation of at least 1 mm in standard leads or at least 2 mm in two adjacent
    precordial leads or new left bundle branch block.
Absolute contraindications:
  Active haemorrhage
  Recent central nervous system surgery or major trauma ($<$ 3 months)
  Known intracranial neoplasm
  Recent central nervous system stroke ($<$ 3 months)
  Suspected or confirmed aortic dissection
Relative contraindications:
  Recent non-central nervous system surgery ($<$ 10 days)
  Recent trauma ($<$ 10 days)
  History of stroke
  Recent gastrointestinal haemorrhage
  Prolonged and/or traumatic resuscitation
  Coagulation disorders and current use of anticoagulants
  Pregnancy or $<$ 10 days postpartum
  Severe hypertension (diastolic BP $>$ 130 mmHg)
  Haemorrhagic retinopathy (e.g. diabetic) or recent retinal laser treatment
  Conditions with potential for central nervous system embolism (e.g. bacterial
    endocarditis)

Management otherwise is supportive (Table 22.11). Relieve any pain. Aim to maintain normal oxygenation, systemic arterial pressures, cardiac output and haemoglobin levels in order to provide adequate oxygen levels to the myocardium. Myocardial oxygen demand can be reduced by measures such as avoiding tachycardia and reducing cardiac afterload. Insertion of a pulmonary artery catheter, particularly in patients with already compromised oxygen demand/supply ratios, may help with titration of drug regimens.

The roles of early β-blockers and calcium channel blockers, have not been determined in the critically ill.

## Cardiogenic shock

Cardiogenic shock reflects failure of the heart as a pump. Its clinical signs are as follows:

1 Hypotension: systolic pressure less than 90 mmHg, or 30 mmHg below the 'normal' systolic pressure.

**Table 22.11.** Management of acute myocardial infarction

---

Oxygen 4–6 L/min may marginally improve myocardial oxygenation

Continuous ECG monitoring for 24–48 hours, if uncomplicated

Pain relief: liberal use of narcotics in the acute stage; morphine 2.5–5.0 mg IV, titrated against pain relief

Nitrates: reduce preload and myocardial oxygen demand and improve collateral flow. They may exacerbate hypotension

Aspirin 150 mg/day

Consider if the patient is suitable for adjunctive treatment of IV β-blocker, IV nitrate, IV heparin or ACE inhibitors

Consider percutaneous coronary intervention

If not available or the patient not suitable consider thrombolysis if no contraindications (Table 22.9)

Observe and treat complications (e.g. unstable angina, heart failure, pulmonary oedema, pericarditis, arrhythmias and mechanical complications such as ruptured papillary muscle, ruptured intraventricular septum or left ventricular aneurysm)

Non-STEMI do not benefit from thrombolysis but do benefit from glycoprotein IIb/IIIa receptor inhibitors, e.g. tirofiban and adjunctive treatment with IV β-blockers, nitrates, heparin and nitroglycerine

---

2 Manifestations of a low cardiac output, such as
- oliguria
- confusion, coma, agitation
- peripheral vasoconstriction
- high systemic vascular resistance (SVR), high PAWP.

The commonest cause is an acute STEMI. Other causes are listed in Table 22.12. Between 4 and 7% of all myocardial infarctions develop cardiogenic shock. Older patients are more likely to develop shock. The infarcted zone is usually greater than 40% of the left ventricle.

## Pathophysiology

The mortality remains high ($> 60\%$) despite many new interventions (e.g. acute angioplasty and drugs).

A large, acute anterior STEMI is the most common cause of cardiogenic shock. The cardiac output decreases, leading to hypotension and decreased end-organ perfusion. Left ventricular end-diastolic pressure rises and pulmonary venous pressure increases, which then leads to pulmonary oedema. This results in hypoxia, decreased lung compliance and increased work of breathing. The myocardial oxygen supply is compromised secondary to low $SaO_2$ and low diastolic BP. Therapeutic options in cardiogenic shock are limited by the basic problem of inadequate pump function.

**Table 22.12.** Causes of cardiogenic shock

Acute coronary syndromes including
  STEMI
  non-STEMI
Cardiomyopathy
Valve rupture
Aortic dissection
Cardiac tamponade
Acute pericarditis

Patients usually have a high PAWP and are severely hypoxic secondary to pulmonary oedema, so that left ventricular preload cannot be increased. However, decreasing the left ventricular preload can cause worsening of the hypotension, as a failing heart usually is very dependent on preload.

The cardiac afterload usually is very high and it would be advantageous to off-load the heart. However, that normally results in hypotension and decreased coronary perfusion. Combinations of inotropes and vasodilators may work.

With limited options in regard to altering preload or afterload, increasing the contractility is the only option. This may increase cardiac output, but at the expense of increasing the myocardial oxygen demand and possible extension of the infarction!

## Management

### Reverse the reversible

Correct hypovolaemia: Patients with acute heart failure are sometimes hypovolaemic. This is related to aggressive diuretic treatment and is secondary to loss of protein-rich pulmonary oedema fluid into the lungs. Furthermore, a high filling pressure is needed for a failing heart. Aim to keep PAWP >18 mmHg (2.4 kPa). Patients with an inferior infarction and right ventricular involvement are especially dependent on a high preload for optimum cardiac output.

Correct electrolyte and acid-base disturbances.

Exclude or correct, where possible:

- acute myocardial infarction
- mitral regurgitation secondary to ruptured papillary muscle
- ventricular septal rupture
- pericardial effusion
- any other surgically reversible lesion
- arrhythmias
- pulmonary embolism
- tension pneumothorax.

### General supportive measures

Pain: Treat pain or anxiety with continuous IV infusion of opiates.

   Oxygenation: Increased oxygen delivered by:

- simple face mask

   or

- continuous positive airway pressure (CPAP), via a mask or endotracheal tube (ETT), especially in the presence of pulmonary oedema, to keep $PaO_2 > 80$ mmHg (10.00 kPa). Continuous positive airway pressure has the unique ability to improve gas exchange and decrease respiratory work, in addition to decreasing preload and afterload. In other words, cardiac function potentially can be improved without increasing myocardial oxygen demand.

Monitoring: Monitor arterial BP, pulse rate and specific indices of organ function, such as hourly urine output, peripheral skin perfusion and level of consciousness. Pulmonary artery catheterisation, with measurement of PAWP and cardiac output, can help to optimise ventricular filling pressures.

### Specific treatment

The outcome of cardiogenic shock is closely linked to the patency of the culprit coronary arteries.

   Thrombolytic agents: Reperfusion with thrombolytic agents will decrease the incidence of cardiogenic shock. Tissue plasminogen activator may be more effective than streptokinase.

   Once shock has developed, thrombolytic agents will not alter the mortality. This is probably related to inadequate coronary thrombolysis with low coronary perfusion pressure.

   Intra-aortic balloon pump: The intra-aortic balloon pump (IABP) can be inserted directly or percutaneously into the femoral artery using the Seldinger technique. Use of the IABP results in increased coronary perfusion and decreased afterload without increasing myocardial oxygen demand. It can temporarily improve cardiac function and may be of benefit in conjunction with revascularisation.

   Revascularisation: Whether patients with cardiogenic shock benefit from acute revascularisation is unclear. Some studies show clear benefit compared to medical therapy (including thrombolytics) and some show no improvement in outcome. It does appear that younger patients are more likely to benefit from revascularisation.

   Principles of drug management: The aim is to increase end-organ perfusion without adversely affecting the remaining cardiac function. This can be difficult. For each beneficial effect of an intervention or drug, usually there will be an adverse effect. The mortality from cardiogenic shock is still high (70%) and is related to the vicious spiral of the underlying pathophysiology and limited treatment options.

Anticoagulation: Consider the use of full dosage heparin, especially if there is a large anterior infarction; otherwise, use 'low' subcutaneous doses of heparin.

Vasodilator therapy: It is difficult to use vasodilator treatment when the arterial pressure is already low, as a further decrease will reduce coronary perfusion and exacerbate myocardial dysfunction. Sodium nitroprusside and nitroglycerine can be cautiously commenced as a continuous infusion. However, further hypotension must be avoided.

Vasopressor and inotropic treatment: Increasing contractility of the remaining heart muscle with inotropes, such as with noradrenaline, adrenaline, and dopamine will also increase peripheral vascular resistance and afterload. This may increase arterial pressure and coronary blood flow, but it will simultaneously increase cardiac oxygen consumption ($VO_2$). An inotrope with mainly $\beta$ activity, such as dobutamine, may be more appropriate. However, it can increase $VO_2$ by increasing the heart rate and it may decrease coronary perfusion and arterial BP as a result of peripheral vasodilatation.

Vasodilators, inotropes and vasopressors must be carefully balanced when treating cardiogenic shock. Careful monitoring and titration of the drugs, with an understanding of their actions, is essential. There may be a drug combination that will be ideal for a given patient. A combination of $\alpha$ effects to increase coronary perfusion pressure and $\beta$ effects to increase cardiac output is often necessary. In the presence of pump failure secondary to severe obstructive coronary artery disease, coronary autoregulation is limited and coronary blood flow becomes dependent on perfusion pressure. It is crucial, therefore, not to decrease BP in these circumstances.

# Aortic dissection

## Pathophysiology

Aortic dissection occurs as a result of a tear in the intima of the aorta, usually against a background of hypertension and atheroma. Pressure within the aorta forces the blood to dissect within the intimal plane. The blood forms a false lumen. It can then rupture back through the intima, further along the aorta, or even rupture through the media and adventitia.

Aortic dissection, intramural aortic haematoma and penetrating aortic ulcers are part of a cardiovascular syndrome called acute aortic syndrome. All three have a similar aetiology and clinical presentation.

## Clinical presentation

Pain is usually a marked feature of sudden dissection. Pain usually begins retrosternally and radiates to the back, as well as to wherever the dissection extends (e.g. legs, abdomen, limbs, face). Branches of the aorta, such as the carotid, subclavian, renal and mesenteric arteries, may be involved, causing a wide range of signs and symptoms, such as stroke, loss of peripheral pulses and bowel ischaemia. Abdominal pain, bloody diarrhoea and oliguria will indicate involvement of the splanchnic and renal circulations. The aortic valve can also be involved, causing aortic incompetence. When coronary arteries are involved, myocardial ischaemia and infarction can occur.

Important considerations in the differential diagnoses are AMI, cholecystitis and pancreatitis.

## Investigations

1 A chest x-ray may show evidence of a widened mediastinum.
2 Monitor with 12-lead ECG recordings.
3 Perform routine haematology and biochemistry tests including CK-CKMB and troponin.
4 Whereas angiography is widely held to be the gold standard investigative tool, contrast-enhanced CT, MRI, and combined transthoracic-transoesophageal echocardiography have all been shown to have similar sensitivities and specificities in the right hands.
5 Certain diagnostic information is required:
   a Confirm the presence of dissection.
   b Determine whether the dissection involves the ascending aorta (type A) or descending aorta (type B).
   c Determine the extent of the dissection, the sites of entry and re-entry, the extent of involvement of other arteries and the presence or absence of thrombus in the false lumen. Information on aortic insufficiency and pericardial effusion should also be obtained.

All four diagnostic techniques have strengths and weaknesses in these areas.

## Management

- The diagnosis must be rapidly confirmed and then the type and extent of dissection must be defined.
- Early cardiothoracic surgical consultation is essential, especially if there are mechanical complications such as aortic valve involvement. Some dissections may be amenable to endovascular repair.
- Propagation of the dissection is dependent on both the level of the BP itself and the velocity of the left ventricular ejection. Therapy needs to be directed at both the BP and the rate of pressure rise. Commonly used agents are β-blockers and SNP.

**Table 22.13.** Causes of pericardial effusion

Haemorrhage
   Cardiac surgery
   Trauma (blunt and penetrating)
   Anticoagulation
   Aortic dissection

Malignancy

Infection
   Tuberculosis
   Viral infections
   AIDS

Pericarditis
   Post-irradiation
   Uraemic

## Outcome

The prognosis is poor with a mortality of 25% within the first hour, 50% cumulative mortality at 1 week and 90% mortality at 1 year in untreated or unrecognised cases.

## Cardiac tamponade

Cardiac tamponade occurs when there is accumulation of fluid or air in the pericardium causing impaired filling of the ventricles and therefore decreased cardiac output.

### Pathophysiology

It is important to distinguish between pericardial effusion and cardiac tamponade. Pericardial effusion is a collection of fluid in the pericardial space that does not necessarily impede cardiac function. The effusion may be blood, transudate or exudate, usually having been accumulated chronically (Table 22.13).

On the other hand, cardiac tamponade occurs when the pericardial fluid or gas impairs cardiac filling and output: both right and left ventricular filling pressures are increased, but filling volumes are decreased. Initially this is compensated for by an increase in heart rate. As the tamponade worsens, cardiac output decreases.

As little as 250 ml of fluid can cause acute cardiac tamponade, whereas under chronic conditions, greater amounts of pericardial fluid can accumulate, as the cardiovascular system can slowly adjust.

## Clinical features

1  Tachycardia and hypotension:
   low volume pulse
   pulsus paradoxus
2  Poor peripheral perfusion.
3  Dyspnoea.
4  Signs of impaired ventricular filling:
   a  Right ventricle:
      increased JVP or CVP
      hepatomegaly (in chronic cases)
      ascites, pleural effusions (in chronic cases)
      peripheral oedema (in chronic cases).
   b  Left ventricle:
      low cardiac output
      high PAWP (classically, PAWP equals CVP, which equals pericardial pressure).
5  Muffled heart sounds.
6  ECG:
   tachycardia
   small complexes
   signs of atrial enlargement.
7  Chest x-ray:
   cardiomegaly (if chronic)
   oligaemic lung fields (if acute).

## Investigations

Echocardiography is diagnostic and not only will detect pericardial effusion but also will document ventricular function.

## Management

Cardiac tamponade is a medical emergency and drainage of the pericardial effusion is a priority. In the first instance, pericardiocentesis should be performed under ultrasound guidance, either by using a Seldinger technique to pass a catheter into the pericardial space or by aspirating the effusion with a needle.

Some patients may require thoracotomy and surgical drainage of the effusion.

A fluid bolus will initially increase cardiac output. Inotropes usually are ineffective.

## TROUBLESHOOTING

### Sinus tachycardia

Sinus tachycardia rarely needs specific treatment. Beware of specifically reducing the rate, as the cardiac output and arterial BP may depend on a high heart rate.
Exclude hypoxia and hypercarbia.
Consider the problem of increased work of breathing (e.g. partially occluded ETT; bronchospasm; pulmonary oedema, or circuit, humidifier or ventilator malfunction).
Consider the possibility of infection (e.g. catheter infection, pneumonia, sinusitis, intra-abdominal sepsis, urinary tract infection).
Ensure that there is no pain, distress or distended bladder.
Consider the possibility of occult bleeding.
Check the use of drugs (e.g. $\beta_2$-agonists, inotropes).
Exclude the possibility of myocardial ischaemia or infarction.
Consider the presence of alcohol or other drug withdrawal.
Often sinus tachycardia is a non-specific accompaniment of MOF.
Often sinus tachycardia is a non-specific accompaniment of severe trauma.

## FURTHER READING

### Arrhythmias

Cain, M. E. Atrial fibrillation – rhythm or rate control. *New England Journal of Medicine* 347 (2002): 1822–23.
Luce, J. M., Trohman, R. G. and Parrillo, J. E. (ed.) Arrhythmias in the critically ill patient. *Critical Care Medicine* 28 (2000): 115–80.

### Hypertensive crises

Beevers, G., Lip, G. and O'Brien, E. The pathophysiology of hypertension. *British Medical Journal* 322 (2001): 912–16.
Varon, J. and Marik, P. The diagnosis and management of hypertensive crisis. *Chest* 118 (2000): 214–27.

### Acute myocardial infarction

Armstrong, P. New advances in the management of acute coronary syndromes: 2. Fibrinolytic therapy for acute ST-segment elevation myocardial infarction. *Canadian Medical Association Journal* 165 (2001): 791–97.
Curzen, N., Haque, R. and Timmis, A. Application of thrombolytic therapy. *Intensive Care Medicine* 24 (1998): 756–68.

Fitchett, D., Goodman, S. and Langer, A. New advances in the management of acute coronary syndromes: 1. Matching treatment to risk. *Canadian Medical Association Journal* 164 (2001): 1309–16.

Maynard, S. J., Scott, G. O., Riddell, J. W. and Adgey, A. A. J. Management of acute coronary syndromes. *British Medical Journal* 321 (2000): 220–3.

The American Heart Association in Collaboration with the International Liaison Committee on Resuscitation (ILCOR). Guidelines 2000 for cardiopulmonary resuscitation and emergency cardiovascular care. International consensus on science. *Circulation* 102 (suppl.) (2000): 1–384. Also at http://www.circulationaha.org

## Cardiogenic shock

Hasdai, D., Topol, E. J., Califf, R. M., Berger, P. B. and Holmes, D. R. Jnr. Cardiogenic shock complicating acute coronary syndrome. *Lancet* 356 (2000): 749–56.

Williams, S. G., Wright, D. J. and Tan, L. B. Management of cardiogenic shock complicating acute myocardial infarction: towards evidence based medical practice. *Heart* 83 (2000): 621–6.

## Tamponade

Spodick, D. Pathophysiology of cardiac tamponade. *Chest* 113 (1998): 1372–8.

## Acute aortic syndrome

Vilacosta I. and San Roman, J. A. (Editorial). Acute aortic syndrome. *Heart* 85 (2001): 365–8.

# 23

# Acute intracranial disasters

- Attention to the basic principles such as airway, breathing and circulation is crucial in the management of all patients with intracranial abnormalities.
- Management of patients with increased intracranial pressure (ICP) must be based on a thorough understanding of intracranial pathophysiology.
- Manoeuvres designed to reduce ICP such as hyperventilation and the use of barbiturates and mannitol, should be reserved for short-term reduction of a high ICP, rather than as part of long-term management.

The complexities of intracranial function remain a mystery. Compared with our knowledge of organs and structures such as the heart, lungs, limbs and gut, our knowledge of the brain is relatively crude.

No matter what the cause of the intracranial catastrophe, there are certain principles of management that are held in common:

- Ensure an adequate supply of well-oxygenated blood under a reasonable head of pressure (e.g. attention to basic details of airway, ventilation, oxygenation and cardiovascular support).
- Reduction of intracranial volume is the most important way of decreasing intracranial pressure. Make more space inside the head if possible (e.g. remove tumour, drain blood or cerebrospinal fluid (CSF), reduce oedema, craniectomy) (Table 23.1).
- Study the basic principles of intracranial pathophysiology and learn how to work with them – for example, the way cerebral blood flow (CBF) varies with metabolic activity and $PaCO_2$, and the concepts of intracranial compliance and autoregulation.

**Table 23.1.** Reducing intracranial pressure

| |
|---|
| Reduce mass, e.g. evacuate blood as a result of SDH, EDH or ICH; surgical removal of tumour or abscess |
| Reduce CSF, e.g. ventriculostomy |
| Reduce cerebral blood volume, e.g. hyperventilate, induce coma |
| Reduce parenchymal volume, e.g. osmotic diuresis; surgical removal of brain tissue |
| Make more space, e.g. craniectomy |

## Pathophysiology

Although the brain contributes only 2% of the total weight of a human body, it receives 15% of the cardiac output and accounts for 15–20% of the total oxygen consumption ($VO_2$). Cerebral ischaemia occurs when there is an inadequate oxygen supply resulting from a critical reduction in CBF, haemoglobin concentration or oxygen saturation in the blood. The brain is heterogeneously vulnerable to ischaemia. The most vulnerable zones are the cerebellum, parts of the hippocampus, the basal ganglia and boundary zones between major intracranial vessels.

Another unique feature of the brain which can make it vulnerable to certain insults is that the intracranial contents are confined within a rigid bony box. That affords considerable protection for the brain, but at the cost of subjecting it to high pressures within its confining box when there is intracranial swelling.

### Intracranial volume

The contents of the cranium are as follows:

| | |
|---|---|
| Cells | 85% |
| CSF | 10% |
| Blood volume | 5% (150 ml) |

#### Cells
Cells account for most of the intracranial content. Apart from removing brain tissue or shrinking it with diuretics, the cell mass cannot be decreased.

#### Cerebrospinal fluid
In the presence of increased ICP, CSF production is decreased and CSF absorption is increased and the remainder that cannot be accommodated is squeezed into the spinal canal. Thus, draining the CSF in an attempt to make more space may not be effective – hydrocephalus being an exception to this principle. Failure to image the ventricles on a CT scan is a common feature in patients with increased

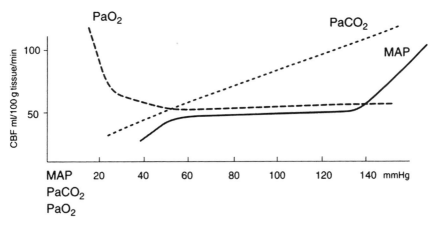

**Figure 23.1.** Effects of PaCO$_2$, PaO$_2$ and mean arterial blood pressure (MAP) on CBF.

ICP. If excessive CSF is present, it can be drained by ventriculostomy. The initial compensation mechanism for increased ICP is displacement of CSF into the spinal cord. Because epidural analgesia involves the use of large volumes of fluid which can interfere with spinal CSF flow, it should be avoided in patients suspected of having increased ICP.

## Blood volume

The volume of intracranial blood is approximately 150 ml and although it is the smallest component of the intracranial contents, it is the most amenable to therapeutic manipulation. The aim is to decrease CBF in an attempt to make more space within the cranium. Altering PaCO$_2$ is the main way of manipulating the CBF (Figure 23.1). However, the CBF must not be reduced below the critical levels necessary for adequate cellular perfusion. An increase in PaCO$_2$ will cause an increase in the CBF, which in turn will increase the ICP and can result in ischaemia. Conversely, a decrease in PaCO$_2$ will reduce the CBF and if that reduction is severe enough, it can also cause ischaemia. This represents a fine therapeutic line. Moreover, reduction of PaCO$_2$ is only a short-term measure, the CBF soon returning to original levels. Intracranial blood volume is normally well controlled over a wide range of systemic pressures by a phenomenon known as autoregulation.

## Cranial vault

Decompressive surgery, i.e. craniectomy, may be the only way of allowing the increased intracranial volume to occupy a greater space – thus decreasing the ICP.

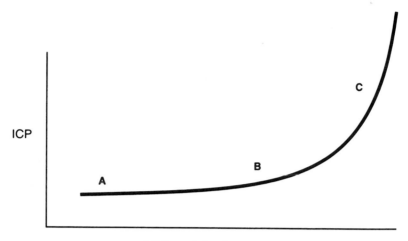

ICP

Intracranial volume

**Figure 23.2.** Relationship between ICP and intracranial volume.
A: As the intracranial volume increases on this part of the curve, compensation occurs and the ICP rises little.
B: Compensation is increasingly ineffective.
C: At this point on the curve, a small increase in intracranial volume causes a great rise in the ICP. For a patient functioning on this part of the curve, meticulous care is mandatory in order to avoid catastrophic ischaemia. Similarly, small decreases in volume will result in large decreases in pressure.

## Intracranial pressure

As the intracranial volume increases, compensation takes place and the ICP remains stable up to a point at which decompensation begins to occur, and then the ICP rises dramatically (Figure 23.2). On that part of the intracranial compliance curve where the pressure suddenly increases, a small rise in volume will cause a dramatic increase in the ICP and will further reduce cerebral perfusion. Similarly, meticulous care of a patient who is functioning on this part of the curve can be rewarding. Any small decrease in intracranial volume that can be achieved (e.g. by sitting the patient up, keeping the head straight, using adequate sedation) can have a dramatic effect in bringing the ICP down. **Meticulous nursing care is crucial to outcomes for patients with increased ICP.**

The cerebral perfusion pressure (CPP) is equivalent to the mean arterial pressure (MAP) minus the ICP. The aim of treatment is to maintain the CPP at more than 60 mmHg (8.0 kPa) with an adequate MAP and a low ICP. If measures aimed at reducing ICP fail to maintain an adequate CPP, then the MAP should be increased. To achieve this, volume loading and vasopressors should be considered.

$$CPP = MAP - ICP$$

**Table 23.2.** Advantages of intracranial pressure monitoring

---

Can be useful as a continuous means of monitoring heavily sedated patients when there is no other means of assessing the level of consciousness.

Any procedures that can cause a severely elevated ICP can be identified and thereafter modified or avoided. This is very useful for assisting the staff in managing these patients.

The CPP can be determined as a guide to cerebral perfusion and should be maintained at more than 60 mmHg (8.0 kPa)

The ICP will track the progression of the cerebral oedema and give an indication as to when to cease sedation, wean from ventilation and assess the neurological status

The ICP is a guide to prognosis. Patients without intracranial haematomas who have ICP values consistently above 40 mmHg (5.3 kPa) have a grim prognosis

If the ICP rises to more than 25 mmHg (3.3 kPa) for more than 5 minutes and the arterial BP is constant, short-term manoeuvres should be employed to reduce the ICP after obvious reversible factors have been attended to (e.g. hypoxia, hypercarbia, intracranial bleeding) and the pressure measurement checked

---

ICP values:

| 0–15 mmHg | (0 to 2.0 kPa) | normal |
| 15–20 mmHg | (2.0 to 2.7 kPa) | equivocal |
| 20–40 mmHg | (2.7 to 5.3 kPa) | moderately increased |
| 40 mmHg | (> 5.7 kPa) | severely increased |

Even in the normal patient, the ICP can transiently rise to high levels. During manoeuvres such as physiotherapy and endotracheal suction, the ICP can rise to very high levels.

**Failure of the ICP to rapidly return to normal levels after a transient rise indicates decreased intracranial compliance.**

Like many aspects in the management of seriously ill patients, ICP monitoring has not been demonstrated to affect outcome. However, it does keep the staff aware of the factors that can affect the ICP for better or worse, in addition to being a guide to CPP (Table 23.2). Moreover, these patients often are rendered unconscious and clinical signs of increased ICP are almost non-existent. There need to be direct measurements of ICP. So long as attention is not focused on any absolute values for ICP, and it is seen in its clinical context, then ICP is as useful as many other forms of invasive monitoring. A good trace usually indicates adequate ICP performance. Changes in ICP should be sought via a Valsalva manoeuvre, coughing or occlusion of the internal jugular veins. An estimate of intracranial compliance can be achieved by bilateral compression of the internal jugular veins and observing the rate of rise and return to the baseline of the ICP.

## Intracranial pressure monitoring

### Indications for ICP monitoring

Monitoring should be considered for patients who are comatose and have CT signs of significantly increased ICP, such as midline shift, third ventricular or cisternal compression and who have a potentially reversible disease, e.g. head injury, subarachnoid haemorrhage (SAH), intracerebral haematoma, meningitis, encephalitis, fulminant hepatic failure, Reye's syndrome or cerebral oedema from other causes.

### Types of monitoring

Intraventricular: Intraventricular monitoring is the gold standard for ICP monitoring. However, it can be difficult to locate the ventricles in the presence of increased ICP and the risk of infection is higher than in the other forms of ICP monitoring. The infection rate increases after 5 days in situ and infection is almost inevitable after 10 days. A decrease in the patient's level of consciousness or clinical state may accompany infection.

Subdural and extradural: Extradural monitoring in the adult is often damped, as compared with subdural monitoring. There are many commercial products available which can measure both extradural and subdural pressures. Alternatively, a narrow catheter, such as an infant feeding catheter, can be inserted into the epidural or subdural space. The column of fluid in the catheter can be transduced and displayed in the most convenient form. Monitoring of both subdural and extradural pressures is damped compared with intraventricular monitoring and in rare cases it can be associated with bleeding.

## Cerebral monitoring

Apart from measurement of the ICP and the use of an EEG, the parameters of cerebral function that one might wish to monitor are relatively inaccessible. It is usually assumed that if well-oxygenated blood with normal haemoglobin is supplied to the brain at a reasonable MAP, that cerebral autoregulation will meet the brain's oxygen needs. This assumes there is no vessel obstruction and no increased ICP. Normal findings on global measurements of cardiorespiratory function usually will guarantee adequate cerebral function. However, more accurate means for monitoring cerebral function are becoming increasingly available and they may provide more than our current assumptions and our relatively crude monitoring of the oxygenation of brain tissue.

Brain electrical activity: Measurement of voltage on a cerebral function monitor (CFM) with biparietal electrodes will give an indication of the general level of the brain's electrical activity. This can be useful in testing for brain death and detecting convulsive activity and it can serve as a general guide to treatment with sedative drugs.

Evoked potentials: An evoked potential provides a measure of the ability of the nervous system to receive and respond to an external stimulus. Evoked potentials can sensitively reveal the quantitative response to auditory, visual or somatosensory stimulation. They are more accurate for predicting outcome for patients in coma than is a CT scan, ICP monitoring or clinical examination. Evoked potentials are particularly useful in assessing cerebral function in the presence of drugs, because, unlike the EEG, evoked potential responses are not altered by the presence of drugs. Assessment of cerebral ischaemia and confirmation of brain death are also feasible with evoked potentials.

Cerebral blood flow: Measurement of CBF usually is based on a technique to determine the clearance of xenon 133 from the brain, as detected by scintillation counters positioned over the scalp after intracarotid injection. Because of technical difficulties, it has mainly been used as a research tool.

Flow velocity: Transcranial doppler (TCD) ultrasound is a commercially available non-invasive technique often used to measure flow velocity in the middle cerebral artery. It is a useful technique for detecting severe stenosis, assessing collateral circulation and evaluating vasospasm after SAH.

Jugular venous saturation: The oxygen content of blood obtained from the jugular venous bulb ($CjvO_2$) is the cerebral equivalent of the oxygen content of mixed venous blood. The cerebral metabolic rate for oxygen ($CMRO_2$), CBF, arterial oxygen content ($CaO_2$) and $CjvO_2$ are related according to the following equations:

$$CMRO_2 = (CBF)(CaO_2 - CjvO_2)$$

$$CjvO_2 = CaO_2 - \frac{CMRO_2}{CBF}$$

Retrograde cannulation of the jugular bulb is technically simple and measurement of $CjvO_2$ or continuous monitoring of jugular venous saturation ($SjvO_2$) is possible. Both measurements offer only global average estimates of the degree of cerebral ischaemia and, as such, have limitations.

Near-infrared spectroscopy: This provides another indirect measure of brain metabolism. Near-infrared light penetrates the skull and during its transmission through brain tissue it will undergo changes in wavelength that will be proportional to the relative concentrations of oxygenated haemoglobin in the tissue beneath the field. This may become a practical, non-invasive technique for continuous cerebral monitoring.

## Cerebral oedema

Cerebral oedema is an abnormal extravascular accumulation of fluid in the brain, in either the intracellular or the interstitial compartment. It should not be confused with other causes of increased intracranial volume, such as vascular

**Table 23.3.** Principles of management of intracranial disasters

1 Ensure adequate airway. Intubate if necessary
2 Ensure adequate ventilation. Use artificial ventilation if necessary
3 Ensure adequate cardiovascular function, oxygenation and haemoglobin concentration. Correct acidosis
4 Reverse any reversible abnormality (e.g. drain intracranial blood, treat seizures, hydrocephalus or infection)
5 Keep the arterial BP within 'normal' limits. Hypotension will cause a decreased CPP and hypertension can cause 'breakthrough oedema', increased ICP and consequently a decreased CPP
6 Avoid hypertensive surges and guarantee sedation with continuous IV narcotics and intermittent boluses of narcotics immediately before procedures such as physiotherapy, turning or suction. Lignocaine (1.5 mg/kg IV) may help to reduce a raised ICP during intubation
7 Facilitate jugular venous drainage:
Sit the patient up at 30° to 45° and maintain arterial BP. Avoid head down position
   Keep the head straight
Avoid hard collars where possible and securing the artificial airway with tape that can cause constriction around the neck
8 In order to avoid the problems of coughing, straining or 'fighting' the ventilator, use continuous IV narcotic infusion and muscle relaxants if necessary
9 Avoid the use of high ventilatory pressures, which would decrease cerebral venous drainage
10 Avoid excessive crystalloid treatment – maintain intravascular volume – so-called euvolaemic dehydration
11 Consider ICP monitoring if high pressures are suspected (on the basis of observing the waveform and whether or not the ICP increases with brief bilateral jugular compression)
12 Avoid drugs that would cause a rise in ICP (e.g. volatile anaesthetic agents, nitrates and ketamine)
13 Use hyperventilation as a short-term manoeuvre; otherwise keep $PaCO_2$ at approximately 40 mmHg (5.3 kPa)
14 Consider diuretics (e.g. mannitol 0.3 g/kg 8-hourly) with or without a loop diuretic as a temporary measure to reduce ICP
15 If measures aimed at reducing ICP fail, consider a further increase in intravascular volume and the use of vasopressors in an attempt to increase the MAP and therefore the CPP
16 Consider the development of reversible intracranial pathological conditions (e.g. a new haemorrhage or hydrocephalus)
17 Consider 'coma therapy' if diuretics fail to halt severe increases in ICP:
Give intermittent boluses or a continuous infusion of thiopentone, phenobarbitone or propofol. The effects may take up to 6–7 days to wear off, especially with barbiturates, so modify the neurological assessment.

congestion, tumour or hydrocephalus. Cerebral oedema is a non-specific accompaniment of many disorders, such as head injury, tumour, and infection. The division of cerebral oedema into vasogenic (vascular damage, or damage to the blood–brain barrier) and neurogenic (direct cellular damage) forms is of little clinical importance, as common insults such as global ischaemia and head injury are accompanied by both forms of oedema and the clinical differentiation is, in any case, impossible.

Cerebral oedema can be detected on CT scan or by monitoring the results of oedema, such as clinical signs or direct measurement of the ICP. The signs of increased ICP seen on CT scan can include reduced CSF, loss of gyri and sulci, loss of grey/white differentiation and flattening of the basal cisterns.

## Principles of management of raised intracranial pressure

The initial assessment and investigation of a patient with increased ICP are discussed in the section on coma. As with all aspects of treating intracranial disasters, attention to basic principles is crucial (e.g. monitoring the airway, ventilation, oxygenation, intravascular volume and blood pressure; Table 23.3).

### Autoregulation

Autoregulation normally operates as an excellent mechanism for maintaining CBF over a wide range of the MAP (approximately 60–160 mmHg). **Remember that in hypertensive patients, the autoregulation curve will be shifted to the right** (i.e. they will maintain a constant flow at a higher than normal MAP, but CBF will decrease at a pressure that would be considered normal in the non-hypertensive patient).

Autoregulation, unfortunately, may be compromised by the underlying intracranial abnormality. The CBF may then passively follow changes in arterial pressure and in the ICP. Therefore, never assume autoregulation offers full protection against a fluctuating BP. **Meticulously avoid hypotension and hypertension.** Hypertensive surges associated with pain, endotracheal intubation and suctioning, procedures that involve turning the patient and so forth, can cause a sudden increase in cerebral blood volume and may increase oedema formation across a damaged blood–brain barrier. An extra bolus of sedation (e.g. 5–10 mg morphine, 25–100 mg propofol) may be required before any of these procedures is performed in order to attenuate the hypertensive response.

Lignocaine (1.5 mg/kg) has been recommended before intubation and tracheal suctioning, in order to prevent hypertensive surges. The BP should otherwise be maintained at 'normal' or premorbid levels.

## Facilitate venous drainage

Occlusion of the cerebral venous drainage can cause acute and dangerous increases in cerebral blood volume and ICP (e.g. coughing, straining and fighting the ventilator can all cause dangerous increases in ICP by impeding venous return).

Depending on how much pressure is transmitted intracranially, intermittent positive pressure ventilation (IPPV) and positive end-expiratory pressure (PEEP) can also cause increases in ICP.

Taping the endotracheal tube (ETT), tracheostomy tube or nasotracheal tube too tight can cause partial occlusion of the jugular veins in the neck and can increase the ICP.

Venous occlusion will be accentuated by allowing the head to turn, even slightly. Keep the head absolutely straight if the patient's ICP is high.

Beware of hard collars as used for patients suspected of having cervical spine injuries, as they can also increase ICP.

As long as the MAP is maintained at a normal value, position the patient sitting up at 30° to 45°, in order to facilitate venous drainage. Avoid the head down position whenever possible, even for medical procedures. It is important to maintain the MAP in the desired range when placing a patient head up in an effort to achieve an adequate CPP.

## Carbon dioxide

The $PaCO_2$ largely determines the CBF and therefore cerebral blood volume, because of its rapid effect on the extracellular fluid hydrogen-ion concentration (ECF $[H^+]$). The cerebral blood volume will change by approximately 4 ml for every change in $PaCO_2$ of 5 mmHg (0.6 kPa). Below a $PaCO_2$ of 25 mmHg (3.3 kPa), there is a danger of causing cerebral hypoperfusion. Therefore, the suggested ideal $PaCO_2$ in these circumstances is 25–35 mmHg (3.3–4.7 kPa). However, normally there is almost full adaptation to the new $PaCO_2$ and a return to the same CBF within 4 hours. If the $PaCO_2$ returns to 'normal' levels, a dangerous increase in CBF can result, as the so-called normal $PaCO_2$ will then be equivalent to hypercarbia. The 'ideal' $PaCO_2$ in patients with elevated ICP values is not known and hyperventilation should be reserved for use as a temporary measure when the ICP rises suddenly. Otherwise, the $PaCO_2$ should be kept at 40 mmHg (5.3 kPa). Similarly, acidosis should be avoided as it can also increase CBF independent of $PaCO_2$.

## Oxygenation

Hypoxia ($PaO_2$ < 50 mmHg [6.7 kPa]) can cause an increase in CBF. Maintaining an airway and guaranteeing ventilation and oxygenation is therefore essential for the management of an elevated ICP.

## Diuretics

Of all the diuretics, mannitol has become the one most frequently used in clinical practice. Like hyperventilation, it can only buy time and certainly is no substitute for the definitive measures needed to reduce intracranial volume, such as drainage of a subdural or extradural haematoma. It should be given as a bolus at 0.3 g/kg over 15 minutes and then no more frequently than 8 hourly. Higher doses cause rapid increases in circulatory blood volume and CBF, yielding a paradoxical increase in ICP. Mannitol should not be used at all if the serum osmolality is greater than 330 mOsm/L. A loop diuretic such as frusemide, will reduce ICP probably by its diuretic effect in addition to reducing CSF formation. It can enhance the action of mannitol. Frusemide should be used in small doses (0.2–0.3 mg/kg), repeated as necessary in order to avoid a sudden diuresis leading to hypovolaemia, hypotension and decreased CPP.

## Fluid restriction

Excessive intravenous (IV) administration of crystalloid can exacerbate cerebral oedema. Achieve 'euvolaemic dehydration' by maintaining the intravascular volume and CPP with blood or colloid and otherwise limit fluids to less than 1500 ml or approximately two-thirds of the patient's normal maintenance fluid intake over 24 hours. Maintain the serum sodium concentration at the upper limit of normal, as hyponatraemia can potentiate cerebral oedema.

## Avoid drugs which cause increases in intracranial pressure

- Most of the volatile anaesthetic agents (e.g. halothane, ethrane but not isoflurorane).
- Nitrous oxide.
- Ketamine.
- Sodium nitroprusside.
- Nitroglycerine.

## Maintain colloid oncotic pressure within normal limits

A low colloid oncotic pressure (COP) theoretically can encourage movement of fluid from the intravascular space and worsen cerebral oedema. Maintaining a normal serum albumin usually will maintain a normal COP.

## Decreased metabolic activity of the brain: 'coma therapy' or 'brain protection'

Although a decrease in metabolic activity is an attractive goal, it is clinically difficult to achieve. 'Coma therapy', using large IV doses of anaesthetic agents, such as barbiturates and propofol has, in the past, been used in order to reduce the ICP. Although the ICP can be reduced in the short term, these drugs often cause cardiovascular depression and immunosuppression and do not appear to have made any impact on outcome. In clinical practice, the metabolic activity of the brain is most effectively influenced by aggressive control of seizures. There may still be a place for drugs that can specifically decrease the ICP, when all other efforts have failed, or in specific conditions such as Reye's syndrome. High fever should be actively treated, as it can increase the cerebral metabolic rate. A relative degree of central hypothermia (35–36 °C) may, in turn, decrease cerebral metabolic rate and oxygen demand. However, excessive hypothermia must be avoided, as it predisposes to unpredictable haemodynamic effects, impairment of drug metabolism and increased rates of infection. It has also been suggested that glucose-containing solutions should be avoided during the early stages of treating head injuries, in an attempt to decrease brain metabolic activity by decreasing the supply of metabolic substrate.

Some of the drugs used to decrease cerebral metabolism and ICP are as follows:

Barbiturates: Intermittent or continuous IV infusions of barbiturates (e.g. thiopentone or phenobarbitone) are sometimes employed to control severe increases in ICP. Their effects of immunosuppression and cardiovascular depression, along with the absence of good data supporting their effectiveness, have limited the use of barbiturates for treating increased ICP. After cessation of treatment, the effects of large doses of barbiturates can take up to one week to wear off and so neurological assessment can be difficult.

Intravenous anaesthetic and sedative agents: Propofol will decrease the CBF and the ICP in certain patients. However, its effects in large doses have not been investigated and studies of its efficacy have not been performed on a large scale in seriously ill patients. Benzodiazepines, while having no specific action on brain metabolic rate, are often used to supplement sedation.

## Other drugs

Corticosteroids have been used extensively for the management of intracranial abnormalities. Their current uses are limited to patients with certain brain tumours, brain abscesses and meningoencephalitis. They have little, if any, place in the acute treatment of head injuries.

The indications for prophylactic anticonvulsants in patients with head injuries are controversial.

## Surgical procedures

Procedures to remove brain tissue or craniectomy are sometimes used to decrease severe elevations in ICP.

## Miscellaneous

- Aggressively control seizures which sometimes may not have an overt motor manifestation.
- Institute prophylaxis for stress ulcer.
- Seek an early return to enteral feeding.
- Give antibiotics for documented infection.
- Neurogenic pulmonary oedema is a rare condition in patients with elevated ICP, possibly associated with a sympathetic storm. It should be treated as for acute respiratory failure (see Chapter 16).
- In patients with diabetes insipidus, match urine output with hypo-osmolar fluids and consider giving desmopressin acetate (DDAVP), 1–5 units IV 4–6-hourly according to control of the polyuria.

## FURTHER READING

Castillo, del M. A. Monitoring neurological patients in intensive care. *Current Opinion in Critical Care* 7 (2001): 49–60.

Eker, C., Asgeirsson, B., Grande, P.-O., Schalen, W. and Nordstrom, C.-H. Improved outcome after severe head injury with a new therapy based on principles for brain volume regulation and preserved microcirculation. *Critical Care Medicine* 26 (1998): 1881–6.

Gisvold, S. W. The Lund concept for treatment of head injuries – faith or science? *Acta Anaesthesiologica Scandinavica* 45 (2001): 399–401.

Grant, I. S. and Andrews, P. J. D. ABC of intensive care: neurological support. *British Medical Journal* 319 (1999): 110–13.

Haitsma, I. K. and Maas, A. I. R. Advanced monitoring in the intensive care unit: brain tissue oxygen tension. *Current Opinion in Critical Care* 8 (2002): 115–20.

Macmillan, C. S. A. and Andrews, P. J. D. Cerebrovenous oxygen saturation monitoring: practical considerations and clinical relevance. *Intensive Care Medicine* 26 (2000): 1028–36.

# 24

# Specific intracranial problems

## Coma

Coma or decreased level of consciousness is a common condition in intensive care. Consciousness depends on both the reticular activating system (RAS), which is responsible for general alertness, and the cerebral cortex, which is responsible for the quality of behaviour. The cause of coma must be localised to one of these two sites – the brainstem, cerebral hemispheres or their connections. Coma is usually defined in terms of a Glasgow Coma Scale (GCS) of $\leq 9$.

### Causes of coma

The causes of coma are many (Table 24.1). A helpful mnemonic in order to assist in diagnosis is outlined:

A lcohol
E pilepsy
I nfection
O verdose
U raemia and other metabolic causes

T rauma, tumour, temperature
I nsulin
P sychiatric
S trokes and other vascular causes.

### Coma in intensive care

Although there are many causes of coma, the commonest in the setting of the ICU usually fall into these categories:

**Table 24.1.** Aetiology of coma

| | | |
|---|---|---|
| Cortical | | |
| | Structural: | Diffuse axonal injury |
| | | Tumour |
| | Vascular: | Cerebrovascular accidents – haemorrhage or infection |
| | | SAH |
| | | Arteriovenous malformation |
| | | Global ischaemic injury |
| | Trauma: | Subdural haemorrhage |
| | | Extradural haemorrhage |
| | | Multiple petechial haemorrhage |
| | | Contracoup injury |
| | Infection: | Cerebral abscess |
| | | Meningoencephalitis |
| | Metabolic: | Hypoxia |
| | | Hypercarbia |
| | | Hypoglycaemia |
| | | Hepatic failure |
| | | Renal failure |
| | | Rapid changes in serum osmolality |
| | | Electrolyte disorders |
| | | Endocrine abnormalities |
| | Others: | Hypothermia |
| | | Hypotension and shock |
| | | Poisons |
| | | Drugs |
| | | Post ictal |
| | | Psychiatric |
| Reticular activating system | | |
| | | Brain herniation |
| | | Tumour |
| | | Haemorrhage |
| | | Cerebrovascular injury |

1 Related to a primary brain lesion, e.g. head injury, global hypoxia.
2 As a result of a systemic illness, e.g. hepatic encephalopathy, multiorgan failure (MOF), shock, sepsis.
3 As a result of drugs, either those used for analgesia or sedation or as a result of poisoning.

The combination of (2) and (3) is common and is often called 'ICU coma'. It affects the elderly more severely than the young, is often exacerbated by MOF and is completely reversible.

## Specific syndromes important in the ICU

*Vegetative state* describes a syndrome of diffuse cortical damage together with brainstem activity, such as eye opening and movements but with no voluntary control of the movements. It is usually a long-term and permanent state associated with primary injuries such as head injury and global ischaemia.

The *locked in syndrome* describes a state of quadriplegia and paralysis of the lower cranial nerves with a normal level of consciousness. Patients can communicate only by blinking and eye movement. It is important to differentiate it from true coma. The syndrome is rare and survival is uncommon.

*Psychogenic coma* is recognised by apparent unresponsiveness with normal electroencephalogram (EEG) and brainstem tests.

## Assessment of coma

**Initial assessment and treatment of coma must occur simultaneously. Assess and control the airway, breathing and circulation and exclude hypoglycaemia.**

### History

History is all-important in the assessment of coma. A diagnosis can often be made rapidly by talking to witnesses. Of particular importance are the circumstances surrounding the onset of coma (e.g. headache, trauma, seizures), together with a history of previous illnesses (e.g. diabetes, drug abuse, epilepsy).

### Neurological assessment

A full neurological examination should be carried out but initial focus should be on diagnosing conditions that need rapid treatment such as:

- localising signs in trauma
- signs of raised intracranial pressure (ICP)
- meningism
- seizures.

Level of consciousness: Firstly assess the level of consciousness. The GCS is widely accepted as the standard method (Table 24.2). Coma is usually defined as a GCS < 9. It is usually documented in shorthand according to eye movement (E), motor response (M) and verbal response (V), e.g. E3M4V3 – giving a total GCS in this patient of 10. Of the components of the GCS, the best motor response gives the most useful prognostic information. Eliciting a painful stimulus in the supraorbital region can cause nerve damage and on the sternum can cause unsightly bruising. Nail bed pressure is more satisfactory.

The advantage of the GCS is that it provides a standardised, easily reproducible assessment of the level of consciousness rather than ill-defined words such as

**Table 24.2.** Glasgow coma scale

| Eye opening: | spontaneous | 4 |
|---|---|---|
| | to speech | 3 |
| | to pain | 2 |
| | nil | 1 |
| Best motor response: | obeys commands | 6 |
| | localises pain | 5 |
| | withdraws to pain | 4 |
| | abnormal flexion | 3 |
| | extensor response | 2 |
| | nil | 1 |
| Verbal response: | oriented | 5 |
| | confused conversation | 4 |
| | inappropriate words | 3 |
| | incomprehensible sounds | 2 |
| | nil | 1 |

semiconscious or rousable. Its disadvantages include the lack of localising signs or documentation of pupil size and reaction. These must be specified separately.

Motor function: Motor examination gives us two important pieces of information: focal signs and positioning. When assessing motor function, it is important to compare left and right sides. Asymmetry in muscle tone, power or reflexes is highly suggestive of a focal lesion. Plantar reflexes are not specific and most comatosed patients will have bilateral upgoing toes regardless of aetiology.

Brainstem reflexes: *Pupils* should be assessed for size, reactivity and equality. Unreactive, but not necessarily dilated pupils suggest a severe brainstem abnormality and a large unilateral pupil indicates tentorial herniation causing a third nerve palsy. Remember that a small percentage of the population normally have unequal pupils and that severe facial injuries can be associated with pupil damage. Small pupils usually result from a pontine lesion or ingestion of opiates.

*Pain* eliciting a painful stimulus below the neck should cause a cranial nerve response such as grimacing above the neck and vice versa. Bizarre spinal reflexes can sometimes occur in response to painful stimuli in the presence of brain death.

*Corneal reflex* when absent indicates deep coma.

*Gag reflex* stimulate the back of the throat or pass a suction catheter down the endotracheal tube (ETT) if the patient is intubated in order to test for a gag or cough reflex. Beware of eliciting a gag reflex in an unconscious patient with an unprotected airway.

*Ocular vestibular (caloric) reflexes* firstly, examine the external auditory canals for patency and an intact tympanic membrane. Ice cold water (20 ml) is then slowly syringed into each canal. Nystagmus should be provoked within 20–30 seconds. The so-called 'dolls eye movement' tests the same pathways in a less

**Table 24.3.** Acute management of coma

Support while making diagnosis
Maintain clear airway – intubate if any doubt
Ventilate if doubt about respiration
Maintain 'normal' BP
Restore intravascular volume
Correct hypoxia and anaemia
Give 50 g of glucose IV if hypoglycaemia cannot be excluded
Give 50 mg IV thiamine

satisfactory fashion and may be dangerous if there is a question of cervical spine injury.

*Abnormal respiratory patterns* such as Cheyne–Stokes are non-specific signs. Complete apnoea is part of the spectrum of total brainstem failure.

General examination: A complete and thorough general examination should be performed on all patients with coma, looking for:

- Needle marks.
- Signs of trauma.
- Signs of chronic disease – alcoholism, renal failure.
- Signs of skin and muscle damage as a result of pressure, e.g. compartment syndrome.

### Investigations

Rapidly exclude:

- hypoglycaemia
- hypoxia
- hypercarbia
- electrolyte abnormalities
- drug overdose.

Further evaluation may require CT scan, lumbar puncture, angiography, EEG or magnetic resonance imaging (MRI).

### Management of coma (Table 24.3)

Keep the patient alive until a diagnosis is made. The general principles of management of the critically ill apply. The management of specific causes of coma are discussed elsewhere, e.g. head injuries, meningitis and poisoning.

### Airway

Maintaining a clear airway and preventing aspiration is the first priority in the management of coma. Lateral posturing and supplemental oxygen is often sufficient if the gag reflex is adequate. If not, intubation is mandatory.

### Ventilation

Ventilation should be performed if there is doubt about adequate respiration or as a short-term measure to decrease ICP by decreasing the $PaCO_2$ and cerebral blood flow (CBF).

### Blood flow and oxygenation

Adequate cerebral perfusion with well-oxygenated blood is essential. Maintain a normal arterial blood pressure where possible and restore the intravascular volume, correct hypoxia and anaemia.

### Drugs

If there is any doubt about whether the coma is related to hypoglycaemia, 50 g of intravenous glucose should be administered. Thiamine and naloxone are often given as first-line drugs in order to exclude the involvement of alcohol or narcotics.

## Prognosis

The best indicators of survival are related to the cause of the coma, age, best motor response, duration of coma, the absence of intracranial haemorrhage and the state of somatosensory evoked potentials. As a general rule, and apart from head injuries or where sedation has been used, when a patient aged more than 20 years has been in a coma for more than 2 weeks the mortality approaches 100%.

## Global ischaemia

This is a term implying generalised cerebral damage due to insufficient blood flow, usually as a result of cardiorespiratory arrest (Table 24.4). The term global ischaemia also implies damage secondary to severe hypoxia, hypotension, anaemia or following insults such as carbon monoxide poisoning.

Some aspects of the pathophysiology of cerebral ischaemia are becoming clearer. For example, while complete functional recovery cannot be expected after more than 7 minutes of normothermic global anoxia, some neurones can survive 1 hour of circulatory arrest. The duration, as well as the degree of ischaemia, will also affect cellular survival.

**Table 24.4.** Summary of management in global ischaemia (see Chapter 23)

| |
|---|
| Protect the airway |
| Prevent hypoxia |
| Prevent hypercarbia |
| Facilitate cerebral venous drainage |
| Maintain a 'normal' BP for that patient |
| Nurse the patient in the 30°–45° head up position, keeping the head straight and avoid constricting tape around the neck |
| Avoid hypertensive surges |
| Avoid drugs which may cause an increase in ICP |
| Maintain 'euvolaemic dehydration', i.e. avoid excessive clear fluid but maintain intravascular volume |
| Treat epilepsy aggressively |

The only effective treatment given after the event that improves neurologic recovery in patients with cardiac arrest is induced hypothermia. Studies showed hypothermia was effective in out-of-hospital arrests in ventricular fibrillation. Caution should be exercised extrapolating this data to in-hospital arrests with asystole!

Brain swelling and raised ICP is not as marked a feature of global ischaemia as it can be, for example, in severe head injury. Therefore, ICP monitoring and osmotherapy are rarely indicated.

The only undisputed therapeutic principle is to improve the cerebral oxygen demand: supply ratio. The rapid restoration and maintenance of cerebral perfusion and arterial oxygenation is crucial. The general principles of management of any intracranial disaster have been outlined previously.

Drugs such as antioxidants, free radical scavengers, steroids, barbiturates, lazaroids, calcium-channel blockers and prostaglandin inhibitors have so far not been demonstrated to influence recovery from global ischaemia.

## Prognosis (Table 24.5)

The most important clinical advances in the management of global ischaemia have been in prognostic guidelines. These have obvious importance as to whether active treatment should be continued or withdrawn. Patients in coma after cardiac arrest and global ischaemia are commonly seen in the ICU. The major dilemma is whether after all the efforts of resuscitation, the patient will remain in a persistent vegetative state (PVS). The indiscriminate salvage of patients in a PVS remains one of the more legitimate criticisms levelled against ICUs. Only approximately 10% of patients regain any sort of independent function after coma resulting from global ischaemia. Many patients remain in a PVS with spontaneous eye opening,

**Table 24.5.** Guidelines for management of global ischaemia based on prognosis

| Time following initial global ischaemia | Best response | Management |
|---|---|---|
| 48 hours | Motor response to pain – extensor or absent | Withdraw and withhold therapy |
| | Motor response to pain – better than extensor | Full ICU support for another 24 hours |
| 72 hours | GCS < 5 | Withdraw and withhold therapy |
| | GCS 5–8 | Tracheostomy for airway support |
| | | Explain very poor prognosis to family. Review in 2 weeks |
| | | Can support own airway – extubate Very guarded prognosis |
| 2 weeks | GCS 6–8 | Withdraw and withhold therapy |
| | GCS >8 | Extubate as own airway can be maintained |

normal brainstem reflexes but without cognition – 'the lights are on but nobody is at home'.

Careful and frequent neurological examination should be performed as a guide to prognosis. One needs to regularly assess pupillary light reflex, motor response, spontaneous eye movement and corneal reflex with regard to prognosis, especially in the first 72 hours after the onset of coma. The rate of clinical improvement should be taken into consideration.

To prevent unnecessary suffering to patients and relatives, it is important not to prolong advanced supportive measures indefinitely where there is little hope.

EEG – although burst suppression and predominately delta patterns are indicators of a poor prognosis, there are no specific features of global ischaemia on EEG.

Sensory evoked potentials (SEPs) – absent cortical response at 8 hours is a bad prognostic sign.

The patient's age, sex, spontaneous eye opening, presence of post-anoxic seizures and myoclonic seizures do not correlate well with neurological outcome. However, status epilepticus and status myoclonus are predictive of a poor outcome.

## Cerebral infarction

Acute cerebrovascular events can lead to infarction or haemorrhage. Cerebral infarction is usually as a result of thrombosis or embolism. Patients with cerebral thrombosis and cerebral embolism are usually not routinely admitted to the ICU because active monitoring and support rarely changes the course of the disease. Brain infarction is not amenable to many interventions in the ICU, apart from special circumstances such as a postoperative complication of carotid artery endarterectomy or craniectomy in malignant middle cerebral artery stroke.

Strokes are very common in our community. An ageing population with a high incidence of hypertension and arteriosclerosis is being treated in our ICUs. These patients can coincidentally develop cerebral infarction, precipitated by events such as hypotension, hypoxia or atrial fibrillation, whilst being treated in the ICU for other conditions. Early mobilisation and rehabilitation in a specialised unit offers the best outcome for patients with cerebral infarction.

## Investigation

The most important investigation in cerebral infarction is a CT scan in order to exclude other pathology such as intracranial haemorrhage, especially if the question of anticoagulation is being considered. However, the evidence for infarction on CT scan may not be seen for several days and there are certain areas of the brain such as the brainstem which are difficult to visualise on CT scan and may be more amenable to screening with MRI.

## Treatment

### Support

General supportive measures such as physiotherapy, maintenance of a good airway, prevention of pressure areas and nutritional support are the mainstay of treatment. Low-dose heparin or 'antithrombotic' stockings may reduce the associated high incidence of deep venous thrombosis. The role of antiplatelet therapy has not, as yet, been established.

### Surgery

Surgical procedures such as carotid endarterectomy are useful as a preventative measure but have no place in the management of acute stroke. There are many doubts about the effectiveness of extracranial–intracranial anastomoses in the prevention of strokes. Decompressive surgery and ventriculostomy for occlusive hydrocephalus may be indicated in certain circumstances.

### Hypertension

Beware of acutely reducing the patient's BP after a stroke unless it is much higher than 'normal' and even then, cautiously. Hypertension is common after stroke and may be a reflex phenomenon which helps to maintain blood flow.

### Other drugs

Drugs such as corticosteroids, 21-amino-steroids, osmolar agents or naloxone should be avoided until evidence for their efficacy is demonstrated. There is currently little evidence for the routine use of thrombolytics for the acute management of stroke. However, trials are currently under way to determine if there is a subgroup of patients who would benefit from thrombolytics. The therapeutic window is very narrow. Tissue salvage is optimal within 45 minutes. After 4 hours the incidence of associated parenchymal haemorrhage is relatively high.

## Spontaneous intracranial haemorrhage

Cerebral infarction secondary to thrombosis or embolism accounts for approximately 85% of strokes and spontaneous intracranial haemorrhage accounts for a further 10–12%.

### Intracerebral haemorrhage

Intracerebral haemorrhage is usually the result of systemic hypertension, but can also result from other forms of intracranial pathology such as arteriovenous malformations, tumours or infection. It can also occur secondary to thrombocytopaenia or a coagulopathy. Diagnosis is best made by CT scan which may also help in deciding whether evacuation of the haematoma is indicated (Figure 24.1). Most cases are treated conservatively but surgical evacuation may be indicated if the haematoma is within the cerebellum or elsewhere causing a mass effect with raised ICP or hydrocephalus. The prognosis largely depends on local destruction due to haemorrhage rather than the level of ICP.

### Subarachnoid haemorrhage

Subarachnoid haemorrhage (SAH) refers to bleeding within the subarachnoid space rather than the brain parenchyma and is usually the result of rupture of a cerebral aneurysm. The peak incidence of SAH occurs in the fourth to sixth decade of life and two-thirds of all cases are women. The classical onset is marked by abrupt onset of headache, a variable period of unconsciousness, vomiting, meningeal irritation and focal signs (Table 24.6). A preceding or 'sentinel headache' occurs in up to 50% of patients. Confirmation is usually by CT scan. Lumbar puncture will often cause an acute deterioration, especially if there is significant intracerebral bleeding. Lumbar puncture should therefore be performed after CT scan unless CT scanning is unavailable and then, only in the absence of signs of raised ICP. Xanthochromia in cerebrospinal fluid (CSF)

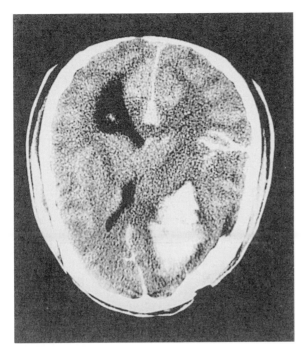

**Figure 24.1.** CT scan head – intracranial haemorrhage with surrounding oedema and midline shift.

**Table 24.6.** Grading of subarachnoid haemorrhage*

|           | Glasgow Coma Scale | Motor deficit       |
| --------- | ------------------ | ------------------- |
| Grade I   | 15                 | Absent              |
| Grade II  | 13 or 14           | Absent              |
| Grade III | 13 or 14           | Present             |
| Grade IV  | 7–12               | Absent or present   |
| Grade V   | 3–6                | Absent or present   |

*Scale developed by World Federation of Neurological Surgeons.

results from the breakdown of haemoglobin and occurs if blood has been present in the CSF for at least 6 hours.

### Outcome
Approximately half of all patients with SAH die, 12% before hospital and 40% within a month of hospital admission. More than one-third of all survivors will

**Table 24.7.** Total mortality associated with subarachnoid haemorrhage

| | |
|---|---|
| Initial haemorrhage | 50% |
| Vasospasm | 20% |
| Rebleed | 13% |
| Surgery | 4% |
| Other | 13% |

have major neurological deficits and cognitive defects are present in many of the so-called good outcomes. The major complications are rebleeding, vasospasm and hydrocephalus (Table 24.7). Wherever possible the patient should be rapidly transferred to a specialised neurosurgical unit. The aim of treatment is to prevent further haemorrhage and to manage the sequelae of the haemorrhage such as vasospasm and cerebral oedema.

## Investigation

Serial CT scan: A CT scan is essential in order to detect the site and extent of bleeding as well as associated oedema, infarction or hydrocephalus. The CT scan is 90–95% positive if the study is performed within 24 hours of the bleed. The pattern of subarachnoid blood on CT scan may suggest the likely location of the ruptured aneurysm. If there is a strong suspicion of SAH in the presence of a normal CT scan, then lumbar puncture should be performed.

Angiography: Angiography is needed to demonstrate the anatomy of the aneurysm and its association with parent vessels, as well as to define the presence of vasospasm and to exclude multiple aneurysms. MRI angiography and helical CT angiography is less invasive but also less sensitive.

## Management

General principles: While there are commonly agreed guidelines for the management of SAH, they are not based on exhaustive Evidence-Based Medicine (EBM) principles. The general principles of care of the unconscious patient and the principles of care associated with raised ICP apply to these patients. However, beware of controlling hypertension too rapidly. Hypertension may herald the onset of further haemorrhage. A high pressure may also be needed to maintain an adequate CBF, especially in the presence of vasospasm. However, hypertension ($\geq$160 mmHg systolic) must also be avoided in order to prevent rebleeding. β-blockers are the drug of choice.

Vasospasm or delayed cerebral ischaemia: Vasospasm is responsible for much of the morbidity and mortality associated with SAH. It generally develops between the 5th and 14th day after the SAH with a peak incidence between days 7 and 10. There is a 30–40% incidence of clinical vasospasm and between 60 and 80%

incidence on angiography. The incidence of vasospasm is correlated with the extent of the haemorrhage. However, the pathophysiology is not well understood. The diagnosis is made on clinical grounds and confirmed by angiography, doppler or CBF studies. Symptoms include an insidious decrease in the level of consciousness and fluctuating focal neurological signs. Angiography can worsen the vasospasm. The calcium-channel blockers, especially nimodipine (60 mg orally 4-hourly for 21 days), are widely used for the prevention and treatment of vasospasm. Dose commences at 15 $\mu g \cdot kg^{-1} . h^{-1}$ IV infusion and, monitoring the BP carefully, increasing to 30 $\mu g \cdot kg^{-1} . h^{-1}$ IV infusion for 7 days, followed by 14 days of oral therapy. Other therapies include endovascular balloon angioplasty and intra-arterial papavarine. After the aneurysm is clipped, induced hypertension, hypervolaemia and haemodilation ('triple H' therapy) can be used to increase cerebral perfusion pressure (CPP). Cerebral autoregulation is impaired in the ischaemic area and blood flow possibly changes with BP. Aim for 20–40 mmHg (2.6–5.3 kPa) higher than the premorbid systolic BP.

Triple H therapy (Hypervolaemia; Hypoviscosity; Hypertension) can be used to reduce vasospasm. There is no definitive evidence for this approach. Moreover, the excess fluid is rapidly excreted as part of a normal physiological response. In other words, hypervolaemia and resulting hypoviscosity are at best short lived and possibly dangerous. Artificial hypertension up to approximately 160 mmHg systolic, may be beneficial in overcoming vasospasm but there is no strong evidence.

Rebleeding: Rebleeding occurs in 15–20% of patients with a rate of 4–20% within the first 24 hours and then between 1 and 2% per day for the first 2 weeks. The mortality associated with rebleeding is approximately 25%. This is related to clot breakdown. Antifibrinolytics such as epsilon aminocaproic acid (EACA) have been suggested in order to reduce the incidence of further haemorrhage. However, EACA can also cause intracerebral and systemic venous thrombosis as well as vasospasm and we await the results of further trials as to its real efficacy. Rebleeding can be prevented by surgical clipping of the neck of the aneurysm or endovascular therapy.

Surgery: Ventriculostomy is commonly required because of blood in the basal cisterns and the high incidence of hydrocephalus. The placement of a clip across the neck of an intracranial aneurysm is the most definitive treatment. As with most other aspects of SAH there is controversy over timing. As a general principle, patients who are grade IV or V are initially treated conservatively and depending on progress are clipped at a later date, while grade I–III patients should have early surgery. However, practice and results vary widely. Emergency surgery is indicated in patients who have a major mass effect as a result of a haematoma. There is an increasing trend to aggressive craniectomy, especially in those patients with cerebral oedema. In these cases the oedema is commonly seen on CT scan in the form of white matter forming 'fingers' towards the periphery of the brain tissue.

Endovascular therapy: This is emerging as a promising alternative to surgical clipping in selective cases such as in aneurysms with narrow necks or in basilar aneurysms. Soft metallic coils which encourage thrombosis of the sac are used.

Other complications: Cardiac arrhythmias, myocardial ischaemia and pulmonary oedema can sometimes occur in SAH. This is probably related to massive catecholamine release. Convulsions occur in about 5% of patients. Cerebral oedema occurs in approximately 20% of patients and may transiently respond to measures such as mannitol or hypertonic saline.

Summary: Management of patients with SAH has been made difficult by the lack of knowledge about pathophysiology and specific management. For example, guidelines on the control of the BP include warnings about hypertension causing further bleeding, as well as suggestions about the possible benefits of induced hypertension in vasospasm. More data are needed on the role of drugs in vasospasm and rebleeding, as well as the timing of surgery.

## Severe head injury

- Defined as GCS $\leq$ 8 after resuscitation and lasting for $>$ 6 hours.
- Meticulous and obsessive intensive care is vital to the outcome of severe head injury.
- It is difficult to achieve consensus on approach to severe head injury management because of heterogeneous population and lack of large randomised controlled trials.

### Primary head injury
Primary head trauma occurs at the moment of impact and includes scalp lacerations, skull fractures and brain injury.

### Secondary head injury
Secondary damage occurs as a result of oedema from injured cerebral tissue, bleeding from torn intracranial blood vessels or exacerbation of primary damage. Some of the causes of secondary brain injury include:

- hypoxia
- hypercarbia/hypocarbia
- hypoglycaemia/hyperglycaemia
- seizures
- hypotension/hypertension.

**Treatment of severe head injury is aimed at limiting the secondary damage which occurs mainly in the first 8 hours.**

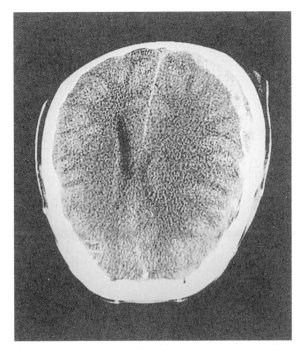

**Figure 24.2.** CT scan head – subdural haematoma and midline shift as a result of trauma.

## Intracranial haemorrhage (Figures 24.2 and 24.3)

*Extradural haematoma* occurs between the dura and inner table of the skull, usually as a result of laceration of the middle meningeal artery.

*Subdural haematoma* occurs between the inner table's dural surface and the thin meninges covering the brain. The bleeding is usually venous in origin and associated with contusion of the underlying brain.

*Intracerebral haematoma* variable in size, number and locations according to the force of impact.

### Initial management

For more details on the principles outlined below see Chapter 14.

#### Airway
The patient's level of consciousness is often impaired leading to airway obstruction. This may be exacerbated by facial fractures and bleeding.

## Intracranial Haemorrhage

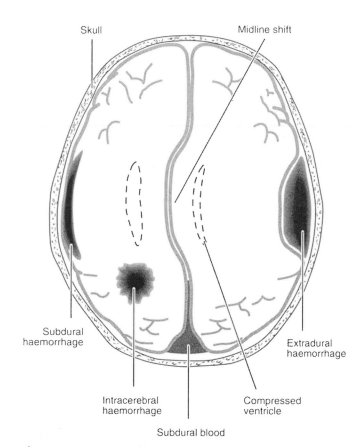

**Figure 24.3.** Intracranial haemorrhage

Initially, attempt chin lift and jaw thrust manoeuvres or insert an oropharyngeal airway. If there is doubt about the airway, *intubate*.
Technique for intubation:

- Keep the head in a neutral position during airway manoeuvres until cervical spine fractures have been excluded. This is achieved by inline immobilisation or a hard collar.
- Avoid nasal intubation, especially if base of skull fractures are suspected.
- Avoid aspiration – always suspect a full stomach and use rapid sequence intubation with preoxygenation and cricoid pressure.

- Sedate the patient adequately in order to prevent hypertensive surges during instrumentation. Hypertensive surges can aggravate intracranial bleeding and cerebral oedema. During intubation, keep the patient well sedated in order to prevent coughing and straining for the same reason. In the short term, an intubating dose of a drug such as thiopentone is useful for preventing hypertensive surges. However, in the presence of hypovolaemia and cardiovascular instability, the dose would have to be modified in order not to decrease the BP and CPP.
- Insert orogastric tube initially. Change to a nasogastric when a base of skull fracture is ruled out.

## Ventilation
All patients with serious head injury require artificial ventilation. This should be rapidly instituted, especially when the injuries are in association with chest injuries or hypercarbia and hypoxia. Aim for a $PaO_2$ of $> 90$ mmHg (12 kPa) and a normal $PaCO_2$ of 40 mmHg (5.3 kPa).

Hyperventilation is a short-term measure which decreases ICP by decreasing CBF. However, CBF rapidly adapts to a lower $PaCO_2$ and returns to a former baseline. This can give a false sense of security. If the $PaCO_2$ then rises to a so-called 'normal' level, this represents hypercarbia with an increase in CBF and ICP. After artificial hyperventilation, care should be exercised when returning to 'normal' levels of $PaCO_2$, so that the CBF can adjust to a new level of $PaCO_2$.

## Cerebral blood flow
Hypovolaemia and hypotension should be reversed as soon as possible in order to establish an adequate CPP and CBF. Acute injury diminishes the brain's ability to withstand changes in $PaCO_2$ and CPP. Hyperventilation causing $PaCO_2$ levels less than 25 mmHg (3.3 kPa) should be avoided as it may cause cerebral ischaemia.

Hypotension in the presence of cerebral trauma is *not* due to the brain injury. The most likely cause is hypovolaemia (exacerbated by mannitol and other diuretics). Other causes of hypotension include concurrent drugs or cardiac dysfunction related to contusion or coincidental infarction.

## Haemoglobin
Significant bleeding should be rapidly treated with blood. Beware of underestimating blood loss from scalp wounds which can account for rapid and early loss of blood at the site of injury.

## Sedation
Sedation during ventilation is often necessary to achieve pain relief and to prevent hypertensive surges, coughing and straining; all of which increase ICP. A continuous infusion of narcotics and benzodiazepines is safe, effective and inexpensive. Muscle relaxants should be avoided if possible.

Routine use of IV anaesthetic agents such as barbiturates, once claimed to offer 'brain protection', is becoming less fashionable because of the dangers of cardiovascular depression and immune suppression. The role of other drugs such as propofol has not been defined.

The argument that sedation obscures neurological signs is offset by the disadvantages of a restless patient on a ventilator with surges of increased ICP.

## Priorities in management

Head injuries often occur in the setting of multitrauma and management priorities need to be established. For example, if the patient is hypotensive despite ongoing blood and colloids they may need a laparotomy/thoracotomy before a head CT scan. If the patient is stable, a head CT may be done before other more definitive treatment.

## Diagnosis, assessment and further treatment (Table 24.8)

**A full and thorough general examination of patients with multitrauma must be performed as soon as possible in order to exclude other injuries (see Chapter 14).**

### Neurological examination

Document the level of consciousness according to the GCS. Examine the external scalp for obvious fractures. Fractures of the orbital and maxillofacial structures can usually be detected by palpation. A bloody discharge from the nose or ear indicates leakage of CSF. Bruising over the mastoid bone (Battle's sign) and periorbital haematoma (raccoon's eyes) suggest a base of skull fracture.

The size and reaction of pupils and evidence of decortication or decerebration and evidence of lateralising signs in the limbs should all be tested. Ongoing neurological assessment should be performed frequently. This should consist of a clinical examination recording GCS, pupil size and reaction, tone, reflexes and cranial nerve function. This can be difficult in severely traumatised patients, especially those with high levels of sedation and muscle relaxation. Pupil dilation is a reliable but late neurological sign. Intracranial pressure monitoring is useful and should be inserted in all patients with severe head injury. The intracranial compliance can be estimated by transiently occluding the internal jugular veins and observing the rate of rise of ICP and return to baseline levels. This should not be attempted when the ICP is moderately raised.

### CT scanning

Any serious head injury should be investigated with a CT scan as soon as the patient is resuscitated and relatively stable (Table 24.9).

**Table 24.8.** Management of severe head injuries

Secure the airway – if in doubt, intubate with in line immobilisation of head and neck
Stabilise the cervical spine with a hard collar until fracture/dislocation is excluded
Sedate and paralyse all patients for intubation. Prevent coughing and gagging which
    causes acute rises in ICP
Artificially ventilate to ensure normal oxygenation and normal $PaCO_2$ of 40 mmHg
    (5.3 kPa)
Maintain normal mean arterial pressure (MAP) and keep CPP >60 mmHg (9.3 kPa)
CPP = MAP – ICP. Hypotension is almost always as a result of blood loss, not
    intracranial pathology. Aggressively lower the ICP. If ICP remains high consider
    vasopressors to maintain CPP in euvolaemia.
CT scan. Clinical signs are notoriously inaccurate in determining intracranial pathology.
    Exclude and treat intracranial haematomas
Facilitate cerebral venous drainage
    Sit patient up $\geq 30°$
    Avoid compressing internal jugulars with ill-fitting hard collars and artificial airway
        fixation
    Avoid high levels of PEEP and high ventilatory pressures unless absolutely necessary
    Avoid high intra-abdominal pressures which can increase right heart filling pressure
        and ICP
Sedate but avoid neuromuscular blockade if possible
Avoid hypertensive surges before procedures such as endotracheal suction and
    physiotherapy, e.g. bolus of sedation plus lignocaine 1.5 mg/kg
Avoid excessive fluid intake – maintain normal intravascular volume and avoid excessive
    oedema
Avoid fever – aim for normothermia
Avoid high intrathoracic or intra-abdominal pressure

**Table 24.9.** Mnemonic for reviewing CT scans

| Blood | – | Blood |
|-------|---|-------|
| Can | – | identify four key Cisterns |
| Be | – | examine Brain |
| Very | – | review four Ventricles |
| Bad | – | bones of Cranium |

As a general guide, all head-injured patients with transient loss of consciousness, post-traumatic amnesia or localising signs should have a CT scan regardless
of the GCS.

A follow-up CT scan within 24 hours of admission reveals new pathology in
about one-third of patients and about one-third of these will require surgery.

Further CT scanning should also be considered for clinical deterioration or a persistently raised ICP.

All patients going to have a CT scan should be accompanied by personnel skilled in advanced resuscitation.

## Monitoring and investigations
- Concurrent monitoring of ICP and mean arterial BP to determine CPP form the basis of monitoring severe head injuries. Aim for a CPP of more than 60 mmHg (9.3 kPa) and an ICP of less than 20 mmHg (2.7 kPa).
- Jugular bulb oximetry ($SjO_2$) – enables assessment of global cerebral oxygen delivery ($DO_2$) and utilisation. The $SjO_2$ may be useful for determining optimum CPP and $PaCO_2$ levels as well as for tracking effects of treatment and as an indication of prognosis. Normal $SjO_2$ levels are 55–75%.
- $SjO_2$ < 55%: may indicate oedema – consider osmotherapy.
- $SjO_2$ >75%: may indicate cerebral hyperperfusion – consider extra sedation, β blockade and use together with transcranial doppler (TCD) to confirm hyperaemia.
- A TCD permits continuous assessment of middle cerebral artery flow velocity which can be a useful indicator of CBF when used in conjunction with other monitoring such as $SjO_2$ and CPP.
- EEG – apart from the detection of seizures may offer prognostic information.
- MRI, single photon emission CT (SPECT), positron emission tomography (PET) and xenon-133 enhanced CT have, as yet, little application in the clinical management of acute head injuries.

## Nutrition
Early enteral feeding is desirable. However, there is often an ileus and excessive gastric aspirates in patients with severe head injuries, even in the absence of abdominal trauma.

## Surgery
Obviously significant intracranial haemorrhage should be surgically evacuated as soon as possible. The delay from injury to operation is the single most important determinant of prognosis. Meticulous management of the patient along the lines already outlined must be maintained during transport to and from the CT facilities, as well as during the operative procedure.

## Skull fractures
Skull x-rays are often performed for head injuries, but the absence or otherwise of fractures has little bearing on outcome except as an indicator of a higher than otherwise incidence of intracranial bleeding.

Depressed fractures may require early elevation, especially if compound or causing a mass effect.

Basal fractures are often complicated by tearing of the dura mater with CSF leak and possible cranial nerve damage. Prophylactic antibiotics are not initially indicated. Surgery may be indicated for persistent CSF leaks.

## Cerebral oedema

Most patients with head injury develop some degree of cerebral oedema. This can vary from minor concussion to rapidly life-threatening generalised oedema. The general principles of treatment of cerebral oedema have been outlined previously (see Chapter 23). They are summarised here.

Ventilation: The length of time that the patient needs to be ventilated is variable. From ICP and CT scan evidence, the acute stage of intracranial oedema causing compression is between 2 and 15 days. The advantages and disadvantages of ventilation for each patient need to be assessed on a daily basis. Remember, reducing $PaCO_2$ is only a short-term measure for reducing CBF and ICP – they both usually return to a baseline value within 4 hours.

It is advisable to keep the $PaCO_2$ normal at 40 mmHg (5.3 kPa) so that hyperventilation can be used as a reserve measure in case of further increases in ICP. As we learn more about head injuries, we may be able to define certain subgroups of patients where hyperaemia is an important feature, in which case hyperventilation may be more effective by reducing CBF and ICP.

Sedation: With continuous IV narcotics, benzodiazepines or propofol. Straining and coughing should be avoided as it causes acute rises in ICP. Boluses of sedation should be tried before procedures such as turning or physiotherapy.

Facilitate venous drainage: sit patient $30°$–$45°$ – make sure BP is maintained in order to guarantee adequate cerebral perfusion.

Head position: Avoid head turning or tying the ETT tightly with a constricting bandage. Hard collars for stabilisation of cervical spines increases ICP, probably by reducing venous drainage and should be removed as soon as the cervical spine is cleared. Keep the patient sitting up at least $30°$.

CSF: Avoid epidural analgesia as it may interfere with CSF drainage from the ventricles and consequently exacerbate a rise in ICP. Consider drainage of CSF if intraventricular catheter is in place.

Temperature: Aim to keep the patient's body temperature normal. Perhaps selective intracranial cooling may become important.

Decompressive craniectomy: There is increasing use of craniectomy for persistently raised ICP.

Mannitol: 0.3 g/kg – only for acute rises in ICP that have a reversible cause.

Intravenous fluids: Maintain normal intravascular volume with colloid or blood plus maintenance fluid.

Seizures: Treat seizures aggressively.

Blood pressure: There are two opposing schools of thought with regard to BP. Some believe increasing the BP to maintain the CPP in the presence of raised

ICP is beneficial. Others suggest that increasing the BP causes an increase in capillary hydrostatic pressure causing increased cerebral oedema. The so-called Lund school believe maintaining normal intravascular volume and not artificially increasing the BP optimises outcome. To complicate matters, lowering the BP too far would cause cerebral vasodilatation and an increase in ICP. Perhaps the best approach is to maintain the patient's normal BP. Another way of thinking about the issue is to attempt to lower the ICP if that is the primary problem and to increase the BP if reversible hypotension is the cause of reduced CPP.

## Outcome

Most head injuries are minor and only admitted for short-term observation. However, many patients with even minor head injuries suffer long-term effects such as headaches, emotional disturbances and personality changes. Other symptoms such as cognitive dysfunction, fatigability, depressive symptoms, anxiety, flattening of affect and slowness of thinking are very common. The more serious the initial head injury is, the more profound these symptoms are.

The facilities and services for rehabilitation of patients with head injuries are usually not as good as for their acute management.

Unfortunately there are few early and accurate predictors of outcome from head injuries. About one-third of patients with severe head injury die, one-third make a good recovery and one-third are variously disabled. Many of the so-called 'good recoveries' have the long-term disabilities mentioned in the previous paragraph. This is an enormous burden on society as well as on the relatives and friends of patients. The increasing age of the patient and severity of the GCS correlate with a bad prognosis. For each year over the age of 35 that a patient is in coma for more than 6 hours, the chance of death or PVS increases by about 3.6% – so that by the age of 75 and after being in coma for more than 6 hours, the chance of dying or being left in a PVS is almost 100%.

## Viral encephalitis

Apart from herpes simplex encephalitis (HSE) most common viral infections of the central nervous system (CNS) tend to be relatively benign. The diagnosis is usually made on history and examination and is often one of exclusion. The specific virus is often difficult to isolate.

Clinical features:

- Headache
- Vomiting
- Fever

- Seizures
- Signs of increased ICP
- Neck stiffness
- Drowsiness
- Focal neurological signs

CSF:

- Often normal
- Raised protein
- Glucose – normal to low
- Raised white cell count – especially lymphocytes.

EEG: non-specific.
CT scan: non-specific changes.

## Herpes simplex encephalitis

Herpes simplex encephalitis is the most common form of sporadic encephalitis and has a very high mortality and morbidity.

### Diagnosis

Herpes simplex encephalitis may have a higher incidence of focal EEG abnormalities and more temporal lobe involvement on CT scan and MRI scanning than other forms of viral encephalitis. However, these findings may be normal in the early stages of the disease. Moreover, abnormalities are not specific for HSE. Specific herpes simplex viral antibody titres are accurate but delayed. Antigen detection using a polymerase chain reaction (PCR) technique is proving a sensitive technique for early detection of HSE infection. Because antiviral agents originally used in HSE had many side-effects, a specific diagnosis by brain biopsy was thought essential. This is no longer thought necessary.

### Treatment

The mortality of HSE approaches 70%. This depressing outcome may be favourably influenced by early administration of acyclovir (10 mg/kg, 8-hourly for 10 days) a specific antiviral agent. The lack of serious side effects of this agent and the high morbidity and mortality associated with HSE suggests that acyclovir should be started in any patient with suspected viral encephalitis who has focal clinical features, while waiting for confirmation with viral antibody tests. The management of raised ICP in association with encephalitis follows the general principles of raised ICP due to any cause and has been outlined elsewhere (see Chapter 23).

## Bacterial meningoencephalitis

### Clinical features

- Fever
- Headache
- Signs of raised ICP
- Photophobia
- Neck stiffness
- Altered level of consciousness
- Excitability and restlessness
- Seizures.

It is important to make a rapid diagnosis of bacterial meningitis as it carries a high morbidity and mortality. These patients can deteriorate and even die within hours of presentation.

### Management

**The sooner antibiotics are started, the better the patient outcome.** There is good evidence to suggest that antibiotics should be commenced as soon as the disease is suspected even in the prehospital setting.

Lumbar puncture: Because of the danger of raised ICP and coning, a CT scan should be performed before a lumbar puncture is attempted. However, a normal CT scan does not guarantee normal ICP. Blind antibiotic therapy should be commenced without an initial lumbar puncture.

Organisms: The causative organisms in children more than 3 months old and adults are usually *Neisseria meningitidis, Haemophilus influenzae* type B, or *Streptococcus pneumoniae*. It is usually a disease of childhood but also occurs in adults.

If antibiotics were given before the organism was identified, pneumococcal or haemophilus antigens may be detected in the urine. Alternatively, PCR may be performed on the CSF at a later time.

Bacterial identification can often be made on Gram-staining. While waiting for identification and sensitivities, the following antibiotic therapy should be commenced.

Cefotaxime 50 mg/kg up to 2 g/kg IV 6-hourly
*plus either*
penicillin 1.8 g IV 4-hourly
*or*
ampicillin 2 g IV 4-hourly.

The antibiotics may need modification when sensitivities are known.

Prophylaxis in the form of rifampicin 20 mg/kg (maximum 600 mg) should be given daily for 4 days to all people who had close contact with patients who have had meningococcal meningitis.

Strains of *Haemophilus influenzae*, resistant to ampicillin and chloramphenicol have been identified. Strains of *Streptococcus pneumoniae* have also been identified which are resistant to penicillin. High doses of third-generation cephalosporins such as cefotaxime or ceftriaxone are indicated in these cases.

The question of optimal length of antibiotic treatment has not been resolved. Most authorities recommend a 7–10 day course.

Corticosteroids: Although the results of trials are equivocal, there is some evidence that corticosteroids may be useful in meningitis, decreasing some neurological sequelae in children. However, this was only in the *Haemophilus influenzae* group and, due to immunisation, they are becoming rare. The recommended dose is dexamethasone (0.15 mg/kg), given 15–20 minutes before antibiotic therapy is commenced.

Complications: Complications of meningitis include seizures, PVS, extensive brain infarction, oedema, brain abscesses and venous sinus thrombosis. A CT scan will identify many of these complications. The mortality for adults who have *Streptococcus pneumoniae* meningitis remains around 20–30% with neurological morbidity affecting over half of all survivors.

### Other CNS infections

Meningitis after neurosurgery: usually caused by gram-negative aerobic bacilli.

Treatment: ampicillin + cefotaxime

Rarer forms of meningitis: tuberculous, pseudomonas, fungal cryptococcus and other rarer organisms should be thought of, especially in the immunocompromised host.

Bacterial brain abscess: usually associated with sinusitis, otitis, cranial trauma or metastatic infection. Appropriate antibiotics, general principles of management of raised ICP and surgical drainage or excision are the mainstays of therapy.

## Status epilepticus

Epilepsy is a chronic disorder or group of disorders, characterised by seizures that usually recur unpredictably in the absence of consistent provoking factors (Table 24.10). Seizures are characterised by excessive and hypersynchronous discharge of cortical neurones. Status epilepticus is a medical emergency. The brain is at risk from cerebral oedema, hypoxia and direct neuronal damage, while the lungs are at risk from aspiration. Status epilepticus is defined as seizures that persist for a prolonged length of time (more than 30 minutes) or occur frequently enough that recovery between attacks does not occur.

**Table 24.10.** Causes of tonic-clonic status epilepticus

First presentation
    Drug overdose, e.g. phenothiazines, theophylline, tricyclic antidepressants
    Drug withdrawal, e.g. after prolonged midazolam use in the ICU
    Metabolic disorder, e.g. electrolyte disturbances, hypoglycaemia, renal and hepatic
       dysfunction
    Global ischaemia
    Head injury
    Cerebrovascular disease
    Infection, e.g. brain abscess, meningoencephalitis
    Intracerebral tumour
    Inflammatory arteritis
    Eclampsia
    Embolism – fat or air
Background of epilepsy
    Inadequate therapy, e.g. non-compliance or drug reduction
    Alcohol or drug withdrawal
    Pseudostatus epilepticus

## Complications of status epilepticus

### Intracerebral

During any form of seizure there is increased electrical activity, increased neuro-transmitter release, increased brain oxygen consumption ($VO_2$), increased CBF and cerebral oedema. Molecular events include an increase in intracellular calcium, arachidonic acid, metabolites, prostaglandins and leucotrienes. The more prolonged the seizure, the worse these effects are. Permanent brain damage can occur after 30 minutes of continuous convulsions.

### Airway

The airway is compromised by extreme muscle activity, increasing intragastric pressure, as well as by the loss of consciousness and decreased airway reflexes. Moreover, the drugs used to treat status epilepticus compromise the airway further. If there is any doubt about aspiration, or airway competence, intubation should be performed early.

### Muscle activity

Excessive muscle activity can significantly increase $VO_2$ and can cause hyperthermia, excessive fluid loss, rhabdomyolysis, hyperkalaemia as well as renal failure.

### Ventilation

Discoordinate muscle activity often impairs ventilation, causing hypoxia and hypercarbia. Paralysis and artificial ventilation may be necessary. While paralysis will prevent muscle activity it will not affect intracerebral epileptic activity. Therefore there is need for either continuous EEG monitoring or only partial paralysis, so that ongoing abnormal muscle activity is detected.

### Other complications

Hyperglycaemia or hypoglycaemia can occur. Autonomic dysfunction, sweating, hypertension and hypotension can all occur in status epilepticus.

## Management of epilepsy (Table 24.11)

**Status epilepticus is a medical emergency.**
The physiological disturbances during epilepsy are life threatening. Urgent treatment is required.

### Resuscitation
**Airway, breathing, circulation.**

As with any other medical emergency, the first priority is to secure the airway. If necessary, intubation should be performed. Hypoxia and hypercarbia should be corrected with adequate ventilation and oxygenation. Vascular access must be secured and hypotension, acid base abnormalities and electrolyte disorders corrected where necessary.

All patients who are having a seizure must be continually observed in an appropriate area. Every precaution needs to be taken against aspiration and, if necessary, the patient's airway must be protected by intubation.

### Diagnosis, monitoring and further management

Restoration of cerebral oxygenation with adequate resuscitation is as important as the use of anticonvulsant drugs and must be performed simultaneously while drugs are being administered.

The cause of epilepsy should be investigated and corrected as soon as possible. A history often gives the diagnosis.

Glucose – 50 ml of 50% glucose IV if hypoglycaemic coma cannot be excluded.

Blood glucose, urea, electrolytes, blood count, osmolality, toxicology screen, anticonvulsant drug levels and arterial blood gases are necessary in the first instance. Thiamine (1 mg/kg IV) if there is a suggestion of alcohol abuse. Monitor respiration, arterial BP, ECG and continuous EEG (where possible).

More definitive tests when stable: lumbar puncture, CT scan and EEG.

### Anticonvulsant therapy

Initial therapy: Midazolam 5–10 mg IV or clonazepam 2 mg/min IV until seizures cease.

**Table 24.11.** Management of epilepsy

---

1 Must be aggressively and rapidly treated – epilepsy is a medical emergency
2 Airway, breathing and circulation
3 Drugs
  midazolam 5 mg IV increments/min up to 50 mg
  *or*
  clonazepam 2 mg bolus, then 0.5–1 mg/min until seizures stop or respiratory
  depression begins
  *plus*
  phenytoin 20 mg/kg IV over 1–4 h (< 50 mg/min), depending on the cardiovascular
  status as a loading dose
  *then*
  phenobarbitone 100 mg/min IV up to 20 mg/kg
  *or*
  thiopentone 25–400 mg IV over 5 min then 2 g in 500 ml titrated as an infusion. Up to
  5 g/day
  *or*
  sodium valproate 200–800 mg rectally every 6 h
4 Exclude and treat reversible causes of epilepsy, e.g. hypoglycaemia, electrolyte
  disturbances, while resuscitation is continuing.
5 Use neuromuscular blocking agents only in the presence of excessive muscle spasm, as
  this may cause complications such as hyperthermia and rhabdomyolysis

---

*Simultaneously* give phenytoin 20 mg/kg IV over 1–4 h (< 50 mg/min) as a loading dose and then 5 mg/kg IV daily as a single dose over 1 hour with monitoring of levels. Beware of cardiotoxicity, hypotension and bradycardia. Give slowly with continuous ECG monitoring. If the patient has been on phenytoin, levels should be measured first.

Further therapy: There are many other drugs recommended for intractable epilepsy including amylobarbitone, paraldehyde and even halothane. The latter should be avoided because it causes an increase in CBF and ICP. As epilepsy has such disastrous consequences, there is a sound argument for using an effective drug such as IV barbiturate (thiopentone or phenobarbitone) as the agent of choice after diazepam and phenytoin have failed.

Intubation, ventilation and IV fluid replacement are indicated at this stage.

Barbiturates: Phenobarbital 100 mg/min IV until seizures cease in a loading dose of up to 20 mg/kg.

Thiopentone (2.5% solution) 25–400 mg IV over 5 minutes or until seizures cease; then 2 g in 500 ml of isotonic saline titrated against effect in a dose of 2–3 mg/kg per h. This should produce isoelectric or extensive short suppression on EEG. Beware of hypotension and accumulation; barbiturates such as thiopentone may take many days to be metabolised. The level of consciousness would be depressed until the drug is metabolised and excreted, making neurological assessment difficult.

Other anticonvulsants may be used in addition to diazepam, phenytoin and thiopentone. These include:

Sodium valproate 200–800 mg can be given rectally every 6 hours.
Propofol infusion 5–10 mg/kg/h until seizures are controlled.

The patient should be loaded simultaneously with long-acting anticonvulsants, so that drugs such as thiopentone can be ceased within 72 hours.

### Other measures

Temperature: Hyperthermia should be aggressively treated with fanning, tepid sponging, axillary icepacks and antipyretics via the NG tube or rectally. For more aggressive measures see Chapter 11.

Excessive muscle movement: Muscle movement should be ameliorated with muscle relaxants if necessary. As little as possible should be used unless continuous EEG recording is available, in order to clinically monitor the effects of anticonvulsant therapy. Otherwise the potentially fatal situation could arise of successfully treating the muscular manifestations while the cerebral epileptiform activity continues unabated.

Supportive measures: Airway, breathing and circulation must be constantly monitored. Prophylaxis against stress ulceration.

Beware of the possibility of supervening nosocomial infection such as pneumonia or sepsis, especially if using large doses of IV barbiturates.

Avoid pro-convulsant drugs: Certain co-existing risk factors such as renal failure, extremes of age, previous history of epilepsy, sepsis and meningitis can interact with drugs commonly used in the ICU such as theophylline, non-steroidal anti-inflammatory agents and high-dose steroids. Antibiotics such as penicillins, cephalosporins, carbapenems, fluoroquinolones and isoniazid also have proconvulsant effects. It is important to note that phenytoin has not been found to be effective for antibiotic-induced convulsions and that benzodiazepines and barbiturates are the first-line drugs of choice.

Re-evaluate: Re-evaluate the cause of epilepsy if it continues. Further investigation may be required, e.g. lumbar puncture or CT scan.

### Non-convulsive status epilepticus

This is a rare variant of status epilepticus and difficult to diagnose and treat. It is seen in patients with an unknown cause of coma on a background of epilepsy and requires an urgent EEG for confirmation. Even though there is no muscular twitching, the dangers to cerebral function are as ominous as normal epilepsy.

## Brain death

Brain death is present when there is irreversible loss of consciousness and loss of brainstem reflexes, including cessation of respiratory centre function. This is associated with irreversible cessation of intracranial blood flow.

Clinical confirmation is all that is legally required in many countries. Angiography may be required if one or more of the clinical tests are unable to be performed.

There are certain essential steps which must be taken before brain death can be established. It is important to be meticulous about these steps as once established, organ donation is contemplated and further treatment is futile.

### Diagnosis of brain death

Preconditions
1  That the patient is deeply comatose.
2  The patient is being ventilated because their spontaneous respiration has ceased.
3  There is no doubt that the patient's condition is due to irremediable structural brain damage and not due to potentially reversible disorders such as Guillain-Barré syndrome or botulism poisoning. A diagnosis is essential. Head injury and intracranial haemorrhage account for approximately 80% of cases. Other causes include global ischaemia, infection or brain tumour.

Exclusion of reversible causes
Drug intoxication: Long-acting drugs such as barbiturates, especially if used in large doses, make neurological assessment difficult. Hypometabolism which often accompanies brain death can also decrease the rate of metabolism of drugs. Adequate time for drug metabolism must therefore be allowed. Drug levels should be measured where possible and sedative drugs must be less than the therapeutic range before testing is contemplated. There must be no residual effect of neuromuscular blocking drugs.

Hypothermia: Patients with brainstem dysfunction often become hypothermic. Testing can only be done when core temperature is $> 35.0\,°C$.

Metabolic and endocrine disturbances: Normal metabolic and endocrine status must be established. Electrolytes, acid base and blood glucose must be within normal range.

Confirmatory tests
The following test brainstem reflexes and respiratory centre function. These should only be performed after the above conditions have been met.

- Pupils not responding to light, direct or consensual.
- No corneal reflex.
- Vestibulo-ocular reflexes absent when 20 ml of ice-cold saline is injected into the patient's external ear after ensuring a clear canal and an intact ear drum.
- No response to painful stimuli within the cranial nerve distribution when stimulated below the neck.
- No gag reflex.
- No respiratory movements after disconnection from the ventilator in the presence of a $PaCO_2$ of more than 50 mmHg (6.7 kPa). In order to avoid hypoxia during testing, the patient should be insufflated with low flow rates of 100% oxygen (3–5 L/min), preferably with 5 cm $H_2O$ positive end-expiratory pressure (PEEP). Because of hypometabolism, the $PaCO_2$ may not rise to adequate levels before 5–10 minutes.

### Definitive diagnosis

A definitive diagnosis of brain death varies between different countries. Angiography, EEG and evoked potentials are not necessary adjuncts for the diagnosis of brain death in most countries. The number of examinations, timing between examinations, the number of separate assessors and their qualifications also vary between countries.

## Relatives

The confidence and trust of the relatives should be gained during this trying period. It must be emphasised that the diagnosis of brain death is equivalent to the diagnosis of death and that the decision to withdraw support is purely a medical one and not one the relatives need bear in any way.

## Transplantation

Consent for transplantation must be gained from the relatives. They should be approached only after the diagnosis of brain death and then given time and, if necessary, further information with which to make the decision.

Keeping the cadaveric organs well perfused once the diagnosis of brainstem death has been made and organ transplantation is being considered, can be a real challenge. Large fluid losses secondary to polyuria as well as hypotension, bradycardia and hypoxia can all compromise potential donor organ function. Adequate perfusion often necessitates large amounts of fluid and inotropes in order to maintain an adequate pressure.

## TROUBLESHOOTING

### Persistently raised ICP unresponsive to standard treatment

- Check ICP measurement.
- Re-CT scan.
- Correct reversible extracranial cause, e.g. high intrathoracic or intra-abdominal pressure.
- Mannitol 0.3 gm/kg IV ± frusemide 40 mg IV.
- Hyperventilation – short term. $PaCO_2$ 30–35 mmHg.
- Artificial elevation of MAP.
- CSF drainage.
- High dose barbiturate – 25–100 mg IV boluses of thiopentone ± continuous infusion of 2 g in 500 ml of isotonic saline titrated against an effect.
- Hypothermia 33–35 °C.
- If hyperperfusion is suspected, β-blockers (metoprolol 5–20 mg IV ± clonidine 75–150 μg IV)
- If post-traumatic vasospasm is suspected – nimodipine.
- Decompressive craniectomy

## FURTHER READING

### Coma

Plum, F. and Posner, J. B. (eds.) *The Diagnosis of Stupor and Coma.* 3rd edn. Philadelphia: F.A. Davis Co, 1980.

Teasdale, G. and Jennett, B. Assessment of coma and impaired consciousness – a practical scale. *Lancet* (1977) ii: 81–4.

### Brain death

Lazar, N. M., Shemie, S., Webster, G. C. and Dickens, B. M. Bioethics for clinicians: 24 Brain death. *Canadian Medical Association Journal* 164 (2001): 833–6.

Wijdicks, E. F. M. Current concepts: the diagnosis of brain death. *New England Journal of Medicine* 344 (2001): 1215–21.

Wijdicks, E. F. M. Brain death worldwide: accepted fact but no global consensus in diagnostic criteria. *Neurology* 58 (2002): 20–5.

### Global ischaemia

Edgren, E., Hedstrand, U., Kelsey, S., Sutton-Tyrrell, K. and Safar, P. BRCT 1 Study Group. Assessment of neurological prognosis in comatose survivors of cardiac arrest. *Lancet* 343 (1994): 1055–9.

Grubb, N. R., Elton, R. A. and Fox, K. A. A. In-hospital mortality after out-of-hospital cardiac arrest. *Lancet* 346 (1995): 417–21.

## Acute cerebrovascular events

Brott, T. and Bogousslavsky, J. Treatment of acute ischemic stroke. *New England Journal of Medicine* 343 (2000): 710–22.
Dorsch, N. W. C. Therapeutic approaches to vasospasm in subarachnoid haemorrhage. *Current Opinion in Critical Care* 8 (2002): 128–33.
Hacke, W., Stingele, R., Steiner, T., Schuchardt, V. and Schwab, S. Critical care of acute ischemic stroke. *Intensive Care Medicine* 21 (1995): 856–62.
Schievink, W. Intracranial aneurysms. *New England Journal of Medicine* 336 (1997): 28–40.
Van Gijn, J. and Rinkel, G. J. E. Subarachnoid haemorrhage: diagnosis, causes and management. *Brain* 124 (2001): 249–78.

## Severe head injury

Bullock, R., Chesnut, R. M., Clifton, G. *et al.* Guidelines for the management of severe head injury. *Journal of Neurotrauma* 13 (1996): 639–731.
Carnall, D. Head injuries. *British Medical Journal* 320 (2000): 1348.
Facco, E. and Munari, M. The role of evoked potentials in severe head injury. *Intensive Care Medicine* 26 (2000): 998–1005.
Gibbons, K. J. Science and surveys in the treatment of head injuries. *Critical Care Medicine* 28 (2000): 256–7.
Kleist-Welch Guerra, W., Piek, J. and Gaab, M.-R. Decompressive craniectomy to treat intracranial hypertension in head injury patients. *Intensive Care Medicine* 25 (1999): 1327–9.
Maas, A. I. R., Dearden, M., Teasdale, G. M. *et al.* EBIC guidelines for the management of severe head injury in adults. European Brain Injury Consortium. *Acta Neurochirurgica* 139 (1997): 286–94.
Munch, E., Horn, P., Schurer, L., Piepgras, A., Paul, T. and Schmiedek, P. Management of severe traumatic brain injury by decompressive craniectomy. *Neurosurgery* 47 (2000): 315–23.
Naredi, S., Olivecrona, M., Lindgren, C., Ostlund, A. L., Grande, P. O. and Koskinen, L. O. D. An outcome study of severe traumatic head injury using the "Lund therapy" with low-dose prostacyclin. *Acta Anaesthesiologica Scandinavica* 45 (2001): 402–6.

## Meningoencephalitis

Hinson, V. K. and Tyor, W. R. Update on viral encephalitis. *Current Opinion in Neurology* 14 (2001): 369–74.
Rosenstein, N. E., Perkins, B. A., Stephens, D. S., Popovic, T. and Hughes, J. M. Medical progress: Meningoccal disease. *New England Journal of Medicine* 344 (2001): 1378–88.

## Epilepsy

Browne, T. R. and Holmes, G. L. Epilepsy. *New England Journal of Medicine* 344 (2001): 1145–51.

Chapman, M. G., Smith, M. and Hirsch, N. P. Status epilepticus. *Anaesthesia* 56 (2001): 648–59.

Durham, D. Management of status epilepticus. *Critical Care and Resuscitation* 1 (1999): 344–53.

Heafield, M. T. E. Managing status epilepticus. *British Medical Journal* 320 (2000): 953–4.

Nashef, L. and Brown, S. Epilepsy and sudden death. *Lancet* 348 (1997): 1324–25.

Newton, D. E. F. Electrophysiological monitoring of general intensive care patients. *Intensive Care Medicine* 25 (1999): 350–2.

# 25

# Critical care neurology

## Myasthenia gravis

Myasthenia gravis is a neuromuscular disorder characterised by weakness and fatigability of voluntary muscles. The weakness is exacerbated by effort and improved by rest and it affects, in order of decreasing frequency, the ocular, bulbar, neck, limb, girdle, distal limb and trunk muscles.

It is a classic autoimmune disease marked by the presence of heterogeneous acetylcholine receptor antibody (IgG) in approximately 90% of symptomatic patients. The antibodies react with the receptor, block its action and accelerate receptor degradation. As a result, fewer receptors can be activated causing muscle weakness.

### Diagnosis

Clinical suspicion and the finding of skeletal-muscle fatigability with repetitive exercise will support the diagnosis. The diagnosis can be confirmed by complete reversibility of muscle fatigue after IV administration of the rapidly acting anticholinesterase drug edrophonium (5–10 mg IV over 1 minute, should produce an effect within 10 minutes).

Electrophysiological testing will demonstrate progressive decline in muscle action potentials with repetitive stimulation of a motor nerve.

### Treatment

Definitive treatment aims to reduce antibody production and/or increase the effect of unaffected acetylcholine receptors.

#### Anticholinesterases
The longer-acting anticholinesterase, pyridostigmine, is titrated against patient response using a starting dosage of 60 mg orally four times daily. Excessive use of anticholinesterases can cause a cholinergic crisis, with progressive muscle

weakness as well as muscarinic effects, such as abdominal colic, diarrhoea, small pupils, lachrymation and excessive salivation.

### Thymectomy

Among all patients with myasthenia gravis, 75% have thymic abnormalities. Most have thymic hyperplasia, but up to 15% have thymomas. It is thought that the thymus may be initiating development of the autoantibodies that attack the post-synaptic acetylcholine receptor. Thymectomy is especially useful in patients who are young at the onset of disease. Complete remission or improvement occurs in about 80% of patients without a tumour of the thymus, although it may take 3–5 years to gain the full benefit.

### Corticosteroids

Corticosteroids can be used in patients for whom thymectomy has not been successful, in patients who are seriously ill before thymectomy and occasionally for those with ocular myasthenia. Steroids may take several weeks to achieve their optimum effects and may even cause an initial deterioration.

### Azathioprine

Azathioprine should be reserved for patients with severe myasthenia who do not respond to other forms of treatment. It should be used in association with plasma exchange.

### Plasmapheresis

Plasmapheresis can produce a dramatic short-term improvement. It should be reserved for use in severely ill patients while other forms of treatment are taking effect.

## Myasthenia gravis in intensive care

Myasthenic patients often are admitted to the ICU for elective ventilation after thymectomy or incidental surgery (Table 25.1). Prolonged paralysis can occur in some patients, even after the use of reduced doses of anticholinesterase drugs and in the presence of neuromuscular drugs. Patients can also be admitted for myasthenic or cholinergic crisis.

In patients with deteriorating myasthenia gravis, it is important to differentiate between myasthenic and cholinergic crisis. This can be determined by the response to IV edrophonium, 5–10 mg IV given in 2 mg increments. Patients in myasthenia crisis will show rapid improvement in terms of their symptoms, whereas those in cholinergic crisis will deteriorate.

Whatever the reason myasthenic patients are in the ICU, they usually have decreased respiratory and bulbar muscle function and many of the aspects of management for myasthenia and cholinergic crises are the same.

**Table 25.1.** Evaluation of the need for respiratory support in patients with neuromuscular disease

| Parameter | Normal | Borderline | Failure |
|---|---|---|---|
| Forced vital capacity | >15 ml/kg | 10–15 ml/kg | <10 ml/kg |
| Negative inspiratory force | >−40 mmHg | −25–40 mmHg | <−25 mmHg |
| Airway integrity | Eats and drinks normally; no difficulty in articulating | Cannot handle fluids well, but manages with oral suctioning; noticeable impairment of speech | Obstruction of airway in certain positions; intermittent aspiration of secretions |
| Chest x-ray | Absence of atelectasis | Presence of subsegmental atelectasis | Major atelectasis or infiltrate |

Reprinted by permission of Williams and Wilkins. Malkoff, M. D. Neuromuscular disease. In *Pathophysiologic Foundations of Critical Care*, ed. M. R. Pinsky and J.-F. A. Dhainaut, pp. 778–88. New York: Williams and Wilkins, 1993.

## Management

Airway: Secure the compromised airway with an endotracheal tube (ETT).

Ventilation: Artificial ventilation will be necessary if respiratory muscles are in-effective. Ventilation should be regularly assessed by measurements of parameters such as peak flow, vital capacity and tidal volume.

Respiratory complication: Atelectasis, pneumonia, aspiration and sputum retention should be prevented or treated aggressively by early physiotherapy as well as early intubation and ventilation, where indicated (see Chapter 19).

Supportive care: A return to enteral feeding, prophylaxis against deep venous thrombosis, and provision of emotional support (see Chapter 5) are essential for these patients.

Anticholinesterases: Each patient should be stabilised on the optimal dosage of anticholinesterases, either with oral pyridostigmine or IV neostigmine, given continuously or intermittently. This should be titrated against muscle strength, especially the bulbar and respiratory groups. Intravenous edrophonium 2–10 mg in between doses can be used as a guideline to the optimal dosage. Give IV edrophonium in 2 mg IV increments, pausing in between, especially if there is a suspicion of cholinergic crisis.

After thymectomy, patients may have markedly reduced anticholinesterase requirements within the first 48 hours.

Cholinergic crisis: Atropine, intravenously or preferably orally, can be titrated against the muscarinic or parasympathomimetic manifestations of a cholinergic crisis.

**Table 25.2.** Pathogens associated with Guillain–Barré

| |
| --- |
| CMV |
| Epstein–Barr virus |
| *Varicella zoster* |
| *Campylobacter jejuni* |
| Mycoplasma |
| Rabies and swine influenza vaccines |

Concurrent drug therapy: If possible, avoid drugs that might make the condition worse, such as non-depolarising muscle relaxants, aminoglycosides, quinine, quinidine, procainamide, lignocaine and propranolol.

Weaning: Carefully assess the strength of bulbar and respiratory muscles during weaning from ventilatory and airway support in order to decide when artificial ventilation can be ceased and the patient extubated. Objective measurements of parameters such as expiratory flow rates and vital capacity can be used to monitor progress. Tracheostomy may be required if intubation is prolonged.

Weaning from the ventilator, for some patients, may be impossible without corticosteroids. Azothioprine or plasmapheresis may be indicated when the response to anticholinesterase drugs is unsatisfactory.

## Guillain–Barré syndrome

### Pathophysiology

Guillain–Barré syndrome is a post-infectious antibody-mediated attack on peripheral nerves. A peripheral neuropathy results with lymphocytes and macrophages surrounding endoneural vessels with adjacent demyelination. The incidence of Guillain–Barré is 2 in 100 000 and it has two peaks, in adolescence and the elderly. In adolescence, it coincides with the peak of infection with cytomegalovirus (CMV) and campylobacter, in the elderly with failing of immune suppressor mechanisms.

Guillain–Barré is an example of molecular mimicry – the immune response against the infecting organism induces antibodies that cross react with neural tissue. Pathogens for which there is convincing evidence of an association are listed in Table 25.2.

### Clinical features

Guillain–Barré syndrome is an acute inflammatory demyelinating polyneuropathy (AIDP) that often presents with dramatic onset of muscle weakness and

**Table 25.3.** Bad prognostic signs for residual disability at one year

---

Age > 60 years
Rapid progress to quadraparesis by 7 days
Need for ventilatory support
Mean distal motor amplitude < 20% of normal
A preceding diarrhoeal illness

---

autonomic signs. Despite the acute nature of this disorder, patients occasionally require ventilatory support for months or even years. Some cases never completely resolve.

Typically, the syndrome is heralded by paraesthesia of the fingertips and toes, followed within days by a progressive, symmetrically ascending, flaccid motor paralysis. This may remain localised to the lower limbs, or it can extend to the trunk and respiratory muscles, as well as to the cranial nerves. Tendon reflexes are absent in the affected areas. Seventy per cent of patients are at their worst by 2 weeks. Pain is common, especially in the large muscles of the upper legs and back. However, usually there is only minimal sensory loss.

The clinical course can be described in four phases:

Prodromal phase: The prodromal phase develops over days or weeks, with over 60% of patients having had a preceding viral illness. Other cases are associated with vaccination or gastrointestinal tract infection.

Extension of neurological deficits: This phase is relatively constant and lasts about 2 weeks.

Plateau phase: The plateau phase can be unpredictable, but usually lasts from a few days to a few weeks, or even longer in about 10% of cases. The maximum effects occur within 2 weeks of onset in about 50% of cases and within 4 weeks in 90% of cases.

Recovery phase: Most patients recover within 6 months. However, about 85% of patients will have no residual deficits. About 65% have persistent minor problems, such as weakness or distal numbness. Permanent disabling weaknesses or other severe neurological deficits occur in about 5–10%. About 5% of patients develop chronic relapsing polyneuropathy, with further bouts of demyelination (Table 25.3).

Clinical variants: Variants of Guillain–Barré include:

- Miller–Fisher syndrome (ophthalmoplegia, ataxia, areflexia with little weakness). This has a different immunological basis to AIDP.
- Weakness without paraesthesia or sensory loss. Acute motor axonal neuropathy (AMAN).
- Pure ataxia.
- Facial paresis with paraesthesia.
- Pharyngeal cervical brachial weakness.

## Diagnosis

The diagnosis of Guillain–Barré syndrome is usually made on clinical grounds. Cerebrospinal fluid (CSF) typically shows normal pressure, few or no cells and an elevated protein concentration. Protein levels may be normal initially, and the cell count is occasionally increased. The major reason for lumbar puncture is to exclude other conditions, not to make a positive diagnosis of Guillain–Barré syndrome. Abnormalities of nerve conduction occur early and demonstrate the characteristic findings of demyelination, including conduction block (causing motor weakness) and spontaneous discharges in demyelinated sensory nerves (causing paraesthesia and pain). However, normal findings on nerve conduction studies do not exclude the diagnosis.

## Management in intensive care

Meticulous supportive care is the mainstay of the treatment of Guillain–Barré syndrome in the ICU. This includes prevention of aspiration and respiratory infections, avoiding the complications of intubation and tracheostomy and commencing prophylaxis for deep venous thrombosis. Because the underlying disease is largely reversible and the complications largely avoidable, successful outcomes can be achieved by excellent supportive care.

The immediate dangers are increasing bulbar weakness and impaired ventilation. Respiratory function must be tracked by serial measurements of parameters such as vital capacity and negative inspiratory effort, rather than by using arterial blood gas analysis. Test and chart three separate groups of muscles (bulbar, limb and respiratory) on a regular basis.

### Airway

If in doubt about the airway, intubate the patient before complications occur. Support the patient's respiration with artificial ventilation before widespread collapse and infection occurs. Approximately 20–30% of patients will require intubation and mechanical ventilation.

**Do not use suxamethonium to facilitate intubation. It is unnecessary and can cause massive release of potassium from denervated muscle, leading to cardiac arrest.**

### Ventilation

Ventilatory failure usually occurs when the vital capacity falls below 20 ml/kg. Patients who need artificial ventilation usually require it for between 4 and 8 weeks and sometimes for several months or even longer.

Tracheostomy should be considered early in order to facilitate nursing care and reduce the complications involved in using an ETT.

Because artificial ventilation is often prolonged, maintain meticulous airway toilet. Regular checking of the airway cuff pressures is required.

### General support

Institute general measures such as enteral feeding, physiotherapy and provision of emotional support.

These patients usually are fully conscious; explain every manoeuvre and discuss the proposed management and progress with them. It is important to provide stimulation directly from the staff and from audiovisual aids, in addition to encouraging frequent and flexible visits from relatives and friends.

Because of the danger of pulmonary emboli, all ventilated patients should receive prophylaxis, either low-dose heparin (5000 units subcutaneously three times daily) or clexane. Other prophylactic techniques, such as compression stockings, may also be useful.

Patients with Guillain–Barré syndrome usually have moderate to severe pain that is muscular in origin. Patients should be carefully questioned about this possibility and given appropriate and generous oral or parenteral pain relief. Up to 50% of patients require IV morphine.

### Cardiovascular complications

Autonomic instability is common in these patients, resulting in tachyarrhythmias and severe blood pressure fluctuations. They are often precipitated by stimulation of the patient. IV sedation, volume loading with fluid and $\alpha$- or $\beta$-adrenoceptor blockade may be necessary to treat these complications. Similar treatment may be required prophylactically before procedures. The same strategies are used for the autonomic instability in patients with tetanus and are discussed in detail under that section.

Other explanations of the cardiovascular manifestations are high levels of circulatory catecholamines or a myocarditis associated with the infecting organism, e.g. CMV, Epstein–Barr and mycoplasma can all cause myocarditis.

### Hyponatraemia

Hyponatraemia, possibly due to inappropriate secretion of antidiuretic hormone (ADH) is sometimes seen. Avoidance of hypovolaemia and excessive water administration usually will correct the abnormality. Rarely, hypertonic saline is needed.

### Other therapy

Corticosteroids: Corticosteroids should not be used as a sole treatment in patients with Guillain–Barré syndrome. They may be advantageous in association with IV immune globulin (IVIG).

Fresh frozen plasma: Use of fresh frozen plasma probably is of no benefit.

Plasmapheresis: Early use of plasmapheresis will reduce the duration and severity of the acute phase of the disease and may accelerate recovery. Albumin, rather than fresh frozen plasma, is the replacement fluid of choice. The optimal number of plasma exchanges and the scheduling of changes are not known. A commonly employed treatment is five courses over 10 days. Several issues remain unresolved: Which group of patients can benefit most from plasmapheresis? Does it reduce overall mortality? Moreover, plasmapheresis is not without complications, such as increased bleeding and activation of complement and fibrinolysis.

Compared with no plasmapheresis, patients who are exchanged have shorter times on the ventilator and walk unaided quicker. It is ineffective if started more than 2 weeks after the onset of symptoms.

IVIG: Use of IVIG may speed recovery and decrease the need for ventilatory support. It is as effective as plasmapheresis with less complications. The amount suggested is 0.4 gm/kg/day, for 5 days. The addition of plasmapheresis to immune globulin confers no additional benefit. The postulated mechanism of action is that added IgG binds to the immunoglobin receptor on the phagocyte and prevents attachment at the autoantibody and hence prevents myelin destruction.

## Critical illness polyneuropathy and myopathy

Critical illness polyneuropathy and myopathy may be another manifestation of multiorgan failure (MOF) (see Chapter 9). It involves impairment of peripheral nerve function, including the cranial nerves. It can affect both motor and sensory function.

While critical illness polyneuropathy and critical illness myopathy are sometimes considered separately, there is good evidence to suggest that both nerve and muscle are affected.

Critical illness polyneuropathy is a difficult diagnosis to make, because as the patients often are unconscious or sedated, testing sensation and motor function is almost impossible. The syndrome can manifest as failure to wean from the ventilator or it may become obvious as the patient recovers. Because it is so difficult to diagnose, the incidence has not been accurately documented but it may affect up to 70% of patients with MOF.

This diagnosis is made after one excludes all other possible causes for the polyneuropathy. It is important to remember that there are many potential causes of polyneuropathy (Tables 25.4 and 25.5). The finding of primary axonal degeneration of mainly motor fibres but also sensory fibres, without inflammatory change and with a relatively normal CSF, can distinguish this neuropathy from Guillain–Barré syndrome. The precise cause remains obscure. Recovery occurs spontaneously. In addition to a thorough clinical examination, studies of nerve conduction and electromyography (EMG) studies may be necessary to document the syndrome. The creatinine phosphokinase (CPK) levels will be normal or only slightly elevated.

There have been increasing reports of motor neuropathy and/or myopathy in patients receiving neuromuscular blocking agents and steroids, especially patients being ventilated for severe asthma. However, there is, as yet, no direct evidence linking those drugs to the observed weakness.

**Table 25.4.** Disorders of neuromuscular function

| Level | Associated clinical features | Nerve conduction | EMG findings |
|---|---|---|---|
| Upper motor neuron | Weakness<br>Hyperreflexia<br>Increased muscle tone<br>May have sensory and autonomic changes | Normal | Normal |
| Lower motor neuron | Weakness<br>Atrophy<br>Flaccidity<br>Hyporeflexia<br>Fasciculations<br>Bulbar involvement<br>No sensory changes | Normal | Denervation potentials of giant motor units |
| Peripheral | Weakness | Reduced | Denervation potentials in axonal neuropathies |
| Neurons | Flaccidity<br>Hyporeflexia<br>Bulbar involvement<br>Sensory and autonomic changes | | |
| Myoneural | Fluctuating weakness | Normal | Change in amplitude of the muscle and response to repetitive nerve stimulation |
| Junction | Fatigability<br>Ocular and bulbar involvement<br>Normal reflexes<br>No sensory changes | | |
| Muscle | Weakness, usually proximal<br>Normal reflexes<br>No sensory or autonomic changes<br>Often have pain | Normal | Small motor units |

**Table 25.5.** Neuromuscular disorders in the seriously ill

| Condition | Clinical features | Electrophysiology | Morphology |
|---|---|---|---|
| Guillain–Barré syndrome | Mainly motor neuropathy | Consistent with primary demyelinating polyneuropathy | Primary demyelination of nerve and inflammation; invariable denervation of muscle |
| Nerve compression due to positioning, plasters, etc. | Motor and sensory features | Consistent with primary degeneration | Fibre atrophy on muscle biopsy |
| Cachectic myopathy | Diffuse muscle wasting | Normal | Type II fibre atrophy on muscle biopsy |
| Critical illness polyneuropathy | None, or else signs of mainly motor neuropathy | Consistent with primary axonal degeneration of mainly motor fibres | Primary axonal degeneration of nerve, denervation atrophy of muscle |
| Neuromuscular blocking agents | Persistent quadriplegia for up to 2–3 weeks | Neuromuscular transmission deficit and/or axonal motor neuropathy | Normal or denervation atrophy on muscle biopsy |

Reprinted by permission of Bolton, C. F. Neuropathies in the Critical Care Unit. *British Journal of Hospital Medicine* 47 (1992): 58–60.

# Tetanus

## Features

Tetanus is caused by *Clostridium tetani*, an anaerobic, gram-positive spore-forming bacillus. Clostridial spores, which are endemic in soil and dirt, develop into the vegetative form of the organism when introduced into the anaerobic environment of devitalised tissue. *Clostridium tetani* itself does not cause tissue damage or evoke an inflammatory response, but rather produces an exotoxin, tetanospasmin.

The exotoxin forms an irreversible bond with synaptosomes, both in the spinal cord and in the central nervous system. The toxin ascends intra-axonally in motor and autonomic nerve fibres. The exact site of action has not been elucidated but some evidence suggests that it mainly depresses the inhibitory influence from Renshaw cells (inhibitory interneurones). This leads to paroxysmal muscle spasm, often triggered by minimal sensory input.

The centripetal spread of toxin is more rapid with increased doses of toxin. A rapid onset of symptoms suggests inoculation by a larger dose of exotoxin and increased severity of disease.

The first symptoms usually are stiffness in the back muscles, abdominal muscles and masseters, followed by dysphagia and eventually generalised muscle spasms. Most muscles are eventually affected. The respiratory pattern and breathing can be compromised by general muscle spasms leading to hypoventilation and even respiratory arrest. Tetanus varies from a very mild disease, with minimal muscle spasm to a fulminant variety characterised by severe recurrent spasms and autonomic overactivity.

The mortality from tetanus remains high (10–50%) despite management in the ICU. Nowadays, death often occurs as a result of autonomic overactivity, with arrhythmias, hypotensive and hypertensive crises and myocardial ischaemia, rather than as a result of respiratory failure.

## Diagnosis

The diagnosis is made on the basis of the clinical history and observation of muscle spasms. The organism can be cultured from the suspected infection site.

## Treatment

### Eradication of the source
- Vigorous drainage and debridement of the suspected site of infection is important.
- Penicillin G, 3–6 million units/day IV, for approximately 10 days.
- Use erythromycin if the patient is allergic to penicillin.
- Immobilisation of the wound area.

## Neutralisation of toxin

There is some doubt about the efficacy of human tetanus immunoglobulin because the exotoxin rapidly becomes fixed on the nervous tissue and therefore will not be modified if symptoms are already present.

However, immunoglobulin is still commonly given: 3000–10 000 units of human tetanus immunoglobulin diluted with saline, as a slow IV solution over 15 minutes.

Human immunoglobulin has been given intrathecally (250 units) in an attempt to neutralise unbound exotoxin but meta-analysis has shown no benefit.

## Supportive care

Airway: The airway must be protected, and intubation performed early if there is any doubt about airway patency. Intubation is often necessary to facilitate ventilation and to prevent aspiration. Tracheostomy usually is considered when the course of the disease is longer than 2–3 weeks.

Ventilation: Some ventilatory assistance (see Chapter 19) will almost certainly be required in most patients because of inefficient respiration resulting from muscle spasms or from the drugs given to control the spasms. As muscle spasms are controlled with sedation and muscle relaxants, total respiratory support may become necessary, rather than the use of modes that employ spontaneous ventilation, such as intermittent mandatory ventilation (IMV) or continuous positive airway pressure (CPAP) (see Chapter 19).

Control of spasms:

Benzodiazepines: A benzodiazepine such as diazepam (intermittent IV doses or infusion of 5–10 mg/h) is often used as a first-line drug because it has muscle-relaxing and sedative properties. Shorter-acting benzodiazepines are equally as effective.

Narcotics: Narcotics should be used liberally, especially in the presence of spasms, which can be quite painful (e.g. intermittent or continuous IV infusion of morphine 2–20 mg/h).

Non-depolarising muscle relaxants: Use these only if other drugs fail to control the spasms. Continue diazepam and/or narcotics during administration of muscle relaxants. Give them either as intermittent IV boluses or as a continuous infusion. **Depolarising muscle relaxants are contraindicated, as they can cause acute hyperkalaemia and cardiac arrest.**

Feeding: Start enteral feeding early. Parenteral feeding is necessary only if enteral food is not tolerated (e.g. as a result of autonomic dysfunction and ileus).

Fluids: Fluid requirements should be met by adequate enteral nutrition. Otherwise, use a maintenance IV regimen. Hypovolaemia should be rapidly corrected. Hypertension, paradoxically, can be caused by hypovolaemia during autonomic dysfunction.

Thrombosis and embolism: Begin prophylaxis against venous thrombi and pulmonary embolism, using subcutaneous heparin (5000 units, two or three times daily). Antithrombotic stockings may also be useful.

Other general supportive measures: Supportive measures such as chest physiotherapy and prophylaxis against stress ulceration (see Chapter 3) are necessary.

Patient and relatives: Patients with tetanus who are not being heavily sedated, often are fully aware. They need constant reassurance from the attending staff and relatives.

## Autonomic overactivity

Cardiovascular instability is characterised by overactivity of the sympathetic and parasympathetic nervous system, including tachycardia, labile and elevated BP, variable skin blood flow, fever, hypersalivation, arrhythmias and even cardiac standstill. It usually presents some days after the onset of muscle spasms. The overactivity can persist for many hours, but more often is intermittent and of short duration. Autonomic overactivity can be associated with mortality of more than 50%.

Management: IV sedative agents such as benzodiazepines and phenothiazines usually are required. General anaesthetic agents have also been used. The aim of treatment is complete inhibition of both somatic and autonomic overactivity without producing hypotension or hypothermia. Suggested regimen: diazepam 20 mg, 4–6-hourly, and additional increments as required. In severe uncontrollable cases, IV diazepam may need to be supplemented with thiopentone at a starting dosage of 25 mg IV hourly by continuous infusion. Sedation is usually required for at least 2–3 weeks. Muscle relaxants usually are necessary only for control of severe spasms and they always must be used in conjunction with sedation.

Increase sedation (e.g. diazepam) before any procedure that can precipitate autonomic dysfunction. Other measures also need to be considered:

Correct hypovolaemia: Paradoxical hypovolaemia is commonly associated with hypertension and a labile BP.

Intravenous β-blockers: Intravenous β-blockers (either intermittent or continuous) must be used with caution and only if sympathetic overactivity is still present after maximum sedation. Use a short-acting agent such as esmolol, and titrate it against an effect. Beware of unopposed α activity when using β-blockers.

Intravenous α-blockers: Intravenous α-blockers (either intermittent or continuous) for hypertension must be used with caution and only after correcting hypovolaemia and after failure of maximum sedation and β-blockers. Chlorpromazine is the most commonly used drug.

Continuous lumbar epidural blockade: Lumbar epidural blockade with local anaesthetic or morphine has also been used to control labile BP. Hypovolaemia should be aggressively reversed with fluid infusion before epidural drugs are commenced.

Magnesium sulphate: Magnesium sulphate by IV infusion can be used if other measures have failed: 70 mg/kg over 5 minutes, then infusion to keep serum magnesium between 2.5 and 4 mmol/L, measuring serum levels every 4 hours. Ventilation is mandatory in these patients.

Atropine: Atropine by IV infusion, titrated against response, can be used if parasympathetic symptoms are predominant.

## FURTHER READING

### General

Davidson, A. and Diamond, B. Advances in immunology: autoimmune diseases. *New England Journal of Medicine* 345 (2001): 340–50.

### Myasthenia gravis

Palace, J., Vincent, A. and Beeson, D. Myasthenia gravis: diagnostic and management dilemmas. *Current Opinion in Neurology.* 14 (2001): 583– 9.

### Guillain–Barré syndrome

Hahn, A. F. Guillain–Barré syndrome. *Lancet* 352 (1998): 635–41.

Plasma Exchange/Sandoglobulin Guillain–Barré Syndrome Trial Group. Randomised trial of plasma exchange, IV immunoglobulin, and combined treatments in Guillain–Barré syndrome. *Lancet* 349 (1997): 225–9.

Yu, Z. and Lennon, V. A. Clinical implications of basic research: mechanism of intravenous immune globulin therapy in antibody-mediated autoimmune disease. *New England Journal of Medicine* 340 (1999): 227–8.

### Critically ill polyneuropathy

Bolton, C. F. Neuromuscular conditions in the intensive care unit. *Intensive Care Medicine* 22 (1996): 841–3.

Hund, E. Critical illness polyneuropathy. *Current Opinion in Neurology* 14 (2001): 649–53.

### Tetanus

Richardson, J. P. and Knight, A. L. The management and prevention of tetanus. *Journal of Emergency Medicine* 11 (1993): 737–42.

# 26

# Acute renal failure

- Most acute renal failure (ARF) in the ICU is potentially preventable.
- Rapid restoration of renal blood flow and arterial blood pressure is crucial.
- Old and 'sick' kidneys (e.g. patients with chronic renal impairment) are particularly vulnerable to acute insults.
- The kidney in the ICU is like the canary in the coal mine. It is an accurate marker of severe disturbances in the body. It also is an early marker of general recovery.

## Acute renal failure in intensive care

### Pathophysiology

Acute renal failure (ARF) occurs when there is a temporary and usually reversible failure of the kidney's ability to excrete the waste products of metabolism.

The kidney is usually an innocent bystander in the critically ill – the common causes of ARF in the ICU are renal ischaemia secondary to hypotension and hypovolaemia and nephrotoxic drugs, sometimes in combination.

The pathophysiology of ARF involves patchy tubular cell necrosis, cell swelling and loss of the brush border. The cellular debris coalesces with protein to form intraluminal casts, which impede tubular flow. However, the glomerulus is also affected. This may be related to pre-glomerular vasoconstriction. The combination of back pressure from tubular obstruction and pre-glomerular vasoconstriction decreases the net glomerular transcapillary pressure gradient to almost zero, resulting in little or no filtrate formation (Figure 26.1). The renal medulla is relatively vulnerable to hypoxic injury as compared with the cortex. Because the tubular workload is determined by the glomerular filtration rate, ARF may be a physiologically based, short-term response, designed to minimise medullary hypoxic damage. The reduced tubular and glomerular functions can be viewed as

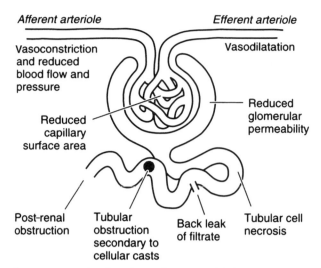

**Figure 26.1.** Pathophysiology of acute renal failure, which is often multifactorial. Some or all of these factors may play roles.

an effort to protect the ischaemic medullary ascending limb from further hypoxic injury. This results in reduced ability to concentrate urine. Water, potassium, acid and urea/creatinine excretion are the four most readily measured markers of renal failure. The acute phase is marked by an unpredictable combination of these four abnormalities. Sometimes one function is impaired more than the other three with many combinations of the four abnormalities also possible.

Following ischaemic damage, usually there is an 'oliguric phase' lasting about 2 weeks, but this can be for shorter periods or occasionally can continue for up to 60 days. The return of renal function is heralded by a 'diuretic phase' marked by increasing urine output. This may be due in part to removal of excess water and salt but it can also be a reflection of impaired tubular function, which sometimes remains for weeks or months. A modified diuretic phase can occur after renal insufficiency and relative oliguria.

## Aetiology of acute renal failure in the setting of an ICU

The causes of renal failure often are divided into 'pre-renal', 'renal' and 'post-renal' causes (Table 26.1). Hypotension in the presence of chronic renal insufficiency or chronic hypertension is a particularly dangerous combination. Post-renal causes of renal failure are uncommon in the ICU. However, a kinked or blocked catheter can be a spurious cause of anuria or oliguria. The commonest 'renal' causes of renal failure in intensive care are related to drugs and toxins. The aminoglycoside antibiotics are the drugs best known for causing direct nephrotoxicity in the ICU,

**Table 26.1.** Major causes of acute renal failure in the ICU

---

*Pre-renal causes*:
Decreased effective circulating volume
Hypovolaemia, e.g.
   Haemorrhage
   Gastrointestinal loss
   Skin loss
   Polyuria
Volume redistribution
Peripheral vasodilatation, e.g.
   sepsis and anaphylaxis
'Third space' loss, e.g.
   peritonitis, pancreatitis, ascites

Decreased cardiac function
Congestive heart failure
Cor pulmonale
Vascular heart disease
Pericarditis, tamponade

Renal vascular disease
Dissecting aortic aneurysm
Thromboembolic disease

*Renal causes*:
Nephrotoxins
Antibiotics
  – aminoglycosides ($\pm$ frusemide)
  – cephalosporins
  – penicillins
  – quinolones
Antifungals – amphotericin B
NSAIDs
ACE inhibitors
Radiocontrast agents
Free haemoglobin and myoglobin
Methotrexate
Cisplatin
Hypocalcaemia, hyperuricaemia
Heavy metals, glycosis, organic solvents
*Septicaemia*
Combination of cardiovascular failure,
   intravascular volume redistribution
   and nephrotoxicity
*Post-renal causes*:
Blocked or kinked urinary catheter
High intra-abdominal pressure from
   any cause
Bilateral ureteric pathology

*Other renal causes*:
Acute interstitial nephritis
Microvascular (e.g. malignant,
hypertension, DIC)
Glomulonephritis secondary to systemic
   disease (e.g. systemic lupus
   erythematosus, vasculitis, endocarditis)
Acute-on-chronic renal failure
Renal vein thrombosis (e.g. hypercoagulable
   states)
Papillary necrosis (e.g. diabetes, sickle cell
   disease)
Hepatorenal failure.
Thrombotic microangiopathy (e.g.
   scleroderma, malignant hypertension)

---

but others have been implicated. Toxins such as those found in patients with septicaemia have also been implicated in ARF.

Acute renal failure in the ICU is often multifactorial. For example, the factors contributing to sepsis can include hypotension, a direct nephrotoxic effect of septicaemia and possibly drugs, especially the aminoglycosides. Whatever their causes, cases of ARF usually have similar pathophysiologies and clinical courses in the ICU. Renal biopsy is indicated only if the cause of the ARF is uncertain. For example, pre-renal and post-renal causes of ARF are excluded and the 'renal' cause is other than toxins or ischaemia.

Ultrasound or nuclear medicine studies may give some idea of renal size if chronic renal disease is suspected. Small kidney size indicates chronic renal disease. Glomerulonephritis is rare in the setting of intensive care. Proteinuria, haematuria and the presence of red cell casts point to that possibility.

Rhabdomyolysis is relatively common in certain groups of critically ill in intensive care and usually is found in association with prolonged immobility following a drug overdose, intravenous narcotic abuse, trauma, alcoholism or an infective process. Obvious limb damage, with muscle necrosis, is common.

Rhabdomyolysis is marked by myoglobinuria, a rapid and profound rise in the serum concentration of creatinine phosphokinase (CPK), and the presence of pigmented casts in the urinary sediment. There will be a grossly increased solute load, combined with decreased renal function. The prognosis for complete recovery in this type of ARF is excellent.

Non-oliguric renal failure: Non-oliguric renal failure is characterised by a urine output of > 400 ml/day in the presence of uraemia. The pathophysiology is similar to that seen in classical ARF but usually involves a lesser result. However, while the production of urine, albeit not of good quality, makes fluid balance easier, the prognosis for patients with non-oliguric renal failure requiring repeated dialysis is the same as for those with oliguric renal failure. There have been suggestions that drugs such as mannitol and frusemide might be able to convert oliguric to non-oliguric renal failure, but as yet it is uncertain which, if any, of these drugs has this action, what dosages should be employed, in which types of renal failure they could be successful and at what stage in the disease process the drugs might be effective. Despite this, frusemide infusions are often used in the early stages of renal failure in order to maintain urine output, with some excretion of other waste products as well.

## Investigations

Routine investigations: The diagnosis of ARF is usually clinical: uraemia in the presence of suggestive clinical circumstances (e.g. sepsis or hypotension). Daily determinations of serum creatinine, urea and electrolytes, including sodium, calcium, phosphate and magnesium should be performed. Routine haemoglobin and blood counts should be done. Because active intervention may be required, more frequent estimations of serum potassium and arterial blood gases may be needed when ARF is suspected.

Urinalysis: There can be higher concentrations of protein in the presence of glomerular disease than in renal failure of pre-renal or post-renal origins.

Glomerular lesions are usually associated with urinary sediment that contains cells, casts and cellular debris.

Drug-induced acute interstitial nephritis can occur in the intensive care setting. It is suggested by the presence of white cells, white cell casts and eosinophils in the urine and can be associated with fever, rash and peripheral eosinophilia.

Urine sodium concentration and osmolality: Classically, renal hypoperfusion is associated with avid retention of sodium by the body, with minimal excretion in the urine (usually less than 20 mmol/L). In patients with intrinsic renal disease, the excretion of sodium in the urine is typically greater than 40 mmol/L.

Similarly, decreased renal perfusion is associated with a high urine osmolality (> 400 mOsm/L), whereas with intrinsic renal disease, the urine osmolality typically is between 300 and 400 mOsm/L. In the presence of diuretics, urinary electrolytes are difficult to interpret.

Other investigations: In patients in whom the causes of ARF are unclear, renal ultrasound is the investigation of first choice, because it provides information about chronicity in terms of kidney size, in addition to excluding obstruction. It is a highly sensitive but non-specific detector of dilatation of the collecting system and it is most useful as a screening method for discriminating between chronic obstruction and acute obstruction. Intravenous pyelography may be useful for defining renal anatomy and ruling out the possibility of obstruction. A CT scan may provide more detail regarding a site of obstruction. The use of contrast medium can exacerbate renal disease. If vascular occlusion is suspected, radionuclide imagining or angiography can be performed. Renal biopsy should be performed only if the cause remains unclear, or if there is prolonged ARF (4–6 weeks).

## Prevention of acute renal failure

The onset of ARF in intensive care usually occurs days after the precipitating event. It is crucial to apply the basic principles of rapid cardiorespiratory resuscitation *outside* as well as *inside* the ICU in order to prevent renal failure. For example, multitrauma victims must be rapidly transfused and perioperative patients must be kept well hydrated. The degree of ischaemic insults that individual kidneys can tolerate will vary considerably. 'Old' hypertensive diabetic kidneys cannot tolerate ischaemic insults as well as young healthy kidneys. **Many cases of ARF could have been avoided if hypovolaemia and hypotension had been corrected within minutes rather than hours.** The management of ARF represents an enormous drain on resources and considerably increases the ICU mortality figures. The aim of preventative manoeuvres is to continually provide ideal homeostatic conditions in which healthy kidneys can operate (Table 26.2).

**Table 26.2.** Prevention of acute renal failure

Maintain renal perfusion
    Begin rapid and efficient resuscitation
    Maintain patient's normal BP
    Correct hypovolaemia
    Avoid hypoxia
    Correct low cardiac output
    Avoid abdominal tamponade
    Diagnose and aggressively treat septicaemia
    Avoid high intrathoracic pressure
Avoid or closely monitor nephrotoxic drugs and contrast
Exclude obstruction of urinary tract
Other possible drugs
    Mannitol
    Frusemide

## Renal perfusion

### Hypovolaemia

In many instances, rapid correction of hypovolaemia is all that is required to prevent ARF. This is best achieved with a rapid infusion of fluids (see Chapter 4). Hourly urine output is a critical measurement for all seriously ill patients and it must always be *monitored and maintained.*

### Cardiac output

Restoring cardiac output depends on manipulating the preload, afterload and contractility of the heart (see Chapter 21).

## Hypotension

Blood pressure must be restored rapidly. This is particularly important in previously hypertensive patients. 'Hypotension' is a relative term. Always note a patient's pre-admission pressure or theoretically 'normal' BP and aim for that level. The blood flow to the kidneys is autoregulated according to the patient's normal BP range and a 'normal' pressure may be too low in previously hypertensive patients. This is often the case with the elderly, when a combination of decreased renal function and a moderate degree of pre-existing hypertension makes them particularly prone to develop ARF during hypotensive insults.

### Inotropes

In some situations such as septicaemia, it is difficult to increase the BP despite an adequate preload and good cardiac function. The use of a drug with vasoconstrictive properties such as adrenaline or noradrenaline often paradoxically increases, rather than decreases, renal blood flow and urine output. This is related to an increase in renal perfusion pressure.

## Low-dose dopamine

The status of low dosage ($1-3\ \mu g \cdot kg^{-1} \cdot min^{-1}$) dopamine is changing. It was thought to stimulate specific dopaminergic receptors, causing renal vasodilatation, promoting diuresis and sodium excretion. However, at such low dosages, dopamine enhances renal plasma flow by a global increase in cardiac output and mean arterial pressure. There is little specific dopaminergic mediated renal vasodilatation and it is no longer recommended specifically for its so-called 'sparing' function related to increasing renal blood flow.

## Abdominal tamponade

Abdominal tamponade due to excessive bleeding, intra-abdominal fluid, severe ileus or intestinal obstruction can cause renal impairment because of the combination of decreased arterial supply and decreased venous drainage.

As a guide to the severity of abdominal tamponade and as a guide to surgical intervention, the intra-abdominal pressure should be measured in all seriously ill patients when the abdomen feels tense. The intravesical pressure is an accurate reflection of intra-abdominal pressure and is easily measured. Decreased renal blood flow and oliguria occur with pressures as low as 20 cmH$_2$O. This will progressively worsen until total anuria eventually supervenes.

There is urgent need to relieve the tamponade by laparotomy. The abdomen may have to be left open with packs, or closed using a Marlex graft. The combination of oliguria and abdominal tamponade due to bleeding is a difficult diagnostic and therapeutic dilemma. It is often assumed that the oliguria is related to hypovolaemia rather than to the tamponade itself. Moreover, relief of the tamponade may be impossible when the intra-abdominal bleeding cannot be controlled by the usual surgical techniques.

## Positive intrathoracic pressure

Positive-pressure ventilation, especially with high levels of positive end-expiratory pressure (PEEP) can reduce renal blood flow by up to 20%. Ventilatory modes using lower mean intrathoracic pressures such as continuous positive airway pressure (CPAP) or pressure-support ventilation (PSV) may result in improved renal perfusion (see Chapter 19).

## Avoid or closely monitor nephrotoxic drugs

Drugs can exacerbate or cause renal failure by direct nephrotoxicity or interstitial nephritis. Drugs that can exacerbate renal failure include those that can contribute to hypotension or hypovolaemia such as diuretics and vasodilators.

### Direct nephrotoxicity

Aminoglycoside antibiotics are the drugs best known to cause nephrotoxicity in intensive care. They are directly toxic to the tubules and levels should be monitored closely when they are used. Once-daily dosing decreases their toxicity. Other drugs that have been implicated in the intensive care setting include the tetracyclines, methotrexate, cisplatin, cephalosporins, ethylene glycol, amphotericin B, radiographic contrast agents and non-steroidal anti-inflammatory agents (NSAIDS). Although the angiotensin converting enzyme (ACE) inhibitors are not directly nephrotoxic, they can predispose to ARF especially in patients with longstanding hypertension or renal artery stenosis. This is related to their pronounced vasodilatory effect on the efferent arteriole of the kidney, reducing the glomerular capillary pressure.

## Drugs for preventing renal failure

One of the great dilemmas in treating ARF is whether or not to use mannitol and loop diuretics. Except in special circumstances such as in the presence of damage due to myogloburia or haemoglobinuria, neither has been shown to prevent ARF and both have certainly been abused. Oliguria is not due to a lack of either drug, and too often the automatic response to oliguria is to use frusemide. The theoretical basis for their use supposedly is related to their ability to increase renal blood flow and encourage tubular fluid flow. Mannitol may encourage necrotic debris to be washed away but it has also been implicated in causing ARF, presumably by exacerbating hypovolaemia as a result of its diuretic effect. The 'diuretic challenge' or 'kick start' with loop diuretics usually is based on the premise that it may do some good and probably will not do any harm. However, both loop diuretics and mannitol have side effects that are exacerbated by their accumulation in patients with renal failure. Furthermore, diuresis will worsen renal insufficiency related to hypovolaemia. At best, diuretics may convert an oliguric renal failure to a non-oliguric one, once all other reversible causes have been excluded. Neither mannitol nor loop diuretics have consistently been shown to alter the course of ARF, or improve survival. Having stated that a frusemide infusion may make the patient's management easier by encouraging fluid and some waste product excretion. A common regimen is to use 250 mg of frusemide diluted in a 50 ml syringe pump and titrate the infusion rate against urine output. Commence with a rate of 1 mg/h and increase accordingly. Remember that frusemide in high doses has side effects, including the development of a metabolic alkalosis and hearing impairment.

## Radiocontrast nephropathy

Patients at risk of radiocontrast nephropathy include those with chronic renal impairment, diabetes, heart failure and those on other nephrotoxic drugs, e.g.

NSAIDs and aminoglycosides. The pathogenesis appears to involve reactive oxygen species causing direct toxic effects on the renal tubular cells and medullary ischaemia. Intravenous hydration precontrast with 0.9% NaCI will help prevent worsening renal function. Adding oral acetylcysteine 600 mg bd on the day before and the day of the study also decreases the incidence of worsening renal function in those patients with chronic renal failure.

## Exclude obstruction

Acute onset of renal failure with total anuria in the absence of shock, should direct the diagnostician's attention to the urinary tract in order to exclude obstruction along its length. Always flush the catheter in order to exclude obstruction. Replace the urinary catheter if there is doubt about obstruction, especially in the presence of blood clot or sediment. Ultrasound or pyelography with computed tomography should be employed to rule out obstruction within the urinary tract. Obstruction should be relieved quickly as recovery of renal function is directly related to the duration of obstruction. Ureteric stenting or percutaneous nephrostomy can relieve the obstruction.

## Management of renal failure

The functions of the kidneys are to maintain fluid and electrolyte homeostasis and to excrete the waste products of metabolism. The following are immediate considerations that precede the decision whether or not and when to use dialysis.

Water retention: Water retention results in peripheral and pulmonary oedema. Fluid restriction should be used only in the presence of established ARF. Restriction of fluid in the presence of hypovolaemia will increase the likelihood of the renal insufficiency becoming established.

Hyperkalaemia: The rate of rise of the potassium concentration will depend on the degree of oliguria, the amount of tissue trauma and the presence and extent of haemolysis, protein catabolism and sepsis.

Acidosis: Acidosis usually is not a problem in the early stages of ARF. If it becomes significant (e.g. hydrogen ion concentration $\geq$ 80 nmol $\cdot$ L$^{-1}$ (pH < 7.1)), then bicarbonate can be given (50 ml of 8.4% solution) as a temporary measure. Dialysis should be started early.

Blood urea: The rate of increase in the urea concentration will depend on the degree of hypercatabolism – usually 5–10 mmol $\cdot$ L$^{-1}$ $\cdot$ d$^{-1}$.

Serum creatinine: The rate of increase will depend on the degree of muscle breakdown – usually 50–200 $\mu$mol $\cdot$ L$^{-1}$ $\cdot$ d$^{-1}$.

Hyponatraemia: Hyponatraemia usually is not a major problem. It is related to water retention, rather than an absolute decrease in body sodium. Sodium-containing solutions are not indicated.

Calcium and phosphorus metabolism: Hyperphosphataemia and hypocalcaemia can occur in ARF.

Neurological complications: Alterations in mental status can occur in patients with ARF, with progression from somnolence to disorientation and coma.

Impaired coagulation: Uraemia is associated with impaired platelet function.

Dialysis: Clearly, the above are all temporary measures, and if the renal failure progresses, dialysis is indicated. Uncontrolled hyperkalaemia, uraemia, acidosis and fluid accumulation are indications for dialysis. Strict indications for the commencement of dialysis can be misleading. The rate of rise of urea and creatinine is more important. A blood urea concentration of 35 mmol/L and serum creatinine concentration of 60–800 μmol/L are guidelines for commencement of dialysis. Aim to keep the blood urea below 30 mmol/L. Dialysis should be instituted earlier, rather than later, and should be carried out more aggressively in hypercatabolic states, such as sepsis, trauma or rhabdomyolysis.

Dialysis should be continued until there is recovery of renal function. Recovery is heralded by increasing urine output, and by a 'plateauing' of urea and creatinine concentrations. The urinary catheter should always be removed if there is significant oliguria, as it is simply an extra source of infection.

## Complications of acute renal failure

Gastrointestinal tract bleeding
This can be a serious problem in patients with ARF and measures should be taken to prevent it.

Septicaemia: The major cause of mortality among patients with ARF is septicaemia. Meticulous attention should be paid to the prevention, detection and treatment of septicaemia (Chapter 13).

Feeding: Where possible, enteral feeding should be encouraged in patients with ARF. The use of peritoneal dialysis (PD) does not interfere with intestinal absorption. If enteral feeding is not possible, parenteral nutrition should be considered as long as there is adequate removal of fluid and urea.

Drug treatment in acute renal failure: Drugs normally handled by the kidney often need to be given in modified amounts during ARF. Consideration should also be given to the efficiency of drug removal by haemodialysis, PD or haemofiltration.

## Recovery and prognosis

Acute tubular necrosis will last less than 2–3 weeks – rarely more than 2 months.

If complete anuria lasts for more than 4–5 weeks, then the likelihood of irreversible cortical necrosis increases and further investigation is necessary.

Patients can rapidly become dehydrated in the polyuric phase of renal recovery. Measure the urinary electrolytes and replace them with an equivalent solution – usually 0.45% saline solution. The mortality from ARF in intensive care remains at about 50%. Despite many advances, the mortality regarding ARF with multiorgan failure has changed little over the past 20 years.

## Mode of dialysis

The mode of renal replacement therapy will be determined by the clinical circumstances and by the hospital facilities available. Intermittent haemodialysis (IHD) is still commonly used but it requires specialised nursing staff and facilities. Increasingly, continuous renal replacement therapy (CRRT) such as continuous haemofiltration and haemodiafiltration are being used in ICUs. Peritoneal dialysis is used infrequently.

### Haemodialysis

Haemodialysis works on the principle of diffusion of molecules across a semipermeable membrane. The movement of molecules occurs largely as a result of a concentration gradient and the nature of the membrane. Haemodialysis is an efficient technique for removing waste products and correcting electrolyte imbalances.

Haemodialysis is less efficient than PD or haemofiltration for removing water but ultrafiltration can be employed in conjunction with IHD for rapid and efficient removal of water. Ultrafiltration involves fluid movement as a result of a pressure gradient.

Hypotension is invariably associated with IHD in the critically ill. Bicarbonate dialysate rather than acetate will decrease this complication. Hypotension decreases the efficiency of dialysis.

Highly trained nursing staff are required for IHD. In these days of decreasing resources and increasing demand for IHD, this poses a problem for hospital renal services. Furthermore, patients in the ICU often require long and difficult dialysis every second day, or even daily.

### Peritoneal dialysis

Peritoneal dialysis works in a manner similar to that of IHD. The capillaries in the peritoneal membranes are used as a semipermeable membrane and exchange occurs as a result of diffusion, according to the concentration gradient between the capillaries and the peritoneal fluid. Movement of water occurs according to the osmolality of the PD fluid.

Peritoneal dialysis is not as efficient as IHD for removing waste products but is more efficient for removing fluid. This has certain advantages in the ICU, as patients commonly have pulmonary and peripheral oedema. Furthermore, with efficient fluid removal, adequate space can be made for parenteral nutrition, blood products and colloid.

It may be an added advantage to use PD for renal failure in the presence of peritonitis or pancreatitis. However, patients in intensive care commonly have concurrent lung abnormalities. Increased abdominal pressure due to the dialysate can cause elevation of the diaphragm and basal atelectasis. This can worsen the existing hypoxia and compromise ventilation. Aggressive physiotherapy, sitting the patient upright, or using CPAP via a mask or cuffed endotracheal tube can be used to help prevent basal atelectasis.

Technique:

1  The peritoneal catheter should be a soft, Silastic 'Tenkhoff' type catheter, inserted in the midline 3 cm below the umbilicus, preferably by a surgeon experienced in the technique under sterile conditions in the operating theatre. Suturing the catheter onto the top of the bladder improves the efficiency of the procedure. Commence PD intra-operatively to prevent blockage: initially, use small volume (500 ml) cycles (20 min to run in, 20 min of dwell time, 20 min to run out), in order to minimise leakage and scrotal oedema.

2  Add heparin, 500 units/L, for the first 48 hours and whenever infection is present in order to decrease the incidence of fibrin formation and catheter occlusion.

3  After 24 hours, conduct hourly exchanges of either 1 or 2 litres of peritoneal dialysate (20 min run in, 20 min dwell time, 20 min run out) for as long as renal failure persists. Continuous PD ensures adequate removal of waste products as well as continuous fine-tuning of fluid removal.

4  Having recently had a laparotomy is not necessarily a contraindication to PD. The wounds usually will not leak if they are made waterproof by suturing with continuous nylon and the volume used is less than 500 ml hourly for the first 48 hours. If drains are employed during the laparotomy, PD is not, of course, possible.

5  Varying concentrations of glucose in the dialysate (usually 1.5%, 2.5%, 4.5%) will determine the rate of removal of fluid. The 1.5% solution usually results in neutrality – no fluid loss. Resulting hyperglycaemia may require an insulin infusion. Potassium can be added in an appropriate concentration to the dialysate (usually 3.5 mmol/L) or directly to the patient in an IV form.

### Troubleshooting

**Poor drainage is the commonest problem with PD.**

Inadequate drainage usually is related to malpositioning of the catheter or fibrin clotting in the catheter lumen. Addition of 500 units of heparin to each litre of dialysate can help prevent fibrin clots and flushing of the catheter can dislodge the fibrin clots. Unfortunately, an occasional 'rogue' catheter will fail to drain whatever is done. This necessitates early surgical replacement.

Infection of the dialysate can present as peritonism, cloudy dialysate, fibrin aggregates or clinical deterioration of the patient. It is relatively common during prolonged PD in intensive care. Gram staining and culturing should be performed daily on the dialysate. In the presence of infection, antibiotics should initially be added to the dialysate; penicillins or cephalosporins (200 mg/L) and/or amino-glycosides (5 mg/L). Heparin (500 units/L) should also be added to the dialysate in the presence of infection, to prevent fibrin aggregation.

Overall PD is infrequently used in intensive care now. Intermittent haemodialysis and CRRT provide better uraemic control in the critically ill.

Disadvantages of peritoneal dialysis:

- Technical problems with fluid drainage.
- Leakage around catheter site.
- Peritonitis.
- Basal atelectasis and interference with ventilation.
- Hyperglycaemia.
- Peritoneal dialysis is not as efficient as IHD for removing waste products of metabolism.
- Peritoneal fluid can leak out of peritoneal space to form oedema.

Advantages of peritoneal dialysis:

- Can be performed by non-specialised staff in the ICU.
- Very efficient for removing fluid.
- Can control metabolic disturbances in most patients.
- No special dialysis equipment required.

## Continuous renal replacement therapy (Figure 26.3)

Techniques of renal support have expanded greatly in intensive care in the last 10 years. Intravascular access can be arterial or venous, mechanisms of solute and water clearance range from ultrafiltration to haemofiltration to haemodiafiltration. Each has its own advantages and disadvantages. The choice of technique should be determined by the needs of the patient and the expertise of that unit. Commercial CRRT machines are available which can do most techniques automatically.

Haemofiltration passes extracorporeal blood across a filter. The filter has a polyacrylnitrile or polycarbonate membrane with a pore size similar to that of a normal glomerulus. A filtrate of blood, similar to glomerular filtrate in composition, is formed from the hydrostatic pressure across the membrane. The movement of fluids and small molecules is due to convection, not diffusion as in IHD. An extracorporeal circuit containing the filter is connected either between a larger artery and vein or between two large veins if a roller pump is used. Prevention of clotting in the system is achieved by heparinisation (500–1500 units/h) by prostacyclin infusion or by a combination of the two.

50-100 ml/min

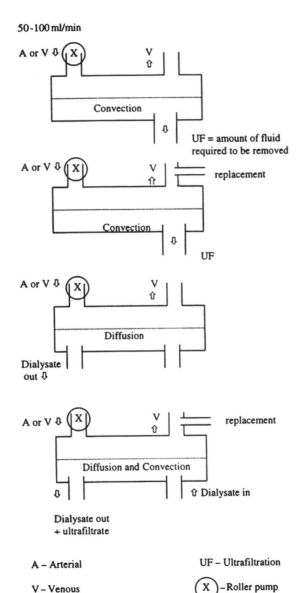

Slow Continuous
Ultrafiltration
(SCUF)
for slow fluid
removal
e.g. 1–3 L/day.
No replacement.

Continuous
Haemofiltration
A-V or V-V.
Ultrafiltrate is replaced.
Solute removal equals
volume of UF.
Removes 'middle
molecules'.

Continuous Haemodialysis
A-V or V-V plus pump.
High flux membrane.
Fluid not lost unless UF
used.
No replacement.
Good urea and small
molecule clearance.

Continuous
Haemodiafiltration
A-V or V-V plus pump.
Volumes of dialysate
and UF can be
controlled.
Small and large
molecules removed.

A – Arterial

V – Venous

UF – Ultrafiltration

X – Roller pump

**Figure 26.2.** Continuous renal replacement techniques.

Whereas the filter acts like an artificial glomerulus, there is no equivalent to a renal tubule in this system. In order to achieve elimination of urea, creatinine and other products of metabolism, the filtrate (blood − [red blood cells + large molecules such as protein]) is replaced by a fluid whose composition is similar to that of the filtrate but without waste products (e.g. Ringer's Lactate). Therefore, to achieve relatively normal levels of urea and creatinine, a large fluid turnover is needed. Depending on the catabolic rate, a fluid turnover of 10−40 L/day may be needed. Haemodiafiltration largely overcomes this problem by employing a filter with a membrane that is capable of dialysis, using diffusion as in conventional haemodialysis, as well as convection as in haemofiltration. Haemofiltration and/or haemodiafiltration are increasingly being used as the dialytic technique of choice in ICUs.

## Dialysis issues

Most units now use veno-venous access with a pump or have automated CRRT machines. The possible choices of dialytic technique for the patient in renal failure are huge. Below are some guidelines. Like ventilators, it is not the flashiness of the machine that saves lives, it is the skill and understanding of the operator!

## Which technique?

Slow continuous ultrafiltration (SCUF): Good for the fluid-overloaded, oliguric, haemodynamically unstable patient who does not have clinically significant uraemia, acidosis or hyperkalaemia who needs 2−3 L/day of fluid taken off to improve pulmonary and interstitial oedema until the kidneys recover.

Continuous haemofiltration: Can be used for all patients in ARF. Good at fluid and middle molecule removal (most mediators of sepsis are this size). If the patient is very catabolic, large volumes of ultrafiltrate will need to be removed and replaced, up to 40 L/day.

Intermittent haemodialysis: The IHD machines have high flux membranes which remove urea and other small molecules very well. Fluid is removed by ultrafiltration if required.

In critically ill patients they are associated with an incidence of 20–30% of severe hypotension. Their episodic use (every second day) means that volume control is difficult particularly 'making room' for nutrition. Uraemic control is difficult and there is some evidence to suggest that the higher the dialysis dose the better the patient outcome.

Renal patients are catabolic and often their dietary intake is compromised as they quickly become uraemic. Continuous techniques allow more nutritional intake.

Having made all these points, at present there is no hard evidence to say that CRRT has a survival advantage over IHD. There is some evidence to suggest that patients on CRRT have better renal recovery. In most units there is no cost difference between the two.

Continuous haemodiafiltration: Adding dialysis to haemofiltration decreases the amount of ultrafiltrate that needs to be removed to get solute clearance and also increases the clearance of small and large molecules. Many aspects of this therapy can be varied to suit the individual patient. For example, patients who are very catabolic can be treated by increasing the dialysate flow, e.g. to 2 L/h, increasing the ultrafiltrate flow and increasing the blood flow rate.

## Which access?

Arterial access techniques are rarely used now as compared with veno-venous access with a roller pump. Arterial access has a higher complication rate due to problems with wide bore arterial access, blood flow in the circuit being dependent on the patient's BP and the circuits frequently clotting.

Access needs to be large, into a straight, high-flow vein. Our preference is for the femoral or internal jugular veins. Double lumen lines work well and have little clinically significant recycling. Large bore, side-by-side catheters may be advantageous.

## Which anticoagulant?

Anticoagulation can be a difficult choice in some patients. Recent surgery, particularly cardiac or neurosurgery may preclude it. The patient may already have a bleeding problem, e.g. a disseminated intravascular coagulopathy (DIC) or open wound. On the other hand some patients clot their circuits no matter what anticoagulation you provide. This can be one of the most frustrating things about CRRT.

No anticoagulation: This is possible with high blood flows (150–250 ml/min), limiting dependent loops in the circuit, predilution (adding replacement fluid before the filter) and limited ultrafiltrate removal. Really good wide IV access is required, e.g. side-by-side catheter in a femoral vein.

Heparin: This is still the commonest anticoagulant used. It has a short half-life, its effect can be measured (activated partial prothrombin time (APPT)) and it can be readily reversed. Aim to keep the circuit anticoagulated (APPT between 60–80) and the patient's APPT normal. Protamine can be added after the filter but is not usually necessary.

If the circuit is primed with heparin then an IV bolus before commencing is not necessary.

Prostacyclin: Prostacyclin is expensive, induces hypotension and its anticoagulant effect can not be monitored. However, for some patients who cannot have heparin and who cannot be dialysed without an anticoagulant, it works well.

Citrate: Citrate is another anticoagulant option but it is very expensive and difficult to monitor.

## Which replacement fluid?

This only applies to haemofiltration and haemodiafiltration (Figure 26.3).

The amount of ultrafiltrate should be empirically adjusted on an hourly basis (e.g. 100–300ml/h) against an estimation of the body's fluid retention status.

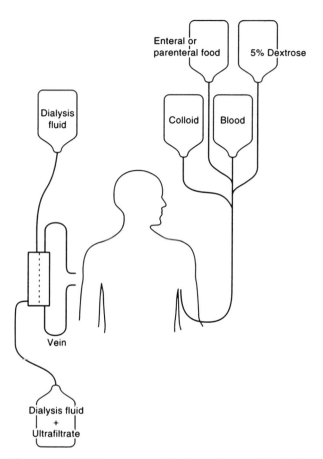

**Figure 26.3.** Fluid management during continuous dialytic therapies.

The other fluids should be titrated separately according to separate end points (e.g. colloid against intravascular measurement, blood against haemoglobin, 5% dextrose against serum sodium and food according to nutritional status). There is little point in adding all of these fluids together when considering fluid balance.

The ideal is a normal person's plasma. Hartman's (lactated Ringer's solution) is commonly used. Normal saline should not be used as a routine as the chloride concentration is too high. Commercial companies produce replacement solutions which are suitable. Some patients who have a high lactate may benefit from a replacement solution with bicarbonate rather than lactate as one of the anions.

### Starting continuous renal replacement techniques
Some patients may become haemodynamically unstable when they start on CRRT. Decide if you are going to use inotropes or fluid to treat their hypotension and get it set up before you start!

Blood flow rate. Start at 150 ml/min.

Start the heparin at 500–1500 units/h.

Decide on the dialysate flow rate.

Decide how much ultrafiltration you want.

Decide what you want the patient's hourly fluid balance to be. Then balance between the ultrafiltrate off and the replacement fluid in.

## Troubleshooting

Poor blood flow: This is related to the vascular access – either the vascath is kinked or has clots in the lumens. Occasionally rotating the vascath helps, as does switching the arterial and venous lines from the vascath. Most of the time this problem is only solved by changing the vascath. This can be done over a wire at the same site if it is 'clean' or the patient is coagulopathic or going to a new site.

Filter clotting: This can be related to the vascular access, the anticoagulation or the state of the patient. Poor flow from the patient and high pressures pushing the blood back into the patient can both clot the filter. Try higher blood flow rates, a different vascular access site and prostacyclin instead of heparin or IHD.

Urea and creatinine not falling: Check the creatinine clearance of the filter. It may need changing despite the fact that the pressures are low.

The patient may be very catabolic so try higher blood flow rates, higher volumes of ultrafiltrate removal and replacement and a higher dialysate flow rate.

Bleeding: Reverse the anticoagulant if bleeding is life-threatening.

Do not remove the circuit in anticipation it will clot. It may keep going!

Try no anticoagulant (see above) or use IHD with no heparin.

Thrombocytopaenia: Low platelet count can have many causes in CRRT. It can be part of the patient's illness or related to the dialysis, e.g. bleeding, frequent circuit changes, a heparin effect or heparin-induced thrombocytopaenic syndrome (HITS).

## When to start

The classical indicators are:

Anuria or oliguria < 200 ml/day.

Urea greater than 35 mmol/L or symptoms of uraemia.

pH < 7.1.

Potassium > 6.5 mmol/L or rapidly rising with arrhythmias.

Fluid overload unresponsive to other therapies.

There is a trend in the critically ill to start dialytic therapies sooner than these criteria suggest. There is also a trend to use dialysis as an adjunct therapy to remove soluble mediators in sepsis. Neither of these trends is supported by evidence as yet.

**TROUBLESHOOTING**

## Oliguria

### Pre-renal
A pre-renal cause of oliguria is the commonest by far.
  Hypovolaemia.

- Intravenous fluid will correct most oliguria in the ICU.
- Give a fluid bolus and increase the rate of fluid infusion.
- Think about possible causes for the hypovolaemia.
- Then give more fluid.

Hypotension.

- Correct hypovolaemia.
- Restore BP to the patient's 'normal' level.
- Vasopressors and/or inotropes may be required.

### Renal
Nephrotoxic drugs.

- Check levels (e.g. aminoglycoside antibiotics).
- Avoid where possible (e.g. radio contrast drug).

Sepsis.
Myoglobin.

### Post-renal
No catheter, kinked catheter, blocked catheter.
Increased intra-abdominal pressure.
Bilateral ureteric obstruction (e.g. trauma, tumour).

## When to stop
This is often decided by when the filter clots!
  Some other indicators to stop CRRT are:

Return of urine output (> 20 ml/h).
Plateauing of the urea and creatinine.
Normalising of pH and potassium.
Encephalopathy improving.
The process that caused the ARF resolving.

Try stopping CRRT for 24 hours and measure the rise in urea, creatinine, potassium and the change in pH.

## FURTHER READING

Bellomo, R. and Ronco, C. Continuous renal replacement therapy in the intensive care unit. *Intensive Care Medicine* 25 (1999): 781–9.

Brady, H. R. and Singer, G. G. Acute renal failure. *Lancet* 346 (1995): 1533–40.

Davenport, A. Anionic bases for continuous forms of renal replacement therapy (CCRT) in the ICU. *Intensive Care Medicine* 25 (1999): 1209–11.

Duke, G. J. Renal protective agents: a review. *Critical Care and Resuscitation* 1 (1999): 265–75.

Galley, H. F. (ed.) *Critical Care Focus. 1. Renal failure.* London: BMJ Books, 1999.

Lote, C. J., Harper, L. and Savage, C. O. S. Mechanisms of acute renal failure. *British Journal of Anaesthesia* 77 (1996): 82–9.

Mehta, R. Anticoagulation strategies for continuous renal replacement therapies: what works? *American Journal of Kidney Diseases* 28 (1996): S8–14.

Thadhani, R., Pascual, M. and Bonventre, V. Acute renal failure. *New England Journal of Medicine* 334 (1996): 1448–60.

# 27

# Critical care gastroenterology

## Fulminant hepatic failure

Fulminant hepatic failure (FHF) is defined as encephalopathy due to massive hepatic necrosis within 8 weeks of the onset of the primary illness, with no evidence of previous liver disease. This excludes subacute hepatic necrosis, acute-on-chronic hepatic failure and chronic hepatic encephalopathy. It is a relatively rare disease.

### Aetiology

- Viral causes: the viruses that cause hepatitis A, B, C, D, E and non-A, non-B, as well as Epstein–Barr virus, herpes simplex virus and cytomegalovirus (CMV). Viral causes account for over 70% of all cases of fulminant hepatic failure.
- Paracetamol poisoning.
- Idiosyncratic drug reactions: antituberculous drugs, methyldopa, monoamine oxidase inhibitors, halothane hepatitis.
- Direct drug toxicity: carbon tetrachloride, yellow phosphorus.
- Ischaemia, hypoxia, heatstroke, shock.
- Budd–Chiari syndrome, lymphoma.
- Acute fatty liver of pregnancy.
- Wilson's disease.

### Clinical features

The diagnosis can be difficult especially in the early stages. Patients usually do not have signs of chronic liver failure such as spider naevi and palmar erythema.

Encephalopathy is the hallmark of this disease and disturbance in the level of consciousness may be the only presenting feature.

The clinical course may be over hours or days.

Encephalopathy: Many factors have been implicated but as yet no definite cause of the encephalopathy has been found. Ammonia, free fatty acids, phenols, bilirubin, bile acids, mercaptans, false neurotransmitters, benzodiazepine analogues and $\gamma$-aminobutyric acid (GABA) are some of the implicated compounds.

Stages of encephalopathy:

Grade I:    mood change and confusion.
Grade II:   drowsiness and increase in muscle tone.
Grade III:  stuperose but rousable.
Grade IV:   unrousable to maximum stimulation.

There are no specific clinical or EEG features that can be used to differentiate this encephalopathy from those associated with other metabolic disturbances.

Encephalopathy is associated with cerebral oedema – **This, together with sepsis, is usually the cause of death.** Over 80% of patients with grade IV encephalopathy have cerebral oedema. If active treatment is planned the sequelae of the cerebral oedema – elevated intracranial pressure (ICP) – should be monitored and attempts should be made to decrease it. One must rule out the presence of hypoglycaemia, intracranial haemorrhage, acid-base or electrolyte disturbances and hypoxia, as these contribute to the severity of the encephalopthy.

Bleeding diathesis: Most of the clotting factors are manufactured in the liver and therefore their levels usually will be decreased.

The prothrombin time is always prolonged – it is a good marker of liver function and clinical course. Platelets are reduced in number and function. Gastrointestinal tract (GIT) or other haemorrhage may occur.

Hepatorenal syndrome: The 'hepatorenal syndrome' is renal failure that occurs in patients with liver disease in the absence of other causes. It usually occurs in patients with chronic hepatic insufficiency, usually in association with ascites and often is associated with a sepsis-like syndrome, with peripheral vasodilatation and increased cardiac output. Hepatorenal syndrome is exacerbated by hypovolaemia and hypotension, especially in association with fluid loss secondary to diuretic treatment and aggressive paracentesis. The so-called syndrome may, in fact, be acute tubular necrosis as a result of hypovolaemia and/or sepsis. Most patients with hepatorenal syndrome die. That it is related to the liver failure is emphasised by the fact that renal function recovers after liver transplantation. Apart from liver transplantation there is no definitive treatment.

Electrolytes: Hypokalaemia occurs early. Hyperkalaemia associated with renal failure may supervene. Hyponatraemia may occur in the latter stages.

Acid-base disturbances: Respiratory alkalosis is common in the early stages. Lactic acidosis occurs in over half of all these patients especially in the latter stages.

Hypoglycaemia: Hypoglycaemia can occur and probably is due to failure of gluconeogenesis.

Cardiovascular failure: Hypotension, with a high cardiac output and vasodilatation, is common. The pathophysiology is similar to that of septicaemia.

Respiratory failure: The airway may be compromised because of coma. Acute lung injury (ALI) may occur and probably is due to increased membrane permeability.

Immunocompromise: Bacteraemia and endotoxaemia are common because of decreases in reticuloendothelial clearance, leucocyte function and complement activity. Spontaneous bacterial peritonitis can occur in patients with ascites.

Jaundice: Jaundice often develops late.

## Investigations

The diagnosis is clinical – based mainly on encephalopathy. Investigations are necessary to find the cause of the FHF, to determine prognosis and to chart the course of the disease and its complications.

- Viral serology.
    HAV IgM anti-HAV.
    HBV HbsAg, IgM anti-Bc, HBV DNA.
    HCV Anti-HCV antibody, HCV mRNA.
    HDV IgM anti-HDV.
    HEV Anti HEV antibody.
    Seriology for other viruses such as CMV, EBV, herpes simplex.
- Autoantibodies/immunoglobulins.
- Ultrasound scan liver and spleen.
- Paracetamol levels if drug poisoning is suspected.
- Coagulation studies: The prothrombin time is probably the most sensitive laboratory indicator of liver function in fulminant hepatic failure. It should be measured daily.
- Liver function tests: The functions of the liver include lipid, protein and carbohydrate metabolism, production of bile acids; storage; and detoxification and excretion of lipid soluble compounds. All of these functions can be compromised, but few are routinely tested in clinical practice. Hepatic enzymes are crude markers of liver destruction rather than function and may appear 'normal' in the presence of massive liver destruction. To date, there are few clinically sensitive and specific laboratory markers of hepatic function.
- Bilirubin determinations have no value for prognosis or treatment. Serum bilirubin and bile acid levels in hepatobiliary disease are related to excretory function.
- Blood sugar levels should be measured regularly.
- Potassium should be measured as indications arise.
- Other serum electrolytes should be measured daily (sodium, calcium, magnesium, phosphate).

- Blood urea is a measure of liver (production) and renal (excretion) functions and therefore is difficult to interpret.
- Creatinine: Measure daily.
- Arterial blood gases: Measure at least twice per day.
- Chest x-ray should be obtained daily.
- EEG should be carried out on admission and regularly thereafter as an indicator of the severity of encephalopathy.
- CT scan and brain stem evoked potentials may be helpful, mainly for prognosis.
- Regular microbiological screenings should be conducted.

## Monitoring

Monitoring is necessary as a guide to patient management while the liver is given an opportunity to regenerate. Because cerebral oedema, with an elevated ICP, is the major cause of death among patients with FHF, the cerebral perfusion pressure (CPP) and mean arterial pressure (MAP) should be continuously monitored to provide a basis for adjustments in the treatment:

$$CPP = MAP - ICP$$

There is a danger of causing intracranial haemorrhage when inserting the ICP monitor. Ideally the prothrombin ratio should be less than 1.3 and platelet count more than $100 \times 10^9$/L before insertion. Monitor:

- Pulse rate.
- Temperature.
- Continuous ECG.
- Continuous blood pressure.
- Central venous pressure.
- Urine output.
- Pulse oximetry.
- Pulmonary artery wedge pressure (PAWP), if needed.
- Cardiac output, if needed.
- Oxygen consumption and delivery, if needed.

## Management

Ideally, these patients should be transferred at an early stage to a specialised ICU with appropriate expertise and monitoring equipment. Early discussions with a liver transplantation unit should be undertaken (Table 27.1). Apart from cases of paracetamol overdose, where drug removal may be possible, the principles of treatment are meticulous monitoring and support until the liver can be given an opportunity to regenerate.

Maintain cerebral perfusion pressure:

**Table 27.1.** Criteria for possible orthotopic liver transplantation (Kings College Criteria)

Paracetamol overdose
    Arterial pH < 7.30 in fluid resuscitated patient
    All the following:
        Prothrombin time >100 seconds
        Creatinine >300 μmol/L
        Grade 3 or 4 encephalopathy
    Non-paracetamol overdose
    A prothrombin time of >100 seconds
    *or*
    Arterial pH < 7.1 in a fluid resuscitated patient
    *or*
    Any three of the following:
        Aetiology non-A, non-B hepatitis, drug-induced hepatitis
        Age < 10 or > 40 years
        Jaundice to encephalopathy time of > 7 days
        Serum bilirubin > 300 μmol/L
        Prothrombin time > 50 seconds

Treat elevated ICP (for details, see Chapter 23).
Position the patient 30°−40° upright.

If the ICP is significantly elevated, prevent hypertensive surges to the non-autoregulated cerebral circulation by giving small amounts of sedation before procedures. Narcotics and other sedatives depend on liver function for metabolism and should be given in only small amounts until the degree of liver damage is assessed.

Keep the patient's head straight and avoid jugular venous compression.
Give mannitol boluses, 0.3 g/kg IV boluses (no more than three times per day), if ICP is consistently raised (ICP > 25 mmHg (3.3 kPa)) and monitor serum osmolality. Keep osmolality < 320 mOsm/L.
Hyperventilation may be useful as a short-term measure.
Phenobarbitone and thiopentone may also help to reduce ICP.
Maintain the MAP with fluids and inotropes.

Cardiovascular system: The cardiovascular abnormalities are very similar to those found in the presence of sepsis. Usually there will be high cardiac output, low MAP and decreased peripheral vascular resistance. It is crucial to avoid hypotension in patients with liver failure. Oxygen delivery to the liver should be optimised by supporting cardiac output, oxygen saturation and haemoglobin levels. Aggressive fluid resuscitation and inotropes are often necessary. The type and dosage of inotrope are dependent on the patient's needs. A suggested starting regimen for hypotension, with normal filling pressures, is adrenaline or noradrenaline titrated against the response.

Nutrition:

Cease dietary protein.
Give oral lactulose (30–50 ml 8-hourly).
Avoid neomycin as it can be absorbed and can cause renal failure.

Blood glucose: Because the liver is a major source of glucose, hypoglycaemia can occur. Measure blood glucose hourly and titrate against levels, with 10% or 50% dextrose IV infusions – large amounts may be necessary.

Electrolytes: Correct hypokalaemia with IV potassium chloride as necessary. Correct hyponatraemia with water restriction – may need to concentrate dextrose solutions and IV drugs in order to decrease the water intake.

Fluids: Often patients will require liberal amounts of fluid or blood products (Chapter 4) because hypovolaemia and hypotension are poorly tolerated. If hypotension persists, despite adequate cardiac filling pressures, use inotropic support.

Acid-base disturbances: Respiratory alkalosis does not require active treatment. For metabolic alkalosis consider giving acetazolamide 500 mg IV 8-hourly. If there is metabolic acidosis, treat the underlying cause.

Gastrointestinal haemorrhage: $H_2$-receptor antagonists, although effective, will reduce blood flow to the liver and antacids may predispose to gastric colonisation. Sucralfate may be preferable.

Coagulation abnormalities: Use fresh frozen plasma and blood and platelets where necessary, to replace coagulation factors and maintain haemoglobin levels.

Respiratory failure: Intubate if airway patency is in question.

Treat ALI or acute hypoxia with an increased concentration of inspired oxygen, continuous positive airway pressure (CPAP) or ventilation with positive end-expiratory pressure (PEEP) if necessary. Encourage spontaneous ventilation, and low pressure ventilation as increased intrathoracic pressure will decrease liver blood flow.

Renal failure: Avoid hypovolaemia and hypotension.

Use loop diuretics and aminoglycosides cautiously as they can contribute to renal insufficiency.

Dialyse early if established renal failure is confirmed. Remember most patients with renal failure and FHF will die unless definitive transplantation is planned.

General measures: Avoid sedation and analgesics unless they are being used to control ICP or to relieve pain. Use very small incremental doses in order to avoid accumulation in the absence of adequate liver detoxification.

## Other forms of treatment
The following will not influence survival:

- Corticosteroids.
- Exchange blood transfusion.
- Cross circulation with humans, animals or excised livers.

- Haemodialysis.
- Branched-chain amino acids.

Charcoal perfusion with prostacyclin may improve survival rates if commenced early. N-acetylcysteine may improve outcome of FHF, even when not caused by paracetamol. Other temporary measures to support liver function include bioartificial techniques such as pig hepatocytes or human hepatoblastoma cells and toxin removal techniques. Liver transplantation may play an increasing role in these patients. The results thus far indicate a survival rate higher than 50% among selected patients and in the absence of cerebral oedema.

### Prognosis
Without transplantation, the mortality from grade IV encephalopathy is more than 80%. With early and aggressive treatment of patients with grade III encephalopathy, mortality can be reduced to about 40%.

## Acute-on-chronic liver failure

Acute-on-chronic liver failure and FHF are, for practical purposes, considered together. Although there are many differences, the management, if not their causes, has some similarities. The diagnosis of acute-on-chronic liver failure is the easier of the two, because in addition to the disturbed level of consciousness, there are the obvious stigmata of chronic liver disease (jaundice, spider naevi, hepatomegaly, ascites etc). Increasing numbers of patients with alcohol-related liver disease are being admitted to ICUs for acute deterioration (e.g. bleeding oesophageal varices) and concurrent acute illnesses.

### Differences between fulminant hepatic failure and acute-on-chronic liver failure

- Infection, surgery, drugs and nitrogenous loads in the GIT can precipitate acute liver failure and hepatic encephalopathy in patients with chronic liver failure. In these patients, lactulose (30–50 ml 8-hourly orally) may be helpful. Avoid or limit sedative drugs.
- The role of cerebral oedema in acute-on-chronic liver failure has not been established.
- Short-term survival is better for acute-on-chronic failure than for FHF.
- However, among those patients with acute-on-chronic liver failure who require ventilation, mortality is about 90%.

## Liver dysfunction in critical illness

Many patients with previously normal liver function will become jaundiced while acutely ill, especially in association with septicaemia, trauma, multiorgan

**Table 27.2.** Clinical features of ischaemic hepatitis and ICU jaundice

| Parameter | Ischaemic hepatitis | ICU jaundice |
|---|---|---|
| Clinical setting | Shock | Sepsis<br>Trauma<br>Following surgery<br>After severe shock<br>MOF |
| Pathogenesis | Reduced liver blood flow | Reduced liver blood flow<br>Inflammatory mediators<br>Bilirubin load<br>Nutritional factors<br>Drugs |
| Time of onset | Within 24 hours | Usually 1–2 weeks |
| Liver function tests | | |
|   Bilirubin | Normal/moderate | 150–800 μmol/L |
|   AST/ALT | >1000 units/L | Normal/moderate |
|   ALP/GGT | Normal/moderate | Normal/moderate |
|   Blood glucose | Hypoglycaemia | Hyperglycaemia |
|   Prothrombin time | Prolonged | Normal |
|   Bile salts | Normal | Markedly elevated |
| Histology | Centrilobular necrosis | Intrahepatic cholestasis<br>Steatosis<br>Increased Kupffer cells<br>Occasionally hepatocyte necrosis |
| Mortality | > 50% | > 50% |
| Clinical course | Resolves if shock is reversed.<br>Predisposes to ICU jaundice | Associated with other manifestations of multi-organ dysfunction, immunosuppression and abnormal intermediary and drug metabolism |

Adapted by permission from Hawker F. Liver dysfunction in critical illness. *Anaesthesia and Intensive Care* 19 (1991): 165–81.

failure (MOF) and shock. This is almost certainly another manifestation of MOF resulting from hypoperfusion (Chapter 9). There are two major syndromes (Table 27.2).

Ischaemic hepatitis: Ischaemic hepatitis is characterised by acute increases in liver transaminases that occur within 24 hours of the onset of shock. It is an indicator of generalised and severe ischaemia, often also involving renal failure. Histologically there will be centrilobular necrosis, presumably as a result of an acute decrease in liver blood flow. The bilirubin will be normal or only mildly elevated. The prothrombin time usually will be prolonged.

ICU jaundice: The syndrome of ICU jaundice is characterised by a rising bilirubin that occurs within days of the onset of the illness that required admission to the ICU. The aetiology is multifactorial and includes:

- Decreased liver blood flow and ischaemia (artificial ventilation can, by itself, decrease liver blood flow and may potentiate liver ischaemia).
- Inflammatory mediators released in response to the systemic inflammatory reaction to insults such as sepsis or trauma.
- Intravenous nutrition (IVN).
- Drugs.
- Blood transfusions.

## Management

Both ischaemic hepatitis and ICU jaundice will resolve spontaneously as the underlying disease resolves and the patient improves. Exclude other causes of liver dysfunction such as hepatitis, post-anaesthetic jaundice, gallstones and acalculous cholecystitis. Ultrasound and CT are useful investigations to exclude biliary obstruction. An iminodiacetic acid (IDA) scan can be used for diagnosing both acute and chronic cholecystitis and acute biliary obstructions and may, in fact, detect biliary tract dilatation before it is seen on ultrasound. Avoid hypotension and hypoxia as well as high intrathoracic pressures from artificial ventilation. Treat any underlying problem such as sepsis aggressively.

## Ascites

### Pathogenesis

Portal hypertension with increased hydrostatic pressure.

Decreases in serum albumin and colloid oncotic pressure (COP).
Sodium retention.
Impaired free water excretion, often resulting in relatively greater water retention than sodium retention, causing hyponatraemia.
Relative hypovolaemia secondary to peripheral vasodilatation with salt and water retention.

### Management

**There is no simple answer to liver-induced ascites. Most manoeuvres only provide temporary relief.**
Bed rest and low sodium diet: A low sodium (40–50 mmol/day) diet will result in control of ascites in about 20% of patients. Sodium restriction can diminish

diuretic requirements. However, many cirrhotics are anorexic and malnourished and that can be worsened by a low sodium diet.

Diuretic: Spironolactone (100–500 mg/day) is effective in most patients who do not have renal failure. A loop diuretic alone produces a satisfactory response in only about 50% of cirrhotics and should be added only after failure of spirono-lactone.

Patients with impaired renal function do not respond well to standard doses of diuretics. Their serum concentrations of potassium and magnesium must be carefully monitored during diuretic therapy.

Peritoneovenous shunt: The LeVeen shunt consists of a perforated intra-abdominal tube connected through a one-way pressure-sensitive valve to empty into the superior vena cava. It provides short-term improvement but is associated with a high rate of complications:

- Obstruction: 30%.
- Infection: usually with *Staphylococcus* (shunt must be removed).
- Coagulation disorders: usually mild and in the immediate postoperative period.
- Pulmonary oedema, pulmonary embolism and endocarditis: the shunt should be reserved for patients with diuretic resistant oedema and preserved hepatic function.

Paracentesis: Paracentesis can predispose to hypovolaemia, hypotension, renal failure, dilutional hyponatraemia and hepatic encephalopathy. It may be temporarily of use in combination with intravascular volume replacement.

Other approaches:

- Albumin infusions: short-term benefits.
- Portacaval shunt: hepatic dysfunction is usually so marked in cirrhotics with refractory ascites that surgery is not an option.
- Liver transplantation: may be considered in selected cases, especially if there is no renal impairment.

Prognosis: Over 50% of patients with ascites from liver dysfunction are dead within 2 years. This puts ascites in the same prognostic category as many terminal malignancies.

## Pancreatitis

### Aetiology

Approximately 80% of patients with acute pancreatitis have either biliary lithiasis or chronic alcohol ingestion. Other causes include hyperlipidaemia, surgery, penetrating peptic ulcer, physical trauma, instrumentation of the pancreatic duct, hypercalcaemia, toxins and drugs. Up to 10–20% of cases are idiopathic.

## Pathogenesis

Acute necrotising pancreatitis is characterised by autodigestion of the pancreas and surrounding issues by proteolytic and lipolytic enzymes. Oedema, haemorrhage and ischaemia of the affected regions of the pancreas will eventually result in focal necrosis.

The massive initial inflammatory reaction characterises the early toxaemic phase. Distant organ damage and MOF often occurs during this phase. These effects are attributed to the local inflammatory reaction activating the kallikrein, complement, coagulation and fibrinolytic systems. Activated leucocytes release a variety of toxic substances, including proteases, phospholipases, lyosomal enzymes, reactive oxygen metabolites and leucotrienes, that result in additional damage to the pancreas and distant organs. Multiorgan failure as a result of non-bacterial pancreatitis is indistinguishable from bacterial sepsis.

The initial phase can last for up to 3 days after the onset of symptoms. That is followed by the necrotic phase. Most (about 70%) patients go on to spontaneous recovery but others can develop complications such as abscesses, haemorrhage or pseudocyst.

## Diagnosis

Pancreatitis will be suspected on the basis of history and clinical features, supported by the finding of an elevated serum amylase. Pancreatitis must be differentiated from other acute abdominal emergencies such as ischaemia, obstruction, cholecystitis, perforation and abdominal aneurysm. Imaging with ultrasound or CT scan can support the diagnosis. Some form of imaging should be performed early in the course of the disease in order to establish a baseline impression of the extent of the disease, in preparation for following its course and detecting complications.

## Clinical features

- Pain is reported by more than 90% of patients – usually near the hypochondrium but sometimes lower abdominal or flank pain. The pain usually is gradual in onset, steady, boring and often relieved by sitting up.
- Nausea and vomiting.
- The abdomen often is slightly distended with diffuse tenderness. Sometimes there is pronounced guarding and, at other times, there will be no signs at all despite severe pain. Cullen's sign (umbilical discoloration) and Grey–Turner sign (flank discoloration) are rare and late signs usually indicating severe necrotising pancreatitis.
- Systemic signs and symptoms include tachycardia, tachypnoea, low-grade fever, hypotension, shock and decreased level of consciousness.

### Prognostic evaluation

There are three main ways to evaluate the severity of acute pancreatitis: the Imrie (Glasgow) system, Ranson scoring or APACHE II. Of these, the APACHE II score is probably the most accurate.

There is no single marker that can be used to predict the severity of pancreatitis. Serial CT scanning with contrast is the most accurate technique for evaluating the extent and site of necrosis and the occurrence of complications. Necrosis of the head of the pancreas is much more severe than necrosis of the tail.

### Laboratory abnormalities

Serum amylase: The serum amylase concentration begins to rise 2–12 hours after onset of the attack, reaches its peak at 12–24 hours and returns to normal within 2–5 days. Peak levels can therefore be missed and so normal levels do not exclude the disease.

- An elevated serum amylase concentration is not specific for acute pancreatitis.
- An elevated serum amylase concentration in the absence of pancreatitis is common in the ICU.
- If the serum amylase remains elevated, suspect a pancreatitic pseudocyst.
- There is no correlation between severity of disease and the serum amylase level.

Serum lipase:

- The test for serum lipase is a difficult test to perform and is not specific for acute pancreatitis, but the lipase concentration is elevated in about 75% of cases.
- The specific serum lipase $A_2$ concentration is shown to correlate well with the severity of pancreatitis. However, the assay is difficult to perform and time-consuming and, at present, is of little clinical value.

Other tests:

- C-reactive protein is an acute-phase protein whose concentration correlates well with the severity of acute pancreatitis. However, the assay is non-specific.
- Serum tyrosine: Protease is found exclusively in the pancreas and is increased in all cases of pancreatitis.
- Elevated concentrations of glucose, urea, lactic dehydrogenase and bilirubin are all non-specific, as is leucocytosis.
- Low calcium, albumin and magnesium concentrations are sometimes found.

### Imaging abnormalities

- A plain abdominal x-ray may show localised ileus, pancreatic calcification or gallstones, but x-rays are insensitive and non-specific. Its diagnostic value is mainly for exclusion of other possible causes of abdominal pain.

**Table 27.3.** Management of acute pancreatitis

| |
|---|
| Aggressive fluid resuscitation of the intravascular space and blood if required |
| Parenteral maintenance fluids |
| Treat hypoxia with |
|    increased $FiO_2$ |
|    maintenance of normal serum albumin levels |
|    restriction of crystalloid fluid |
|    early CPAP |
| Early (within 24 hours of diagnosis) enteral nutrition |
| Correction of electrolyte and glucose abnormalities |
| Pain relief |
| Stress ulceration prophylaxis |
| Early prophylactic antibiotics for acute necrotising pancreatitis |
| Investigate suspected local complications with CT scan |
| Aggressive surgical intervention for local infection or deterioration not responding to other measures |
| Peritoneal lavage may be useful |

- Chest x-ray: In all but minor cases of pancreatitis there will be radiologically observable changes such as basal atelectasis, decreased lung volume, pleural effusions and pulmonary infiltration.
- Ultrasound: Findings are normal in about one-third of patients with mild pancreatitis. Its greatest value is as a tool for detecting pseudocysts and assessing gallstones and underlying biliary disease. An inflamed pancreas often will be hidden behind dilated loops of bowel, making visualisation difficult.
- CT is important in diagnosing, defining severity and following the complications of pancreatitis. It is superior to ultrasound. CT should be performed with both oral and IV contrast. Apart from transport issues, the limitations of CT scanning include the difficulty in using it to distinguish between solid necrosis and fluid collections and to predict which lesions will require surgery and which will resolve spontaneously. The changes seen with contrast-enhanced CT correlate well with the severity of the disease.
- Magnetic-resonance imaging (MRI): Its place is yet to be defined in regard to pancreatitis and its images can be difficult to interpret because of artefacts associated with respiratory movement and bowel peristalsis.

## Management (Table 27.3)

### Supportive treatment
In 85–95% of patients recovery occurs, without complications, within 1 week. However, among the complicated cases, 20–50% of patients die.

**The mainstays of treatment in these patients are meticulous supportive care in an intensive care environment, aggressive fluid replacement and early operation for patients with intra-abdominal complications.**

Fluid replacement: Hypovolaemia and hypotension are common with acute pancreatitis and may predispose to renal failure and MOF. Fluid losses can be extremely high and large amounts of replacement fluid may be necessary. Pancreatitis can be equivalent to a severe internal burn in regard to fluid loss. Fluid treatment should be carefully titrated against intravascular measurements such as urine output, arterial BP, CVP and, if necessary, PAWP. Maintenance fluid should be hypotonic saline solution (1000–3000 ml/day).

Respiratory complications: Patients often are hypoxic because of basal atelectasis and reduced lung volume, as a result of increased intra-abdominal pressure (IAP) and bilaterally raised diaphragms. Hypoxia can also occur as a result of ALI. Measures to alleviate hypoxia include:

- Increasing $FiO_2$.
- Sitting the patient upright.
- Physiotherapy.
- Maintaining normal serum albumin and COP.
- Limiting sodium-containing clear fluid (crystalloids) in order to avoid interstitial oedema.

If those measures fail, consider the following:

- Give CPAP or BiPAP via a mask. This has the advantage of improving oxygenation and increasing lung volume without necessitating intubation of the patient.
- CPAP or pressure support ventilation (PSV) via an endotracheal tube (ETT) will be needed if the airway is compromised or if the patient is unable to tolerate the mask.
- Early tracheostomy should be considered for severe cases.

The general approach to respiratory failure is covered elsewhere (see Chapter 16).

Pain relief: Pain relief is very important during the acute stage. Continuous IV infusion of an opiate is a cheap and effective technique for titrating analgesia to the patient's requirements. Continuous epidural block with either a local anaesthetic or a narcotic or a combination of both, is an alternative if there are no contraindications such as a coagulopathy, thrombocytopaenia or hypotension.

There are theoretical reasons for avoiding the use of morphine in patients with pancreatitis, such as stimulation of the sphincter of Oddi. However, there does not appear to be any clinical problem with its use.

Fasting and nasogastric (NG) suction: The concept of 'resting' the pancreas has traditionally been employed, without any evidence that it affects outcome. Though fasting still is often employed, NG suction is less commonly used.

Stress ulceration: It seems advisable to use some form of prophylaxis against stress ulceration.

Nutrition: Early (< 24 hours of onset) enteral nutrition is associated with improved outcome. A jejunal tube, placed at the time of laparotomy for other reasons, increases effectiveness of feeding. Parenteral nutrition should only be considered after sustained failure of enteral feeding.

Metabolic considerations: Correct magnesium, phosphate, and calcium concentrations as necessary – daily measurements are required. An insulin infusion may be necessary to control hyperglycaemia. A suitable technique is to use 50 units of short-acting insulin (e.g. Actrapid) in 50 ml of fluid and titrate against blood glucose measured hourly.

## Definitive treatment

There is no universal agreement on definitive treatment for acute pancreatitis. However, the following have been advocated.

Peritoneal lavage: The role of lavage is controversial. It is believed that lavage may help to remove toxic substances released from the pancreas and reverse some of the systemic effects of the early phase mediated by circulating toxins. Lavage is more successful in reducing early systemic complications than later local complications.

As yet, the subgroups of patients who would benefit from lavage have not been precisely defined. They may include patients with severe pancreatitis or early shock and marked clinical deterioration. If it is to work, it should be instituted early (i.e. within the first 48 hours). The response to peritoneal lavage usually is immediate and dramatic. If there is no response, one should consider an error in diagnosis or the presence of associated biliary or systemic sepsis. Continuous percutaneous peritoneal dialysis with an isotonic solution such as warm Ringer's lactate can be used. The catheter should be inserted in the midline just below the umbilicus. The technique is similar to peritoneal dialysis. Depending on the flush rate, peritoneal lavage will have the same effects as peritoneal dialysis. A fluid should be used with approximately the same electrolyte concentrations as plasma, and electrolytes measured frequently. Heparin should be added to each bag of fluid (500 units/L). One litre cycles (20 min run in, 20 min of dwell time, 20 min to run out) allow for adequate lavage without causing excessive abdominal distension and diaphragmatic elevation. If renal failure supervenes, the isotonic solution can be replaced by dialysate fluid. Lavage should be performed for 2–5 days or until the systemic effects of pancreatitis are reversed.

Endoscopic papillotomy: Endoscopic retrograde cholangiopancreatography and papillotomy if impacted stones are present is suggested for severe acute pancreatitis related to gallstones. In mild pancreatitis the risks probably outweigh the benefits.

The role of surgery: The role of surgery in acute pancreatitis remains controversial. Accepted indications include when a diagnosis is in doubt, persistent biliary pancreatitis, infected pancreatic necrosis and pancreatic abscess.

Infected pancreatitic necrosis is a definite indication for surgery. Necrosis is documented by contrast enhanced CT scan and infection proven by percutaneous aspiration.

Pancreatic abscesses commonly occur at more than 4 weeks after onset and are differentiated from necrosis on CT scan.

Percutaneous catheter drainage is usually unsuccessful, even for localised pancreatic abscesses. Extensive debridement and gravity lavage is usually required. The role of procedures such as repeated laparotomies, closed lavage of the lesser sac and open or closed abdominal operations remains to be established.

Other controversial areas include indications for surgery in the presence of sterile pancreatic necrosis; clinical deterioration; and MOF not responding to conservative measures. There are no firm conclusions based on sound data at present about definite indications in those areas. However, there is perhaps an argument that severe cases such as these should be treated in units that have extensive experience.

Drugs: Drugs which inhibit pancreatic secretion such as calcitonin, glucagon, atropine, cimetidine and fluorouracil do not alter the course of the disease. Similarly octreotide and somatostatin, despite sound theoretical justification, so far have not been shown to improve the outcome of pancreatitis. Protease inhibitors such as aprotinin also do not alter the course of this disease. Bacterial infection of necrotic pancreatic tissue occurs in approximately 40–70% of patients. Early administration of prophylactic high-dose antibiotics such as a quinolone, cefuroxime or a carbapenem to patients with demonstrated acute necrotising pancreatitis has been demonstrated to be beneficial.

Prognosis: Pancreatitis has many complications (Table 27.4). The overall mortality for pancreatitis is 10% but acute necrotising pancreatitis is associated with a mortality of 27–45%. Long-term follow-up suggests that those who survive, maintain a good quality of life, although some suffer permanent exocrine and/or endocrine failure.

## Acute stress ulceration

Acute stress ulceration is defined as acute upper GIT bleeding associated with mucosal abnormalities of the oesophagus, stomach or duodenum. It is usually found in the critically ill. The mucosal abnormalities range from hyperaemia and small petechial haemorrhages to deeper ulceration and, rarely, perforation.

### Pathogenesis (Figure 27.1)

Decreased gastric blood flow and tissue anoxia: These are the most important factors, though many other factors can contribute to cellular ischaemia and hypoxia:

- hypotension
- hypoxia

**Table 27.4.** Complications of acute pancreatitis

Local
    Plegm
    Abscess
    Pseudocyst
    Fat necrosis
    Obstructive jaundice
    Ascites
    Local necrosis of surrounding structures (e.g. vessels, bowel)

Systemic
    Respiratory
        Pleural effusions
        ALI
        Atelectasis
    Cardiovascular
        Hypovolaemia and shock
        Pericardial effusions
    Haematological
        Disseminated intravascular coagulation
        Coagulopathies
    Gastrointestinal
        Acute stress ulceration
        Ileus
    Central nervous system
        Decreased level of consciousness and coma
        Renal insufficiency or failure
    Metabolic
        Hyperglycaemia
        Hypertriglyceridaemia
        Hypoalbuminaemia
        Hypocalcaemia
        Hypomagnesaemia

- sepsis
- anaemia
- increased intrathoracic pressure
- shock
- drugs.

Decreased mucosal barrier. This can be secondary to:

- bile salts
- non-steroidal anti-inflammatory agents

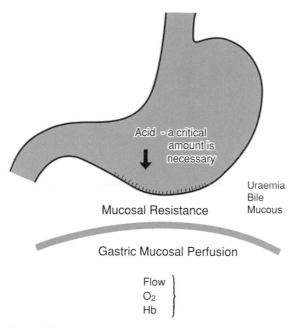

**Figure 27.1.** Pathogenesis of acute stress ulceration.

- uraemia
- alcohol.

Increased acid and pepsin: This can occur particularly in patients with burns or as a result of neurogenic causes.

### Clinical features and diagnosis
Microscopic quantities of blood are found in up to 40% of patients.

Macroscopic bleeding usually occurs 4–10 days after the initial insult. Only 2% of patients have clinically important bleeding.

Endoscopy is indicated in all patients with significant bleeding to exclude other causes such as a bleeding ulcer or oesophageal varices, which will require a different approach to management.

### Management
Prevention (Figure 27.2):

- Begin aggressive management of the underlying disease (e.g. sepsis, liver failure, multitrauma).
- Rapidly reverse abnormalities which may accompany the critical illness and that decrease gastric blood flow and oxygen delivery to the GIT mucosa (e.g. hypotension, hypoxia). This is the most important preventative measure.

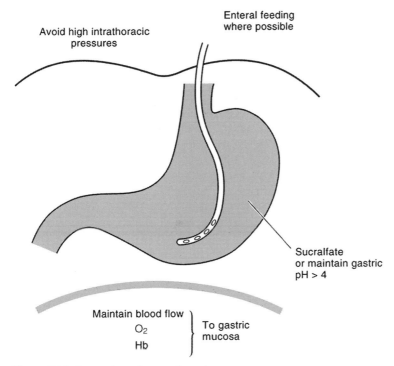

**Figure 27.2.** Prevention of stress ulceration.

- Institute enteral feeding if possible. This is as effective as neutralising gastric acidity with drugs.
- Prophylactic drugs: There is some evidence that if the above measures are instituted there is little need for prophylactic drugs. However, in patients at risk of clinically important bleeding (e.g. respiratory failure and/or coagulopathy), $H_2$-receptor antagonists are probably more effective than sucralfate or antacids.

  Definitive measures for active bleeding: Resuscitation:

- Replenish the circulating volume.
- Ensure adequate haemoglobin.
- Ensure adequate oxygenation.

Aggressively treat precipitating factors such as sepsis.

Urgent endoscopy and, if necessary, angiography to exclude surgically treatable causes of bleeding. Manoeuvres such as selective embolisation or angiographic injection with vasopressin, and IV vasopressin infusions have been used with varying degrees of success, but not in a controlled fashion.

Somatostatin (continuous IV infusion at 250 μg/h for 72 hours) may be of some benefit.

Surgery should be a last resort for diffuse bleeding as it is associated with a high mortality.

## Upper gastrointestinal tract bleeding

Apart from stress ulceration, other causes of upper GIT bleeding include

- peptic ulcer
- Mallory–Weiss tears
- oesophagitis
- neoplasm
- vascular malformations
- oesophageal varices.

Multiple lesions are found in 15–30% of these patients.

### Clinical presentation
Upper GIT bleeding usually presents as haematemesis, melaena or sudden cardiovascular collapse.

### Aetiology and clinical course
- Among patient with upper GIT bleeding, 75% will stop bleeding shortly after admission and will never rebleed.
- Of the remaining 25% with continued or recurrent bleeding, more than 30% will require immediate surgery or other advanced therapeutic manoeuvres. More than 30% will die.
- Severe episodes of bleeding are almost always due to ulcer disease (40–50%), oesophageal varices (4–8%) or diffuse gastritis (10–15%).
- Elderly patients (> 65 years) and those with severe underlying disease have poor prognoses.

### Management
Resuscitation: The circulating volume must be restored immediately. Transfuse blood after cross-matching according to the degree of hypovolaemia and haemoglobin levels. Urine output should always be closely monitored and maintained.

Diagnosis: Once the patient is stable, and while resuscitation continues, the cause of bleeding should be sought. Diagnostic evaluation is not an urgent matter for patients in whom the bleeding stops within 1 hour of admission and who are at a low risk of recurrent bleeding.

Endoscopy: Endoscopy will reveal the site and nature of bleeding in approximately 80–95% of patients, even in the presence of brisk bleeding. It is the examination of choice for patients with persistent or recurrent bleeding and for those with a high risk of recurrent haemorrhage. It should be performed within the first 24 hours.

Angiography: Mesenteric angiography may be useful if endoscopy fails to establish the site of bleeding. For it to be successful, the rate of bleeding usually must exceed 1.0 ml/min and be from a discrete site.

Radionuclide imaging: Like angiography, this examination requires that there be active bleeding.

Barium meal: A barium radiograph is inappropriate as an early investigation for acute bleeding.

Controlling the blood loss: There are many anecdotal reports and unproven techniques in this area. One of the difficulties with proving the effectiveness of any technique is that many patients will stop bleeding spontaneously.

- Endoscopic coagulation, with laser photocoagulation, bipolar diathermy, or heated probes, may be successful in selected cases. Endoscopic injection at the bleeding site is also successful.
- Somatostatin (continuous IV infusion, 250 μg/h for 72 hours) may decrease bleeding by decreasing splanchnic blood flow and gastric acid secretion.
- $H_2$-receptor antagonists and omeprazole are often used for active bleeding from gastric and duodenal ulcers. However, there is no conclusive evidence that they influence active bleeding.
- Vasopressin (antidiuretic hormone) (10–20 units/h, IV infusion) may be effective in patients with oesophageal varices, but IV vasopressin does not influence bleeding in patients with other causes of upper GIT bleeding. Selective arterial vasopressin infusion may be more effective. As the action of vasopressin is generalised vasoconstriction, beware of ischaemia in vital organs – especially in the presence of ischaemic heart disease.
- Embolisation during angiography may be effective in cases of significant bleeding from a discrete point.
- Surgery: The indications for surgery are still controversial. It should be seriously considered early for patients with severe haemorrhage (more than 2 L/24 h) and for patients with active arterial bleeding from chronic ulcers, especially elderly patients. Compulsive monitoring and replenishment of intravascular volume and steps to maintain renal function are critical in these patients.

## Bleeding varices

It is important to suspect this as a cause of upper GIT bleeding and to confirm it with endoscopy, because the approach to its management is different from the approach to other causes of upper GIT bleeding. Moreover, such a patient usually will have associated liver dysfunction, often alcoholic in origin. Other causes of upper GIT bleeding are common in the presence of oesophageal varices. Immediate endoscopy is essential to exclude those causes and to determine the site of the varices – oesophageal or gastric.

More than two-thirds of patients with oesophageal varices are dead within 1 year. The overall prognosis is related more closely to the underlying liver disease, rather than the actual bleeding varices and has not changed in spite of more sophisticated ways of controlling bleeding in the short term.

### Supportive therapy

Replenishment of the intravascular volume is most efficiently achieved with colloid or blood (Chapter 4). There must be compulsive monitoring of the intravascular volume.

Reduce the potential nitrogen load from the bleeding varices by active NG suction and oral lactulose (20–30 g, three or four times per day) if encephalopathy is suspected. Because neomycin is absorbed and contributes to renal failure, it should no longer be used in this setting.

Nutrition: Supplements such as vitamin K, folic acid and thiamine should be given early if nutritional depletion or alcoholism is suspected.

Clotting factors must be monitored and replaced as necessary.

### Control of bleeding

There are many unanswered questions concerning the best ways to control variceal bleeding. Firstly, should it be treated at all? Among those patients with severe impairments of liver function (e.g. with encephalopathy and coagulopathy), the immediate mortality is greater than 70%. More than half of all patients with variceal bleeding will stop bleeding, no matter what measures are used. Outcome must be looked at in the light of control of the acute bleeding, prevention of further bleeding and long-term prognosis. Interpretation of the data from clinical trials is difficult. There are problems with entry of patients, limited numbers, lack of randomisation and whether outcome was measured in the short-term or long-term.

The usual approach after resuscitation is variceal banding or sclerotherapy, with or without prior balloon tamponade. If that fails, a vasoactive drug (e.g. vasopressin) can be tried or a surgical procedure such as oesophageal transection, devascularisation or an emergency shunt procedure. All of these techniques and combinations thereof have their proponents.

Propranolol is useful long-term to prevent further bleeding.

Endoscopic variceal sclerotherapy: Sclerotherapy with ethanolamine oleate or sodium tetradecyl sulphate can be used alone or in combination with tamponade to control acute bleeding. Retrosternal discomfort and fever sometimes accompany sclerosis. The decision to undertake sclerotherapy at the time of initial endoscopy depends on the rate of bleeding and the expertise of the endoscopist.

Sometimes balloon tamponade is initially needed to control bleeding, and that is followed by sclerotherapy. Sclerotherapy can control bleeding for the short term in up to 90% of patients but overall survival is not increased.

Endoscopic banding of oesophageal varices is also possible and may be technically easier.

Balloon tamponade: A modified Sengstaken–Blakemore tube or Minnesota tube with a fourth channel for oesophageal aspiration is probably ideal. These are now available in a disposable plastic form.

Insertion technique:

Ensure the patient's airway. Intubation is almost always required in these patients. Check the balloon before insertion.

A pre-lubricated stiffening wire will aid insertion.

To check placement, insert 50 ml of air into the gastric balloon and take an x-ray.
  If the balloon is in the stomach, insert 300 ml of air into the gastric balloon; 20 ml of 25% Hypaque can improve radiological visualisation of the gastric balloon.

Draw the gastric balloon towards the cardia by gentle traction.

The tube can be taped to the face or placed on gentle traction.

The oesophageal balloon usually is not inflated, because bleeding often is controlled by the traction of the gastric balloon alone. Up to 120 ml of air to produce a pressure of 30–50 mmHg (4.5–6.65 kPa) in the oesophageal balloon, may sometimes be needed to control the bleeding. With both balloons clamped, their positions should be checked radiologically.

Continuous gastric and oesophageal low pressure suction should be applied.

The pressure in the oesophageal and gastric balloons should be regularly monitored.

Complications such as aspiration pneumonia are common and patients should be monitored in the ICU.

The tamponade should be applied for 12–24 hours, then reassessed by deflating the balloon in situ and observing for further blood loss. If the oesophageal balloon has been inflated, it should be deflated first, followed approximately 2 hours later by the gastric balloon. Balloon tamponade is only a holding procedure and rebleeding occurs in almost half of all patients. Longer-term measures such as sclerotherapy should be considered as soon as the bleeding has been controlled with balloon tamponade.

Vasopressin infusion: Vasopressin has been largely superseded by sclerotherapy and tamponade. However, an IV infusion of 10–20 units per hour can control bleeding in over half of these cases. Its disadvantages include ischaemia of the heart, skin and intestine. Rebleeding is common.

Somatostatin: Somatostatin may be as efficacious as balloon tamponade and can be used alone or in conjunction with balloon tamponade (continuous IV infusion, 250 µg/h for 72 hours).

Embolisation: Embolisation at angiography may achieve haemostasis in many cases. However, rebleeding is common.

Surgery: Surgery should be considered after these less radical approaches have failed. Transoesophageal ligation and portocaval shunting are the most common procedures. Varices in the cardia of the stomach, as opposed to oesophageal varices, often require shunt procedures. Liver transplantation should be considered in selected patients. Mortality for this type of surgery is high.

## Lower gastrointestinal tract bleeding

### Clinical presentation
- Colon: usually bright rectal bleeding.
- Caecum and small intestine: maroon melaena (e.g. diverticular disease, polyps, angiodysplasia, trauma).

### Management
Resuscitation: Rapid replacement of intravascular volume and clotting factors (see p. ) is essential. Investigation of the site of intestinal bleeding is limited by several factors:

- Bleeding is notoriously intermittent.
- Blood travels in an antegrade and retrograde direction from the site of bleeding.
- Blood can travel long distances from the site of bleeding.

Diagnosis:

- Sigmoidoscopy can be used to exclude lower colon lesions.
- Fibreoptic colonoscopy can exclude lesions up to the caecum.
- Enema and intestinal lavage may be necessary to improve observations.
- Isotope scanning with $^{99m}$Tc-labelled red cells can detect bleeding rates as low as 0.1 ml/min. A specific compound, $^{99m}$Tc-pertechnetate, is necessary to detect a Meckel's diverticulum.
- Angiography can detect bleeding rates as low as 0.5 ml/min in over half of these patients.
- Barium enema and small bowel series should be considered *after* the bleeding has ceased and where the diagnosis is uncertain.

Treatment: Definitive measures for stopping the bleeding depend on the site and nature of the lesion. The available methods include

- Coagulation via endoscopy.
- Vasopressin infusion.
- Embolisation.
- Early surgery should be performed for massive uncontrolled bleeding.

# Acute abdominal disorders in the critically ill

It is important that the abdomen be given careful attention as part of the normal daily examination of each patient in the ICU. Because these patients often are unconscious, sedated or paralysed, there may be few symptoms and blunted signs. Nevertheless, the abdomen plays a key role in many seriously ill patients.

Many GIT manifestations of MOF, such as non-occlusive small bowel ischaemia, ischaemic colitis, stress ulceration and hepatocellular dysfunction, can be mediated by ischaemia related to activation of the renin-angiotensin axis.

## Specific abdominal disorders in the critically ill

### Intestinal hypomotility

The GIT is often hypoactive in seriously ill patients especially in the elderly, even without abdominal surgery. There may be decreased bowel sounds, abdominal distension and increased NG aspirate. This can simulate acute obstruction of the bowel with life-threatening increases in IAP. The cause may be related to opiate or other sedative use or electrolyte disturbances and the condition often accompanies MOF.

Pseudo-obstruction is not a contraindication to enteral feeding, but it may have to be facilitated by a nasojejunal or nasoduodenal tube in order to prevent aspiration of gastric contents.

Hypomotility is not a contraindication to enteral feeding but it may have to be facilitated by a nasojejunal or nasoduodenal tube in order to prevent aspiration of gastric contents.

Drugs to increase motility and enemas do not appear to have much effect on the GIT stasis and the ileus invariably resolves as the patient's underlying condition improves. However, abdominal tamponade with high IAP can result. Gaseous distension may decrease in response to small increments of neostigmine (0.25 mg IV increments slowly) (monitor heart rate). An infusion of 2.5 mg neostigmine in 50 ml of fluid can also be titrated against an effect as the ileus can recur. A plain abdominal film should be taken before neostigmine to exclude massively dilated large bowel and/or signs of obstruction. Giving neostigmine in this circumstance may lead to perforation. More aggressive measures such as rectal flatus tubes, colonoscopic gas deflation and even surgical decompression are sometimes necessary.

### Acute acalculous cholecystitis

Acute acalculous cholecystitis can occur spontaneously in the critically ill. It can be associated with IVN, intermittent positive-pressure ventilation (IPPV), hypoperfusion of the gall bladder or increased biliary stasis.

Acalculous cholecystitis manifests as a site of intra-abdominal infection and/or occult sepsis, with all of the attending features and complications. Often there is a tender mass in the right upper quadrant. Ultrasound is more accurate than CT scan and may show enlargement of the gall bladder, a thickened gall bladder wall (> 3.5 mm), a layering effect in the wall of the gall bladder or a pericholecystic collection due to perforation. Laparotomy is the only way to definitively diagnose acalculous cholecystitis.

It can present as peritonitis in association with peritoneal dialysis or with ascites (e.g. in patients with cirrhosis or nephrotic syndrome).

Although antibiotics should be commenced, surgery is the only definitive treatment – cholecystectomy and/or a drainage procedure.

Enteral feeding rather than IVN may decrease the incidence of acalculous cholecystitis.

## Mesenteric ischaemia

Associated factors: Hypotension, raised IAP, postoperative surgical complications, sepsis and vasoconstrictive drugs (e.g. adrenaline) can all cause mesenteric ischaemia. Despite these factors being relatively common in the critically ill, the incidence of clinically significant splanchnic ischaemia is low. Perhaps subclinical episodes are common and overt complications such as bloody stools, abdominal distension, perforations and peritonitis occur, leading to circulatory shock and metabolic acidosis. The diagnosis in a sedated, ventilated patient is very difficult. The creatinine phosphokinase (CPK) levels are often raised.

Local factors: Local arteriosclerosis, colonic distension, emboli, bowel strangulation and venous occlusion can predispose to mesenteric ischaemia. Aggressive surgery is indicated in all cases of non-viable gut. The mortality remains very high.

## Coincidental abdominal disorders in the critically ill

Remember that patients in an ICU can coincidentally develop acute abdominal disorders such as

- appendicitis
- cholecystitis
- tooth abscess and sinusitis
- pancreatitis
- perforation of a viscus
- volvulus.

Diagnosis: Careful examination of the abdomen at least once each day is mandatory in all seriously ill patients as the symptoms often are non-existent and the signs blunted. Hypotension, shock and the signs of sepsis can accompany any acute abdominal disorder. Girth measurements are not reliable indicators of increasing intra-abdominal contents.

Intravesical pressure should be measured in all patients suspected of having high IAPs. An upright chest x-ray should be obtained to exclude pneumoperitoneum and to elicit other signs such as a pleural effusion, that may be secondary to the pathological abdominal condition.

Abdominal x-rays are difficult to obtain and interpret in the ICU because of the limitations of portable equipment.

Contrast studies: Apart from simple tests to exclude perforation or to identify a fistula, contrast studies have little place in the management of the acutely ill.

Ultrasound is a rapid technique involving portable equipment, but it is limited by the experience of the user and the difficulty of obtaining good images in the presence of excessive gas and in patients who have recently had surgery.

A CT is useful for detecting the site and extent of abdominal sepsis and for trauma.

Diagnostic laparotomy should be considered earlier, rather than later, for patients in whom serious intra-abdominal abnormalities are suspected and for whom other tests have not been helpful.

## Abdominal tamponade

Abdominal tamponade can be due to many causes in the intensive care setting, including intra-abdominal bleeding, ascites or pneumoperitoneum. Increasingly it is also associated with gaseous distension, particularly of the large intestine. The condition is called Ogilvy's syndrome or intestinal pseudo-obstruction and usually occurs in elderly patients. Ogilvies syndrome is perhaps part of a spectrum of causes of ileus in the critically ill and may be another manifestation of MOF. Ileus in the critically ill is also associated with drugs such as opiates and electrolyte dysfunction. Gaseous and faecal retention may also be related to the fact that rectal evacuation is actively controlled by striated muscle around the anus and this is, of course, compromised in the semiconscious patient.

Abdominal tamponade from any aetiology can cause ischaemia of the intra-abdominal organs. This is related in part to a decrease in cardiac output secondary to decreased venous return, as well as direct pressure effect on the intra-abdominal organs. The ischaemia can be marked and will affect all intra-abdominal organs. The degree of ischaemia will be proportional to the severity of the IAP. One of the earliest manifestations of decreased organ blood flow is oliguria and eventually anuria related to decreased renal blood flow.

### Assessment of intra-abdominal pressure

Because of inherent inaccuracies, abdominal girth measurements are of no use for assessing the degree of IAP and should be discarded from our clinical practice. If there is concern about a tense abdomen, the IAP should be assessed by directly measuring the intravesical pressure. One needs only a low index of suspicion to consider this measurement, as it is simple to perform and provides valuable information.

There are several techniques for measuring intravesical pressure. One of the simplest involves inserting a T-piece connector with a three-way tap at the end of the urinary catheter: urine is allowed to drain normally until a measurement is required. Then 50 ml of isotonic saline is instilled into the bladder. The distal drainage from the urinary catheter is clamped and the three-way tap is turned to connect to a water manometer device for measuring CVP. The height of the column taken from the pubic symphysis represents the intravesical pressure. The bladder acts as a passive container at volumes of 50–100 ml and intravesical pressure closely correlates with IAP over the range of 0–70 mmHg (0–9.3 kPa).

Decreased renal blood flow and oliguria will begin to occur at pressures above 25 mmHg (3.3 kPa) and will progressively become worse as the pressure increases.

Increased abdominal tamponade causes decreased lymph and venous drainage from the lower limbs; decreases lung volume, sometimes to a life-threatening degree; and increases ICP secondary to decreased cerebral venous flow.

Management includes general supportive measures, especially aggressive fluid replacement to counteract decreased venous return to the thorax. Reversible causes of raised pressure such as gaseous distension and pneumoperitoneum should be corrected.

Consideration should be given to early surgical decompression of abdominal tamponade. This can be achieved either by laparotomy, leaving the wound packed and open, or by closing the wound with material such as a Marlex graft. Surgery in these circumstances can be a challenge, especially if the tamponade is related to intra-abdominal bleeding. The bleeding may become uncontrollable if the tamponade is relieved. On the other hand, intra-abdominal organs become more ischaemic as the IAP increases. Non-invasive techniques such as embolisation should be considered if the source of the bleeding is from the pelvis. The intravesical pressure should be monitored regularly in all patients suspected of having raised IAP (> 20 mmHg (2.6 kPa)).

The raised IAP in Ogilvy's syndrome or intestinal pseudo-obstruction can be life-threatening. Aggressive measures should be taken to decrease the pressure. Encouraging bowel action is one technique, but if the raised IAP is associated with gaseous distension which is not amenable to normal NG tube drainage, IV neostigmine can be trialled; either a single dose of neostigmine (0.25 mg increments) or a neostigmine infusion of 2.5 mg diluted in 50 ml commencing at 1 ml/h (0.05 mg/h) and increasing to achieve an effect. The neostigmine will encourage peristalsis, bowel constriction and passage of gas and faeces. The major side effects are abdominal pain and bradycardia, reversed by atropine. A continuous infusion is often necessary as the distention often recurs (see Precautions. If this fails, then regular colonoscopy may empty the large intestine allowing a reduction of intraluminal pressure of the bowel and return to normal function. Occasionally surgical decompression with a colostomy is necessary in order to prevent life-threatening raised IAP and bowel ischaemia and rupture.

Fistula

A fistula joins two epithelial surfaces and can be a challenging complication when involving a tract between a hollow abdominal viscus and the skin.

Investigation: Defining the fistula can be achieved by imaging radio-opaque liquid injected from the skin surface or methylene blue down the NG tube. Defining the patency of the GIT above and below the fistula is also important.

Management: Supportive treatment is the most important approach. Fluid and electrolyte homeostasis needs to be maintained. Measurement of the total output and electrolyte composition of the fistula fluid helps in this regard.

$H_2$-receptor blocking drugs may decrease the acid content of the fistula, if high in the GIT and somatostatin may decrease the total fluid volume.

The effluent from the fistula needs to be managed particularly with regard to maintaining skin integrity. A stoma nurse may provide useful advice.

Enteral feeding should be maintained. In this regard, the fistula should be considered merely as a poorly formed stoma. Depending on the site of the fistula, it can even be used as a source of enteral feeding. Intravenous nutrition should only be considered as a last resort.

Up to 80% of fistulas spontaneously close. Factors prolonging closure need to be excluded. These include uncontrolled local infection, distal obstruction, a foreign body, epithelialisation of the fistula tract and local complications such as carcinoma or radiation damage.

Definitive surgical management is difficult but diversions of the bowel contents proximal to the fistula can sometimes promote spontaneous healing.


# Diarrhoea

Diarrhoea can be a problem in up to 40% of patients in an ICU. It is usually related to the underlying disease or treatment, rather than a specific cause such as pelvic abscess. The presence of diarrhoea represents a large workload for nurses, adds to the risks of cross infection and, when infective, can cause systemic signs and fluid loss.

## Non-infective diarrhoea

Diarrhoea is a common and non-specific precursor of generalised sepsis or infection. Non-infective diarrhoea is the most common form of diarrhoea in an ICU and it is mainly related to enteral feeding. The diarrhoea is as a result of hypersecretion from the gut and can result in significant protein loss. Diarrhoea is then exacerbated by hypoalbuminaemia. It can be decreased by using iso-osmolar enteral feeds, by commencing feeding at low rates, by using lactose-free feeds or possibly by adding liquid bulking agents. However, enteral feeding should be continued in the presence of diarrhoea. Agents that will encourage bacterial action, which in turn enhances salt and water absorption with 'drying' of the stool, are useful for reducing the incidence of diarrhoea. Imodium (4 mg initially, and 2 mg prn up to 20 mg daily) and octreotide (dose is dependent on effect) can sometimes decrease intractable diarrhoea.

Diarrhoea may be a non-specific manifestation of MOF.

### Antibiotic-associated diarrhoea

Antibiotic-associated diarrhoea should always be suspected in the critically ill.

Pseudomembranous colitis: Most antibiotics, especially clindamycin, can predispose to pseudomembranous colitis, caused by the toxin produced by the *Clostridium difficile* bacteria. The treatment of choice is oral vancomycin. Pseudomembranous colitis can also occur in patients who are not on antibiotics.

Methicillin-resistant *Staphylococcus aureus* enterocolitis: This also occurs in association with broad-spectrum antibiotics, particularly in critically ill patients or immunocompromised hosts. It can cause systemic septicaemia and MOF.

Infective diarrhoea: Other pathogens such as *Salmonella* spp., *Shigella* spp., *Campylobacter* spp. and *Escherichia coli* are only rarely the causes of diarrhoea in the ICU.

### Management

Diarrhoea is a relatively common accompaniment of MOF and infection.

Always perform a rectal examination to exclude abnormalities such as impaction and spurious diarrhoea.

Adjust the enteral feeding regimen:

- Use iso-osmolar solutions.
- Avoid lactose-containing solutions.
- Add faecal bulking agents.

Replace water and electrolyte losses.

Culture stools, especially for:

- *Clostridium difficile* and its cytotoxin.
- *Staphylococcus aureus* (Gram-stain and culture).
- Treat both pseudomembranous colitis and *Staphyloccocus aureus*-related diarrhoea with oral vancomycin, 250–500 mg 6-hourly for 10 days. Relapses can occur in both cases.

Employ barrier nursing if the diarrhoea is infective in origin.

## FURTHER READING

### General

Ponec, R. J., Saunders, M. D. and Kimmey, M. B. Neostigmine for the treatment of acute colonic pseudo-obstruction. *New England Journal of Medicine* 341 (1999): 137–41.

Schmidt, H. and Martindale, R. 2001. The gastrointestinal tract in critical illness. *Current Opinion in Clinical Nutrition and Metabolic Care* 4 (2001): 547–51.

Takala, J. Determinants of splanchnic blood flow. *British Journal of Anaesthesia* 77 (1996): 50–8.

### Fulminant hepatic failure

Eckardt, K.-U. Renal failure in liver disease. *Intensive Care Medicine* 25 (1999): 5–14.

Gimson, A. E. S. Fulminant and late onset hepatic failure. *British Journal of Anaesthesia* 77 (1996): 90–8.

Rahman, T. and Hodgson, H. Clinical management of acute hepatic failure. *Intensive Care Medicine* 27 (2001): 467–76.

Schafer, D. F. and Sorrell, M. F. (ed.) Power failure, liver failure. *New England Journal of Medicine* 336 (1997): 1173–4.

### Pancreatitis

Wyncoll, D. L. The management of severe acute necrotising pancreatitis: an evidence-based review of the literature. *Intensive Care Medicine* 25 (1999): 146–56.

### Acute gastrointestinal tract bleeding

Lewis, J. D., Shin, E. J. and Metz, D. C. Characterization of gastrointestinal bleeding in severely ill hospitalized patients. *Critical Care Medicine* 28 (2000): 46–50.

### Acute stress ulceration

Cook, D., Guyatt, G., Marshall, J., Leasa, D., Fuller, H., Hall, R., Peter, S., Rutledge, F., Griffith, L., McLellan, A., Woods, G., and Kirby, A., for the Canadian Clinical Trials Group. A comparison of sucralfate and ranitidine for the prevention of upper gastrointestinal bleeding in patients requiring mechanical ventilation. *New England Journal of Medicine* 338 (1998): 791–7.

Mantamis, D. Prevention of upper gastrointestinal bleeding in patients requiring mechanical ventilation. *Intensive Care Medicine* 25 (1999): 118–9.

### Oesophageal varices

Harry, R. and Wendon, J. Management of variceal bleeding. *Current Opinion in Critical Care* 8 (2002): 164–70.

Shara, A. I. and Rockey, D. C. Medical Progress: Gastrointestinal variceal hemorrhage. *New England Journal of Medicine* 345 (2001): 669–81.

## Acute abdominal disorders in the critically ill

Evans, H. L., Raymond, D. P., Pelletier, S. J., Crabtree, T. D., Pruett, T. L. and Sawyer, R. G. Diagnosis of intra-abdominal infection in the critically ill. *Current Opinion in Critical Care* 7 (2001): 117–21.

## Abdominal tamponade

Sugrue, M. and Hillman, K. M. Intra-abdominal hypertension and intensive care. In *Update in Intensive Care and Emergency Medicine*, ed. J.-L. Vincent, pp. 667–76. Berlin: Springer-Verlag, 1998.

Sugrue, M., Jones, F., Janjua, K. J., Deane, S. A., Bristow, P. and Hillman, K. Temporary abdominal closure: a prospective evaluation of its effects on renal and respiratory physiology. *Journal of Trauma* 45 (1998): 914–21.

## Ileus

Bauer, A. J., Schwarz, N. T., Moore, B. A., Turler, A. and Kalff, J. C. Ileus in critical illness: mechanisms and management. *Current Opinion in Critical Care* 8 (1998): 152–7.

# 28

# Critical care haematology

## Blood transfusion

### Indications for blood transfusion

Fresh whole blood remains the ideal fluid for resuscitation following acute haemorrhage. However, it is rarely available today. Whole blood usually is fractionated into red cell concentrates, plasma protein solutions and platelet concentrates.

Blood is given to restore oxygen-carrying capacity and intravascular volume. The haemoglobin level is an important contributor to the oxygen carrying capacity: 1.34 ml of oxygen combines with every gram of haemoglobin (Hb).

$$\text{Oxygen carrying capacity} = \text{Hb} \times 1.34 \text{ ml O}_2/\text{g} \times \text{oxygen saturation of Hb} \times \text{cardiac output.}$$

Critically ill patients require optimal oxygen delivery ($DO_2$). The ideal haemoglobin level in normals is uncertain. It is probably greater than 10 g/dL. Otherwise we would all have lower haemoglobins than we do and would not suffer symptoms such as tiredness and lassitude when the levels drop to around 10 g/dL. The ideal balance is between increased $DO_2$ for each extra haemoglobin molecule and the increased viscosity caused by that extra haemoglobin molecule, which can decrease blood flow and $DO_2$. The ideal haemoglobin of 10 g/dL is meant to take into account its oxygen-carrying capacity and viscosity. However, viscosity in these circumstances is an artificial concept based on false assumptions such as laminar flow and a constant diameter of the vessels. In fact, viscosity is rarely a significant factor in vivo, even with levels towards the upper limits of normal.

Critically ill patients often require transfusion secondary to frequent blood tests, haemodilution and extracorporeal blood losses (e.g. during haemofiltration). However, the exact level where transfusion is required in the critically ill is difficult to define. One randomised study in a heterogeneous group of critically ill patients demonstrated that maintaining a haemoglobin of more

**Table 28.1.** Blood transfusion guidelines

If the patient is haemodynamically stable and the bleeding has stopped, consider
supplemental iron, vitamin $B_{12}$, folate and erythropoietin, rather than blood

If the patient is haemodynamically stable, but symptomatic (e.g. dyspnoea, palpitations,
malaise), use packed red cells to restore oxygen-carrying capacity

If the patient is haemodynamically unstable, but the bleeding is controllable, use packed
red cells and fluid volume replacement

If the patient is haemodynamically unstable and bleeding rapidly, use the freshest blood
available as well as
FFP
platelets
and liaise with haematology services

than 9.0 g/dL did not affect outcome, except for patients with acute coronary
syndromes.

Guidelines for transfusion are given in Table 28.1.

## Cross-matching

Serological safety of blood

| | Probability of Compatibility |
|---|---|
| ABO compatibility | 99.4% |
| ABO and Rh compatibility | 99.8% |
| ABO and Rh compatibility with negative antibody screen | 99.94% |
| Complete pre-transfusion compatibility testing | 99.95% |
| Autologous | 100% |

It is important to institute blood replacement rapidly in cases of significant haemorrhage. From the foregoing information it can be seen that uncrossed matched
blood that is ABO compatible can, if necessary, be administered in an emergency.
However, a saline cross match can be performed by most blood banks within
10 minutes. Thus, it is rarely necessary to give group O non-cross-matched blood,
as resuscitation with colloid usually is satisfactory until group and saline cross
matches are performed.

## Blood products

The term 'ultrafresh blood' implies collection within 4 hours without refriger-
ation. If it is practical, there is an argument for using ultrafresh blood when
more than the patient's own blood volume has been lost, as additional blood
components will not be needed.

Fresh blood is blood that has been stored for less than 7 days. If it is not possible to use ultrafresh blood, then fresh blood is preferred for massive blood transfusion.

Stored blood is blood that has been stored for more than 7 days and it is associated with a gradual decrease in the concentration of 2,3-diphosphoglycerate (2,3-DPG) that interferes with the oxygen-delivering capacity of haemoglobin. Platelet and granulocyte functions also deteriorate.

Microaggregates of platelets and white cells gradually accumulate with time and can cause obstruction of the pulmonary microcirculation. There has been no evidence that these microaggregates are clinically significant and microfilters probably are not required.

## Red cell concentrate (packed cells)
- Haematocrit 70–80%.
- Volume 200–300 ml (red cells 150–200 ml).
- Citrate phosphate dextrose (CPD): packed cells with a maximum storage time at 4 °C of 21 days.
- CPD with adenosine (CPD-A): can be stored at 4 °C for 21 days.

Storage changes of red cell concentrate (CPD-A):

|  | 0 days | 35 days |
|---|---|---|
| pH | 7.6 | 6.98 |
| hydrogen ion concentration (nmol/L) | 25.1 | 106.1 |
| sodium (mmol/L) | 169 | 155 |
| potassium (mmol/L) | 4.0 | 30.0 |
| adenosine triphosphate (ATP) (%) | 100 | 55 |
| plasma haemoglobin (% lysis) | 0.05 | 0.1 |
| 2,3-DPG (%) | 100 | 0 |

## Complications of blood transfusion

### Pyrexia
Pyrexia is relatively common and usually has an immunological basis.

### Serological incompatibility
Most of these problems are now due to errors in identification of the patient to receive the transfusion. Initial symptoms and signs of a haemolytic transfusion reaction include rigors, nausea, vomiting, flushing, pain and circulatory collapse. Other features include haemostatic failure, oliguria, renal failure, anaemia and jaundice. Minor incompatibility usually occurs as a result of reaction to white cells, platelets or plasma proteins and often results in fever, rash and urticaria.

### Blood-borne infections associated with transfusion

Bacteria: Bacterial infections are very rare after blood transfusion in developed countries. Contaminants that have rarely been reported as causing bacteraemia include *Pseudomonas* spp., coliforms and *Staphylococci* spp. More recently, the possibility of infection with *Borrelia burgdorferi*, causing Lyme disease, has become a concern.

Fungi and parasites: These also are very rare in developed countries. Transfusion transmitted malaria poses a problem, because there is no simple and sensitive screening test.

Viruses: Hepatitis viruses, including hepatitis A, B, C and D, can be transmitted by blood transfusion. Currently, screening tests exist for hepatitis A, B and C viruses.

Cytomegalovirus (CMV), Epstein–Barr virus (EBV) and human herpes virus 6 (HHV-6) can contaminate blood. They are often associated with a syndrome that includes severe pyrexia, with or without atypical mononucleosis, 7–10 days post transfusion. This can be confused with an occult source of sepsis. It usually settles spontaneously over 2–3 weeks.

Retroviruses: Human immunodeficiency virus, type 1 and 2 (HIV-1, HIV-2), human T-cell lymphotropic virus, types I and II (HTLV-I, HTLV-II) were of great concern in the early 1980s. Screening is now routinely carried out for anti-HIV-1 and 2, as well as anti-HTLV-I and II.

Other viruses: Other viruses, including Colorado tick fever virus, Lassa fever virus, Rift Valley virus, Creutzfeldt–Jakob disease and Ebola virus, are only very rarely found as contaminants.

Immunosuppression: There is some evidence that blood transfusion can decrease graft tolerance, increase susceptibility to infection and predispose to recurrence of cancer.

## Massive blood transfusion

This is usually defined as replacement of more than the patient's circulating blood volume within a 24-hour period.

In this situation, the circulating volume and red blood cells should be replaced rapidly with either whole blood or red blood cells and plasma solution. The blood should be as fresh as possible. **Blood should be used earlier, rather than later, in order to prevent a decrease in the oxygen-carrying capacity and to allow time for the red blood cells to regenerate 2,3-DPG.** Avoid inflexible rules for replacement of platelets, potassium, calcium and coagulation factors during massive blood transfusion. It is better to regularly measure the end-points of transfusion and adjust therapy as necessary.

- Give haemoglobin in the form of blood cell transfusion as necessary.
- Platelets: Give 8–10 units when the platelet count drops below $30 \times 10^9/L$ and/or when there is an indication for their use on clinical grounds.

**Table 28.2.** Abbreviations used in the context of critical care haematology

| | |
|---|---|
| WBCT | whole blood clotting time |
| TCT | thrombin clotting time |
| PT | prothrombin time |
| APPT | activated partial thromboplastin time |
| PTT | partial thromboplastin time |
| FDPs | fibrinogen degradation products |
| TT | thrombin time |
| DIC | disseminated intravascular coagulation |
| FFP | fresh frozen plasma |
| SPPS | stable plasma protein solution |
| PPF | purified protein fraction |

- Coagulation profile: The need for fresh frozen plasma (FFP) (Table 28.2) or cryoprecipitate is gauged by screening tests such as the activated partial thromboplastin time (APPT), prothrombin time (PT), thrombin times (TT) and fibrinogen levels. Because of delays in screening tests, FFP can be given on a qualitative basis (e.g. two FFP units for each six units of blood).

## Complications of massive blood transfusion
Impaired oxygen transport: Impairment of oxygen transport during transfusion can be related to:

- Defective red cell function.
- Impaired haemoglobin function.
- Microaggregates.
- Fluid overload or hypovolaemia.
- Decreased lung function and acute lung injury (ALI).

Haemostatic failure: Haemostatic failure can be related to

- Dilution and/or depletion of platelets and clotting factors.
- Disseminated intravascular coagulation (DIC).
- Hypocalcaemia.

Electrolyte and metabolic disturbances:
Hyperkalaemia: Although stored blood has a high level of potassium, hyperkalaemia usually is not a problem, even with rapid transfusion. Potassium moves intracellularly in the higher pH environment of the body.
Hypokalaemia: Delayed hypokalaemia is more common than hyperkalaemia.
Citrate toxicity: Despite theoretical considerations, this is rarely a problem.
Hypocalcaemia: Hypocalcaemia is also a rare problem and it is now suggested that calcium should be given according to clinical signs, ECG evidence or concentration of ionised calcium, rather than as a routine.

Hypernatraemia: Infusion of multiple units of blood can result in hypernatraemia.

Hypothermia: Efficient blood warmers should be used to keep the temperature of infused blood above 32 °C. Even mild hypothermia has a marked effect on clotting.

Jaundice: Up to 30% of transfused red blood cells may not survive. This presents a large bilirubin load. In combination with liver hypoperfusion as a result of blood loss, the normally unconjugated bilirubin may be conjugated, giving a cholestatic picture. Haematoma may also contribute to the jaundice.

## Platelets

- Volume of 1 unit: 20—50 ml ($70 \times 10^9$ platelets).
- Duration of activity: 2–7 days at 20 °C (optimum storage duration 2 days).

If transfusion is indicated, an adult usually receives $300 \times 10^9$ platelets (about 4–5 units) or approximately 1 unit/10 kg. The platelet count should rise by 5 – $10 \times 10^9$/L for each unit transfused. Platelets should be transfused through a standard blood filter, not a microaggregate filter. Ideally, platelets that are group compatible and compatible with the patient's leucocyte antigen (HLA) should be used. Rhesus-negative (Rh-negative) platelets should be used for Rh-negative patients, as platelet concentrates are often contaminated by red blood cells.

The best measure of platelet function is bleeding time but the platelet count at 1 hour postinfusion reflects viability and correlates with bleeding time.

Indications for platelet transfusion in intensive care:

- Platelet count $< 10$—$20 \times 10^9$/L.
- Low ($20$—$50 \times 10^9$/L) platelet count, with clinically significant bleeding.
- Qualitatively defective platelets and spontaneous bleeding (e.g. drug induced).

## Granulocytes

- Volume 300—500 ml ($2$—$4 \times 10^{10}$ granulocytes).
- Viable for up to 12 hours.
- HLA-compatible granulocytes should be used.

Indications for granulocyte transfusion in intensive care: There has been a reduction in the use of granulocyte transfusions in clinical practice. The safety, efficiency and cost-effectiveness of transfused granulocytes are being questioned. They are sometimes still employed as a short-term basis for neutropaenic patients, either prophylactically or for established bacteraemia. Granulocyte colony stimulating factor elevates neutrophil numbers and is used mainly for neutropaenia following chemotherapy. Its role in the critically ill is, as yet, unclear.

## Fresh frozen plasma

- Volume of 1 unit: 200–300 ml.
- One unit contains approximately 10% of an adult's total clotting factors.
- Maximum storage duration is 6 months when kept below $-30\,^\circ$C. It should be used within 6–24 hours after thawing.
- Contains all the coagulation factors.
- Fresh frozen plasma also contains approximately
    - sodium 172 mmol/L
    - potassium 3.5 mmol/L
    - protein 5.5 g/dL.
- Fresh frozen plasma should be ABO compatible.
- Commence with 10 ml/kg.

## Cryoprecipitate

- Volume: 15 ml.
- Stored below $-30\,^\circ$C, will remain stable for about 6 months.
- Contains
    - factor VIII
    - fibrinogen
    - von Willebrand's factor
    - fibronectin
- Use for a fibrinogen deficiency, e.g. DIC.

# Blood substitutes and colloids

Colloids are fluids that because of their oncotic pressure, are confined mainly to the intravascular space. Colloids derived from blood exert their oncotic pressure via protein particles (e.g. plasma and albumin solutions), whereas artificial colloids contain other particles (e.g. dextrans and gelatin solutions).

Plasma expanders are colloids that contain higher concentrations of colloid particles than does plasma and therefore they cause fluid to move from the interstitial space to expand the intravascular space (e.g. concentrated albumin, high molecular weight (MW) dextrans).

## Blood derivatives

### Human plasma protein solution
Human plasma solutions are available as fractionated and pasteurised iso-oncotic (4–5%) or hyperoncotic (20% or 25%) solutions. The iso-oncotic solution has protein and electrolyte concentrations approximately the same as those of

circulating plasma. Other characteristics of human plasma protein solutions include the following:

- Half-life of circulating protein is about 5–10 days.
- Long shelf life.
- Free from transmittable disease.
- Allergic reactions are very rare.

## Artificial colloids

### Dextrans
The dextran solutions contain polysaccharide molecules. These are classified according to their MW:

- Dextran 70 (MW 70 000) – intravascular half-life approximately 6 hours.
- Dextran 40 (MW 40 000) – intravascular half-life approximately 3 hours.

Both solutions are isotonic using either saline or dextrose.

Other characteristics include a small but significant incidence of serious anaphylactoid reactions. Dextran 40 particles are excreted in the kidneys and can block small renal tubules. There is no interference with blood cross-matching techniques using currently available dextrans. The total maximum dosage is limited to less than $1.5 \text{ g} \cdot \text{kg}^{-1} \cdot \text{d}^{-1}$, or less than a total of 1500 ml. This limits the usefulness of these solutions for plasma volume replacement.

### Modified gelatins
These are solutions containing modified gelatin and isotonic saline, with potassium and calcium. They are eliminated mainly by kidneys, as well as via the gastrointestinal tract (GIT) and by catabolism. The intravascular half-life is approximately 4 hours. The solutions do not interfere with cross matching, haemostasis or renal function. They cause a very low incidence of anaphylactoid reactions.

### Hydroxyethyl starch
This is a macromolecular polymer from hydrolysed corn in a solution similar to isotonic saline. It is eliminated by catabolism and excretion in urine and faeces. It has a very low incidence of anaphylactoid reactions. It does not affect renal function but can interfere with haemostasis.

### Artificial blood
Either stroma-free haemoglobin or perfluorochemicals act as a colloid but also have the potential to carry oxygen.

They are commercially available in some countries but their place in clinical practice awaits evaluation.

# Disorders of white cells

## Neutrophilia

Neutrophilia is commonly seen in critically ill patients. An acute increase may indicate a new source of infection – bacterial, viral or fungal. However, neutrophilia is also a non-specific accompaniment of many non-infectious factors such as steroids, surgery, stress, inflammation, diabetic ketoacidosis, asthma and acute myocardial infarction.

## Neutropaenia

Neutropaenia can be an ominous sign especially when associated with severe sepsis. It is probably due to a combination of bone-marrow suppression and increased adherence and utilisation of white cells at the site of infection.

There is a long list of drugs that can cause neutropaenia. They include captopril, hydralazine, procainamide and quinidine. Primary bone marrow disorders, such as leukaemia, also can result in decreased white cell production. It may be very difficult in the critical care setting to determine the exact cause of the neutropaenia.

# Disorders of haemostasis

## Diagnosis

Normal clot formation requires

- An intact vascular wall.
- A normal clotting cascade.
- Normal platelet numbers and function.

Abnormalities of haemostasis in critically ill patients commonly involve

- Damage to a vessel (i.e. surgical bleeding) or endothelial cells.
- An abnormality of the clotting cascade.
- Decreased platelet numbers.

or a combination of these. The process of haemostasis is generally described in terms of primary haemostasis (platelet activation, platelet vessel wall and platelet–platelet interactions), secondary haemostasis (coagulation cascade) and antithrombotic mechanisms (e.g. fibrinolysis). One scheme for approaching the disorders of haemostasis is as follows.

### Approach to bleeding

Surgical bleeding: Rule out the possibility of surgical bleeding.

History: Does the patient have renal failure, liver failure or sepsis? Was there a recent operation? Is the patient being given drugs that can predispose to bleeding?

Initial coagulation tests: Check PT, APPT, TT and platelet count (see Table 28.2 for abbreviations).

Coagulation cascade abnormalities:

Prolonged PT:

- Test the extrinsic pathway.
- Factor VII abnormality.

Causes include:

- Vitamin K deficiency.
- Warfarin therapy.
- Mild liver disease.

Prolonged APPT:

- Tests the intrinsic pathway.
- Factor VIII the most important factor.

Causes include:

- Haemophilia A or B.
- Von Willebrand's disease.
- Heparin.
- Blocking inhibitor (e.g. lupus anticoagulant, acquired anti-factor-VIII antibody).

Prolonged PT and APPT:

- Mainly due to diseases affecting the common pathway.

Causes include:

- Liver disease.
- DIC
- Warfarin.
- Primary fibrinolysis.
- Renal disease.

Platelet abnormalities: A decrease in platelet number is a more common cause of coagulation disorders in the ICU than decreased function. The possible causes of decreased platelet numbers include:

- Failure of production.
- Increased destruction (e.g. DIC, loss in extracorporeal circuits).
- Dilution via massive transfusion.

A prolonged bleeding time will show a defect in platelet function.

This scheme should help with the diagnosis. Each of the three components of clotting will now be looked at in detail.

## Vascular disorders

Apart from a hole in a vessel, major bleeding secondary to a vascular disorder is rare. Vascular endothelial damage can be associated with infections, drug reactions and hypersensitivity reactions (e.g. hereditary haemorrhagic telangiectasia).

## Thrombocytopaenia

The causes of thrombocytopaenia include:

- A decrease in production (e.g. aplastic anaemia, acute leukaemia).
- An increase in destruction (e.g. idiopathic thrombocytopaenic purpura (ITP), DIC, the use of extracorporeal circuits such as continuous diafiltration).
- Dilution (e.g. after massive blood transfusion).
- Splenic pooling or trapping in association with hypersplenism.

The management of thrombocytopaenia depends on the cause, the manifestations of bleeding and platelet function and number.

Guidelines for platelet transfusion:

1 Active bleeding in conjunction with platelet count $< 50\,000/\text{mm}^3$ or abnormality of platelet function (bleeding time more than twice the upper limit of normal).
2 Prophylaxis:
platelet count $< 20\,000/\text{mm}^3$
*or*
preoperative platelet count $< 50\,000/\text{mm}^3$
*or*
abnormality of platelet function.
3 Massive transfusion: platelet count $< 50\,000/\text{mm}^3$ and abnormal bleeding.

Drug-induced thrombocytopaenia: Many drugs can interfere with platelet function and numbers. Platelet function – aspirin, NSAIDs, ticlopidine and clopidigrel all irreversibly inhibit platelet aggregation. Ticlopidine and clopidigrel are often taken as prophylaxis following a stroke. Following angioplasty, drugs are often given which bind the platelet IIb/IIIa receptor and inhibit platelet aggregation, e.g. abciximab. All of these drugs can cause prolonged bleeding.

Important drugs that can cause thrombocytopaenia include chloramphenicol, high-dosage penicillin, thiazide diuretics, quinine, antituberculous drugs and antiepileptic drugs.

Heparin-induced thrombocytopaenic syndrome: Thrombocytopaenia is a common complication of heparin treatment, occurring in 1–30% of patients 6–12 days after commencement of treatment. As heparin is a commonly used drug in the ICU, both as a therapeutic agent and as a flushing agent in order to maintain patency of vascular catheter, a high index of suspicion is needed for the diagnosis of heparin-induced thrombocytopaenic syndrome (HITS). There are two types of HITS:

Type I:
Early onset.
Mild thrombocytopaenia.
Probably due to the platelet pro-aggregating effect of heparin.
Treatment may involve:
    continuing the heparin and monitoring platelet count
    changing to warfarin
Type II:
Late onset.
Severe thrombocytopaenia.
Thrombotic complications can cause severe ischaemia.

Caused by an immune mechanism: heparin antibody complexes bind to platelets, resulting in reduced survival, thrombocytopaenia and, in some cases, thrombosis.

Heparin should be stopped immediately. If anticoagulation is required, consider:

warfarin
aspirin
dextrans
thrombolytic agents.

Usually the diagnosis is made on a clinical basis but a heparin-dependent antibody test, using either platelet aggregometry or the $^{14}$C-serotonin-release method as the end-point, can be used in patients suspected of having type II HITS.

Low molecular weight heparins (LMWH) are not useful in the setting of HITS as they are antigenically similar to heparin in the presence of preformed antibodies.

Renal disease: Uraemia causes both platelet dysfunction and factor VIII abnormalities. Dialysis and desmopressin (DDAVP) will help correct the defect.

## Coagulation disorders

Except for factor VIII, all coagulation factors are produced in the liver. The coagulation cascade has been classified into the intrinsic and extrinsic systems. The two systems are not mutually exclusive, however, as several activated factors react in both systems. The classical model of the two pathways is also changing (Figure 28.1). For example, factors VIII, IX and XI, formerly part of the intrinsic pathway, should be considered also as amplification factors of the extrinsic pathway.

Hypothermia strongly inhibits the enzymatic reactions of the coagulation cascade and causes significant pro-coagulation of PT and APPT. This can be overlooked when interpreting coagulation profiles, especially when tested at 37 °C.

### Congenital disorders

Haemophilia A is caused by factor VIII deficiency. If there is less than 5% of the normal factor VIII, there will be spontaneous bleeding. If there is less than 50% of normal factor VIII levels, then factor VIII transfusion will be needed after surgery or trauma. The circulation half-life of factor VIII is 10–14 hours. Factor VIII is available from FFP, cryoprecipitate or as a specific concentrate.

Haemophilia B, or Christmas disease, is caused by factor IX deficiency. The circulation half-life of factor IX is 24 hours. Factor IX is available as FFP or factor IX concentrate.

Von Willebrand's disease is the commonest congenital coagulation defect, caused by a deficiency in factor VIII quality and/or function, plus a qualitative platelet defect. Both deficits can be corrected with FFP or cryoprecipitate. Desmopressin (DDAVP) may be used for mild cases.

### Vitamin K deficiency

Vitamin K is required by the liver for synthesis of factors II, VII, IX and X. Vitamin K deficiency is seen in long-term dietary disturbances (e.g. poor oral intake) and is exacerbated by antimicrobial gut sterilisation. Inhibition of vitamin K is seen with the use of oral anticoagulants, coumarin or indanedione derivatives.

Vitamin $K_1$ 10 mg twice-weekly subcutaneously, should be given to long-term patients in the ICU. Some preparations of vitamin $K_1$ are based in cremophor, which can cause anaphylaxis, especially when given intravenously. Vitamin $K_1$ takes 6 hours before coagulation factor synthesis begins. Thus, FFP would have to be used initially for bleeding related to vitamin K deficiency.

### Liver disease

Clotting factor synthesis is one of the most accurate indicators of liver function. The vitamin K related factors decrease first. As all of the factors produced in the liver have short circulating half-lives, their levels will eventually decrease. The

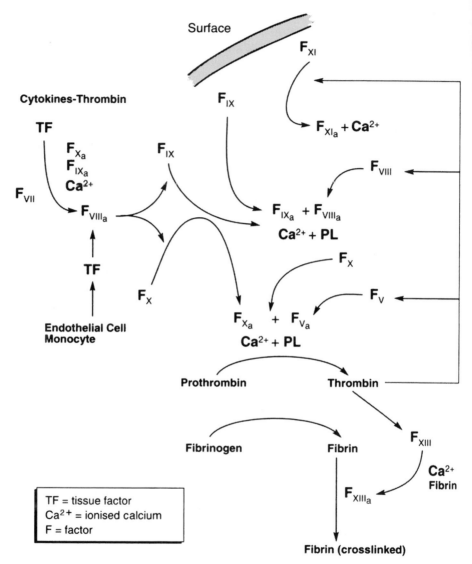

**Figure 28.1.** Coagulation cascade: This diagram represents a revised version of the traditional coagulation cascade. There is more interaction and overlap between the so-called intrinsic and extrinsic pathways.

liver's ability to degrade activated clotting factors can be compromised, causing DIC.

## Massive blood transfusion

Dilution of coagulation factors, platelet loss and hypothermia all add to the coagulopathy in massive transfusion.

## Cardiopulmonary bypass

Cardiopulmonary bypass surgery causes damage to red cells, decreases platelet number and function and activates factor XII.

## Disseminated intravascular coagulation

Disseminated intravascular coagulation is not so much a separate disease as an exaggeration of the normal haemostatic processes in response to a wide variety of insults. The usual clinical manifestation of DIC is bleeding. Widespread intravascular activation of clotting and deposition of fibrin lead to consumption of platelets and clotting factors. Microvascular obstruction and varying degrees of end-organ damage may result. Secondary fibrinolysis then occurs, which accentuates the bleeding.

Some conditions associated with DIC:

- Tissue damage (e.g. burns, heatstroke, dissecting aortic aneurysm, drowning, head injury and crush injury).
- Severe infections (bacterial, viraemia, parasites).
- Immunological (allograft rejection, immune complex disorders, incompatible blood transfusion).
- Obstetric (abruptio placentae, amniotic fluid embolism, retained foetal products, eclampsia, hypertonic saline abortion).
- Metabolic (diabetic ketoacidosis).
- Neoplastic (mucin secreting adenocarcinoma, promyelocytic leukaemia).
- Miscellaneous (envenomation, fat embolism, venous thrombosis).

Diagnosis: The diagnosis is based on (1) clinical evidence of bleeding from many sites and (2) laboratory tests.

Screening tests:

- Prolonged PT.
- Prolonged APPT: more sensitive than PT.
- Hypofibrinogenaemia ($< 1$ g/L): poor sensitivity.
- Thrombocytopaenia ($< 100 \times 10^9$/L): poor specificity.

Rarely will all four of these tests show normal findings in the presence of DIC. More specific tests are needed for confirmation.

Confirmatory tests – these are to show the following:

- A clot has been formed.
- The fibrinolytic system is activated (formation of plasmin) and has lysed the clot (formation of fibrin products).
- Fibrin monomer: Detection of fibrin monomer indicates that plasmin has been formed.
- Fibrin degradation products (FDPs): Their presence also indicates that plasmin has been formed but does not distinguish between primary and secondary fibrinolysis. In some patients with severe DIC there may be no elevation in FDPs, because of inhibition of the fibrinolytic response.
- Fragment E and *d*-dimer: These distinguish secondary fibrinolysis – i.e. a clot has been formed and then lysed. Although the *d*-dimer assay is more *specific* than the FDP assay, it is less *sensitive*:

|  | Sensitivity | Specificity |
|---|---|---|
| FDP | 100% | 56% |
| *d*-dimer | 85% | 97% |
| Combined | 100% | 97% |

Abnormalities in three or more of the screening tests constitute presumptive evidence for DIC. Fibrin degradation products and *d*-dimer assays provide confirmatory evidence in the proper clinical setting. Other laboratory studies do not improve diagnostic accuracy.

Disseminated intravascular coagulation in ICU: Many patients in intensive care have thrombocytopaenia, abnormal coagulation and equivocally raised FDPs, especially in association with multiorgan failure and sepsis. It is debatable that this condition deserves the label DIC. These patients rarely require any specific treatment and the 'DIC' resolves as the precipitating disease process resolves.

## Management of disseminated intravascular coagulation

1 **Remove the precipitating cause of the DIC – this is by far the most important principle** (e.g. urgent delivery of the foetus in cases of abruptio placentae or eclampsia, drainage and/or antibiotics for infection). Because DIC is not a specific disorder but rather a pathophysiological process caused by a variety of underlying diseases, treatment has to be tailored toward the underlying condition.
2 Maintain:
     Circulation – important to correct hypovolaemia.
     Oxygenation.
3 Fluid replacement: Despite objections about 'fuelling the fires', most clinicians will replace platelets, blood and clotting factors as necessary and until the underlying disease process is controlled. Moreover, there are sufficient inhibitors present in the replacement fluids to prevent amplification of the system. Apart

from FFP, cryoprecipitate may also be necessary to replace factor VIII and fibrinogen. Regular laboratory measurements must be used to guide replacement. Guidelines for platelet transfusion:

For surgery or brain injury, maintain the platelet count higher than $100 \times 10^9/L$.

For mild bleeding into the GIT, maintain the platelet count higher than $50 \times 10^9/L$.

4  Heparin: Despite theoretical attractions, heparin is rarely used for DIC. A possible exception may be acute promyelocytic leukaemia. Start with an IV bolus of 500–1000 units, followed by 500 units per hour and increase the dosage depending on laboratory and clinical data. Other possible indications include purpura fulminans and retained dead foetus. Low molecular weight heparin may prove more useful.

5  Future directions may involve specific inhibition of the extrinsic pathway and neutralisation of the triggering factors such as tissue factor and factor VIIa.

## Primary fibrinolysis

This is a rare disorder of which the major component is fibrinogenolysis (i.e. lysis before a stable clot is formed). Burns, certain types of surgery (neurosurgery, prostatic surgery) and malignancy can release inappropriately large quantities of plasminogen activator which is converted to circulating plasmin. This attacks fibrinogen and factor VIII. It can present as sudden catastrophic haemorrhage.

Diagnosis: Excessive fibrinolysis is recognised on the basis of

- Prolonged TT.
- Decreased serum fibrinogen.
- Raised FDPs.
- Decreased euglobin clot lysis time.

Management: Treat the precipitating factors. Antifibrinolytic agents such as $\epsilon$-amino caproic acid (EACA) and tranexamic acid may prove effective in these circumstances.

## Lupus anticoagulant

Despite giving a prolongation of the APPT, the lupus anticoagulant is rarely associated with bleeding, mainly thrombosis. Also, despite its name, it is rarely associated with systemic lupus! The lupus anticoagulant is an antiphospholipid antibody that interferes with the clotting cascade at sites where phospholipid is required.

## Anti-factor VIII antibody

This is autoantibody against the patient's own factor VIII molecule.

# Anticoagulants

## Heparin

Actions:

- Heparin binds to, and potentiates antithrombin III, which is the main physiological inhibitor of the coagulation cascade.
- Heparin enhances platelet aggregation.

Uses:

- For deep vein thrombosis (DVT) prophylaxis, give heparin 5000 units subcutaneously, 8–12-hourly. No monitoring required.
- For systemic anticoagulation:
    loading dose 5000 units IV
    continuous infusion 20 000–40 000 units/24 h

Monitoring:

- No single test is an accurate measure of heparin activity.
  Heparin activity is usually monitored by prolongation of APPT.

Reversal:

- Protamine sulphate 1 mg/100 units heparin, or 50 mg empirically and assess effect.
- Protamine itself can cause coagulation problems and anaphylactoid reactions. Give slowly intravenously.

## Low molecular weight heparin
Compared with heparin, LMWH has these features:

- Lower MW!
- Longer half-life.
- More predictable dose response.
- Not possible to reverse effects.
- Smaller dose for the same antithrombotic effect.
- Less thrombocytopaenia.
- Neutralises Xa as opposed to the action of unfractionated heparin which neutralises both thrombin and Xa.
- Can be partially reversed by protamine (1 mg/100 units Fragmin).
- Not routinely monitored by laboratory test.
- Less frequent incidence of HITS.

Uses:

- Deep vein thrombosis prophylaxis. No monitoring required.
- Systemic anticoagulation.

## Warfarin

Actions:

- Warfarin is a vitamin K antagonist that prevents the vitamin K dependent clotting factors II, VII, IX and X from becoming active.
- The rate of anticoagulant action is determined by the half-lives of the clotting factors, from factor VII (5 hours) up to factor II (60 hours).
- Larger doses will not hasten the onset of anticoagulation.

Uses:

- Can be given when heparin is commenced. Takes approximately 1 week to achieve stability.

Monitoring:

- Initially PT will become abnormal (factor VII).
- Full anticoagulation is not achieved until APPT is abnormal.
- Usually monitored with INR (two–three times normal).

Reversal:

- Fresh frozen plasma will replace clotting factors in an emergency.
- Vitamin K 10 mg will take approximately 6 hours to work.

Special points:

- Drugs that are highly protein-bound will displace warfarin and may exacerbate bleeding.
- Patients may become hypercoagulable initially because of decreased protein C levels.

## Thrombolytic agents

All thrombolytic agents act directly or indirectly as plasminogen activators. They can be given systemically or locally to lyse arterial or venous thrombi. The commonly used agents and their properties are listed in Table 28.3. Optimal dosing regimens are known for patients with myocardial infarction but are less certain for those with pulmonary emboli, strokes and peripheral venous and arterial thrombi.

Common complications include bleeding, haemorrhagic stroke and allergic reactions (streptokinase and anisoylated plasminogen streptokinase activator complex [APSAC]).

Contraindications to the use of thrombolytics:

- Active haemorrhage.
- Recent CNS infarction, haemorrhage, surgery, trauma, malignancy ($< 3$ months).

**Table 28.3.** Properties of thrombolytic agents

| Properties | Streptokinase | Urokinase | Tissue Plasminogen Activator | APSAC |
|---|---|---|---|---|
| Source | Streptococcal culture | Heterologous mammalian tissue culture | Heterologous mammalian tissue culture: recombinant bacterial product | Streptococcal culture |
| Molecular mass (daltons) | 47 000 | 37 000 | 68 000 | 131 000 |
| Type of agent | Bacterial proactivator | Tissue plasminogen activator | Bacterial proactivator | Tissue plasminogen activator |
| Plasma half-life (min) | 23–29 | 15–18 | 6 | 90 |
| Fibrinolytic activation | Systemic | Systemic | Systemic | Systemic |
| Fibrin specificity | Minimal | Minimal | Moderate | Minimal |
| Antigenicity | Yes | No | No | Yes |
| Allergic reactions | Yes | No | No | Yes |
| Cost | Cheapest | More expensive | Most expensive | More expensive |

[a]APSAC, anisoylated plasminogen streptokinase activator complex.

Relative:

- Recent surgery (within 10 days).
- Recent trauma.
- Recent gastrointestinal haemorrhage.
- Recent external cardiac massage.
- Coagulation disorders.
- Pregnancy or 10 days postpartum.
- Severe hypertension (diastolic >130 mmHg).
- Conditions with a potential for CNS embolism (e.g. bacterial endocarditis).

As yet there is no reliable monitor to assess the thrombolytic effect or the risk of bleeding. Fibrinogen levels and FDPs have poor sensitivity and specificity.

## Other drugs
Aprotinin is used mainly with cardiopulmonary bypass to decrease perioperative bleeding. The mechanism of action is uncertain (probably inhibits the increased fibrinolysis secondary to the use of extracorporeal circuits).

Desmopressin (DDAVP) is used clinically in haemophilia, von Willebrand's disease and uraemia and to reduce blood loss during surgery. It increases the circulating levels of factor VIII coagulant activity and von Willebrand factor and will shorten bleeding time.

## FURTHER READING

Aguilar, D. and Goldhaber, S. Z. Clinical uses of low-molecular weight heparins. *Chest* 115 (1999): 1418–23.

Chong, B. H. Heparin-induced thrombocytopaenia. *British Journal of Haematology* 89 (1995): 431–9.

Clinical Practice Guidelines. Appropriate use of blood components. National Health and Medical Reserch Council of Australia. http://www.health.gov.au/nhmrc/publications/ynopsis/cp775syn.htm

Corwin, H. L. and Krantz, S. B. Anemia of the critically ill: "Acute" anemia of chronic disease. *Critical Care Medicine* 28 (2000): 3098–9.

Gawaz, M., Dickfeld, T., Bogner, C., Fateh-Moghadam, S. and Neumann, F. J. Platelet function in septic multiple organ dysfunction syndrome. *Intensive Care Medicine* 23 (1997): 379–85.

Hebert, P. C., Wells, G., Blajchman, M. A., Marshall, J., Martin, C., Pagliarello, G., Tweeddale, M., Schweitzer, I., Yetisir, E. and the Transfusion Requirements in Critical Care Investigators for the Canadian Critical Care Trials Group. A multicenter, randomized, controlled clinical trial of transfusion requirements in critical care. *New England Journal of Medicine* 340 (1999): 409–17.

Heffner, J. E. Platelet-neutrophil interactions in sepsis – platelet guilt by association? *Intensive Care Medicine* 23 (1997): 366–8.

Krafte-Jacobs, B. Anemia of critical illness and erythropoietin deficiency. *Intensive Care Medicine* 23 (1997): 137–8.

Levi, M. and Ten Cate, H. Disseminated intravascular coagulation. *New England Journal of Medicine* 341 (1999): 586–92.

# 29

# Critical care endocrinology

## Severe uncontrolled diabetes

### Pathophysiology

Most diabetic emergencies arise as a result of insulin deficiency, either absolute or relative, that causes decreased uptake of glucose into the cells and via increased glucagon secretion, an increase in hepatic glycogenolysis and gluconeogenesis (Figure 29.1). Increased amounts of regulatory hormones such as catecholamines and cortisol, are released in response to glucagon excess. These hormones, along with the decreased insulin concentration, stimulate lipolysis and generation of fatty acids. Oxidation of these fatty acids in the liver results in ketone body formation and metabolic acidosis. Hyperosmolar hypoglycaemic non-ketotic coma (HHNKC) occurs as a result of relative insulin deficiency or resistance but with minimal counter-regulatory hormonal activation.

An increased serum glucose concentration will lead to osmotic diuresis with extensive water losses, equally from all of the body's fluid compartments. Poor tissue perfusion will eventually lead to lactate formation which, in turn, will exacerbate the metabolic acidosis. The metabolic acidosis will also lead to decreased total body levels of potassium and magnesium as these ions not only are exchanged for extracellular hydrogen ions but also are lost in the urine as a result of the osmotic diuresis, along with sodium, water, phosphate and glucose.

### Clinical features

A wide spectrum of biochemical and clinical abnormalities can occur in acute uncontrolled diabetes (Table 29.1), extending from pure hyperglycaemia without ketosis or HHNKC to pure ketosis without hyperglycaemia (euglycaemic ketoacidosis). Between the ends of this spectrum of presentation there is a mixture of both ketoacidosis and hyperglycaemia that is the classic diabetic ketoacidosis, accounting for about 70% of admissions for diabetes.

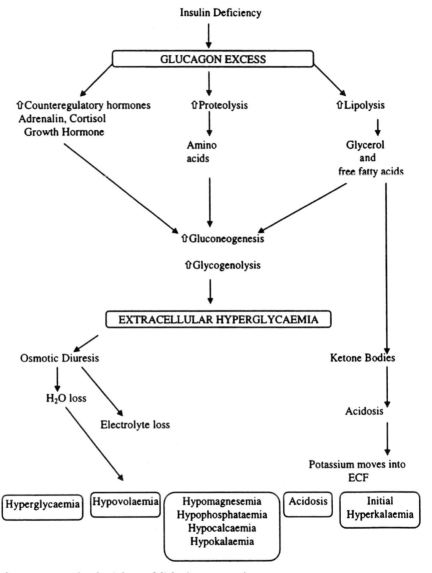

**Figure 29.1.** Pathophysiology of diabetic emergencies.

The clinical features can include:

- Fatigue, thirst, nausea and abdominal pain.
- Decreased level of consciousness, irritability and confusion.
- Hyperventilation (Kussmaul respirations) as a response to the metabolic acidosis.

**Table 29.1.** Features of diabetic emergencies

| Parameter | Euglycaemic Ketoacidosis | Diabetic ketoacidosis | Hyperosmolar non-ketotic coma |
|---|---|---|---|
| Age | Usually young | Any age | Usually old |
| Previous history | Insulin dependent | Known or new diabetic | Insulin dependent or on oral hypoglycaemics |
| Prodromal period | Hours | Days | Days to weeks |
| Acidosis | +++ | +++ | 0/+ |
| Fluid loss | 0/+ | ++ | +++ |
| Change in level of consciousness | 0 | ++ | +++ |
| Blood sugar | 0/+ | ++ | +++ |

- Clinical dehydration as a result of large water and electrolyte losses. Signs such as dry mucous membranes, sunken eyes and loss of tissue turgor may be seen.
- Varying degrees of hypovolaemia occur in all patients with shock occurring in the more severe cases. Because of the osmotic diuresis induced by glycosuria, urine output may be maintained in spite of decreased renal blood flow.
- Ketones can be smelled on the breath of ketotic patients.

Precipitating factors: Although there may be no obvious reason for the sudden deterioration in an otherwise stable diabetic, there are some possible precipitating factors:

- Infection.
- Poor patient compliance due to inadequate instruction.
- Acute illness (e.g. surgery, myocardial infarction).

## Investigation and monitoring

- Intravascular fluid replacement must be monitored in terms of blood pressure (BP), pulse rate, peripheral perfusion, central venous pressure (CVP) and, if necessary, pulmonary artery wedge pressure (PAWP) and cardiac output. Urine output is an unreliable indicator as it is affected by the osmotic diuresis.
- Take hourly Dextrostix readings confirmed by regular blood sugar measurements. Dextrostix are not accurate when the blood sugar levels are over 20 mmol/L, in which case laboratory determinations of blood sugar should be made.
- Determine the serum potassium concentration hourly until stable.
- Initial and then daily serum sodium, magnesium, calcium and phosphate levels.
- Daily measurements of serum osmolality, urea, creatinine, haemoglobin and white cells and obtain a chest x-ray.

**Table 29.2.** Summary of management in diabetic emergencies

1 Aggressive control of airway – ETT if necessary
2 Aggressive resuscitation from hypovolaemia and shock. Colloid is more efficient than crystalloids for this purpose. Avoid rigid regimens and use measurements of the intravascular space (e.g. BP, pulse rate, CVP, peripheral perfusion) as guidelines for resuscitation
3 Replace total body water losses with 5% dextrose or hypotonic solutions, 100–300 ml/h, depending on degree of dehydration
4 Replace fluid losses with half-normal saline or other suitable dextrose/saline solution if there is no evidence of hypovolaemia
5 Replace potassium, magnesium and phosphate according to measured levels
6 Commence IV infusion of short-acting insulin at 1 unit/h for diabetic ketoacidosis and 0.5 units/h for HHNKC and adjust the infusion according to regularly measured blood glucose concentrations
7 Correct acidosis with bicarbonate, 1 mmol/kg, only if arterial pH < 6.9 or is persistently less than 7.2
8 Concurrently treat the underlying cause of the diabetic emergency
9 Give low-dosage prophylactic heparin

- Carry out blood culture, urine microscopy and culture, sputum culture and 12-lead ECG on admission and then as indicated.
- Use plasma Ketostix and determine the serum lactate if necessary, to exclude a source of acid other than ketosis.
- Urinary electrolyte concentrations may help in the selection of a replacement fluid.

## Management

Mortality from severe diabetic ketoacidosis remains around 5% and from hyperosmolar coma around 50% – treatment must be aggressive and meticulous (Table 29.2).

The principles of treatment to be outlined next, apply to classic diabetic ketoacidosis. Hyperosmolar hypoglycaemic non-ketotic coma and euglycaemic ketoacidosis are discussed separately.

### Fluid resuscitation

1. Correct hypovolaemia and reverse shock.

Initially, 2 litres or more may have to be infused rapidly, then 50–300 ml/h, with boluses of 200 ml as necessary, until the circulating volume is restored.

Many recommendations for fluid treatment are based on inflexible recipes that may be irrelevant to a patient's individual needs. The approach to fluid loss in a patient with glycosuria is the same as for a patient with hypovolaemia or shock. It

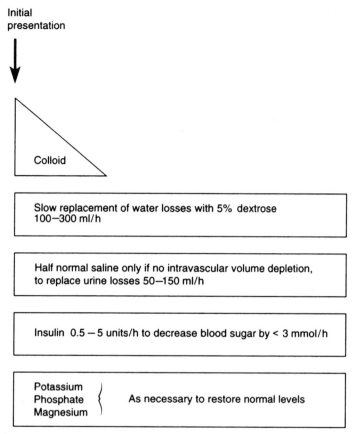

**Initial
presentation**

Colloid

Slow replacement of water losses with 5% dextrose
100–300 ml/h

Half normal saline only if no intravascular volume depletion,
to replace urine losses 50–150 ml/h

Insulin 0.5 – 5 units/h to decrease blood sugar by < 3 mmol/h

Potassium
Phosphate     As necessary to restore normal levels
Magnesium

**Figure 29.2.** Management of acute diabetic emergencies. Colloid is initially used to
resuscitate the circulating volume. Simultaneously, 5% dextrose is used to replace water
losses. If there is no intravascular volume depletion, half-normal saline can be used to
offset polyuria. Insulin is commenced at a low rate and increased as necessary.
Electrolytes are replaced according to frequently measured levels.

would be equally illogical to recommend an inflexible fluid regimen for shock as a
result of a ruptured spleen. Each patient's fluid needs must be assessed individually
and then continuously reassessed (Figure 29.2). Body water follows glucose into
the cells when insulin administration is commenced and this can exacerbate any
underlying hypovolaemia. Fluid should be titrated against regularly measured
end-points reflective of circulating volume, such as BP, pulse rate, CVP and
peripheral perfusion. Colloid probably is more efficient than isotonic saline for
correcting hypovolaemia but isotonic saline is still widely used.

The disadvantage of isotonic saline is that it is ultimately distributed mainly
to the interstitial space, which does not need urgent resuscitation and is not

responsible for hypovolaemia or shock. Moreover, isotonic saline, as a first-line fluid for resuscitation is inefficient in correcting hypovolaemia and inappropriate for correcting the water loss. The average urinary sodium losses as a result of the osmotic diuresis are approximately 50–70 mmol/L and will be adequately replaced by the sodium in the colloid needed for initial resuscitation.

2. Correct water losses.

If there has been minimal fluid loss and there is no hypovolaemia, one can use a solution approximating the sodium concentration in the fluid lost as a result of the polyuria. This would be approximately equivalent to half normal saline.

Although the first priority is to correct hypovolaemia, the total losses of body water should be concurrently and slowly corrected with 5% dextrose or a hypotonic dextrose/saline solution. The extra sugar added in the form of the dextrose-containing solutions is only a small amount and is easily controlled by adjusting the insulin infusion. The amount of fluid given will depend on the degree of dehydration. As a guideline, 2–6 litres (100–300 ml/h) should be given in the first 24 hours, with infusion continuing until the patient is tolerating oral fluids.

**Water losses from the interstitial and intracellular spaces are not immediately life-threatening, but rapid correction can be. It is important that the water losses be corrected slowly (over 24–72 hours), to allow for gradual osmotic equilibration between the body fluid spaces.**

If a patient is severely hypovolaemic, the urine output may be low despite glycosuria. Once the intravascular space has been restored, the urine output will rise driven by glycosuria. It is important that the total fluid infused be greater than the urine output.

### Electrolytes

Potassium: The serum potassium concentration should be measured on admission and hourly until it stabilises and then 2–4-hourly for the first 12 hours. Almost half of all diabetic patients are hyperkalaemic on admission. Some diabetic patients will have compromised renal function and difficulty in excreting potassium.

After checking the initial serum potassium concentration, commence giving potassium 5–40 mmol/h for the first 2 hours and adjust rate according to subsequent serum potassium concentrations measured every hour until stable.

Average requirements:

- 20 mmol/h for 6 hours.
- 10 mmol/h for next 12 hours.

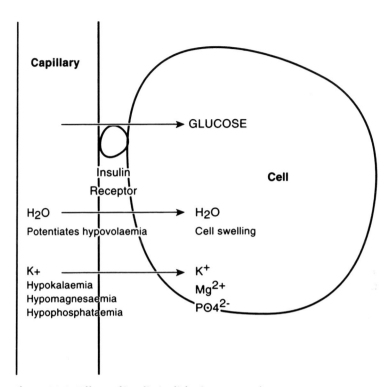

**Figure 29.3.** Effects of insulin in diabetic emergencies.

Phosphate: Initial and daily measurements of phosphate are necessary during the acute stage. Hypophosphataemia can have many complications, including respiratory failure.

If the concentration is low on admission, commence phosphate replacement at a rate of 5 mmol/h until corrected. Because phosphate solutions also contain potassium, the rate of potassium replacement may have to be adjusted.

Magnesium: Depending on the initial and daily measurements, magnesium may also have to be given.

Guideline: 20 mmol of magnesium intravenously over 1 hour and repeat as necessary.

Sodium: Sodium losses are usually corrected by the initial fluid used for re-suscitation. Measurement of serum sodium will be affected by the blood glucose and will appear lower.

$$\text{Real serum sodium} = \text{measured Na} + \frac{\text{blood glucose (mmol/L)}}{4}$$

## Hyperglycaemia

Insulin: Use short-acting insulin (Figure 29.3). The use of human insulin is recommended. Use a continuous intravenous insulin infusion system for better control of glucose. Hourly Dextrostix measurements and routine checks against blood sugar determinations are essential.

Insulin causes potassium, magnesium and phosphate, as well as water, to move intracellularly. **It is essential not to reduce the blood glucose rapidly, as these osmolar fluid and electrolyte shifts can cause severe complications.** Some patients are very sensitive to insulin. An initial loading dose of insulin is unnecessary; it could exacerbate hypovolaemia and cause cell swelling and hypokalaemia.

Guidelines:

Commence insulin 1–2 units/h until the rate of decrease in glucose can be estimated.

Blood glucose should be allowed to decrease by no more than 3 mmol/h, to allow osmotic gradients time to equilibrate gradually.

If higher infusion rates are needed; double, then quadruple the infusion rate and keep on doubling the rate periodically until control is achieved.

A rate of 0.5–3 units/h usually will maintain the blood glucose concentration when it has dropped to below 10 mmol/L.

Insulin adsorption on plastic syringes and giving sets is not a clinical problem, as infusion rates are titrated against regularly measured blood sugar levels. Special carrier solutions usually are not necessary.

Poor responses to insulin often are related to uncorrected hypovolaemia and inadequate resuscitation. Also check the insulin delivery mechanism.

The insulin infusion must continue until the patient has no ketones in their urine. If the blood sugar drops below 10 mmol/L continue the insulin infusion and add 50–10% dextrose to keep the blood sugar level normal.

Acidosis: The acidosis usually will correct itself if the foregoing management principles are followed.

Consider giving $HCO_3$ 1 mmol/kg if the initial arterial pH is less than 6.9 and repeat pH measurement in 30 minutes. Otherwise, consider giving $HCO_3$ 1 mmol/kg if the pH is persistently less than 7.2. Check the adequacy of intravascular volume replacement and the insulin delivery mechanism.

Overcorrection of acidosis with $HCO_3$ is associated with

- Sodium overload and exacerbation of hyperosmolality.
- Paradoxical increase in intracellular acidosis.
- Exacerbation of hypokalaemia.

Treat the underlying cause

- Concurrently, infection should be excluded by Gram stain and cultures.
- Exclude myocardial infarction.

- Better patient education and ready access to medical advice and outpatient and hospital facilities have proved to be significant advances in the management of diabetes mellitus and, when applied effectively, they have largely prevented acute diabetic emergencies.

## Hyperosmolar hyperglycaemic non-ketotic coma (HHNKC)

The same basic principles as for diabetic ketoacidosis should be used for HHNKC, with the following differences:

- Coma and decreased level of consciousness are more common in HHNKC. Aggressive airway control with an endotracheal tube (ETT) is often necessary.
- Because of larger fluid losses, it is even more important to avoid isotonic saline in patients with HHNKC. Use colloid initially for resuscitation and concurrently commence 5% dextrose solution. These patients can be very sensitive to undertreated hypovolaemia and shock, because of their greater age and incidence of associated conditions such as ischaemic heart disease.
- Because the fluid losses are usually higher, more colloid may be needed for initial resuscitation, followed by more 5% dextrose to replace the gross water deficit. **While rapidly reversing shock with colloid, aim to correct water losses over 24–72 hours** (average infusion rate, 100–300 ml/h). The rate is empirical and will depend on clinical assessment of fluid depletion and the time since onset. The slower the onset and the more severe the dehydration, the more severe the osmotic and metabolic disturbances. In order to enable these complex derangements to adjust, correction of water deficits should occur slowly in these patients.
- Resuscitation of the intravascular space should occur rapidly.
- The patients are older and require careful monitoring of fluid replacement (Chapter 4).
- Insulin requirements in these patients usually are lower than those for patients with diabetic ketoacidosis. **Slow infusion is essential to allow osmotic equilibration and to prevent rapid fluid and ion shifts: Aim to slowly reduce blood glucose over at least 24–72 hours.** The rate of reduction of blood glucose will depend on the onset of hyperglycaemia – the slower the onset, the more carefully the blood sugar should be reduced.
- Potassium requirements are usually higher. Phosphate and magnesium losses may also be high.
- Drowsiness, disorientation and coma often are prolonged and can occur up to 6 days after the commencement of treatment. If there is no specific intracerebral lesion, total recovery can be expected.
- Prophylactic heparin should be given – the incidence of venous thrombosis is high among patients with HHNKC.

### Euglycaemic ketoacidosis

The same principles of management as for classic diabetic ketoacidosis apply, with the following differences:

- Minimal fluid loss – may need only 5% dextrose, not colloid.
- Insulin infusion is the mainstay of management.
- Acidosis usually will correct itself.
- Because of the lack of dehydration and the presence of normal blood sugars, the diagnosis often can be overlooked. Beware of the confused unco-operative young diabetic with relatively normal blood sugar.

### Alcoholic ketoacidosis

Alcoholic ketoacidosis is not related to a lack of insulin. Indeed, these patients are very sensitive to insulin. It is typified by hypoglycaemia and ketoacidosis. It usually resolves with fluid resuscitation and IV glucose infusion.

## Thyroid gland disorders

### 'Sick-euthyroid' syndrome

Up to 70% of critically ill patients will have altered thyroid function and yet will be clinically euthyroid. The sick-euthyroid state is a response that prevents hypermetabolism when the body is stressed. It is important to differentiate this syndrome from true hypothyroidism. It requires no treatment.

Low $T_3$ syndrome is very common in the seriously ill:

- Low serum concentration of $T_3$ caused by decreased peripheral conversion of $T_4$ to $T_3$ and reduced protein binding.
- Serum thyroid stimulating hormone (TSH) low or normal, with thyroid releasing hormone (TRH) stimulation producing a normal or blunted TSH response.

High $T_4$ syndromes are less common:

- Elevated $T_4$, usually as a result of increased concentration of thyroid binding globulin (TBG).
- Free $T_3$ is low and $rT_3$ high.

Low $T_4$ and $T_3$ syndrome is a variant of low $T_3$ syndrome, but is less common:

- Hyposecretion of $T_4$ from the thyroid gland and decreased protein binding of $T_4$.
- The TSH is usually decreased and the TSH response to TRH stimulation blunted.

Thyroid function tests can be difficult to interpret in the seriously ill. Provided the patient is not receiving glucocorticoids, dopamine or $T_4$ replacement, a normal TSH assay is a reliable predictor of euthyroidism.

## Hypothyroidism

### Clinical features of myxoedematous coma
- Coma or decreased level of consciousness.
- Cardiovascular collapse (bradycardia, hypotension, hypovolaemia and pericardial effusion).
- Hypothermia and reduced metabolic rate.
- Hypotonia and delayed relaxation of tendon reflexes.
- Respiratory failure (may be due to collapse, atelectasis, aspiration, pleural effusion, hypercarbia, hypoventilation).
- Features of other endocrine disturbances (e.g. hypopituitarism, hypoparathyroidism).
- External features of coarse hair, a large tongue, loss of the external one-third of the eyebrows, yellow coarse skin, hoarse voice, non-pitting oedema and possibly signs of thyroid enlargement or atrophy, depending on the cause.

Many non-thyroid serious diseases mimic hypothyroidism, especially in the intensive care setting. The extreme of hypothyroidism usually known as myxoedematous coma, is the profound physiological expression of lack of thyroid hormone.

### Diagnosis
The diagnosis of true hypothyroidism depends on:

- An accurate history of previous thyroid abnormalities or symptoms associated with hypothyroidism, such as cold intolerance, hoarse voice, lethargy, constipation, alopecia, weight gain despite appetite loss and amenorrhoea.
- Physical findings such as bradycardia, a neck scar, dry skin, hypothermia, respiratory failure and those clinical features mentioned under myxoedematous coma.

### Laboratory findings
- Low $T_3$ and $T_4$ concentrations.
- High TSH if hypothyroidism is primary, or low TSH if it is secondary to pituitary disturbance.
- Elevated serum cholesterol.
- Anaemia.
- ECG: may show low amplitude QRS complex and/or features of ischaemia.
- Chest x-ray: may show pericardial or pleural effusion.
- Metabolic, hyponatraemia, respiratory acidosis and hypoglycaemia.

Further investigations may include a thyroid scan, CT scan and investigation of pituitary and parathyroid functions.

Hypothyroidism may be differentiated from sick-euthyroid states on the basis of the presence of low concentrations of free $T_3$ and $rT_3$, as well as an exaggerated response of TSH to TRH. Treatment should be commenced on clinical grounds.

## Management
- Secure the airway.
- Use oxygenation and ventilation if necessary.
- Fluid replacement and circulatory support with inotropes are often necessary, as for other seriously ill patients.
- Excessive water replacement should be avoided, as these patients usually experience water retention.
- Slowly and passively rewarm.
- Correct other metabolic disorders such as hyponatraemia.
- Treat hypoglycaemia with 50% dextrose intravenously.
- Treat pericardial and pleural effusions as necessary.
- Exclude complications such as skin necrosis, compartment syndrome, rhabdomyolysis and renal failure as a result of coma.

Monitoring: These patients need careful monitoring of their cardiorespiratory status, especially after commencement of hormone replacement, as there can be:

- A rapid increase in oxygen consumption.
- An increase in cardiac output.
- Myocardial ischaemia.

Drug treatment: Initially, only very small doses (e.g. 2.0 μg increments) of $T_3$ should be administered orally, except in the presence of paralytic ileus, where it should be given in even smaller doses intravenously and monitored carefully (IV infusion of 20 μg/day). $T_3$ theoretically is preferable to $T_4$, because it crosses more rapidly from the serum to the cerebrospinal fluid, does not depend on a converting enzyme and has a shorter half-life than $T_4$.

Hydrocortisone, 100 mg IV 6-hourly, is often given as well.

## Thyroid storm

Thyroid storm is a life-threatening clinical extreme of hyperthyroidism. It is very rare nowadays because of better long-term control. It usually occurs in a patient with known hyperthyroidism who has an intercurrent acute illness such as a severe infection, myocardial infarction or diabetic ketoacidosis, or undergoes surgery or childbirth.

## Clinical features
- Hyperthermia (can be extreme).
- Cardiovascular collapse (related to arrhythmias, cardiomyopathy and fluid loss). Initially there is hyperdynamic circulation.
- Restlessness, confusion, tremor and coma are common.
- Hyperventilation.
- Nausea, vomiting, diarrhoea, epigastric pain, cachexia and liver dysfunction are often found.
- Hypokalaemia and hyponatraemia.
- Hypercalcaemia and hyperglycaemia.

## Diagnosis
Treatment should be initiated on clinical grounds. The hormone levels cannot be determined rapidly and will be no different from levels found in uncomplicated hyperthyroidism. Ultrasound examination of the thyroid gland and TSH assays may help with the diagnosis.

## Management
General supportive measures:

- Treat any precipitating factor.
- Secure the airway.
- Correct hypovolaemia and other fluid losses.
- Correct metabolic abnormalities.
- Support the circulation.
- Ventilate and oxygenate if necessary.
- Cool with tepid sponging and fanning.

Drugs treatment aims to:

- Inhibit the effects of circulating hormones ($\beta$-blockers are usually used for this purpose).
- Inhibit the release of thyroid hormone (iodine).
- Block synthesis of and inhibit peripheral conversion of $T_4$ to $T_3$ (propylthiouracil).
  1 $\beta$-adrenergic blockade should be administered cautiously to suppress the signs and symptoms of thyrotoxicosis. Give propranolol 40 mg orally 8-hourly, or 1 mg intravenously, as required. However, $\beta$-blockers by themselves are not effective for thyroid storm.
  2 Give propylthiouracil 1 g orally stat, then 150 mg orally 6-hourly.
  3 Give potassium iodide: 500 mg orally 8-hourly, or 200 mg in 500 ml of isotonic saline intravenously over 2 hours, twice daily, 1 hour after propylthiouracil. Iodine inhibits the release of thyroid hormone.

4 Plasmapheresis, dialysis and resin haemoperfusion have been used successfully in cases that were refractory to the foregoing measures.
5 Dexamethasone 2 mg IV 6-hourly is sometimes used.

## Adrenal gland disorders

What constitutes normal adrenocortical function in the seriously ill remains unclear. For example, cortisol levels can be up to 20 times the 'normal' level in the seriously ill.

### Adrenal insufficiency

In the intensive care setting, adrenal insufficiency occurs most commonly in patients treated with glucocorticoids. Less often it can occur where adrenal tissue has been destroyed by autoimmune disease, tuberculosis, meningococcal or other infection (e.g. AIDS), haemorrhage or infiltration by malignancy. Absolute adrenal insufficiency in the seriously ill is unusual and may result from severe infections, severe hypotension, coagulopathies or severe thrombocytopaenia, suppression after steroid withdrawal or drugs such as etomidate or ketoconazole. Addisonian crisis usually occurs as a result of bilateral destruction of the adrenal cortices and usually is precipitated by an intercurrent catastrophe such as severe infection or surgery.

#### Clinical features
- Weakness, malaise, abdominal discomfort, fasting hypoglycaemia, skin pigmentation (if long term).
- Dehydration, weight loss, hypotension and tachycardia may occur simultaneously with high cardiac output and low systemic vascular resistance.
- Hyponatraemia, hyperkalaemia and metabolic acidosis.
- Hypoglycaemia.

#### Diagnosis
- Low plasma cortisol concentration with a high concentration of adrenocorticotrophic hormone (ACTH).
- In the seriously ill, a single plasma cortisol determination can be helpful. Increased levels are expected in acutely ill patients with normal adrenal function. Up to 25% of all seriously ill patients have low plasma cortisol levels and abnormal responses to ACTH. Abdominal CT may demonstrate the cause of adrenal abnormality.

#### Treatment
- Isotonic saline (approximately 6–8 litres in 24 hours) to correct the hyponatraemia and fluid loss.
- Hydrocortisone 100 mg IV 6-hourly.

- Aldosterone 0.5 mg IM. This is unnecessary when large amounts of hydrocortisone are used.
- Treat the precipitating cause.

## Steroid withdrawal

Corticosteroids are widely used in medicine and their withdrawal can cause an Addisonian-type picture within 24 hours:

- General malaise, anorexia, abdominal discomfort.
- Postural hypotension, pyrexia and Addisonian crisis.

  Treatment:

- Hydrocortisone, 100 mg IV, 6-hourly.
- Isotonic saline

Adrenal suppression is increasingly likely after long-term use (approximately 2–10 years). Therefore, withdrawal of steroids must be gradual. After steroid treatment for more than 8 years, adrenal cortical suppression may be permanent.

If there is doubt about adrenal suppression, an ACTH stimulation test (Synacthen test) can be performed. This can reveal a lack of adrenocortical reserve, as opposed to total absence of activity. Administration of ACTH to these patients should result in diminished cortisol response:

- Short ACTH test – give tetracosactrin (synthetic 1–24-ACTH (synacthen)) 250 μg IM.
- Take blood samples at 30 and 60 minutes post-injection and measure for cortisol. A rise of 250 nmol/L or two–three times the baseline and levels more than 550 nmol/L are considered normal.

## Phaeochromocytoma

Phaeochromocytoma is a rare catecholamine-secreting tumour originating from the chromaffin cells of the sympathetic nervous system:

- 90% develop in the adrenal medulla.
- 10% are malignant.

### Clinical presentation
The symptoms range from mild to severe and can be sustained or paroxysmal. They include:

- Sweating attacks.
- Tachycardia.

- Headaches.
- Hypertension.
- Autonomic dysfunction.
- Possibly arrhythmias, angina and pulmonary oedema can also occur.

## Diagnosis

Determination of urinary metanephrine is a good screening test.
Determination of urinary vanillylmandolic acid is a less sensitive screening test.
Determination of urinary catecholamines is also a good screening test.
Plasma catecholamine measurement is technically difficult to perform.
Localisation:

- CT scan of the abdomen.
- [$^{131}$I] metaiodobenzylguanidine scintigraphy.

## Management

Surgical removal is the only definitive treatment. Careful preoperative preparation is essential and must include:

- α-blockers (usually phenoxybenzamine) commenced 2–3 weeks before operation.
- β-blockers only after α-blockade has been commenced.
- Fluid replacement usually is necessary as the circulation vasodilates.
- Potassium replacement.

## FURTHER READING

Adrogue, H. J. and Madias, N. E. Medical progress: Management of life-threatening acid-base disorders: First of two parts. *New England Journal of Medicine* 338 (1998): 26–34.

Gibson, E. A. M. and Hinds, C. J. Growth hormone and insulin-like growth factors in critical illness. *Intensive Care Medicine* 23 (1997): 369–78.

Hunter, J. D. and Noble, D. Thyroid function in the critically ill. *Anaesthesia* 51 (1996): 508.

Masterson, G. R. and Mostafa, S. M. Adrenocortical function in critical illness. *British Journal of Anaesthesia* 81 (1998): 308–10.

Scherpereel, P. Critical Care Focus Volume 4: Endocrine disturbance. *European Journal of Anaesthesiology* 18 (2001): 417.

# 30

# Obstetric emergencies

- Obstetric emergencies involve young patients who are at the limits of normal physiological adaptation, because of late pregnancy and who can develop catastrophic multisystem disease.
- One must understand the normal physiology of both the mother and foetus and be aware of how these two patients interact with each other and with the underlying disease.
- The obstetrician, neonatologist and intensivist must work closely together in managing these patients.

Physicians dealing with critically ill obstetric patients are encouraged to familiarise themselves with the normal physiology (Table 30.1, Figure 30.1) and pathophysiology of pregnancy. There are many rare and spectacular presentations of critical illness such as fulminant hepatic failure of pregnancy, ovarian hyperstimulation syndrome (OHSS) and postpartum cardiomyopathy. More common complications such as pre-eclampsia, eclampsia, postpartum haemorrhage (PPH), abruptio placentae and amniotic fluid embolism will be discussed here.

Often there is doubt about the most suitable place to manage these emergencies – in an obstetric environment or an intensive care environment. All hospitals should develop their own policies, depending on their respective experiences and the severity of illness. A suggested policy is in Table 30.2. If there is any doubt, the patient should be managed in an intensive care environment until the threat to life abates. Severely ill obstetric patients are amongst the most challenging in intensive care.

**Table 30.1.** Some physiological changes during pregnancy

Increased pulse rate (to 85–90 beats/min)
Decreased BP in second trimester (by 5–15 mmHg)
Cardiac output increases (by 1–1.5 L/min)
Reduction in peripheral resistance
Maternal blood volume increases by 25–50% by late pregnancy
Uterine blood flow increases from 50 to 500 ml/min at term (10% of cardiac output)
Supine hypotension syndrome in the third trimester; lying supine will cause the uterus
   to compress the vena cava, decreasing venous return and cardiac output
Renal blood flow and glomerular filtration rate increases
Tidal volume increases by 40%
Respiratory rate unchanged
Respiratory alkalosis
Delayed gastric emptying
Hypercoagulability

**Table 30.2.** Guidelines for ICU admission in pregnancy-induced hypertension

| | |
|---|---|
| Airway: | Severe facial or laryngeal oedema |
| Breathing: | Pulmonary oedema, acute lung injury, aspiration |
| Circulation: | Continuous infusions of vasoactive drugs |
| | Intra-arterial monitoring |
| Neurology: | Seizures |
| Other: | Coagulation abnormalities – bleeding, thrombosis |

## Eclampsia and pre-eclampsia: pregnancy-induced hypertension

### Definition
Eclampsia and pre-eclampsia are parts of the spectrum of pregnancy-induced hypertension (PIH). Hypertension during pregnancy is defined as a systolic BP $\geq$ 140 mmHg and/or a diastolic BP $\geq$ 90 mmHg, or alternatively, a rise in systolic BP of more than 25 mmHg or a rise in diastolic BP of more than 15 mmHg from the pressure recorded before conception or during the first trimester. Pregnancy-induced hypertension affects approximately 15% of primigravidas.

Hypertension during pregnancy is usually classified as follows:

Pre-eclampsia
   mild
   severe

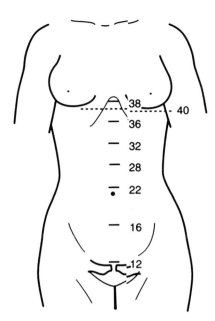

**Figure 30.1.** Uterine size at various stages of pregnancy (in weeks).

Chronic hypertension
  essential
  secondary
Pre-eclampsia superimposed on chronic hypertension.

Recognising pre-eclampsia may be difficult as the signs can be non-specific and there is no reliable diagnostic test. The classic triad of hypertension, proteinuria and oedema does not always occur simultaneously, can occur alone, in other disease states and can even be present during normal pregnancy.

Pre-eclampsia: Pre-eclampsia is also known as PIH. It is associated with proteinuria, oedema and high BP occurring after the 20th week of gestation and usually abating within 24–48 hours of delivery. The patient should have no history of hypertension or renal disease and a normal BP before pregnancy. It is usually a disease of primigravidas. The more severe the proteinuria, the more severe the pre-eclampsia. Oedema is of uncertain significance.

Eclampsia is PIH with superimposed convulsions. It can occur in patients with mild or severe forms of pre-eclampsia.

## Pathophysiology

The pathophysiology of PIH probably has an immunogenetic basis beginning at the time of conception. The result is widespread maternal vasospasm and

**Table 30.3.** Diagnostic criteria for severe pregnancy-induced hypertension

Cardiac
   Diastolic BP $\geq$ 110 mmHg
   Pulmonary oedema
Neurological
   Visual disturbances
   Convulsions
   Hyperreflexia with clonus
Renal
   Serum creatinine > 100 $\mu$mol/L
   Proteinuria > 2 + on dipstick testing
   Oliguria
   Serum uric acid > 0.40 mmol/L
Hepatic
   Epigastric pain
   Elevated plasma bilirubin
   Elevated aspartate transaminase
Haematological
   Thrombocytopaenia
   Haemolysis
Foetal
   Growth retardation
   Abnormal cardiotocograph

Reprinted by permission from Brown, M. A. Pregnancy induced hypertension. *Anaesthesia and Intensive Care* 17 (1989): 185–97.

intravascular volume contraction leading to organ hypoperfusion and ischaemia. Dysfunction occurs in uteroplacental, renal, hepatic, haematologic and neurological vascular beds secondary to thrombosis and vasospasm.

In untreated severe pre-eclampsia there may be low cardiac filling pressures, a high systemic vascular resistance and a low cardiac output. Capillaries may be leaky and oncotic pressure low, leading to decreased intravascular volume and an expanded interstitial space.

Renal dysfunction is usually from a pre-renal cause and can progress to acute tubular necrosis.

## Monitoring and investigation

Exclude other possible causes of hypertension such as essential hypertension, primary renal abnormalities, phaeochromocytoma and coarctation of the aorta.

The initial assessment of patients with severe PIH (Table 30.3) must include neurological assessment, cardiorespiratory evaluation and laboratory determinations of haematological, renal and hepatic functions.

Routine monitoring: The following are only guidelines. The extent and frequency of repeated monitoring will depend on the severity of the illness, the gestational age of the foetus and the timing of the delivery:

| | |
|---|---|
| • BP | 4 hourly |
| • Pulse rate and pulse oximetry. | continuous |
| • Arterial blood gases. | daily |
| • Full blood count. | daily |
| • Clotting studies and platelet count. | daily |
| • Liver function tests, plasma proteins and serum uric acid. | daily |
| • Midstream urine specimen for urinalysis and microscopy. | daily |
| • Creatinine, urea and urine output. | daily |

- Central venous pressure (CVP) and pulmonary artery wedge pressure (PAWP) may be helpful in severe cases.
- Foetal growth and well being: foetal movements and serial ultrasound of foetal size.
- More intensive foetal monitoring in severe PIH, such as cardiotocography (CTG), biophysical profile, Doppler velocimetry and amniocentesis to determine maturation of foetal lungs.

## Management

### Prevention

Low-dose aspirin does not reduce the incidence of pre-eclampsia but delays the onset of the clinical syndrome until later in the pregnancy. Small trials show that supplemental calcium may reduce the incidence of pre-eclampsia; larger trials are needed.

### Fluid balance

The paradox of pre-eclampsia is the simultaneous presence of peripheral oedema and hypovolaemia. The average plasma volume deficit is 400–600 ml. To address this problem, give minimal amounts of crystalloids and hypotonic solutions in order to reduce excessive salt and water retention. Excessive fluid can cause peripheral and pulmonary oedema by passing through leaky capillaries. Colloid solutions may be preferable to crystalloid solutions, as they will maintain the intravascular volume without exacerbating oedema and at the same time will increase rather than decrease the colloid oncotic pressure (COP). Left ventricular compliance may be reduced so give small aliquots of colloid, 200–300 ml and assess the effect on intravascular volume and tissue perfusion. It is particularly important to give fluid prior to using antihypertensive drugs, as the underlying hypovolaemia will be exacerbated by vasodilatation. Avoid diuretics, as they could exacerbate the relative hypovolaemia. Complex monitoring, e.g.

pulmonary artery catheterisation or transoesophageal echo may be required in severe cases to guide fluid and antihypertensive therapy.

## Control of hypertension

Hypertension can result in complications such as cerebral haemorrhage and placental abruption. Medical intervention is necessary when the systolic or diastolic pressure exceeds 170 or 110 mmHg, respectively. Attempt to maintain the diastolic BP between 90 and 110 mmHg. Vasodilators are the drug of choice.

**Avoid rapid decreases in BP, which could compromise placental perfusion. Placental blood flow is not autoregulated and is totally dependent on maternal BP.**

**To avoid hypovolaemia, intravenous fluid is almost always necessary, especially when vasodilatation occurs as a result of antihypertensive agents (Chapter 22).**

**The BP should be continuously monitored during antihypertensive therapy, either invasively or non-invasively.**

The first-line drugs for treatment:

Hydralazine: Give hydralazine 5–10 mg IV over 15 minutes with frequent BP measurements. Alternatively, a continuous IV infusion can be used: 5–20 mg/h, titrated against response. The mechanism of action is through direct relaxation of arteriolar smooth muscle.

Labetalol: Give labetalol by IV infusion, 200 mg in 200 ml of saline, titrated to the BP.

Nifedipine: Titrate nifedipine carefully to avoid hypotension. Give 5 mg initially, with repeated doses of 5–10 mg, no more frequently than every 30 minutes.

The second-line drugs for treatment:

Sodium nitroprusside: Give sodium nitroprusside as a continuous infusion (50 μg/50 ml), commencing at 5 μg/min, up to a maximum of 500 μg/min, *slowly* and *smoothly*, to prevent precipitous falls in BP. Measure plasma cyanide levels when using prolonged high-dosage infusions.

Diazoxide has been used extensively for severe hypertension in patients with pre-eclampsia (15–30 mg every 10–15 minutes). However, it can cause rapid drops in BP that can be dangerous for maternal and foetal perfusion.

Avoid diuretics and angiotensin converting enzyme (ACE) inhibitors, as the circulating volume is low and precipitous falls in BP can result. The ACE inhibitors have also been associated with foetal retardation. Non-steroidal anti-inflammatory drugs (NSAIDs) should also be avoided, as they can precipitate a hypertensive crisis and renal failure.

## Epidural analgesia

For many years the fear of systemic hypotension and foetal distress as a result of sympathetic blockade and peripheral vasodilatation resulted in avoidance of

**Table 30.4.** Guidelines for delivery in pre-eclampsia

Maternal
    Inability to control BP
    Deteriorating liver function
    Deteriorating renal function
    Progressive thrombocytopaenia
    Neurological complication
Foetal
    Non-reactive, positive spontaneous or induced contraction stress test
        with deceleration
    Intrauterine growth retardation

epidural anaesthesia. However, with careful fluid administration to prevent hypovolaemia, it is now becoming the technique of choice for labour and Caesarean section.

Epidural analgesia helps to control maternal BP and increase placental perfusion. The intravascular volume must be maintained and only small doses should be given to achieve a satisfactory block while monitoring the BP. Epidurals are contraindicated in the presence of a coagulopathy and local infection.

## Coagulopathy

A full blood count, platelet count and coagulation profile should be performed at least daily for all severely ill patients with pre-eclampsia. The basis of treatment consists of correction of the underlying disorder and replacement of coagulation factors as necessary.

## Timing of delivery

After the patient has been resuscitated and stabilised, delivery should be considered in severe cases, no matter what the gestational age of the foetus, as this is the only definitive way of arresting pre-eclampsia. The indications for delivery are outlined in Table 30.4. Each case must be considered individually and the indications viewed as guidelines only.

In the meantime, nurse the mother in the left lateral position, when possible, in order to decrease caval compression and maintain uterine blood flow.

Most cases of severe pre-eclampsia require Caesarean section. Adequate analgesia is important both during and after delivery. Oxytoxin, not ergometrine, should be used in order to avoid excessive hypertension.

Close monitoring must be maintained for at least 48 hours postpartum.

Epidural analgesia will provide pain relief and help to control the BP. If it is not possible to use an epidural, a continuous IV narcotic infusion will provide analgesia.

## Prevention of convulsions

This is a controversial area. Magnesium therapy is commonly used in North America as seizure prophylaxis, whereas in Europe and Australasia, phenytoin (20 mg/kg as a loading dose and then according to levels) and other, more standard anticonvulsants such as benzodiazapines are used. As yet, controlled comparative trials have not demonstrated which, if any, of the drugs are most efficacious in preventing seizures.

Magnesium therapy: Magnesium has been used with success in patients with severe pre-eclampsia in order to prevent convulsions. It has been shown to be the drug of choice to prevent recurrent seizures in eclamptic patients.

Its mechanism of action may be via cerebral vasodilatation or a calcium channel blocking action on neuronal cells. Unlike other antiepileptic drugs, it has the advantage of not being detrimental to foetal function in therapeutic doses.

Before commencing treatment, assess renal function and determine the plasma magnesium concentration. Magnesium is excreted by the kidneys so its use in the presence of renal insufficiency is hazardous.

Use a continuous IV infusion of magnesium, preferably via a central vein. The infusions should be continued for 24–72 hours postpartum:

- Magnesium sulphate
  Loading dose, 4 g over 20 minutes (20 ml of 20% magnesium or approximately 16 mmol magnesium)
  Infusion 1 g/h (4 mmol magnesium/h).
*or*
- Magnesium chloride
  Loading dose, 2 g over 20 minutes (20.8 mmol magnesium)
  Infusion 0.5 g/h (5.2 mmol magnesium/h)

These are only guidelines to achieve plasma levels of magnesium within the therapeutic range of 2.0–3.5 mmol/L. Clinically, the rate should be titrated in order to avoid effects such as decreased reflexes and muscle weakness. Beware of prolonged actions of neuromuscular blocking agents, even when magnesium is in the therapeutic range.

Effects of increasing plasma magnesium levels:

|  | Plasma magnesium (mmol/L) |
| --- | --- |
| Normal | 0.8–1.1 |
| Therapeutic range | 2.0–3.5 |
| ECG changes (increased PR interval and widening QRS complex) | > 3.0 |
| Drowsiness | > 4.0 |
| Absent deep tendon reflexes | > 4.0 |

| | |
|---|---|
| Respiratory arrest | > 5.0 |
| Heart block | > 7.5 |
| Cardiac arrest | > 10.0 |

Determine magnesium levels hourly until stable levels are achieved. The myocardial and skeletal muscle effects of magnesium can be partially reversed by IV calcium.

## Eclampsia

The exact causes of seizures in patients with pre-eclampsia is unknown, but hypertensive encephalopathy, vasospasm, ischaemia, haemorrhage and cerebral oedema may be responsible. The standard treatment is rapid control of the seizures, control of the airway if necessary and delivery of the foetus. **Convulsions must be rapidly controlled as they can be life-threatening.**

- Midazolam 5–10 mg or diazepam 2–5 mg increments IV.
- Phenytoin 20 mg/kg IV over 20 minutes (< 50 mg/min) as a loading dose, then 5 mg/kg IV daily as a single dose over 1 hour. Track levels.
- Thiopentone 25–50 mg increments IV – only use if the above measures fail.

All these drugs can cause hypotension which should respond quickly to IV fluids.
Clear and control the airway.
Administer oxygen.
Endotracheal intubation and ventilation may be necessary.
Prevent aortocaval compression and pulmonary aspiration.
Continually assess foetal state. An emergency Caesarean section may be necessary.
Exclude other possible causes of seizures (e.g. cerebral oedema or intracerebral bleed) if they are not being controlled.

## HELLP syndrome

The term 'HELLP syndrome' is derived from the combination 'Haemolysis, Elevated Liver enzymes and Low Platelet count'. The term is being used less frequently as it is only a manifestation of severe pre-eclampsia. It can even occur without overt hypertension. Haemolysis and thrombocytopaenia are the results of peripheral cellular destruction. The elevated liver enzymes result from changes in the liver including periportal ischaemia, necrosis and haemorrhage. Hepatic infarction, haemorrhage and even rupture can occur with severe pre-eclampsia and the HELLP syndrome.

Its management is similar to that for pre-eclampsia and ultimately depends on delivery of the foetus. Complete recovery may be delayed in some cases, even after delivery.

## Postpartum haemorrhage

Postpartum haemorrhage is empirically defined as loss of more than 500–1000 ml of blood following delivery. A PPH remains a significant cause of maternal morbidity and mortality.

### Aetiology

Early causes (< 24 hours)
- Uterine atony continues to be the most common cause of PPH.
- Lower genital tract tears are also common causes associated with interventions or prolonged and precipitous delivery.
- Uterine rupture is a rare cause and is associated with previous uterine surgery, operative vaginal delivery and high parity.
- Uterine inversion is rare and usually obvious.
- Retained placental products can be associated with early or delayed PPH.
- Coagulopathies can directly cause PPH or exacerbate existing PPH (e.g. in association with sepsis, amniotic fluid embolism and PIH).

Delayed causes (> 24 hours)
- Infection
- Retained products of conception.

### Management

Prevention
Predisposing factors such as multiple gestation, high parity, previous Caesarean section, polyhydramnios, previous history of PPH, PIH and uterine polyps should be identified early.

- Avoid premature administration of agents such as Pitocin that are used to facilitate placental delivery.
- Carefully inspect the placenta for intact delivery.
- Manual removal of placenta may be appropriate if it has not been delivered within 10 minutes of birth.
- Oxytocin infusion is commonly employed in order to optimise uterine tone after placental delivery.

Active management
1 Determine the cause and treat it at the same time as the patient is being resuscitated.

2 Early recognition and aggressive treatment of blood loss are essential.
3 Establish IV access and begin replenishment of the intravascular volume early. Give high-flow oxygen via mask.
4 Monitoring:
  a Vital signs.
    • BP
    • Pulse rate.
    • Respiratory rate.
    • Pulse oximetry.
    • Urine output.
  b Estimation of blood loss.
  c More complex monitoring such as ECG and CVP may be necessary in severe cases.
5 Rapidly perform:
  a Blood cross match.
  b Complete blood count.
  May also need:
  a Coagulation screen.
    • Prothrombin time.
    • Partial thromboplastin time.
    • Fibrinogen level.
    • Fibrin split products.
  b Arterial blood gases.
6 Rapidly replace lost blood with fluid according to vital signs. Blood losses tend to be underestimated. Fresh frozen plasma and other components may also be needed.
7 Specific causes:
  a Uterine atony:
    • Fundal compression.
    • Oxytocin infusion (10–40 units in 100 ml of isotonic saline).
    • Other measures (e.g. prostaglandin $F_2\alpha$ by intrauterine or intramuscular injection).
  b Other:
    • Examine the perineum, vagina and cervix for tears and for material in the cervix.
    • Manual examination and removal of these products should be conducted if necessary.
8 If bleeding persists, consider:
  • Curettage of the uterus.
  • Ligation of pelvic arterial vessels.
  • Angiographic embolisation.
  • Hysterectomy.

## Abruptio placentae

Abruptio placentae is characterised by complete or partial separation of the placenta prior to birth. It is usually as a result of bleeding into the decidua basalis.

### Causes
- There is no unifying theory.
- Associated with a high incidence of maternal hypertension.
- As many as 10% of patients with severe PIH have abruption.
- Other causes can include blunt trauma.

### Diagnosis

Abruptio placentae is divided into three grades:

Grade I
- About 40% of cases.
- Slight vaginal bleeding.
- Normal maternal BP and no coagulopathy.
- No foetal distress.

Grade II
- About 45% of cases.
- Greater amount of vaginal bleeding.
- Maternal hypofibrinogenaemia.
- Foetal distress.

Grade III
- About 15% of cases.
- Heavy vaginal bleeding.
- Uterine tenderness.
- Maternal coagulopathy and thrombocytopaenia.
- Foetal death usually occurs.

### Common signs and symptoms

- Vaginal bleeding in the third trimester. Haemorrhage is overt in 80% of cases and concealed in the remainder.
- Pain in about 50% of cases.
- Uterine tenderness and contractions in about 20% of cases.
- Signs of maternal blood loss.
- Perinatal ultrasound may assist in the diagnosis.
- Foetal distress and death.

The differential diagnosis must include uterine rupture, placenta praevia and polyhydramnios.

## Investigations and monitoring

There should be regular monitoring of maternal vital signs:

- BP
- Pulse rate.
- Urine output.
- Respiratory rate.

More complex monitoring may be needed if blood loss is severe. The following investigations and determinations are necessary:

- Full blood count and cross match.
- Coagulation tests.
- Arterial blood gases.
- Urea, creatinine and electrolytes.

Foetal monitoring:

- Foetal heart rate.
- Determine gestational age, foetal weight and viability and placental location with ultrasound examination.

## Management

- The major problems are maternal blood loss, coagulopathy and foetal distress or death. Assessment and resuscitation should be carried out simultaneously. Fluid resuscitation is much the same as for PPH. Establish an IV line and replenish the intravascular volume with colloid or crystalloid solution and blood if necessary. Blood losses are often underestimated.
- Disseminated intravascular coagulopathy is seen in about 10% of cases. It usually occurs only after massive blood loss or when the foetus is dead. It should be clinically suspected when bleeding is excessive or when oozing is seen from venous puncture sites. Coagulation factors and platelets may also be needed.
- The definitive treatment is delivery of the foetus and placenta. This will depend on the maternal and foetal condition, as well as gestational age.

## Amniotic fluid embolism

Amniotic fluid embolism is a rare complication of pregnancy, labour and the postpartum period. It is characterised by sudden and severe hypotension, hypoxia and coagulopathy. The mortality is as high as 80%, with half of all patients dying within 1 hour.

Current reviews suggest there are no identifiable maternal risk factors.

The amniotic fluid probably enters the circulation through a tear in the membranes in the lower uterine segment. It can occur during abortion in the first or second trimester, or as a result of abdominal trauma, amniocentesis or hysterotomy or even in the postpartum period. However, most episodes occur during labour.

## Pathogenesis

The pathogenesis of this condition is still not completely understood. It has similarities to sepsis and anaphylaxis; a foreign substance enters the circulation and causes release of inflammatory mediators. A new name has been suggested: 'anaphylactoid syndrome of pregnancy'.

Amniotic fluid in the pulmonary circulation causes:

- Pulmonary vascular obstruction with sudden decreases in left atrial pressure and cardiac output associated with hypertension and cardiac arrest.
- Acute cor pulmonale.
- Gross ventilation/perfusion inequality and severe hypoxia.

## Clinical features

Respiratory distress and pulmonary oedema.
Cyanosis.
Cardiovascular collapse.
Convulsions and coma.
Bleeding diathesis and haemorrhage.
Foetal distress.

## Diagnosis

- The diagnosis is one of exclusion and is usually on clinical grounds.
- Elements of amniotic fluid and foetal cells occasionally are found in the maternal circulation but their exact clinical significance is unknown.
- At postmortem examination, amniotic fluid material is often found in the lungs, coronary arteries, kidney and brain.
- The differential diagnosis should include septic shock, aspiration pneumonitis, acute myocardial infarction, pulmonary or air embolism, placental abruption and an accidental high spinal block during epidural analgesia or local anaesthetic toxicity.

## Management

Treatment is aimed at resuscitation and support.

## Cardiovascular support
- Give IV fluids to restore circulatory balance.
- Monitor left and right side pressure via pulmonary artery catheter in severe cases.
- Inotropic support may also be necessary.
- Careful pulmonary vascular dilatation with drugs such as prostacyclin or sodium nitroprusside, with appropriate pressure monitoring, may be indicated. The pulmonary hypertension is usually transient.

## Respiratory support
Increases in the inspired oxygen, positive end-expiratory pressure, continuous positive airway pressure, intermittent positive-pressure ventilation and other general measures may be needed to correct hypoxia.

## Haematological support
Blood and component therapy should be given to correct the coagulopathy.

## Foetal management
The foetus will also suffer from the effects of anoxia and hypotension and should be closely monitored and delivered rapidly with full resuscitation facilities.

## FURTHER READING

Davies, S. Obstetrical and pediatric anesthesia. Amniotic fluid embolus: a review of the literature. *Canadian Journal of Anesthesia* 48 (2001): 88–98.

Dekker, G. and Sibai, B. Primary, secondary, and tertiary prvention of pre-eclampsia. *Lancet* 457 (2001): 209–14.

Linton, D. M. and Anthony, J. Critical care management of severe pre-eclampsia. *Intensive Care Medicine* 23 (1997): 248–55.

Mushambi, M. C., Halligan, A. W. and Williamson, K. Recent developments in the pathophysiology and management of pre-eclampsia. *British Journal of Anaesthesia* 76 (1996): 133–48.

Sibai, B. M. Treatment of hypertension in pregnant women. *New England Journal of Medicine* 335 (1996): 257–65.

Walker, J. J. Pre-eclampsia. *Lancet* 356 (2000): 1260–5.

# 31

# Economics, outcome and ethics in intensive care

> - Clinicians in the ICU often need to make a diagnosis of dying.
> - Management is then about supporting the friends and relatives and ensuring a pain-free death with dignity.

No book should discuss critically ill patients without addressing the issues of economics, outcome and ethics. Certain questions must continuously remain on the agenda: For whom is intensive care appropriate? Is the cost justified? How long should treatment be continued? In what manner should treatment be withdrawn? Economics and ethics can no longer be considered separately from clinical practice. No matter how wealthy a society is, it has a finite health budget. Economic considerations will therefore increasingly dictate the limits of therapy and ethical considerations must be evaluated within those limits. Similarly, inherent cultural attitudes and legal pressures interact with ethics.

## Costs of intensive care

The cost of providing intensive care is high – at least three times the cost of providing normal hospital care. Approximately 15% of hospitalised patients account for as much of the health budget as do the other 85%. Among that 15% of patients, treatment for chronic diseases outside of intensive care, accounts for most of the budget.

## Cost containment

There is no longer a blank cheque for medical care. We all have to become aware of the increasing costs of medical care and the limitations they impose upon our practice. Spending money in one area of health decreases the opportunity to spend it in other sometimes less visible areas. In certain cases we can no longer assert our traditional right to do what we think is best for our patients regardless of cost. Rather than become self-righteous about these limitations, we must responsibly meet the practical challenge of a finite health budget. Some of the measures required are discussed next.

## Management principles

Many doctors working in intensive care are familiarising themselves with the principles of good management, including how best to manage manpower within the ICU, how to apply cost–benefit concepts to patient treatment and how to manage budgets efficiently. These and other principles will become increasingly important in our everyday practice (see Chapter 1).

## High technology. The 'latest' drugs

Unless a technology has been shown to be effective and to be justified by economic appraisal, it might be regarded as unethical to use it. This can raise difficult dilemmas in the face of physicians' traditional obsession with clinical freedom and their often naive attitude towards more aggressive marketing strategies. Many commercial strategies exploit the human desire to have the latest complex piece of machinery, or to be seen using the latest drug. Physicians are becoming more sceptical and better educated about these matters, but unless we take an informed initiative in this area, decisions will be indirectly or directly imposed on us by people who are less well informed.

### Efficiency

Labour costs account for the greater part of an ICU budget. As this is a relatively constant feature, strategies such as rapid turnover of patients and more efficient work practices can enable a greater number of patients to be dealt with by the same number of staff.

### Drugs and equipment

Continuous monitoring and appraisal of one's own practice in intensive care can reduce costs.

Invasive monitoring: Invasive monitoring is expensive in terms of both the labour and material cost. In the future there will be more reliance on non-invasive and simpler continuous monitoring (see Chapter 20).

Ventilatory techniques: Intensive care ventilators are increasingly sophisticated and expensive. Early respiratory support with continuous positive airway pressure (CPAP) and non-invasive ventilation may prevent intubation and ventilation.

Materials: Many volumetric infusion devices utilise dedicated plastic giving sets that are very expensive. Infusion syringe pumps perform the same function and utilise inexpensive and universal plastic giving sets.

Drugs: Clinicians and nursing staff should be aware of the costs of individual drugs as well as the amounts of drugs used by their own ICU. Areas of high cost can then be examined.

The 'latest-is-best phenomenon': Money for research is becoming increasingly difficult to find. It is no surprise, therefore, that research is often financed by companies that are marketing new devices or drugs. Publications and marketing associated with newer drugs and equipment tend to focus one's alternatives in that direction. In other words, commerce can set the agenda for our research and therefore influence the current interests of practising clinicians. Often an older and cheaper drug may be just as effective; morphine is much cheaper than fentanyl. It is of little surprise that we do not see drug displays at conferences which market 'adrenaline' or free pens advertising 'morphine'. Similarly, antibiotics account for a large part of the budget in intensive care and the newer ones are not necessarily better, but almost invariably are more expensive.

Preventive medicine: It is sobering to consider that the presence or absence of medical care accounts for only 10% of the differences in mortality among all societies. Genetics, health habits and social class account for the majority of the differences.

Although many clinicians in intensive care tend to see a strict boundary between preventive medicine and their own practice, it does not take much imagination to see the enormous impact of preventable diseases in our own specialty: alcohol-related admissions (e.g. self-poisoning, road traffic trauma, oesophageal varices), smoking-related diseases (coronary artery disease, peripheral vascular disease, respiratory disease) and other forms of drug abuse.

## Severity scoring and outcome prediction

The basic question of whether or not ICUs are justified is difficult, if not impossible, to answer. Randomised controlled trials involving critically ill patients are almost impossible to perform because, like many areas of modern medicine, the practice in question has become an accepted and standard mode of treatment. Attention has been focused, therefore, on scoring the severity of illness. Such measurements are used to predict outcome, as a form of quality assurance, and to describe patient populations for clinical trial.

There are many ways of measuring illness severity. They can be simple and descriptive such as if the sum of the days on a ventilator + age >100, the patient has little hope of recovery. One of the first and most commonly used is the Glasgow Coma Scale (GCS) which measures a patient's level of consciousness. There are other scores that specifically measure the severity of trauma. Two main types of scoring systems have been developed for intensive care patients, those that focus on one end-point – survival – and those that describe morbidity as it evolves – organ dysfunction scores.

## Outcome prediction models.

APACHE score: The Acute Physiology and Chronic Health Evaluation (APACHE) scoring system probably is the one most widely used in ICUs throughout the

**Table 31.1.** APACHE II: A severity of disease classification system

| Acute physiology points |
| --- |

Temperature (rectal)
Mean BP
Heart rate (ventricular response)
Respiratory rates (total non-ventilated or ventilated rate)
Oxygenation (A-a)$DO_2$ or $PaO_2$
Arterial pH
Serum sodium
Serum potassium
Serum creatinine
Haematocrit (%)
White blood cell count
Neurologic state (Glasgow Coma Scale)

A   Total acute physiology score (APS)
    Sum of the 12 individual variable points

B   Age points
    Assign points as follow:
    AGE (years)  Points

| | − |
| --- | --- |
| ≤ 44 | 0 |
| 45–54 | 2 |
| 55–64 | 3 |
| 65–74 | 5 |
| ≥ 75 | 6 |

C   Chronic health points
    If the patient has a history of chronic disease (i.e. a history of severe insufficiency) or
       is immunocompromised, then assign points as follows:
    (a) for non-operative or emergency postoperative patients, 5 points
    (b) for elective postoperative patients, 2 points

world. Currently, the APACHE II system is most commonly used. A more recent and more complicated version, APACHE III, is also available but requires payment of a fee.

The APACHE II system uses basic physiological data to assess the severity of illness and to stratify patients prognostically on the basis of risk of death. It uses 12 physiological variables that are weighted for the severity of the abnormality to yield an acute physiological score (APS) (Table 31.1). The APS is derived from the worst physiological values either on admission or during the first 24 hours after admission. This score is then added to a chronic health evaluation (CHE) which attempts to score the state of health of the patient just before admission.

This takes into account age and the presence of any chronic health problems. The assumption is that age and chronic health problems reflect a diminished physiological reserve.

There is a direct relationship between the total APACHE II scores and hospital death rates. However, this risk of death also varies according to various disease categories. For example, diabetic ketoacidosis is associated with severe acute physiological abnormalities and a high APACHE II score. However, the same score in a patient with severe trauma would indicate a higher risk of death. Therefore, a diagnostic category weight reflecting the risk of death for each disease category must also be taken into account. The APACHE II score and diagnostic weight are used to derive the risk of death.

The figure predicting death can be used as an estimate only for large groups; it is not accurate enough to predict death in an individual patient.

The use of these scores can be quite valuable in comparing standardised mortality rates (SMRs). The SMRs can be used by ICUs to compare their own performance at various points in time and to compare SMRs between units. This is currently one of the best ways of measuring a unit's performance.

SAPS system: The simplified acute physiology score (SAPS II) was derived from a large, heterogeneous patient population using logistic regression. It incorporates age, the presence of chronic disease and the type of admission, as well as data from 12 physiological measurements and investigations. The worst value during the first 24 hours is considered and weighted points are assigned according to severity and the particular variable (e.g. 0 to 3 for temperature abnormalities and 0 to 26 for GCS abnormalities). An equation based on the multiple logistic regression model is then used to predict hospital mortality. Unlike the APACHE scores, the SAPS II score is not weighted for individual diagnosis. It is also easy to calculate.

MPM II system: The mortality probability model (MPM II) is based on a series of models rather than a single model that is applied repeatedly over all ICU admissions. It is used to estimate hospital mortality and it is also a quality assurance tool to compare outcomes between various ICUs.

## Organ dysfunction scores

Multiple organ dysfunction score (MODS): This score uses six organ systems, each given a score between 0–4 (0 being normal function). The worst score for each system is taken in each 24-hour period for the aggregate score. A high initial score correlates with ICU mortality, as does the change in score over time compared with the initial score.

Sepsis related organ failure assessment (SOFA): It has the same organ systems and scoring as the MODS score but uses slightly different parameters to score each organ system. Initially devised for septic patients it can also be applied to non-septic patients. Like the MODS, high scores do correlate with mortality, but the main function of an organ failure score is to describe organ failure, not prognosticate.

Therapeutic intervention scoring system (TISS): Initially devised as a severity of illness score, TISS evaluates staffing needs and the utilisation of ICU facilities. The initial score used 76 variables, a simplified form uses 26 and the easier alternative, the nine equivalent of nursing manpower score (NEMS), uses 9. These scores correlate well with ICU costs and may be useful in planning nursing staffing but they are not useful for assessing severity of illness.

Long-term outcome: Probably even more important than survival is the quality of that survival. It is now becoming possible to quantify a patient's quality of life and to use that measurement to determine the efficiency of an intervention.

The measurement of a patient's quality of life (QOL) is in its infancy and there is, as yet, no universally accepted and validated scale. Measurement of QOL takes into account factors such as physical capabilities, pain, ability to work and social interactions. A QOL rating is usually expressed as a fraction between 0 and 1, where 0 is death and 1 is a full life. Interestingly, there are some states of ill health that are considered worse than death and they are assigned negative values. From the QOL we have derived the concept known as the quality of life adjusted year (QALY). This is calculated as the total number of years over which a particular health intervention is used multiplied by the QOL fraction. For example, if a patient lived for 10 years with a full QOL score of 1, then the intervention is said to have generated 10 QALYs (10 × 1.0). If the patient lived for 10 years, but was racked with pain and confined to bed with a QOL score of, say, 0.5, the intervention is said to have generated 5 QALYs (10 × 0.5).

If the cost of the intervention can be determined then the ratio cost/QALY can be determined. Thus, various health interventions can be compared for effectiveness. The concept of QOL measurement adds another dimension to the field of outcome measurements.

## Who should receive intensive care?

This is never an easy decision and it is not amenable to strict rules. Some of the factors which need to be considered are discussed next.

Underlying diseases: Incurable cancer is often cited as a contraindication to admitting a patient to intensive care. However, at the time of such consideration it is not always known whether or not the cancer is incurable and, even if it is, a short stay in intensive care after a palliative operation may guarantee that the patient will at least be able to leave the hospital.

Age: An age limit could preclude many of the world's current political leaders from admission to an ICU. Whether that would be a good thing or a bad thing is another matter. A strict age limit probably would be as irrelevant as many other single factors in assessing anyone's right to intensive care. Some elderly patients can benefit from a short, effective stay in intensive care. On the other hand, there is often enormous pressure to admit young patients who are hopelessly ill. This is related more to emotive reasons than to logic.

Reversibility of illness: It could be argued that anyone with an acute, reversible pathological condition should be admitted to an ICU. The problem is that the reversibility of such conditions often is not known at the time of admission. A practical approach then, depending on the availability of beds and the staffing situation, is to admit most patients for a 'short, sharp burst' of intensive care. Thereby, acute physiological abnormalities can be reversed while the staff observes rate of response of the patient.

Depending on the slope of this empirical response curve and together with other factors, such as age and underlying disease, a decision can be made to:

1  continue management without reservation,
2  continue management with reservations, or
3  discontinue treatment and allow the patient to die with dignity.

This flexible policy will allow efficient use of scarce ICU resources on the understanding that if the patient is not responding rapidly and has other adverse features, then treatment can be ceased at any point. A careful assessment should be made at least daily, involving all relevant parties in the decision-making process. That will preclude a mindless policy of blindly continuing treatment and support until the patient dies in spite of every effort.

## Discontinuation of treatment

It has become clear that when a patient is brain dead active management should be ceased as there is no hope of survival. Although this is no longer a problem in intensive care, we now recognise that there is a group of patients with an irreversible disease for whom we are prolonging the dying process. At the same time we have to accept that we will never be 100% sure of a given patient's probability of death. In the past, that consideration prompted us to sustain the lives of all patients with every available means until death finally supervened. That approach caused suffering for both patients and relatives, in addition to attracting criticism from many of our colleagues and from society.

Increasingly we are coming to realise that keeping one patient alive in such a manner is at some cost to another patient. Economic pressure is forcing a wider ranging ethical debate. The desirability of attempting to restore health does not imply that it is ethically justified to prolong life at any cost. 'Dying' is a diagnosis commonly overlooked or evaded. The decision to withhold life-sustaining treatment from hopelessly ill patients involves an ethical dilemma and legal uncertainties. Each ICU has to solve these problems in its own way. Some guidelines used within our own unit are as follows:

1. No matter how many people or committees are involved in the decision to make a diagnosis of dying, we attempt never to make the relatives feel that it is their decision. We take complete responsibility for that decision while involving them fully in all other aspects of the dying process.

2. The next challenge is to engage the medical diagnosis of dying with the decision to cease active management.

3. Engage relatives with full information, explained simply, balancing chances of survival with likelihood of long-term serious disability and death.

4. Procedures to deal with conflict about withdrawing and withholding treatment need to be in place. Behind these procedures is a respect for relative's wishes and the patient's autonomy but at the same time no obligation by attending clinicians to continue life in the face of futility. A good grasp of the cultural and religious beliefs of the family is important when dealing with this conflict.

5. All members of the medical and nursing team in the ICU looking after a given patient are involved in the decision to withdraw active management. The relatives and, if possible, the patient should also be involved. The challenge is to not let them feel the burden of guilt involved with them having to make the decision alone but to allow them to be involved with the obvious implications of a person who is dying, even if this involves some degree of uncertainty.

6. The patient must be allowed as much dignity in the dying process as during the living process. The challenge is to ensure that the patient dies pain free and that the needs of the relatives are attended to, and meeting that challenge can be as rewarding as any other aspect of intensive care medicine.

7. Because of the controversies surrounding the use of life support machines, we usually continue ventilatory support in most patients. Usually this is not a major problem as many seriously ill patients can breath spontaneously. If the brain stem is intact, the terminal event usually is cardiovascular collapse or hypoxia rather than hypoventilation. When it is decided that active management is no longer appropriate, all support measures are ceased and every attention paid to the patient's comfort during the dying process. If the patient is unconscious, feeding is stopped, drugs (apart from sedation and pain relief) are discontinued, observations and monitoring are stopped and the patient's appearance is attended to. Pain is treated without causing cessation of breathing. The patient is made to look comfortable and at peace. Dignity is preserved. Where possible privacy is ensured so that the relatives can, if they wish, be with the patient when death occurs. Every effort must be made to learn the cultural aspects of the dying process in different groups in your society and to incorporate respect for these in your practice.

Where a patient is conscious and able to communicate, the prognosis must be discussed openly and honestly. The principles of palliative care and management of the dying process for these patients are the same as for other terminally ill patients.

8. If possible, we prefer to manage the dying process within the ICU. However, often there are constraints involving staffing levels and bed status. When it is

## TROUBLESHOOTING

## Management of the dying patient

Periodically in any ICU it will become obvious that further active management of a given patient is futile. The following are some guidelines for dealing with that difficult situation.

### The diagnosis of dying

The medical and nursing staff responsible for the patient's management must reach a consensus that further active management is futile – this is part of the process of making the diagnosis of dying.

### Involvement of the relatives

Various ICUs will have different policies with regard to the involvement of relatives. Our own policy is to be honest about the hopelessness of continuing treatment, but not to hint in any way that the decision is one that the relatives must make by themselves.

### Change in management direction

Once it has been decided that there is no point in continuing active treatment, several principles become clear:

- Every effort must be made to guarantee that the patient can die with dignity and without pain.
- Careful consideration should be given to cessation of all support, apart from pain relief and basic procedures related to cleanliness and appearance.
- Ventilatory support can often be continued under these circumstances, even if the FiO₂ is reduced. This allows large amounts of narcotics to be used, without directly impairing the patient's airway or respiration.
- Nursing and medical efforts should be redirected toward supporting the patient's relatives and friends.

expected that the dying process may be prolonged, the patient may have to be transferred to a general ward.

## FURTHER READING

Brooks, R., Bauman, A., Daffurn, K. and Hillman, K. Post-hospital outcome following intensive care. *Clinical Intensive Care* 6 (1995): 127–35.

Brooks, R., Kerridge, R., Hillman, K., Bauman, A. and Daffurn, K. Quality of life outcomes after intensive care. Comparison with a community group. *Intensive Care Medicine* 23 (1997): 581–6.

Goldhill, D. R. and Sumner, A. Outcome of intensive care patients in a group of British intensive care units. *Critical Care Medicine* 26 (1998): 1337–45.

Le Gall, J. R., Lemeshow, S. and Saulnier, F. A new simplified physiology score (SAPS II) based on a European-North American multicentre study. *Journal of the American Medical Association* 270 (1993): 29057–8.

Lemeshow, S. and Teres, D. The MPM II system for ICU patients. In *Yearbook of Intensive Care and Emergency Medicine*, ed. J. L. Vincent, pp. 805–15. Berlin: Springer Verlag, 1994.

Nelson, J. E. and Danis M. End-of-life care in the intensive care unit: where are we now? *Critical Care Medicine* 29 (Suppl.) (2001): N2–9.

Skowronski, G. A. Bed rationing and allocation in the intensive care unit. *Current Opinion in Critical Care* 7 (2001): 480–4.

Tinker, J., Browne, D. R. G. and Sibbald, W. J. (ed.) In *Critical Care Standards, Audit and Ethics*. London: Edward Arnold, 1996.

Vincent, J.-L., Ferreira, F. and Moreno, R. Scoring systems for assessing organ dysfunction and survival. *Critical Care Clinics* 16 (2000): 353–63.

# Appendix 1. SI units

Basic and derived units

| | | | |
|---|---|---|---|
| Metre | m | unit of length | (L) |
| Kilogram | kg | unit of mass | (M) |
| Second | s | unit of time | (T) |
| Kelvin | K | unit of temperature | |
| Candela | cd | unit of luminous intensity | |
| Bel | b | unit of sound intensity, 1 decibel $= 0.1$ bel | |
| Ampere | A | unit of electrical current $1\,A = 2 \times 10^{-7}$ N/m | |
| Hertz | Hz | unit of frequency (one cycle per second) | |
| Mole | mol | unit of amount of substance in grams | |
| Newton | N | unit of force that will give 1 kilogram of mass an acceleration of 1 metre per second ($1\,N = 1\,kg \cdot m \cdot s^{-2}$) | |
| Pascal | Pa | unit of pressure expressed as force per unit area ($1\,Pa = 1\,N \cdot m^{-2}$) | |
| Joule | J | unit of energy or work (force through a distance) ($1\,J = 1\,N \cdot m$) | |
| Watt | W | unit of power: (energy per second) ($1\,W = 1\,N \cdot m \cdot s^{-1} = 1\,J \cdot s^{-1}$) | |
| Coulomb | C | unit of quantity of electric charge ($1\,C = 1\,A \cdot s$) | |
| Volt | V | unit of electrical potential difference ($1V = 1\,W \cdot A^{-1} = 1J \cdot A^{-1} \cdot s^{-1}$) | |
| Ohm | Ω | unit of electrical resistance ($1\,\Omega = 1\,V \cdot A^{-1}$) | |

Prefixes to SI units to indicate fractions or multiples

| | | | | | |
|---|---|---|---|---|---|
| $10^{12}$ | tera | T | $10^{-15}$ | femto | f |
| $10^{9}$ | giga | G | $10^{-12}$ | pico | p |
| $10^{6}$ | mega | M | $10^{-9}$ | nano | n |
| $10^{3}$ | kilo | k (K) | $10^{-6}$ | micro | μ |
| $10$ | deca | da (D) | $10^{-3}$ | milli | m |
| | | | $10^{-1}$ | deci | d |

# Appendix 2. Normal biochemical values

'Normal' values vary between laboratories. The figures are representative of normal values but should be checked with individual laboratories.

Blood specimen tube:

| | |
|---|---|
| C | Clotted sample |
| L | Lithium heparin tube |
| H | Heparinised whole blood |
| * | Seek lab advice |
| EDTA | Sequestrone tube |

| Name | Values in old units | Values in SI units | Blood specimen required and comments |
|---|---|---|---|
| Adrenaline | 0.01 μg/dL | 0.546 nmol/L | * |
| Alanine-aminotransferase (ALT) | | 5–35 U/L | C |
| Ammonium | 20–50 μg/dL | 12–31 μmol/L | L (to lab without delay) |
| Amylase | 0–180 Somogyi U/dL | 70–300 U/L | L |
| Aspartate-aminotransferase (AST) | | 5–35 U/L | C |
| Bicarbonate | | | |
| actual | 24–30 mEq/L | 24–30 mmol/L | L |
| standard | 21–25 mEq/L | 21–25 mmol/L | L |
| Bilirubin | | | |
| total | 0.2–1.0 mg/dL | 3–17 μmol/L | C |
| conjugated | < 0.4 mg/dL | < 7.0 μmol/L | C |
| Caeruloplasmin | 30–60 mg/dL | 300–600 mg/L | C |
| Calcium | | | |
| total | 8.5–10.6 mg/dL | 2.25–2.65 mmol/L | C |
| ionised | 4–5 mg/dL | 1.0–1.25 mmol/L | C |

| Name | Values in old units | Values in SI units | Blood specimen required and comments |
|---|---|---|---|
| Catecholamines | 1 μg/dL | < 54.6 nmol/L | * |
| Chloride | 95–105 mEq/L | 95–105 mmol/L | L |
| Cholesterol | 150–300 mg/dL | 3.9–7.5 mmol/L | L |
| Cholinesterase | | | |
| acetyl | – | 9–25 μmol · ml$^{-1}$ · min$^{-1}$ | C |
| plasma | 40–100 U/dL | – | |
| Complement | | | |
| C3 | | 0.7–1.8 g/L | * |
| C4 | 0.16–0.45 g/L | | |
| Copper | 76–165 μg/dL | 12–26 μmol/L | EDTA |
| Cortisol | | | |
| 0900 h | 10–25.3 μg/dL | 280–700 nmol/L | L |
| 2400 h | < 5–10 μg/dL | < 140–280 nmol/L | L |
| Creatinine | 0.7–1.7 mg/dL | 70–150 μmol/L | L |
| Creatinine phosphokinase (CPK) | | | |
| male | | 0–150 U/L | C |
| Creatinine clearance | 120 ml/min | 1.24–2.08 mL/s | * |
| Fibrinogen | 200–500 mg/dL | 2.0–5.0 g/L | * (citrate bottle) |
| Folate | 2–10 ng/ml | 4–22 nmol/L | C |
| Glucose | | | |
| fasting | 72–108 mg/dL | 4.0–6.0 mmol/L | Fluoride bottle |
| postprandial | < 180 mg/dL | < 10 mmol/L | |
| Gamma glutamyl transferase | | 0–30 U/L | |
| Growth hormone | | | |
| male | | 0.5 μg/L | * |
| female | | 0–10 μg/L | * |
| Insulin (fasting) | | 35–145 pmol/L | |
| Iodine, total | 3.5–8.0 μg/dL | 273–624 nmol/L | C |
| Iodine, protein bound | 4.0–7.5 μg/dL | 300–600 nmol/L | C |
| Iodine 131 uptake | 20–50% of dose in 24 h | | C |
| Iron | 80–160 μg/dL | 14–30 μmol/L | C |
| Total iron binding capacity (TIBC) | 302–420 μg/dL | 54–75 μmol/L | C |
| Ketones | 0.8–2.4 mg/dL | 80–140 μmol/L | L |
| Lactate | 3.5–15 mg/dL | 0.4–1.6 mmol/L | * |
| Lactate dehydrogenase | | 50–150 U/L | C |
| Lead | 10–40 μg/dL | 0.5–2.0 μmol/L | EDTA |
| Lipids, total | 400–1000 mg/dL | 4.0–10.0 g/L | C |

(*cont.*)

| Name | Values in old units | Values in SI units | Blood specimen required and comments |
|---|---|---|---|
| Low density cholesterol | 50–190 mg/dL | 1.30–4.90 mmol/L | C |
| High density cholesterol | | | |
|     Male | 30–70 mg/dL | 0.80–1.80 mmol/L | C |
|     Female | 30–90 mg/dL | 0.80–2.35 mmol/L | C |
| Magnesium | 1.4–2.8 mEq/L | 0.8–1.2 mmol/L | C |
| Manganese | 2.2 μg/L | 40.0 nmol/L | * |
| Methaemoglobin | 0.01–0.5 g/dL | 0.1–5 g/L | EDTA |
| Mercury | 0–5 μg/dL | 0–0.25 μmol/L | * |
| Nitrogen (non-protein) | 18–30 mg/dL | 12.8–21.5 mmol/L | C |
| Noradrenaline | 0.05 μg/ml | < 2.95 nmol/L | * |
| Osmolality | 280–300 mOsmol/kg | 280–300 mOsmol/kg | L |
| Phosphate (inorganic) | 2.0–4.5 mg/dL | 0.8–1.4 mmol/L | C |
| Phosphatase | | | |
|   acid | 1–5 KA U | 1–7 U/L | C |
|   alkaline | 3–13 KA U | 30–100 U/L | C |
| Phospholipids | 5–10 mg/dL | 1.6–3.2 mmol/L | C |
| Potassium | 3.5–5.0 mEq/L | 3.5–5.0 mmol/L | L |
| Protein, total | 6.0–8.0 g/dL | 60–80 g/L | C |
|   albumin | 3.5–5.0 g/dL | 35–50 g/L | C |
|   globulin | 2.4–3.7 g/dL | 24–37 g/L | C |
|   IgA | 80–500 mg/dL | 0.8–5.0 g/L | C |
|   IgG | 700–1900 mg/dL | 7–19 g/L | C |
|   IgM | 50–200 mg/dL | 0.5–2.0 g/L | C |
| Pyruvate | 0.4–0.7 mg/dL | 45–80 μmol/L | * |
| Sodium | 135–145 mEql/L | 135–145 mmol/L | L |
| Sulphate | 1–1.8 mg/dL | 0.31–0.56 mmol/L | C |
| Thyroid stimulating hormone (TSH) | 2–11 μU/mL | 1–11 mU/L | * |
| $T_3$ | 7–220 ng/dL | 1.3–2.9 nmol/L | * |
| $T_4$ | 5.0–12.0 μg/dL | 69–150 nmol/L | C |
| Triglycerides | 30–150 mg/dL | 0.34–1.7 mmol/L | C |
| Transferrin | 120–200 mg/dL | 1.2–2.0 g/L | C |
| $T_3$ uptake | 95–115% | 95–115% | C |
| Urate | 2–7 mg/dL | 0.1–0.4 mmol/L | C |
| Urea | 15–40 mg/dL | 2.5–6.5 mmol/L | L |
| Urea nitrogen | 10–20 mg/dL | 1.6–3.3 mmol/L | L |
| Uric acid | | | |
|   male | 3.5–8.0 mg/dL | 0.21–0.48 mmol/L | C |
|   female | 2.5–6.5 mg/dL | 0.15–0.39 mmol/L | C |
| Zinc | 1–2 mEql/L | 11.5–18.5 μmol/L | C |

# Appendix 3. Normal haematology values

Haemoglobin (Hb)
    male                               130–180 g/L
    female                           115–165 g/L

Red blood cell count (RBC)
    male                               $4.5$–$6.5 \times 10^{12}/L$
    female                         $3.5$–$5.0 \times 10^{12}/L$

White blood cell count (WBC)      $4.0$–$11.0 \times 10^9 L$
    Neutrophils (40–75%)      $2.5$–$7.5 \times 10^9/L$
    Lymphocytes (20–45%)    $1.5$–$3.5 \times 10^9/L$
    Monocytes (2–10%)        $0.2$–$0.8 \times 10^9/L$
    Eosinophils (1–6%)       $0.04$–$0.44 \times 10^9/L$
    Basophils (0–1%)          $0$–$0.1 \times 10^9/L$

Platelet count                    $150$–$400 \times 10^9/L$
Reticulocyte count            0–2% of RBCs

Sedimentation rate (ESR)
    male                               0–5 mm/h
    female                           0–7 mm/h

Haematocrit (HCT)
    male                               0.40–0.54
    female                           0.37–0.47

Mean corpuscular volume (MCV)   76–96 fL (femtolitre)
Mean corpuscular haemoglobin   330–370 g/L
    concentration (MCHC)
Mean corpuscular haemoglobin (MCH)  27–32 pg (picogram)

Routine clotting screen
    Activated partial thromboplastin time   21–36 secs
      (APPT)
    Bleeding time                  <9 minutes
    *d*-dimers                       <0.25 mg/L
    Fibrin degradation products (FDP)    <10 µg/ml
    Fibrinogen                   1.5–4.0 g/L

*(cont.)*

| | |
|---|---|
| International normalised ratio used to control warfarin therapy (INR) | 2–2.5 as prophylaxis for deep venous thrombosis (DVT) |
| | 2–3 as treatment for DVT and pulmonary embolism. |
| | 3–4.5 recurrent DVT and pulmonary embolism, arterial disease and grafts, cardiac prosthetic valves. |
| Prothrombin index (PI) | 80–100% |
| Prothrombin time (PT) | 10–14 seconds |
| Prothrombin ratio (*PT /control*) (PTR) | 1.0–1.3 |

# Appendix 4. Normal urine values

| Name | Values |
|------|--------|
| Adrenaline | <100 nmol/24 h |
| Aldosterone | <50.0 μmol/24 h |
| Ammonium | 18–60 mmol/24 h |
| Amylase | 100–1000 units/24 h |
| Calcium | 2.5–7.5 mmol/24 h |
| Catecholamines | |
|   Hydroxymethoxymandelic acid (HMMA) or VMA | 15–75 μmol/24 h |
|   Noradrenaline | 30–592 nmol/24 h |
| Chloride | 100–300 mmol/24 h |
| Cortisol | 0.2–1.0 μmol/24 h |
| Creatinine | 10–20 mmol/24 h |
| Creatinine clearance | 120 ml/min |
| Copper | 0.2–1.0 μmol/24 h |
| Coproporphyrin | 50–300 nmol/24 h |
| Folic acid | 3.5–23.5 μg/24 h |
| Glomerular filtration rate | 105–140 ml/min |
| Glucose | 0–11 mmol/24 h |
| Hydroxyproline | 0.08–0.25 mmol/24 h |
| 5 Hydroxyindole acetic acid (5HIAA) | 15–75 μmol/24 h |
| 17 keto steroids | 34–100 μmol/24 h |
| Lead | < 0.40 μmol/24 h |
| Magnesium | 3.3–5.0 mmol/24 h |
| Oestriol (after 30-week pregnancy) | 30–140 μmol/24 h |
| Oestrogens | |
|   pregnant | 14–86.7 μmol/24 h |
|   non-pregnant | 14–347 μmol/24 h |
| Osmolality | 300–1000 mOsmol/24 h |
| Oxalate | < 300 μmol/24 h |

(*cont.*)

| Name | Values |
|---|---|
| Phosphate | 15–50 mmol/24 h |
| Potassium | 40–120 mmol/24 h |
| Protein (albumin) | 0.02–0.1 g/24 h |
| pH (hydrogen ion) | 10–30 000 nmol/24 h (pH 4.5–8.0) |
| Phosphatase, acid | |
| male | 164 KA units/24 h |
| female | 217 KA units/24 h |
| Porphobilinogen | 1–10 μmol/24 h |
| Renal plasma flow | 500–800 ml/min |
| Sodium | 50–250 mmol/24 h |
| Specific gravity | 1003–1030 |
| Urea | 50–500 mmol/24 h |
| Urea clearance | 60–95 ml/min |
| Urate | 2–6 mmol/24 h |
| Urobilinogen | 0–6.7 μmol/24 h |
| Uroporphyrin I and II | 0–30 nmol/24 h |

# Appendix 5. Normal CSF values

|  | Values in SI units |
|---|---|
| Pressure | 7.0–15.0 cmH$_2$O (0.93–2.0 kPa) |
| Volume | 120 –140 ml |
| Hydrogen ion | 50–54 nmol/L (pH 7.30–7.35) |
| Specific gravity | 1007 |
| Osmolality | 306 mOsmol/kg |
| Calcium | 1–1.5 mmol/L |
| Chloride | 120–130 mmol/L |
| Glucose | 2.7–4.5 mmol/L (1.0 mmol/L less than blood sugar) |
| Lactate | < 2.8 mmol/L |
| Magnesium | 0.36–3.2 mmol/L |
| Sodium | 140 mmol/L |
| Phosphate | 0.13–0.23 mmol/L |
| Potassium | 3–4 mmol/L |
| Lymphocytes | 0–5 × 10$^6$/L |
| Protein | 0.15–0.45 g/L |
|   globulin | 0–20 mg/L |
|   IgG | < 0.05 g/L |
| IgG: Total protein ratio | 5–15% |

# Appendix 6. Respiratory physiology and blood gases

Blood gases
Arterial

| | |
|---|---|
| H$^+$ concentration (pH) | 36–44 nmol/L (7.35–7.44) |
| PaO$_2$ | 11.3–13.3 kPa (85–100 mmHg) |
| PaCO$_2$ | 4.8–5.9 kPa (36–44 mmHg) |
| O$_2$ content | 8.9–9.4 nmol/L (20–21 volumes/dL) |
| CO$_2$ content | 21.5–22.5 nmol/L (48–50 volumes/dL) |

Venous

| | |
|---|---|
| H$^+$ conc (pH) | 38–46 nmol/L (7.34–7.42) |
| PvO2 | 5–5.6 kPa (37–42 mmHg) |
| PvCO2 | 5.6–6.7 kPa (42–50 mmHg) |
| O$_2$ content | 6.7–7.2 nmol/L (15–16 volumes/dL) |
| CO$_2$ content | 23.5–24.0 nmol/L (52–54 volumes/dL) |

pH conversion to nanomoles

| pH units | H + concentration (nmol/L) |
|---|---|
| 6.0 | 1000.0 |
| 6.1 | 794.2 |
| 6.2 | 630.9 |
| 6.3 | 501.2 |
| 6.4 | 398.1 |
| 6.5 | 316.3 |
| 6.6 | 251.2 |
| 6.7 | 199.5 |
| 6.8 | 158.5 |
| 6.9 | 125.9 |
| 7.0 | 100.0 |
| 7.1 | 79.4 |
| 7.2 | 63.1 |
| 7.3 | 50.1 |
| 7.4 | 39.8 |
| 7.5 | 31.6 |

| 7.6 | 25.1 |
|-----|------|
| 7.7 | 19.9 |
| 7.8 | 15.8 |
| 7.9 | 12.6 |
| 8.0 | 10.0 |

Pressure conversion
1 kPa = 7.5 mmHg
1 mmHg = 0.133 kPa
1 mmHg = 1.36 cm $H_2O$

Ventilatory abbreviations
Primary symbols

| C | concentration of gas in the blood |
|---|---|
| D | diffusing capacity |
| F | fractional concentration of a dry gas |
| f | frequency of respiratory (breaths/min) |
| P | gas pressure or partial pressure |
| Q | volume of blood |
| $\dot{Q}$ | volume of blood per unit time |
| R | respiratory exchange ratio |
| S | saturation of haemoglobin with oxygen or carbon dioxide |
| V | gas volume |
| $\dot{V}$ | volume of gas per unit time |

Secondary symbols

| A | alveolar gas |
|---|---|
| a | arterial gas |
| B | barometric |
| c | pulmonary capillary blood |
| c′ | pulmonary end capillary blood |
| D | dead space gas |
| d | difference |
| E | expired gas |
| I | inspired gas |
| i | ideal |
| jv | jugular vein |
| L | lung |
| tc | transcutaneous |
| T | tidal gas |
| $\bar{v}$ | mixed venous blood |

Respiratory measurements
These are only approximate figures for adults and they are subject to age and weight variations.

| Airways resistance | 0.5–3.4 cm $H_2O \cdot L^{-1} \cdot s^{-1}$ |
|---|---|
| Alveolar ventilation ($\dot{V}^A$) | 4.2 L/min (2–2.5 L $\cdot$ min$^{-1}$ $\cdot$ m$^{-2}$) |
| Alveolar air equation | 13.3 kPa (100 mm Hg) approximately |

Alveolar-arterial oxygen difference
   breathing air                   5–20 mmHg (0.7–2.7 kPa)
   breathing 100% oxygen      10–60 mm Hg (1.3–8.0 kPa)
Compliance
   chest wall                   200 ml/cm $H_2O$
   lung                        200 ml/cm $H_2O$
   lung and chest wall        100 ml/cm $H_2O$
Dead space ($V_D$)             150 ml (2.2 ml/kg)
Diffusing capacity of carbon monoxide   17–20 ml CO $\cdot$ min$^{-1}$ $\cdot$ (mmHg)$^{-1}$
   (DCO)
Forced expiratory volume in 1 second   70–80% of VC
   ($FEV_1$)
Maximum ventilatory volume (MVV)   120 L/min (35 × $FEV_1$)
Minute volume                5000–6000 ml/min (100 ml/kg)
Peak expiratory flow rate (PEFR)    300–700 L/min
Peak inspiratory flow rate (PIFR)    200–700 L/min
Pulmonary capillary blood flow ($\dot{Q}c$)   5400 ml/min
Pulmonary capillary blood volume   60 ml
   ($Qc$)
Respiratory quotient           0.8 (on normal diet)
Respiratory rate               12–14 bpm
Venous admixture             5–10% of cardiac output
Work of breathing
   maximum                98 J/min
   quiet                   4.9 J/min
Oxygen consumption         115–165 ml $\cdot$ min$^{-1}$ $\cdot$ m$^{-2}$
Oxygen delivery              900–1000 ml $\cdot$ min$^{-1}$ $\cdot$ m$^{-2}$

LUNG VOLUMES
Tidal volume ($V_T$)             400–600 ml (7–10 ml/kg)
Total lung capacity (TLC)      5000–6500 ml
Vital capacity (VC)          4200–4800 ml (52 ml/kg)
Inspiratory capacity (IC)      3600–4300 ml
Inspiratory reserve volume (IRV)   3100–3750 ml
Expiratory reserve volume (ERV)   950–1300 ml
Functional residual capacity (FRC)  2300–2800 ml
Residual volume (RV)         1200–1700 ml

Normal partial pressure of gases
A bar above a symbol indicates a mean value
A dot above a symbol indicates a value per unit time

| Inspired air | | Expired air | |
|---|---|---|---|
| $PIO_2$ | 158 mmHg (21.06 kPa) | $PEO_2$ | 116 mmHg (15.47 kPa) |
| $PICO_2$ | 0.3 mmHg (0.04 kPa) | $PECO_2$ | 28 mmHg (3.73 kPa) |
| $PIN_2$ | 596 mmHg (79.46 kPa) | $PEN_2$ | 568 mmHg (75.73 kPa) |
| $PIH_2O$ | 5 mmHg (0.67 kPa) | $PEH_2O$ | 47 mmHg (6.27 kPa) |

Arterial blood gases

| | |
|---|---|
| $PaO_2$ | 90–110 mm Hg (12.0–14.67 kPa) |
| $PaCO_2$ | 34–46 mm Hg (4.53–6.13 kPa) |
| $PaN_2$ | 573 mm Hg (76.39 kPa) |
| pH | 44–36 nmol/L (7.35–7.44) |

Alveolar gas

| | | |
|---|---|---|
| $PAO_2$ | 103 mmHg | (13.73 kPa) |
| $PaCO_2$ | 40 mmHg | (5.33 kPa) |
| $PAN_2$ | 570 mmHg | (75.99 kPa) |
| $PAH_2O$ | 47 mmHg | (6.27 kPa) |

Mixed venous blood gases

| | |
|---|---|
| $P\bar{v}O_2$ | 37–42 mmHg (4.93–5.60 kPa) |
| $P\bar{v}CO_2$ | 40–52 mmHg (5.53–6.93 kPa) |
| $P\bar{v}N_2$ | 573 mmHg (76.39 kPa) |
| pH | 38–46 nmol/L (7.34–7.42) |

# Appendix 7. Cardiorespiratory abbreviations

| | |
|---|---|
| $(a-\bar{v})DO_2$ | arterial-mixed venous oxygen content difference |
| BSA | body surface area |
| BP | blood pressure |
| CI | cardiac index |
| CO | cardiac output |
| HR | heart rate |
| LVSW | left ventricular stroke work |
| LVSWI | left ventricular stroke work index |
| MAP | mean arterial pressure |
| PAP | pulmonary artery pressure |
| $P\bar{A}P$ | mean pulmonary artery pressure |
| PAWP | pulmonary artery wedge pressure |
| $P\bar{A}WP$ | mean pulmonary artery wedge pressure |
| $PEO_2$ | partial pressure of $O_2$ in expired gas |
| $PECO_2$ | partial pressure of $CO_2$ in expired gas |
| PVR | pulmonary vascular resistance |
| RAP | right atrial pressure |
| RQ | respiratory quotient |
| SI | stroke index |
| SV | stroke volume |
| SVR | systemic vascular resistance |
| $\dot{Q}_S/\dot{Q}_T$ | venous admixture or pulmonary shunt |
| $\bar{V}O_2$ | oxygen consumption |
| $DO_2$ | oxygen delivery |

Cardiorespiratory equations

Body surface area (BSA)
$$BSA = (\text{weight in kg})^{0.425} \times (\text{height in cm})^{0.725} \times 71.84 \times 10^{-4} m^2$$

Cardiac output (CO)
$$CO = \text{heart rate (HR)} \times \text{stroke volume (SV)}$$

Cardiac index (CI)
$$CI = \frac{CO}{BSA} \ ml \cdot min^{-1} \cdot m^{-2}$$

Stroke volume index (SVI)

$$SVI = \frac{SV}{BSA} \; ml \cdot beat^{-1} \cdot m^{-2}$$

Left ventricular stroke work index (LVSWI)

$$LVSWI = (MAP - PAWP)\,(SVI) \times (0.0136)$$
$$g \cdot m \cdot m^{-2}$$

Right ventricular stroke work index (RVSWI)

$$RVSWI = (PAP - RAP)\,(SVI)\,(0.0136)$$
$$g \cdot m \cdot m^{-2}$$

Systemic vascular resistance (SVR)

$$SVR = \frac{MAP - RAP}{CO} \times 80 \; dyn \cdot s \cdot cm^{-5}$$

Pulmonary vascular resistance (PVR)

$$PVR = \frac{P\bar{A}P - P\bar{A}WP}{CO} \times 80 \; dyn \cdot s \cdot cm^{-5}$$

Respiratory quotient (RQ)

$$RQ = \frac{CO_2 \; produced}{O_2 \; consumed}$$

Alveolar air equation

$$P_AO_2 = PIO_2 - \frac{PaCO_2}{RQ}$$

OR

$$P_AO_2 = PIO_2 - P_ACO_2 \frac{PIO_2 - PEO_2}{PECO_2}$$

Alveolar-arterial difference in partial pressure of oxygen

$$= P_AO_2 - PaO_2$$

Physiological dead space (Bohr's equation)

$$\frac{VD}{VT} = \frac{PaCO_2 - PECO_2}{P_ACO_2} \quad or$$

$$\frac{VD}{VT} = \frac{PaCO_2 - PECO_2}{PaCO_2}$$

Venous admixture

$$\frac{QS}{QT} = \frac{Cc'O_2 - CaO_2}{Cc'O_2 - C\bar{v}O_2}$$

Oxygen consumption ($VO_2$)

$$VO_2 = (CI)\,(CaO_2 - C\bar{v}O_2) \; ml \cdot min^{-1} \cdot m^{-2}$$

Oxygen delivery ($DO_2$)

$$DO_2 = (CI)\,(CaO_2) \; ml \cdot min^{-1} \cdot m^{-2}$$

Cardiovascular measurements

| | |
|---|---|
| Cardiac output | $4-7 \; L \cdot min^{-1}$ |
| Cardiac index | $3.5-4 \; L \cdot min^{-1}$ |
| Stroke volume | 42–52 ml/beat |
| Stroke index | $36-48 \; ml \cdot m^{-2}$ |
| Ejection fraction | 0.55–0.75 |
| End diastolic volume | $60-95 \; ml \cdot m^{-2}$ |
| End systolic volume | $18-32 \; ml \cdot m^{-2}$ |
| Right atrial pressure | 1–8 mmHg (0.13–1.06 kPa) |
| Pulmonary artery wedge pressure | 5–15 mmHg (0.67–2.0 kPa) |
| Right ventricular systolic pressure | 15–25 mmHg (2.0 -3.3 kPa) |
| Right ventricular diastolic pressure | 0–8 mmHg (0–1.06 kPa) |
| Pulmonary artery systolic pressure | 15–25 mmHg (2.0–3.3 kPa) |

| | |
|---|---|
| Pulmonary artery diastolic pressure | 8–15 mmHg (1.06–2.0 kPa) |
| Pulmonary artery mean pressure | 10–20 mmHg (1.3 -2.7 kPa) |
| Left ventricular stroke work index | $44$–$55 \; g \cdot m \cdot m^{-2}$ |
| Right ventricular stroke work index | $7$–$10 \; g \cdot m \cdot m^{-2}$ |
| Systemic vascular resistance | $1500$–$3000 \; dyn \cdot s \cdot cm^{-5}$ |
| Pulmonary vascular resistance | $100$–$250 \; dyn \cdot s \cdot cm^{-5}$ |

# Appendix 8. Toxicology

These data are only approximations. Allowances must be made for individual responses. If in any doubt, contact your Local Poison Centre.

| Drug | Normal or therapeutic Range | Toxic levels |
|---|---|---|
| Amitriptyline | 0.05–0.2 mg/L | >0.40 mg/L |
| Aminophylline (theophylline) | 10–20 mg/L | >20 mg/L |
| Amphetamine | 0.1–3.0 mg/L | >3 mg/L |
| Arsenic (blood) | <30 μg/L | >1.0 mg/L |
| Barbiturates | | |
|   Amylobarbitone | 2–4 mg/L | >8 mg/L |
|   Barbitone | 5–15 mg/L | >20 mg/L |
|   Butobarbitone | 2–4 mg/L | >8 mg/L |
|   Cyclobarbitone | 2–4 mg/L | >8 mg/L |
|   Heptabarbitone | 2–4 mg/L | >8 mg/L |
|   Hexabarbitone | 2–4 mg/L | >8 mg/L |
|   Pentobarbitone | 2–4 mg/L | >8 mg/L |
|   Phenobarbitone | 5–20 mg/L | >25 mg/L |
| Bromide | 50 mg/L | >500 mg/L |
| Cadmium (blood and urine) | <10 μg/L | >50 μg/L |
| Carbamazepine | 3–13 mg/L | >15 mg/L |
| Carbon monoxide | 1% saturation | >15% saturation of Hb |
| Chloral hydrate | 10–50 mg/L | >50 mg/L |
| Chloramphenicol | 2–6 mg/L | >10mg/L |
| Chlordiazepoxide | 3–7 mg/L | 8 mg/L |
| Chlormethiazole | 0.5–2.0 mg/L | >6 mg/L |
| Chlorpromazine (free drug) | 0.2–0.5 mg/L | >0.8 mg/L |
| Copper (serum) | 0.8–1.5 mg/L | >5.0 mg/L |
| Cyanide | 0.15 mg/L | >2 mg/L |

(*cont.*)

| Drug | Normal or therapeutic Range | Toxic levels |
|---|---|---|
| DDT | 10 μg/L | >50 μg/L |
| Desipramine | 0.5–1.4 mg/L | >5 mg/L |
| Dextropropoxyphene | 0.2–0.8 mg/L | >1.0 mg/L |
| Diazepam | 0.5–2.5 mg/L | >5 mg/L |
| Digitoxin | 20–35 μg/L | >50 μg/L |
| Digoxin | 1–2 μg/L | >2.5 μg/L |
| Diphenhydramine | 0.5 mg/L | >1.0 mg/L |
| Ethambutol | 3–5 mg/L | >6 mg/L |
| Ethanol | 0.05 g/l (legal Australian driving limit) | 0.3 g/L (clinically drunk) |
| Ethchlorvynol | 10–20 mg/L | >20 mg/L |
| Ethosuximide | 40–80 mg/L | 100 mg/L |
| Ethylene glycol | – | >1.5 g/L |
| Fenfluramine | 0.1–0.15 mg/L | >0.2 mg/L |
| Fluoride | 0.5 mg/L | >2 mg/L |
| Gentamicin (once daily dosing) | <0.5 mg/L | >15 mg/L |
| Glutethimide | 2–4 mg/L | >8 mg/L |
| Imipramine | 0.1–0.3 mg/L | >0.5 mg/L |
| Indomethacin | 0.7–1.3 mg/L | – |
| Iron | 500 mg/L (erythrocytes) | 6 mg/L (serum) |
| Lead | 0.05–1.0 mg/L | >1.5 mg/L |
| Lignocaine | 2–5 mg/L | >5.0 mg/L |
| Lithium | 0.8–1.2 mmoL/L | >1.5 mmoL/L |
| Meprobamate | 5–20 mg/L | >25 mg/L |
| Mercury (blood) | <15 mg/L | >40 μg/L |
| Methadone | 0.05–1.0 mg/L | >1.0 mg/L |
| Methaqualone | 2–4 mg/L | >5 mg/L |
| Methsuximide | 10–40 mg/L | >40 mg/L |
| Methanol | – | >100 mg/L |
| Morphine | 0.1–0.5 mg/L | >1.0 mg/L |
| Nortriptyline | 0.05–0.15 mg/L | >0.25 mg/L |
| Oxazepam | 1–2 mg/L | >2 mg/L |
| Paracetamol | 5–25 mg/L | >30 mg/L |
| Pethidine | 0.2–0.8 mg/L | >2.0 mg/L |
| Phenacetin | 5–25 mg/L | >30 mg/L |
| Phenylbutazone | 50–100 mg/L | >100 mg/L |
| Phenytoin | 10–20 mg/L | >20 mg/L |
| Procainamide | 3–8 mg/L | >10 mg/L |
| Propranolol | 0.025–0.2 mg/L | >8 mg/L |
| Quinidine | 3–5 mg/L | >6 mg/L |
| Salicylate | 150–250 mg/L | >300 mg/L |
| Sodium valproate | 50–100 mg/L | >100 mg/L |

| Drug | Normal or therapeutic Range | Toxic levels |
|------|------------------------------|--------------|
| Strychnine | – | >2 mg/L |
| Thallium (blood) | <10 | >50 mg/L |
| Tobramycin | 5–8 mg/L | 10–12 mg/L |
| Tricyclics | 50–200 μg/L | >400 μg/L |
| Warfarin | 1–10 mg/L | >10 mg/L |

# Index